Philosophy of Neurological Surgery

AANS Publications Committee
Issam A. Awad, MD, Editor

Neurosurgical Topics

American Association of
Neurological Surgeons

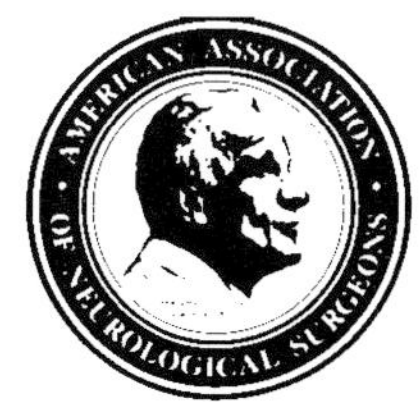

ISBN: 1-879284-32-4

Neurosurgical Topics ISBN: 0-9624246-6-8

This publication is published under the auspices of the Publications Committee of the American Association of Neurological Surgeons (AANS). However, this should not be construed as indicating endorsement or approval of the views presented, by the AANS, or by its committees, commissions, affiliates, or staff.

Daniel L. Barrow, MD, Chairman
AANS Publications Committee

Joanne B. Needham, AANS Staff Editor

AANS1.75M1294

Forthcoming Books in the *Neurosurgical Topics* Series

1995

Contemporary Management of Spinal Cord Injury
  Edited by Edward C. Benzel, MD, and Charles H. Tator, MD

Benign Cerebral Glioma, Volume I
  Edited by Michael L.J. Apuzzo, MD

Benign Cerebral Glioma, Volume II
  Edited by Michael L.J. Apuzzo, MD

Endovascular Neurological Intervention
  Edited by Robert J. Maciunas

Dedication

*To my son Armand,
whose youthful vigor, innocent determination,
enquiring eyes, and splendid promise embody
the essence of neurosurgical philosophy.*

Contents

List of Contributors

Issam A. Awad, MD, MSc, FACS
Professor of Surgery (Neurosurgery)
Head, Neurovascular Surgery Program
Yale University School of Medicine
New Haven, Connecticut

Michael L.J. Apuzzo, MD
Edwin M. Todd/Trent H. Wells, Jr. Professor
Department of Neurological Surgery and
    Radiation Oncology
University of Southern California
    School of Medicine
Director of Neurosurgery
Kenneth R. Norris Jr. Cancer Hospital
    and Research Institute
Los Angeles, California

W. Ben Blackett, MD, JD
Tacoma, Washington

William F. Collins, MD
Harvey and Kate Cushing Emeritus
    Professor of Neurosurgery
Yale University School of Medicine
New Haven, Connecticut

**William Feindel, MDCM, DPhil,
    FRCSC, FACS**
Neurosurgical Service
Montreal Neurological Institute
Professor of Neurosurgery
Department of Neurology and Neurosurgery
McGill University
Montreal, Quebec, Canada

Samuel H. Greenblatt, MA, MD, FACS
Associate Professor of Neurosurgery
Brown University
Chief of Neurosurgery
Memorial Hospital of Rhode Island
Pawtucket, Rhode Island

Oliver Woodhouse Grin, MD, FACS
Chief, Division of Neurosurgery
Blodgett Memorial Medical Center
Grand Rapids, Michigan

J. Peter Gruen, MD
Associate Professor of Neurological Surgery
Head, Peripheral Nerve Service and
    Neurotrauma
Los Angeles County/University of Southern
    California Medical Center
Los Angeles, California

M. Peter Heilbrun, MD
Joseph J. Yager Professor and Chair
Department of Neurological Surgery
University of Utah School of Medicine
Salt Lake City, Utah

Julian T. Hoff, MD
Professor of Surgery
Head, Section of Neurosurgery
University of Michigan Medical Center
Ann Arbor, Michigan

Howard Kaufman, MD
Professor and Chairman
Department of Neurosurgery
West Virginia University
Morgantown, West Virginia

Don M. Long, MD, PhD
Professor and Director
Department of Neurosurgery
Johns Hopkins University School of Medicine
Baltimore, Maryland

Joseph C. Maroon, MD
Chairman, Department of Neurosurgery
Allegheny General Hospital
Professor of Neurosurgery
Medical College of Pennsylvania
Pittsburgh, Pennsylvania

Robert E. Maxwell, MD, PhD, FACS
Professor of Neurosurgery
Department of Neurosurgery
University of Minnesota
Minneapolis, Minnesota

Robert G. Ojemann, MD
Professor of Surgery
Harvard Medical School
Visiting Neurosurgeon
Massachusetts General Hospital
Boston, Massachusetts

Charles Plante, PhD
Washington Representative for AANS/
    CNS Joint Washington Committee
Washington, D.C.

**Jeffrey V. Rosenfeld, MBBS, MS,
    FRACS, FRCS(Ed)**
Deputy Director
Department of Neurosurgery
Royal Melbourne Hospital
Consultant Neurosurgeon
Royal Children's Hospital
Parkville, Australia

Michael Salcman, MD
Clinical Professor of Neurological Surgery
George Washington University
Towson, Maryland

Dennis Spencer, MD
Nixdorff-German Professor of Neurosurgery
Chief, Section of Neurological Surgery
Yale University School of Medicine
New Haven, Connecticut

George T. Tindall, MD
Professor and Chief
Department of Neurosurgery
Emory University School of Medicine
The Emory Clinic
Atlanta, Georgia

Jeffrey Evan Thomas, MD
Resident
Department of Neurological Surgery
Los Angeles County/University of Southern
    California Medical Center
Los Angeles, California

Clark Watts, MD, JD
Ford & Ferraro, Attorneys at Law
Austin, Texas

Robert H. Wilkins, MD
Professor and Chief
Division of Neurosurgery
Duke University Medical Center
Durham, North Carolina

AANS Publications Committee

Daniel L. Barrow, MD, Chairman
Michael L.J. Apuzzo, MD
Issam A. Awad, MD
Edward C. Benzel, MD
John A. Jane, MD (ex officio)

Howard H. Kaufman, MD
Christopher M. Loftus, MD
Robert J. Maciunas, MD
J. Gordon McComb, MD
Setti S. Rengachary, MD

Preface

*Now then to know what properties and conditions this man must have before he
be a perfect Chirurgien. I doe note four things most especially that every Chirurgien ought so
to have: the first, that he be learned; the second, that he be expert; the third,
that he be ingenious; the fourth, that he be well mannered.*
>—Thomas Vicary, in *The Englishman's Treasures* (1633)

Nuestro modo de proceder (Our way of proceeding).
>—St. Ignatius Loyola, founder of the Jesuit Order

*While ours is perhaps the most arduous and responsible of the many surgical specialties,
we can have the great satisfaction of knowing that only men of a certain type will venture to
make it their life work and that, so far at least, both in this country and abroad,
its devotees have not only shown the kind of sympathetic and encouraging interest in
one another's activities that binds men closely together but have at the same time held the
respect of the Profession as a whole. May this continue for all time to be true.*
>—Harvey Cushing, Address at his 70th birthday party, April 8, 1939

Who are the neurosurgeons? As a profession, are they shaped by common knowledge, common duties, and common hopes? If so, then according to Immanuel Kant, they have a philosophy.

There have been many definitions of philosophy, differing through the ages and by philosophers themselves. As in Kant's question-centered definition, philosophy has embodied the love of wisdom as leading to the search for it and, hence, the knowledge of general principles—elements, powers, causes, and laws—as explaining facts and existences. Another dimension of philosophy includes the articulation of general laws that furnish rational explanations, and the calm judgment and equable temper resulting from studies of causes and laws. In the broadest sense, philosophy is a reasoned science (*Encyclopedia Britannica*).

While ancient civilizations have articulated their philosophies with varying impact on subsequent generations, it is largely agreed that modern philosophy of civilized man finds its roots among the Greek thinkers of the millennium before Christ. Pre-Socratic philosophers proposed simple answers to questions of morality. Socrates (470?–399 BC) introduced the theory of knowledge, with logic as a method of tackling moral and practical problems. In the Philosophy of the Academy, Plato (428?–348? BC) introduced intuitional philosophy, which has been immortalized in his *Dialogues*, as recorded by his students. In the Philosophy of the Lyceum, Aristotle (384–322 BC) introduced the first elements of empirical philosophy. During this age of splendid ideas, Hippocrates (460?–377? BC) articulated the first elements of a philosophy of medicine. Later, Galen of Pergamum

(AD 130?–201?) synthesized medical knowledge into numerous treatises incorporating practical and philosophic considerations, guiding the teaching and exercise of medicine for over a millennium.

Philosophy, medicine, and the philosophy of medicine have remained entwined throughout the evolution of thought and civilization. In the Islamic empires, a physician was known as "Hakim," or wise man, a title still in common use in the Middle East today. Indeed, the giants of Arabian medicine were also philosophers. Al-Rhazy (Rhazes, AD 841–926) and Ibn-Sina (Avicenna, AD 900–1037) re-examined current thinking about health and illness, and interpreted them within the context of religious thinking. They tackled questions of metaphysics, the philosophy of the mind and knowledge, and the clarification of concepts. Rhazes introduced experiential observations as a basis for measured medical decisions. For example, he chose the site for a major state hospital by comparing the rate of petrification of meat at the various locations; he was the first to use animal gut in surgical sutures, following the systematic comparison of different materials. Avicenna used medicine as a background for universal philosophic discussions about existence, intelligence, the soul, and the nature of being.

During the European Renaissance, the fundamental elements of the philosophy of science were introduced. René Descartes (1596–1650), Francis Bacon (1561–1626), and Blaise Pascal (1623–1662) consolidated the concepts of cartesianism, the philosophy of nature, and what will later be better described as the "scientific method." At the threshold of the 19th century, science was emerging as a philosophic tool for tackling questions of eternal truths, higher purpose, and empirical uniformities first evoked by Plato. Auguste Comte (1798–1857) formulated the philosophy of positivism. He described a biologic state, mostly fictitious, provisional, and preparatory; a metaphysical state, essentially abstract, absolute, and inherent, but also transitional; and finally, a positive or real state, a *definitive one.* Comte's positivism classified the sciences into a determined hierarchy, with mathematics/astronomy, physics/chemistry, and biology/sociology in a historical, dogmatic, scientific, and logical order. For Comte, philosophy became the "theory of science."

Nineteenth-century scientists and physicians further refined Comte's ideas. Claude Bernard (1813–1878) introduced the principles of experimental medicine and tackled basic issues of the normal and the pathological. Observation of disease became a fundamental principle of understanding normal physiology, and hence the principles of homeostasis (or equilibrium of forces in health). While such ideas were also espoused by ancient philosophers, Bernard and the scientists of his generation encased these concepts into a framework of hypotheses and mechanisms. Henri Poincaré (1854–1912) emphasized the role of hypothesis in the unity of nature. He emphasized that "all generalization is an hypothesis; it ought always, as soon as possible, as often as possible, to be subjected to verification. If it does not stand this test, it ought to be abandoned without reserve." Doing so with an "ill humor" is not justified. To Poincaré, there were dangerous hypotheses, those that were tacit, unconscious, and multiple, and the "natural hypotheses" (rather than neutral ones) that led to erroneous and unjustified conclusions and generalizations. Norman Campbell (1880–1949) emphasized the potential practical value of science, but also its limitations: science was "a choice of means, not a choice of ends," and certainty of scientific knowledge was inherently limited by the narrow angle of "previous experience."

The birth of modern neurological surgery at the turn of the 20th century occurred during this background of maturing scientific philosophy which has so influenced the evolving field of medicine. As the first century of neurological surgery is drawing to an end, the philosophy of science is being further revolutionized by an explosion of information and technology never before witnessed by mankind. Ideas and hypotheses are being tackled by the scientific community in small steps, but in a definitive and deliberate fashion as never before. As ants in a colony succeed exhaustingly at individual small tasks, science and medicine are now challenged to integrate these tasks into a common purpose. In the "Decade of the Brain" (the 1990s in North America), neurosurgeons are being challenged to further advance their work, and also to integrate it within a purpose beneficial to mankind. Metaphysical questions of mind and consciousness are being adopted by molecular biologists (as illustrated in Frances Crick's book *The Astonishing Hypothesis: The Scientific Search for the Soul* [1994]).

Neurosurgeons were an integral part of the scientific medical revolution (notably Harvey Cushing and Wilder Penfield), and also at the heart of applying modern technology (such as the operating microscope, image-guided neurosurgery, and computer-assisted therapeutic planning) for the betterment of man. They are now being challenged to assess the impact of these contributions in socioeconomic terms, and also in a global human context.

The neurosurgeons of today are facing the fundamental philosophic questions articulated by Kant: "What can I know?" "What should I do?" "What may I hope?" These questions can only be answered through system building, the formulation of general notions, and the organization of substance and causality, i.e. *metaphysics*. Also, they must be tackled within a theory of knowledge, a dialectic clarification of concepts, and by relating it to experience, i.e. *epistemology*. Lastly, these challenges must be undertaken within a framework theory of moral judgment, i.e. *ethics*. Such are the elements of any philosophy, and these are the philosophic challenges of neurosurgeons. In the perspective of metaphysics, we must articulate the notions of the neurosurgical system. We should do so by carefully examining our identity and our purpose. These are not known or imposed a priori, but must be formulated by neurosurgeons themselves as no one else can shape and impose such identity. In an epistemologic context, we are challenged to formulate and defend our scientific concepts and our methods of neurosurgical practice. We should define neurosurgery's place among human knowledge, and also its value. We should articulate and defend our ways of posing questions, of raising doubt, and of tackling these issues with mechanistic, experimental, and statistical tools. The strengths and weaknesses of these tools must also be evaluated, lest they themselves become the purpose of our intellectual endeavors. Neurosurgeons must define neurosurgical disease, the framework of our knowledge, and the methods of investigation, and we must articulate the purpose of treatment. We must seek to define and evaluate the line between normal and pathological in neurosurgical disease, and interpret this line in biologic and human terms. Lastly, neurosurgeons are challenged to reflect on our work within a moral and ethical context. We must justify what we take from patients and society in return for our "contribution." Neurosurgical altruism cannot be accepted a priori, nor can it be universally demanded per se. To paraphrase Plato, "While we cannot teach moral values directly, it is not a waste of time to reflect on moral excellence." These are the challenges from society and mankind. These are the defining questions of our purpose and our mission. Hence, the importance of a dialog on neurosurgical philosophy.

As a profession, we have not always agreed on the importance of such a task. A book or compilation of ideas on the subject has not before been published. Yet, neurosurgeons have always been drawn to philosophy. The Cushing Orations and Presidential Addresses at our professional gatherings have represented an important philosophic focus for our profession. Yet, these have not always had a lasting or coherent impact. The Publications Committee of the American Association of Neurological Surgeons (AANS) has sought to integrate current neurosurgical philosophic thinking into a text to be read and reflected upon by our profession. While writings have never solved philosophic problems, they have stimulated discussion and laid the framework for the progress of ideas. As neurosurgeons, we are challenged to do at least this much at this phase of our existence.

The Editor undertook the task of compiling such a manuscript, well aware of its difficulties and limitations. As a first attempt to formulate a neurosurgical philosophy, it was our challenge to raise the defining questions, and not necessarily to answer them. It is our hope that we have done this much. The Publications Committee of the AANS called upon a number of neurosurgical leaders to tackle individual aspects of our identity, method, and purpose. Each has embraced the task and has carefully synthesized important thoughts on the subject. It is hoped that individual neurosurgeons, the daily thinkers of the field, will benefit from this compilation of ideas. Some will hopefully apply questions of roots and identity to their own careers. Others may use methodologic approaches to clinical decisions in the care of individual patients. Non-physician philosophers, non-neurosurgeon colleagues, and aspiring neurosurgeons may hopefully catch an inspiring glimpse of our profession. To all who read the book, may the ideas represent mere seeds for future growth and for additional questions and discussions in our intellectual quest. The Editor apologizes that this preliminary compilation could not include all major forces in current neurosurgical thinking, nor the profound philosophic analysis of any individual problem. The neurosurgical subspecialties have evoked unique and profoundly relevant questions of identity and purpose, which were also beyond the general scope of this book. As in all multiauthored texts, the contributions reflect vastly different styles, perspectives, and presentations. The Editor chose to preserve such individualism, as a reflection of the eclectic dynamism within our profession.

The Editor is grateful to the Publications Committee of the AANS for guidance and support through all phases of preparation of this book, and for the opportunity to tackle the task. The staff of the AANS Publications Office, notably Ms. Linda Miller, Ms. Joanne Needham, and Ms. Gay Palazzo performed an admirable task of processing the material through the various phases of publication. Their professionalism was evident throughout. Ms. Patti Guerra is acknowledged for superb administrative and secretarial skills in compiling and word processing the manuscript. Lastly, my family, colleagues, and patients provided much needed inspiration and encouragement, without which many of the ideas and concepts of this work would not have crystallized.

Issam A. Awad, MD, MSc, FACS
New Haven, Connecticut
1994

Foreword

Neurosurgery is a tapestry. Interwoven in the fabric of this specialty are the physicians, the mentors, the patients, the craft itself. The historic context has interspersed a roughened texture of bleak prognosis and a smooth ribbon of triumph over disease and suffering. Technologic innovations and molecular breakthroughs are brilliant trappings. The piece still is being created, formed by a collective of individuals marked by tremendous drive and focus. The contributors to this book represent some of this talent, and their respective chapters should help to pinpoint the aspects of practice that pertain to us all. Although the rich heritage of neurosurgery now occupies an arena that is marred somewhat by a confusing economic scenario, we need to look to these basic tenets that link us as individual practitioners to our forebears and to those who will claim our legacy. In so doing, we may be able to review, refresh, or even reformulate a personal philosophy that can sustain as well as inspire.

The philosphy of neurosurgery, for me, has a lot to do with hero worship. Osler. Cushing. These names invoke a sense of inspiration, of great gifts for inspiring excellence and perseverence. The style of our mentors also shapes us and thus our philosophy. Mine were Odom and Woodhall. Taskmasters with admirable qualities and not-so-admirable traits. Through them and their programs, I have gained expertise in vascular neurosurgery, in head injury, and in pituitary surgery.

I believe what you enjoy doing most in neurosurgery also helps to formulate your personal philosophy. I love to operate, particularly the dual challenges of control and precision, of a good outcome. I focused on transsphenoidal pituitary surgery because it was a relatively new operation that I enjoyed learning and teaching, and it had good results. I love the puzzle work associated with diagnosis. I believe you have to speak to patients, touch them, listen to them, watch them. This is far more important initially than looking at the imaging studies and coming to early conclusions about diagnosis, and I have tried to impress this on my residents.

My philosophy of neurosurgery has a lot to do with hard work. The rigors of the research lab and the labors of writing all have driven me in my profession. I believe whether you are a resident or attending, an academic neurosurgeon or in private practice, you have to work hard. Cushing said once: "The only way to endure life is to have a task to complete." This sums up my view toward my specialty. Whether in the form of clinical activities, research, writing, or surgery, the neurosurgeon is shaped by the next task at hand. Our training years teach us discipline and focus. We become task-oriented and the expected rewards for completing these tasks successfully have been significant in this society.

At this juncture in the history of neurosurgery, however, what many have perceived as the rewards are being challenged. In today's current economic climate, many neurosurgeons are unhappy, concerned with loss of autonomy, with threatened economic status. The dark side of neurosurgery is a self-serving nature. It is where the fabric does not hold and weakens the construct of the specialty. I would ask: Why, then, do we practice neurosurgery? What personal gain is there? If your answers have more to do with earning a living than serving the living, then your altruism is misplaced. Osler once said that medicine is an art, not a trade. Managed care presents significant challenges to the philosophic basis of our profession. Hero worship and hard work seem to pale in the face of these challenges. The chapters in this book should help each of us to formulate an updated, workable version of our philosophy. Ultimately, however, we cannot lose focus of the drive, the mentoring, the hard work, and the compassion—the enduring fibers of our specialty's tapestry.

—George T. Tindall, MD

The satisfaction of being able to relieve pain and restore function, the intellectual challenge of solving clinical problems, and the variety of human issues we confront in daily clinical practice will remain the essence of doctoring, whatever the changes in the organizational and economic structure of medicine.

—C. Eisenberg, in *On Doctoring*

CHAPTER 1

The Founding Philosophy of Neurosurgery

Don M. Long, MD, PhD

The Neurosurgical Heritage

There are a number of great men in many countries who played important roles in the genesis of the field of neurosurgery, but only two are universally known to be truly instrumental in founding the specialty which we now practice. Harvey Cushing and Walter Dandy defined neurosurgery and their philosophies clearly dominate our field today. To understand Dandy, it is necessary to understand Cushing and Halsted. To understand Cushing, one must know Osler, Welch, Halsted, Gilman, and Kocher.[2,5,6] To understand these great men and their contributions to the philosophy of medicine, it is necessary to know something about the enormous changes that occurred in American medicine around the turn of the century and how these changes impacted upon the ancient philosophy of medicine.[6] The philosophy of neurosurgery cannot be considered apart from the philosophy of medicine, to which too little attention has been paid in the past century. To some extent, the problems now confronted by medicine relate to the lack of a coherent philosophy for the new field of medicine which has been in existence for barely 100 years.[1]

The philosophic basis for medicine is discussed widely, but I believe the indispensable components are found in the healing relationship. The physician must guarantee to every patient that only individual welfare will dictate any choices the physician may make. The healing relationship is diminished when any other motives play a role. The physician is committed to the most accurate diagnosis, a prognosis that must include the natural history of the disease, and a therapeutic plan that has the potential for improving the natural

history. The patient also has responsibilities in the relationship. Patients must trust the physician implicitly, be assured that only their welfare dictates advice and treatment, and place themselves in the hands of physicians for things that may be unpleasant, dangerous, even life-threatening. If the patient does not have this trust, the healing relationship is diminished.

The interactions of doctor and student, and colleague with colleague also represent important parts of medical philosophy. Since the time of Hippocrates, it has been assumed that physicians learn throughout life and apply that increased knowledge for the benefit of their patients. Consultations are freely sought and freely given. Only charlatans employ secret treatments or withhold vital details from other physicians. When any factor diminishes the ability to give and receive consultation or impedes the doctor in teaching a student, the healing relationship is diminished.

Before the revolution in medical education, which began about 100 years ago, the fundamental basis of medicine had continued without much change since the time of Galen (130?–201?).[1] The doctrine of signatures dominated medical thinking. Diagnoses were made by recognizing patterns that occurred in the natural history of a disease, and treatments were devised by observing factors that naturally or logically accompanied those patterns. Not much was done of direct value when compared to what is available today, for prognostication was more developed than therapeutics. The scientific revolution in medicine, which began at Johns Hopkins and then was institutionalized in the Flexner Report, changed the ancient formula, and medicine was reborn as a new field.[2] In my view, medicine is one of the youngest of the scientific disciplines, not the oldest, and as yet has no articulated philosophy to substitute for the centuries-old doctrines that governed medicine previously. The lack of an articulated philosophy makes it important to examine the philosophies of the founders of modern medicine. This is particularly important for neurosurgery, which is one of the most specialized aspects of medicine. Neurosurgeons deal almost exclusively with urgent, life- and function-threatening problems. The neurosurgeon's task is dangerous and unpleasant. We neurosurgeons are as yet unable to modify significantly the natural history of many of the diseases we treat. As neurosurgeons, and thus neurosurgical departments, tend to be highly individualistic, we have no unifying philosophy in neurosurgery. In fact, the subject has been virtually undiscussed.

The philosophic changes that occurred in medicine in the latter half of the 19th century were profound, and represent the most radical departure from the past in the development of science. It was not spontaneous, but developed because of need and as a natural consequence of an even greater revolution in university education. Until the middle of the 19th century, universities had changed little since they were founded in medieval times. Mastery of the trivium could be supplemented by graduate programs in four fields (the *quadrivium*). It was possible to study philosophy, theology, law, or medicine on a graduate level, and these faculties existed in most medieval universities. However, the doctors in the faculty of medicine were only vaguely related to the practicing physicians, for whom degrees certainly were not required. The universities were viewed as repositories of knowledge, much of the great scientific research was done independently, and university appointments usually came as a reward for great work. Many physicians learned by preceptorials; medical schools generally were unrelated to universities, and medicine was commonly regarded as an undergraduate curriculum. There was no specialization, no formal postgraduate training, and most medical education was by lecture and observation only, without any chance to learn practical skills. Learning clinical medicine from patients had been suggested by

Sydenham at least 100 years earlier, but had never been put into practice.

Two signal events changed the philosophic basis of medical education. In the early part of the 19th century, concern about the status of education, particularly in the sciences, led to the formation of a commission chaired by the great German academician Wilhelm von Humboldt. The report of this commission suggested a change in the mission of the university and emphasized the need for a research-oriented faculty. A new university in Berlin was founded on the principals delineated by the report. A short time later, one of its students, Daniel Colt Gilman, was chosen to organize a new university in Baltimore under terms outlined by its founder, Johns Hopkins. Thus, Gilman had the opportunity to choose and organize a faculty with the twin goals of education and the generation of new knowledge. The first research university was born.[6]

There was another important factor in the generation of this new philosophic basis for education. Charles Elliott, president of Harvard, was instrumental in liberalizing the undergraduate curriculum, especially stressing science and biology. The success of Elliott's reforms led to the enormous diversity of potential college experiences in the United States, forever separating the American under- and postgraduate experiences from the traditional forms of Europe.

Today, when every major university follows the model of a research institution and virtually the entire government program for the support of higher education uses this model, it is hard to remember that the research university as a concept is just over 100 years old. The spectacular growth of this educational venture has occurred within the past 50 years.

Equally dramatic changes followed in medical education. Although Johns Hopkins intended to found a medical school, establishing the university and hospital exhausted the available funds.

The gap in financing, however, was filled by an endowment from four young women in Baltimore led by Mary Alice Garrett, heir to a famous railroad fortune. William Welch had already been chosen dean, and Halsted and Osler had joined the faculty, but there was no money to complete the faculty or support the first class in medicine. Miss Garrett and her friends, with the support of

Welch, demanded specific conditions for the new medical school before the endowment would be forthcoming: 1) that women be allowed to compete equally with men for positions in the new school; 2) that all medical students were to have an undergraduate degree; 3) that competitive merit was to be the determining factor in selection; and 4) that regular assessment of performance by formal examination was required. No one would question these concepts now, but at the time they were controversial and were rejected by most educators. The new concepts were hotly debated and still considered to be of questionable merit when Cushing and Dandy began their careers.[2]

Practical changes in education implemented by the founders of the new school were of equal importance. These concepts have been the fundamental basis for medical education for the past 100 years. Therefore, it is sometimes difficult to remember how revolutionary they were a century ago. At that time, medical schools were not regulated in any way, and there were enormous differences in quality. Most medical education was a form of preceptorship and was delivered by lecture. There was little practical experience and patients were not a part of the educational process. William Osler and William Halsted together produced our current model of medical education. Osler took the education of the medical student from the lecture hall to the clinic and bedside. He emphasized clinical diagnosis and the requirement to see many patients with diverse problems. In a way it can be said that Osler returned to Galen's doctrine of signatures. Osler also stressed that the physician must be humanistic and caring, and re-emphasized the healing relationship and the interactions among physicians as fundamental to satisfactory medical practice. Our entire system of medical education comes from Osler's formulations.

In surgery as well, most education was by observation. Operating rooms were large amphitheaters in which students watched a famous surgeon in action. Training in surgery was a form of indentured servitude with no formal curriculum, no specified period or content of training, and little opportunity for the would-be surgeon to do any more than assist, so that most surgeons were self-taught by what they did to patients after training. This lack of formality in surgical training is best understood by remembering that surgery as we know it is also a new field. The introduction of anesthesia at the Massachusetts General Hospital, Koch's discovery of bacteria, and Lister's introduction of measures to prevent surgical infections allowed surgery to be developed after 1850. Even today it is a new field; at the time Harvey Cushing began his training, it was so new as to be undefined. Certainly no philosophy for the practice of surgery had yet evolved.

Halsted developed the field of surgery as we know it today. Even though anesthesia and antisepsis had allowed elective surgery to become a reality, the slash-and-burn technique of surgery practiced since ancient times was slow to disappear. Halsted changed all this with his emphasis upon meticulous hemostasis, anatomic dissection, and reconstruction with gentle tissue handling. The surgical techniques that are now the basis of all operative therapy did not exist before Halsted. The concept of subspecialization in surgery also was developed by the father of modern surgery. Halsted was the first to understand that the enormous potential developments in elective surgery would rapidly exceed the capacity of a single surgeon to master them. He created the fields of orthopedics, urology, and otolaryngology, and was a strong supporter of the development of gynecologic surgery as a separate field. He allowed Harvey Cushing to develop neurosurgery, although he expressed his skepticism about the viability of this aspect of surgery.

Halsted and Osler conceived the concept of formal residency training, which Halsted put into practice. The entire organization of postgraduate specialty education in medicine is based on Halsted's surgical training program, in which the best students were chosen competitively, the training was of a specified length, and the content was defined. Research was made a part of surgical training, and extensive laboratory preparation for surgery on humans was required. The training was of escalating responsibility and culminated with 1 year of supervised practice before completely independent surgery by the student was allowed. This revolutionary change was what Cushing encountered when he moved from Boston to Baltimore.[5]

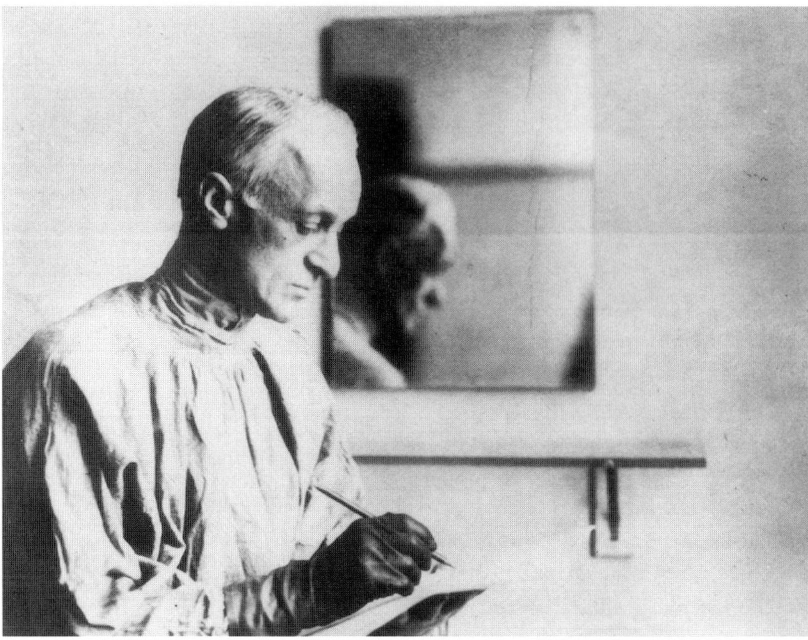

Figure 1. Harvey Cushing, the clinician/scientist and the writer. (Reproduced courtesy of the American Association of Neurological Surgeons Archives.)

In order to understand the practice and philosophy of our founders, it is very important to recognize the meaning of these changes that I have summarized. Over a period of no more than 25 years, there was such a fundamental change in medicine that a new field of study and practice really can be said to have developed. The entire basis of medical education changed. A new field of surgery was born. A medical heritage going back thousands of years was so radically altered that the new field of medicine decidedly can be related only historically to those earlier centuries. These changes were institutionalized in American medicine by the events following the Flexner Report, but all of the reforms of Flexner were in place at Johns Hopkins and influenced the founders of neurosurgery in their formative years.

Harvey Cushing and the Foundations of Neurosurgery

Harvey Cushing was a remarkable man, probably the only true genius American medicine has produced (Figure 1). He founded two medical specialties, neurosurgery and endocrinology. With Halsted, he established the concept of the clinician/scientist in academics. In addition, Cushing established the underlying philosophy of neurosurgery which is still in existence. I believe his philosophy can best be described through understanding these enormous contributions and how they influence our practice today.[4]

The Ether Chart

The key to understanding Cushing's contributions to the practice of medicine is to understand his philosophy of immediate, practical, logical solutions to serious problems in the practice of surgery. While still a medical student, Cushing experienced the dangers of administering anesthesia, at that time a haphazard enterprise dependent upon the experience of the anesthetist. Immediately thereafter, he developed a record of pulse and respiration, which aided the determination of the depth of anesthesia and is now fundamental for every form of anesthetic administered throughout the world. The principal of recognizing a problem and promptly implementing a universal solution is central to Cushing's career. Observing the sphygmomanometer while taking his postresidency European tour a few years later, he immediately recognized the importance of blood pressure measurement during surgery and returned to Baltimore to add the regular determination of such to the ether chart. This application of technology was rejected not only by most surgeons but also by some of the most prestigious medical institutions in the United States. Cushing, the newest surgical staff member at Johns Hopkins, refused to be daunted, and persisted in writing and talking about this important advance until it was accepted and became standard practice.

Technology Transfer: The Use of X-Rays in Surgical Practice

Another key to Cushing's approach to the practice of medicine is seen in his adaptation of x-rays to surgical practice. Soon after the x-ray machine was invented, he saw its advantage for surgeons and had an intraoperative x-ray taken for the localization of a bullet in the cervical spine. The recognition of technologic advances and immediate application of those advances to practice was fundamental to Cushing's philosophy and has remained an integral part of neurosurgery since.

Neurosurgery as a Specialty

Long before Harvey Cushing, there were adventurous surgeons who carried out neurosurgical operations of many kinds. Primitive efforts are found in the origins of recorded human history. Before Cushing, neurosurgery was performed by a few general surgeons. Still fewer did enough neurosurgery to be known even for an interest in the field. Mortality and morbidity were extremely high. In the surgical texts available prior to Cushing, neurosurgery was virtually limited to the treatment of intracranial and spinal infections or trauma.

It is probable that William Osler was the originator of Cushing's interest in the nervous system. Osler's experiences in pathology had led him to conclude that operations on the brain and spinal cord should be possible. It is clear that Cushing was thinking about neurosurgery before he finished training and was encouraged to develop this new field by Osler. Cushing's surgical heritage, however, was Halstedian. Even as a student, he was dissatisfied with the way surgery was practiced and commented before he left the Massachusetts General Hospital, "These men operate about the way a commercial traveler grabs breakfast at a counter." This understanding that a new form for surgery was required brought him to Halsted. He was a leading proponent of Halsted's careful technique as applied to the nervous system, without which it is probable that neurosurgery never could have developed.

Cushing spent a year with Kocher in Bern, during which time he traveled in Europe and participated in his first serious research experience. Kocher's laboratory was famous for research in head injury, and although Cushing never again worked with trauma patients, he recognized the value of research and conceived the idea of including it in the training of all surgeons. Returning to Baltimore, he joined the surgical faculty at Johns Hopkins to direct the Hunterian Laboratory where students and residents learned living anatomy and the techniques of surgery. To these, Cushing added high-quality laboratory research.

The Concept of the Clinician/ Scientist

Cushing, during his tenure as director of the Hunterian Laboratory, developed our modern concept of the clinician/scientist as the fundamental role in academic medicine. He did so by recognizing the similarities between his patients with hypopituitarism secondary to tumors, and hypophysectomized dogs. Thus, he discovered the master hormonal nature of the pituitary gland and established the new field of endocrinology. In so doing, he proved that a busy surgeon could do competitive research. The other great men of Johns Hopkins at that time were eminent clinicians and scholars, and they did clinical research. However, Cushing was unique in the quality and extent of his laboratory commitment. At the origin of our specialty, it was established that the leaders in the field should be capable researchers. However, the impact of Cushing's contribution goes far beyond the field of neurosurgery. With Halsted, he established the model of the clinician/scientist that is now universal in academic medicine throughout the world.

The Hunterian Laboratory established elitism as another feature of Cushing's philosophy. Cushing chose the best student interested in surgery to be his Hunterian fellow and then to work with him in clinical neurosurgery. Thus, the principal that neurosurgery should attract the best students was established early. Years later, Cushing donated $25,000 to the Department of Surgery at Johns Hopkins to support postgraduate training for the best student in the country interested in surgery, and commented about the great value that a similar endowment had been to him at Harvard. He had little interest in training a large cadre of surgeons, preferring to focus on an elite group to carry on his tradition.

Cushing as a Clinical Surgeon

Few men ever revolutionized so completely a field as William Halsted did surgery. Halstedian technique with its emphasis upon tissue handling and anatomic dissection is now the basis of every surgical discipline. Despite this, surgery was still a frightful experience only 100 years ago. Anesthesia was problematic, hemostasis was difficult, and speed was the hallmark of most surgeons. Even as a medical student, Cushing saw the shortcomings of this approach, but he was challenged rather than repelled by what he saw. Just as a catastrophe during ether anesthesia challenged him to produce the ether chart and thus improve the techniques of administering anesthesia, the same was true of his experience in surgery. He learned Halstedian surgery and then applied it to the nervous system. He rapidly determined that the surgical techniques employed by the European general surgeons who performed neurosurgery were unsatisfactory. Even so, his first attempts at intracranial surgery were uniformly bad, but in typical fashion he persisted and soon was able to present mortality and morbidity data that startled the surgical world. Throughout his career he remained a meticulous surgeon, bold for his day, but always mindful of the patient's condition. He strove persistently to reduce the mortality and morbidity of neurosurgery and was incredibly successful for his time. Only in the past 20 years have other surgeons surpassed his results.

Cushing the Writer

It is clear that Harvey Cushing knew his place in history. He saved everything, although his papers have not received the literary treatment they deserve. He wrote extensively, and inspired others who had talent, but perhaps less creativity, to help him collate his extensive clinical collections. He documented everything he did and wrote about it extensively. To this day neurosurgeons maintain this heritage, honoring prolific surgeons who write about their experiences, and innovative surgeons who develop new techniques.

Cushing the Academic Leader

An excerpt from a diary of William Welch epitomizes Harvey Cushing. Having met Cushing in Paris to begin a European junket, Welch commented in his diary that Cushing arrived amidst great fanfare—his arrival known to everyone in Paris. The cost of the evening's festivities destroyed Welch's budget.

Harvey Cushing was a writer as few are and had a keen sense of history. Not many neurosurgeons will ever write as he did, but an historical sense is strong in the field. He encouraged neurosurgical organization, as well as development at the administrative level nationally. Even though he rejected the idea of leading the birth of yet another new field—i.e. the neurosciences in 1911—he remained a strong champion of all things related to neurology. While he did no research after he went to Harvard, he remained a strong advocate for neurologic research and research training for neurosurgeons. Both tendencies are clearly visible in neurosurgery today.

Walter Dandy

Walter Dandy was a surgeon! Although he made great contributions in all aspects of neurosurgery, it is his philosophy of surgery that makes him such a giant in the field (Figure 2).[3] Dandy began his career as Cushing's Hunterian fellow, and his work was key to much of Cushing's success with the early pituitary research. The ideas were Cushing's, of course, but the execution was for the most part Dandy's. Dandy was prepared to

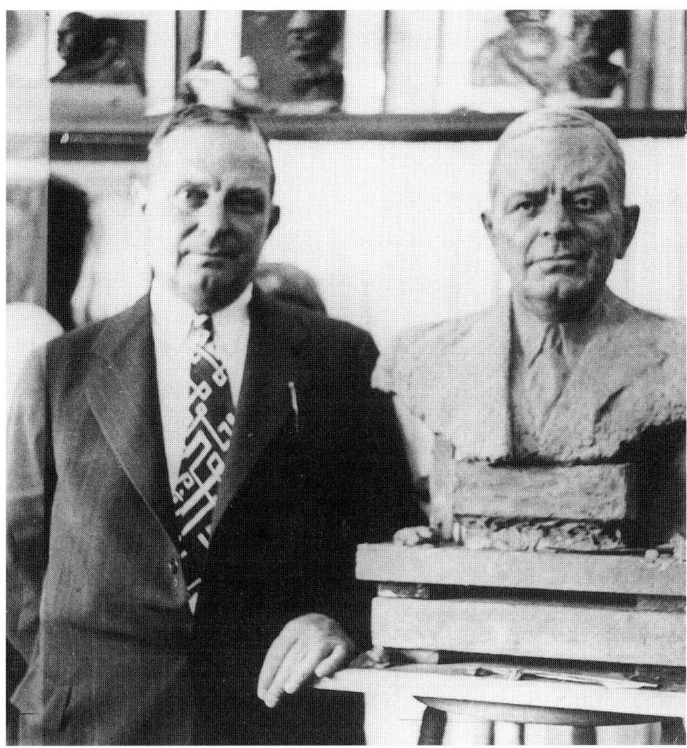

Figure 2. Photograph taken by Dr. Emil Seletz of Walter Dandy with the bust of Dandy created by Dr. Seletz. (Reproduced courtesy of the American Association of Neurological Surgeons Archives.)

leave Johns Hopkins at the conclusion of medical school to join Cushing's house staff at Harvard. The famous break that occurred between the precocious young faculty member and his pupil has been well publicized, but in my view, its fundamental effect upon the development of the field of neurosurgery has been neglected. Had Dandy gone to Harvard, he would have undergone the traditional training program and probably followed the Cushing model. The losses to neurosurgery would have been great. Cushing was careful, precise, and methodical. Dandy was inspired and intuitive. An entire generation of neurosurgery professors worldwide followed Cushing's surgical techniques while Dandy independently developed a brilliant surgical style not matched before or since, setting technical standards that still excite neurosurgeons. Dandy maintained strong ties with general surgery, which was alienated by Cushing and his men. The separation meant that Johns Hopkins, the pioneering medical school and the dominant research university, never entered the mainstream of neurosurgical development, and the revolutionary influences the institution might have brought were never realized in the specialty.

What did Walter Dandy do? Remember that he was left without a job when his offer of a house staff position at Harvard was withdrawn by Cushing. Winford Smith, the director of the Johns Hopkins Hospital, recognized Dandy's enormous potential and took it upon himself to offer Dandy a position in the face of Halsted's prolonged absence. His judgment was immediately confirmed by Halsted upon his return to Baltimore. Dandy and the pediatrician Kenneth Blackfan entered the laboratory to study the poorly understood entity, hydrocephalus. We do not know why Dandy chose this difficult topic. Louis Weed, the Johns Hopkins neuroanatomist, was certainly the leading authority on the circulation of cerebrospinal fluid and the anatomy of the third circulation. The choice demonstrates one of the keys to Dandy's philosophy. He was willing to choose an extremely difficult subject for study, one with a high risk of failure. Many famous anatomists and pathologists had failed in their attempts to understand spinal fluid circulation and the genesis of hydrocephalus. This willingness to attack difficult questions through the use of advanced surgical techniques is fundamental in the specialty today. The success story is well known to everyone. Dandy created what many medical historians believe to be the best piece of applied surgical research ever done through technical feats of surgery that none of the pathologic anatomists studying the problem could match. His combination of physiologic and anatomic studies was a masterpiece, bringing him instant fame even before he joined the house staff.

The next important contribution was the discovery of air encephalography, which alone was one of the major medical advances of the century. Several stories suggest that the discovery was serendipitous, but I think it is probable that this theory was promulgated by Cushing's men, who did not want to credit Dandy with anything. Dandy's writings make it clear that he was convinced, even when he was still in training, that the key to advances in neurosurgery was to be found in precise imaging for localization of abnormalities.

Dandy the Surgeon

The other historical aspect of great interest pertaining to the origins of neurosurgery is that Cushing's departure left Dandy without a mentor. We don't know when Dandy decided to be a neurosurgeon. Neurosurgery as we now know it did not exist at Johns Hopkins during Dandy's training, being carried out at that time by general surgeons. This meant that Dandy was largely self-taught in neurosurgery, but also learned from a mature Halsted and his best, most experienced students. He also had the advantage of watching the fruits of both the residency training program and subspecialization. Rather than learning Cushing's techniques, Dandy entered a surgical field that was much more aggressive and radical in nature than Cushing had experienced. All who knew him recognized his enormous technical skills. Without ties to Cushing's surgical dogma, he was able to develop a new philosophy of surgery which is fundamental in neurosurgery today. Dandy planned to cure, not palliate.

Dandy also expanded neurosurgery to its current broad applications. He was the first to clip an intracranial aneurysm and to successfully treat arteriovenous malformations, and opened the entire field of vascular diseases. He understood the use of neurosurgical procedures to treat functional diseases (tinnitus and vertigo), and made neurosurgeons aware of their ability to manipulate the nervous system to improve its function. He was the first to recognize and remove a herniated intervertebral disc, although for some reason his paper was not cited in the subsequent report by Mixter and Barr. Dandy's isolation from much of the rest of the neurosurgical community may very well account for this. The later paper came from Cushing's institution.

Cushing was the first neurosurgeon and established the field. Dandy was the first *modern* neurosurgeon, and his techniques are only now being supplanted through the use of magnification and technology.

Another feature of Dandy's surgical practice that has remained important in neurosurgery was his enormous capacity for work. It has been estimated that he carried out 500 to 700 major operations per year for most of his career. Dr. Frank Otenasek, his partner when Dandy died, told me he thought that estimate was low. This work ethic begun by Cushing and exaggerated by Dandy has remained an important part of the neurosurgical mystique.

Dandy the Academician

Walter Dandy was clearly an elitist when it came to neurosurgery. He only trained residents in the late stages of his career. There was no administrative designation for neurosurgery, the "Brain Team" simply being a part of general surgical training. A staunch supporter of neurosurgery's place within general surgery, his participations were with the American College of Surgeons, not the newly emerging neurosurgical organizations. This meant that his newly evolving philosophies for practice and research were not a part of neurosurgery in its early stages.

One other feature of Dandy the scholar has remained an integral part of neurosurgery. Cushing wrote from experience, but detailed that experience exhaustively. Dandy wrote his personal philosophy of managing patients as derived from his vast experience. It is interesting that Dandy's philosophy of medical writing became more important than Cushing's for many years in neurosurgery.

The Founding Philosophy of Neurosurgery

The impact of these two great men upon our specialty cannot be over-emphasized. No other field of medicine has been established—nor so dominated—by two such personalities and philosophies. Harvey Cushing was probably the only true genius produced by American medicine. He is the most famous surgeon in history, with the possible exceptions of Halsted and Lord Lister. Walter Dandy, in turn, became the most famous surgeon of his day. Cushing and Dandy demanded outstanding assistants and set a standard of performance that is almost impossibly high. All serious practitioners of our field must feel compelled to maintain that standard. The two men shared an incredible work ethic which persists in the specialty today. The concept of the clinician/scientist, fundamental to academic medicine worldwide, was developed by Cushing, and Dandy became one of its principal examples. Neurosurgeons retain a strong belief that research is an integral part of training, yet both Cushing and Dandy, for all their successes in research, gave up investigations for practice. This habit also persists in neurosurgery. It is clear that research accomplishments are important for the foundation of a neurosurgical academic career, but it is equally clear that it is the clinician who is most honored.

Cushing and Dandy were so dramatically different that it is not surprising they did not remain friends and colleagues. The origins of their quarrel were never specified and are now forgotten. Cushing was well organized, methodical in his approach to clinical medicine, catalogued extensively, wrote beautifully, and approached everything with a great sense of history and propriety. He wished to leave a legacy of devoted followers and did so. Knowing that he was founding a new specialty, he wanted it clearly set apart from general surgery. Dandy was personally and intuitively brilliant, but never organized his clin-

ical material. He depended upon unmatched surgical skills to do things no one had tried before and that were generally considered to be impossible. He rarely recognized previous accomplishments that might have contributed to his success, and he made no effort to found a school of neurosurgery at Johns Hopkins, clearly preferring neurosurgery to remain small and elite. He was not convinced there was a need for an organization separate from surgery and generally considered the national political issues trivial and a waste of his time. He was unconcerned with hierarchy and protocol. These great differences in style and function meant that two very strong, very distinct role models were available in neurosurgery. Cushing was obviously the dominant force, but when Dandy supplanted Cushing (after retirement) as the most famous surgeon in America, this dual personality of neurosurgery was accentuated further. It is interesting to speculate as to what would have happened had these two men been compatible, and had their combined talents rather than their separate personalities become the model for neurosurgeons. The availability of a choice between these disparate styles has reduced cohesiveness in neurosurgery.

The personal differences between the two great founders of neurosurgery are probably not as philosophically important as the fact that the antipathy between them kept the medical reforms that originated at Johns Hopkins out of neurosurgery. Dandy does not appear to have been particularly interested in education except on a personal level with his small number of trainees. Cushing did not even maintain the teaching tenants of Osler and Halsted. Residencies and examinations were not formalized for years and neurosurgical training remained unstructured for much longer than in the other surgical specialties.

The Neurosurgical Philosophy

No philosophy for neurosurgery has been articulated before now. This is not surprising since no serious philosophy for medicine has been proposed since Osler, whose writings are fragmented and do not purport to be all-encompassing. Medicine as we know it today is a new field, barely

100 years old in theory and substantially less than that in practice. No articulated philosophy to guide medical practice has been developed in this short period of time. Yet if we examine the characteristics of neurosurgical behavior and think about the styles of the two great neurosurgeons whom we all emulate, we can outline a rudimentary structure for a philosophy of neurosurgery.

Since the time of Cushing and Dandy, there has been great emphasis on technical skill in neurosurgery. The nature of the specialty requires it, as great harm can be done by minor lapses in technique. No neurosurgeon who is not technically excellent should be satisfied with either training or practice. Neurosurgery requires that the practitioner be a skilled neurologist, neuropathologist, and neuroradiologist. The least that is required in these fields is competency. Cushing emphasized meticulous neurology, Dandy the importance of interpreting the subtleties of imaging, and both men stressed the importance of understanding neuropathology in order to accurately prognosticate for patients. Neurosurgeons maintain arduous schedules both in the operating room and out, a heritage of both our founders, and are quick to recognize the value of new technology and bring it into practice. Individualism is strong in the specialty, and there is an ambivalent tendency to separate from the rest of surgery and to proliferate new neurosurgical societies. Neurosurgeons have been unable to determine whether the field is based in the neurosciences—a separate entity—or remains strongly tied to the field of surgery. The importance of the role of research in medicine remains a firm part of neurosurgical training, and neurosurgeons believe in research. However, as the great men of neurosurgery mostly have been clinicians, few practice research even at the academic level. But neurosurgeons are compelled to write and talk about what they do. This small specialty generates an enormous amount of literature and presentation. This is in keeping with the heritage of our two founders as well.

We are a young specialty that, in its brief existence, has undergone three quantum changes—Halstedian surgery, the imaging era, and microsurgery. We do not have a philosophic tradition on which our field is based. But the qualities brought to the specialty by our founders are hon-ored. Neurosurgeons believe the specialty is unique, practiced by an elite few. Clinicians are honored and great technicians revered, but while research is honored as fundamental to training in neurosurgery, an outstanding research career is not enough. An arduous work schedule is expected, both during a long period of training and after. Neurosurgeons pride themselves on maintaining a large clinical volume, writing and talking about what they do and how they do it. We adapt to new things quickly and are serious about ongoing postgraduate education. As a specialty, we are not afraid to take on difficult clinical challenges or to deal with death and disaster.

There have been other great men in neurosurgery and many have left some aspect of themselves in our field. This is particularly true in countries other than the United States, where pioneers in the new specialties adapted the ideas of Harvey Cushing to a new country and a different medical culture. In no field of medicine, however, have two such dominant personalities had the impact that Cushing and Dandy have had in neurosurgery. There is something challenging to those who follow when such high standards have been set. The philosophy of our new field is of necessity derived from the beliefs and practices of these two men, and it is a sign of maturation of the specialty that we begin to think about our origins philosophically rather than only historically. As modern medicine examines itself a century after the revolutionary ideas that gave it birth, it is time for a serious evaluation of the principals in which we all believe. The ideas of Gilman, Welch, Osler, Halsted, and Cushing were never examined in the way the Federalist papers examined the origins of American democracy. They have never been debated seriously. The practice of neurosurgery is discussed practically, but the basis of that practice is rarely mentioned.

Modern medicine is a new field of science. The radical ideas from which it arose also founded neurosurgery. Cushing and Dandy were the logical fruition of these new ideas. Yet their contributions are fundamentally within the ancient healing relationship. Cushing's detailed clinical material greatly improved prognosis. Dandy's imaging revolutionized diagnosis. But their principal impact was in therapeutics, the goal of all that both men did. It is not surprising that the most important attribute of neurosurgery remains a constant striving to improve outcome for our patients.

Cushing was fond of saying neurosurgery was 20% science, 75% artistry, and 5% community service. We have markedly increased the science. We hope the artistry remains the same. The expansion of our field also has multiplied the value of our community service many times. Giving more than 100% is appropriate to the legacy of our great founders, and is the basis of modern neurosurgery.

References

1. Buchanan SM. *The Doctrine of Signatures.* 2nd ed. Urbana, Ill: University of Illinois Press; 1991.
2. Chesney AM. *The Johns Hopkins Hospital and the Johns Hopkins University School of Medicine.* Baltimore, Md: Johns Hopkins University Press; 1943.
3. Fox WL. *Dandy of Johns Hopkins.* Baltimore, Md: Williams & Wilkins; 1984.
4. Fulton JF. *Harvey Cushing.* Springfield, Ill: Charles C Thomas; 1946.
5. Harvey AM. *Science at the Bedside.* Baltimore, Md: Johns Hopkins University Press; 1981.
6. Muller SM. Wilhelm von Humboldt and the University in the United States. *Johns Hopkins APL Digest.* 1985;6:253-256.

CHAPTER 2

Neurosurgery's Ideals in Historical Perspective

Samuel H. Greenblatt, MA, MD, FACS

It can be argued that neurosurgery is a distinct profession, albeit within the larger professions of surgery and medicine. To whatever extent this is true, it follows that neurosurgery should be distinguishable from other related professions by a distinct set of goals and ideals. Hence, the identification and analysis of these ideals constitutes an important act of self-definition. In some measure, we are what we stand for.

I submit that neurosurgery has at least three sets of goals and ideals that have been transmitted from its founders to the present. They can be described under the rubrics: 1) manual/technical, 2) scientific, and 3) humanistic. None of these is entirely unique to neurosurgery, of course. But taken together, with the particular nuances that our pioneers gave them, they have made us uniquely what we are. Although they guide our thoughts and actions as practitioners and especially as teachers, these ideals have seldom been well articulated. More to the present point, they have not been systematically analyzed historically or in any other way. The present chapter will offer a partial analysis through an historical approach.

By "manual/technical" ideals, I mean primarily the goal of pushing our manual and technical skills to the limits of what human beings can accomplish by those means. The "scientific" ideal refers to our tradition of always trying to improve our clinical practices by drawing upon relevant advances in our sister neurosciences and the broader fields of surgery and medicine. As part of the same ideal, one of our most explicit goals has been to contribute to neuroscientific knowledge through the unique opportunities afforded to us by the privilege of operating on the human ner-

vous system. In sum, we try to push our science to the limit. Finally, the "humanistic" ideal refers to our early leaders' belief in the importance of humanistic scholarship, which allows us to see our individual and corporate selves in the larger context. Its persisting influence is attested by the very existence of this book.

The present chapter centers on the history of the scientific ideal in neurosurgery, because I sense that our particular interpretation of that ideal is most important in defining our distinctiveness as a profession. Indeed, we have been scientifically based from the beginning, because modern "brain surgery" became possible only when experimental cortical localization data became available in the 1870s.[13,14] But even while the scientific ideal has been the centerpiece of neurosurgery's "philosophy," it is connected to the manual/technical ideal since scientific advances have laid the necessary groundwork for improvements in neurosurgical techniques. At the same time, the scientific ideal is connected to the humanistic ideal because neurosurgery's experience seems to show that good scholarship involving the nervous system frequently leads to the scholars' asking larger questions.

An Outline of Neurosurgery's Gestational Period

In a chapter of another book,[14] I have presented an historiographic framework for interpreting the overall development of neurosurgery. Without repeating that entire argument, suffice it to say that modern neurosurgery began with

William Macewen in 1879, when he performed the first successful craniotomies that combined the new technologies of anesthesia, antisepsis, and cerebral localization. The next 40 years were "gestational"—the period when neurosurgery developed into a recognizably distinct profession. The advent of full-blown, modern neurosurgery can be dated to Harvey Cushing's delivery of a major paper on improved brain tumor statistics to the American College of Surgeons in 1919. A direct consequence of that triumphal presentation was the founding of the Society of Neurological Surgeons—the world's first neurosurgical society—in 1920.[26(p68)]

The gestational period breaks down conveniently into two phases: a first phase in Britain and Germany from approximately 1880 to 1900 and a second in America from 1900 to 1920. Since neurosurgery as we know it emerged from the totality of these events, it follows that the ideals of its pioneers were formulated and impressed upon the profession at that time. For choosing which early leaders to include in this analysis, I decided that the criteria for selection should be the extent of the individual's influence through his example and especially through his direct teaching of successors.

During the first phase, the early leaders in Britain were William Macewen (1848–1924) and Victor Horsley (1857–1916), and in Germany, they were Ernst von Bergmann (1836–1907) and Fedor Krause (1856–1937). Macewen set a superb example, but he remained a general surgeon throughout his career. More importantly, he trained no one in neurosurgery. Horsley was truly the world's first neurosurgeon because he devoted his later career to the field, and his devotion to science was legendary. Although he had an important influence on several general surgeons who performed some neurosurgery in Britain, his most important trainee was an American, Ernest Sachs, who founded the early and influential program in neurosurgery at Washington University in St. Louis.

Von Bergmann and Krause were both part and parcel of the great flowering of the German-speaking university system in the late 19th century. Von Bergmann was a leading general surgeon who advocated Listerian principles and applied them early on to the nervous system.[15]

He is especially important to us, because he had a direct impact on American neurosurgery through Charles H. Frazier of Philadelphia. Krause was a great technical pioneer, whose influence in Germany was achieved more through his example than through training of successors.[28] As we shall see, neurosurgery's scientific ideal was derived in major measure from the model of the German university system.

In retrospect, the focus of neurosurgery's development shifted from Europe to North America in 1901, when Harvey Cushing (1869–1939) returned to Baltimore and joined the faculty at Johns Hopkins after a *wanderjahr* in Europe. During the period from July 1900 to August 1901, Cushing traveled and visited throughout Britain and the Continent, but he worked mainly with the surgeon Theodor Kocher and the physiologist Hugo Kronecker in Berne, Switzerland, and with the physiologist Charles Sherrington in Liverpool, England. He initially paid a visit to Horsley, intending to work with him, but Cushing was put off by Horsley's eccentricities and especially by his fast and furious surgical techniques.[10(p163)] Cushing's early acquaintance with Sherrington grew into a friendship that eventually had great implications for neurosurgery's scientific orientation.

Since Cushing was and is the most important single individual in the history of neurosurgery, his professional ideals must necessarily be a major focus of this investigation. The more difficult task was to pick the other candidates for analysis from among the early American pioneers, because our view of neurosurgery's ideals would surely be incomplete if we were limited to those of Cushing. Somewhat arbitrarily, I have chosen Charles H. Frazier (1870–1936) of Philadelphia, Ernest Sachs (1879–1958) of St. Louis, and Walter Dandy (1886–1946), Cushing's trainee and successor at Johns Hopkins. These choices are based largely on the selection criteria given above, in addition to my perception that the neurosurgical centers in Boston, Philadelphia, and Baltimore were the major fonts of neurosurgical innovation and training during the early period. For the same reason, I will also give some attention to the contributions of Wilder Penfield (1891–1976) of Montreal. Although he did his major work later (in the middle of the 20th century), much of his education and training occurred in the period of interest. Especially because his numerous trainees carried his approach throughout the world, Penfield is an appropriate representative of the era that followed the gestational period.

European Science and Medicine in the Late 19th Century

In the first half of the 19th century, Paris was the leading center of cultural and scientific life in Europe. But in the second half of the century, Germany and Great Britain achieved more prominent roles. Because of its large and far-flung empire, London was the center of world affairs toward the end of the century, but in science Germany was significantly ahead of Britain, and it retained a unique position in the field until the calamity of the First World War. Since the model of German science in the German universities was the paradigm for the development of the American system of research universities, we can look to some of its ideals for clues to the nature of our own.

Modern German science began to emerge in the mid-19th century, as the country came out of its romantic period quite abruptly. Biology and medicine played leading roles in this process, partly because their scientific basis in strictly materialistic physiology was explicitly proclaimed by a group of brilliant young researchers in 1848, including du Bois-Raymond and Helmholtz.[31] Their goal was to reduce all biological phenomena to physics and chemistry. Hence, in their view, genuine biomedical science must be laboratory-based. These events coincided with the political and industrial rise of modern Germany under the shrewd and ruthless Otto von Bismark, starting in 1862. In that environment of burgeoning aspirations, generous support was lavished on the university system, especially for laboratories and specialized institutes. In a relatively short time, German science in the German universities became the model for the rest of the world.[12(pp86-87)]

An important point about the "German universities" of the late 19th century is that the term really refers to *German-speaking* universities, which existed in a large area of central Europe including

Austria, Germany, the majority of Switzerland, and parts of several other eastern European countries. Since this somewhat loose system was transnational, it was decentralized in terms of power and prestige. Although the relatively young University of Berlin (founded in 1810) was probably the most prestigious single entity, it was not the national equivalent of Paris or "Oxbridge" (Oxford and Cambridge). The universities at Leipzig and Vienna, for example, were not about to concede anything! This situation arose because the universities were supported by local and regional political entities, and the communities took great pride in their universities.[7]

Within this large geographical domain, students moved from one institution to another with relative ease, and worthy professors were competitively recruited. In any academic field, a full professorship carried financial security and social prestige. The early German pioneers of neurosurgery, von Bergmann and Krause, lived and worked within this stimulating environment. Von Bergmann is an especially appropriate exemplar of how the system worked at its best because he gradually made his way from the relative obscurity of the University of Dorpat (Tartu) in Estonia to a professorship at the University of Berlin on the basis of his considerable merits.[15] By then, of course, he was a very senior professor of *surgery*, and so he did not promote neurosurgery as a distinct entity nor articulate a set of ideals for its separate existence. Indeed, this caveat applies to all of the early German pioneers.[22] In Britain, the same conclusion can be drawn for Macewen, but not exactly for Horsley.[8]

On the British Isles, the long period of relative peace and increasing prosperity known as the "Victorian Age" began with the ascent of young Queen Victoria to the throne in 1837 and ended with her death in 1901. The middle of the century has been characterized as the "Age of Equipoise"—a prosperous but still ungilded era when the idea of progress was assumed to be valid, noble, and uncomplicated. As the century wore on, however, progress seems to have engendered less equanimity. British society became richer and more secularized later in the century, and the increasingly urbanized middle and upper classes seem to have developed an outlook that was an unsettling combination of mild anxiety and ennui.[35]

In the realm of scientific research and education, Oxford and Cambridge were poorly receptive to anything new for an overly long time. In an English tradition that dates back to Sir Isaac Newton (1642–1727) and even earlier in the 17th century, modern science was conducted outside of the formal university structures, although often in the university towns. In the 19th century, Charles Darwin accomplished his epoch-making work largely on a private basis. Until very late in the century, the only type of formal scientific training in the British universities was in the faculties of medicine. Part of the reason for this pattern of recalcitrant behavior is found in the corporate structure of the old universities. The real power—and the money—was vested in the individual colleges at Oxford and Cambridge. As universities, they were less than the sum of their parts. This collegiate arrangement works well for the tutorial study of the classics or mathematics, but it is inimical to the creation of large enterprises such as scientific laboratories, which require expenditures that cannot be duplicated by each college.[12(pp45-47)]

Some progress in this regard was made at the younger and reformist University of London (founded in 1827), but the power structure of British society was such that definitive action had to take place at Oxbridge. Laboratories for physics were created at both universities around 1870. In 1873, Michael Foster obtained his first small but separate facility for physiology at Cambridge, thus initiating the Cambridge School of Physiology.[12(p163)] This event turned out to be highly significant for neurosurgery because of its connection to Sherrington and thence to Cushing and Fulton. By the time Sherrington arrived at Cambridge in 1879, Foster's enterprise was flourishing. Sherrington worked in the physiology laboratory with Walter Gaskell and John Langley from 1880 to 1883. It was through his association with Foster and Langley that Sherrington first became involved in neurophysiological research on cortical localization.[30]

In both physics and physiology, the founding of these British facilities was due in large measure to the correct perception by a few individuals that the Germans were running away with pre-eminence because of the strength of their universities and research institutes.[12(pp86-87)] In science, as in other human affairs, imitation is a form of both flattery and competition.

In the United States, the German example was also attracting attention and envy, but the social and political environment was different. The seeds of imitation took root in different soil, and the result was a distinctly different product.

American Society at the Turn of the Century

Around 1880, the United States emerged from a prolonged period of self-absorption. We had survived the horrific experience of the Civil War and Reconstruction in the 1860s and a mild but tenacious economic depression in the 1870s. On the international scene, we were not yet a major player, but it was obvious that we were destined to become one. Our sheer physical size and economic potential could lead to no other conclusion, partly because the steam engine and the telegraph were reducing the impediments of physical distance in a manner that is strikingly similar to the present effect of jets and computers.

The driving force in all of this was the complex phenomenon of accelerating industrialization. Many of its benefits and its ill effects were as apparent then as now. The population shift from farm to city is the most obvious example. But some of the deeper social consequences have been appreciated by historians only more recently. Robert H. Wiebe has perceived that during the period from 1877 to 1920, there was a fundamental change in the focus of the individual citizen, from a strictly local orientation to a partly national one.[34] Prior to this time, a person's sense of moral authority, political consent, and especially personal dignity was derived entirely from the local community. During this period, a whole congeries of socioeconomic forces conspired to weaken the centrality of the local community, and in the end the focus of these essential attitudes shifted to the national level.

The societal group that simultaneously emerged from this cauldron and led the way out of it was "a 'new middle class'—largely urban professional men and women—who developed the new values of 'continuity and regularity, functionality and rationality, administration and management' in order to cope with twentieth-century problems."[6] From the perspective of American neurosurgery, this societal change occurred during its gestational period and the rise to pre-eminence of Harvey Cushing. American neurosurgery and we who practice it are therefore products of the social process that Wiebe described.[34] From this conclusion, it follows that the goals and ideals of that era were probably incorporated into the specific ideals of our profession, both broadly for medicine as a whole and specifically for neurosurgery. Indeed, this was and is the case, because the idea of progress is a truth that we still hold to be self-evident.

In its modern form, the idea of progress can be traced back to the Enlightenment of the 18th century. However, the American version of approximately 1890 to 1920 had some particular characteristics. Historians use the term "progressive" to describe the philosophically connected set of economic, political, and social movements of that time. Especially in the economic sphere, American progressivism was a reaction against the social Darwinism that had prevailed in the preceding decades. That approach claimed that economic forces are part of the natural world, so complete laissez faire can be the only valid attitude toward them. But the obvious downsides of industrialization and the excesses of the robber barons led many reasonable people to question that assumption, especially after the terrible depression of 1893 to 1896. The Progressives claimed that economic forces are created by human beings and should therefore be subject to control through the application of human reason.[17]

One intriguing aspect of American progressivism that is important to us is its expansive outlook. That is, true Progressives thought that all manner of human problems can be solved if they are approached with rationality, so the field of application of progressive ideas was potentially enormous. The real optimists felt that there was a whole world of difficulties out there, just waiting to be conquered by a rational approach. In that sense, the predominant intellectual mood of the burgeoning American middle class was expansively progressive. There were "frontiers" still to be conquered.

Although the federal government officially declared the western frontier to be closed in 1890, it was a powerful metaphor that shaped the ideals of the nation. The pre-eminent historian of the frontier, Frederick Jackson Turner, perceived this clearly in 1914, when he said in a commencement address:[32(p306)]

> . . . we shall do well . . . to recount our historic ideals, to take stock of those purposes . . . and fundamental assumptions that have gone to make the American spirit and the meaning of America in world history.
>
> First of all, there was the ideal of discovery, the courageous determination to break new paths, indifference to the dogma that because an institution or a condition exists, it must remain. All American experience has gone to the making of the spirit of innovation; it is in the blood and will not be repressed.

It was exactly in this spirit that Cushing and his generation felt they were working on the frontiers of science and medicine.

Cushing and the German Model on American Soil

To understand how the German model of a research university was modified by the American experience, it is necessary to go back a few decades before 1900. The seminal and intriguing events of this period in American medical education have been definitively described by Kenneth Ludmerer.[20] For the purposes of this brief chapter, I will emphasize only those aspects that are immediately relevant to neurosurgery and its scientific ideal.

Isolated but serious efforts to import the German model to American universities began in the 1870s, before the full advent of the Progressive Era. But those efforts were philosophically "progressive" in the historians' sense. They began to succeed widely in the 1890s, just in time to catch the oncoming wave of progressivism and contribute to it. In the 1870s, the most important event in this sphere was the opening of the nation's first real research university, the Johns Hopkins, in 1876. That university was explicitly modeled on its German counterparts, and many budding Progressives did graduate work at Johns

Hopkins.[34] However, the opening of the Johns Hopkins School of Medicine was delayed until 1893. By then, reforms based on the German model had already begun in the medical schools at Harvard and the universities of Pennsylvania and Michigan.[20]

The historian Thomas Bonner has pointed out that the scientific model, which traveling American physicians saw in Germany in the late 19th century, was not the mold in which most German physicians were actually trained.[1] The majority of German medical students received their scientific educations largely from lectures and from private instruction by university-sanctioned tutors, *privatdozenten*. They got very little practical instruction in the laboratory. Only an elite few who were destined for research and academic careers were afforded the chance to work there. But most American physicians who went to Germany during this period had already earned their medical degrees from American schools. They went to learn laboratory science in the research institutes of famous professors. That is what they did and what they saw. Hence, that is what they brought back.

A generation before the Flexner Report of 1910, the young leaders of the new wave in American medical education were deeply influenced by this version of the German model. But they were, after all, American in spirit, and the American spirit takes practicality very seriously. In comparison to Europe, it is also rather fiercely egalitarian. Therefore, if the best way to learn something as important as the new biomedical sciences is to experience them firsthand, then every medical student should have extensive bench-top instruction. In essence, the most elite aspect of German medical education was brought to these shores and eventually made available to all medical students on an equal basis.

Harvey Cushing was the direct beneficiary of these events. Indeed, he participated in them at the peak of the excitement. A brief outline of some selected milestones in Cushing's life[10] shows that the dates of his formative period fell exactly into the timeframe that I have been discussing:

American Progressivism—1890–1920
Cushing's MD at Harvard—1895
Residency at Johns Hopkins—1896–1900
Wanderjahr in Europe—1900–1901
Return to Johns Hopkins faculty—1901
"The special field of neurological surgery"—1904
Move to the Brigham/Harvard—1912
Founding of the Society of Neurological Surgeons—1920.

There can be no doubt that Harvey Cushing was thoroughly imbued with the American progressive ideal of conquering the unknown. How much of that spirit came out of the milieu of his time and place and how much from some inner source is impossible to know. Presumably, Cushing's personal version of this ideal is attributable to both sources. What we want to investigate here is how he proposed to carry out the quest. Fortunately for the erstwhile historian, Cushing told us quite explicitly how he planned to do it.

At the beginning of his career as an independent surgeon and investigator, Cushing made a public plea for the independence of his chosen work, "The special field of neurological surgery."[4] After a few polite acknowledgments, Cushing started out by saying that neurology had been the *"pons asinorum"*—the bridge of asses—in his medical school experience. Very few of his fellow students tried to cross the bridge, and there were formidable obstacles for those, like himself, who proposed to do so. He outlined the numerous contemporary difficulties in the study and treatment of the nervous system, and then went on to explain how he proposed to overcome them.

In essence, Cushing proclaimed that a proper neurological surgeon must be a master of all of the relevant neuroscience, both clinical and experimental. The pattern that he had seen in both Europe and America, with the neurologist telling the surgeon when and where to operate, was worse than unsatisfactory because it would not lead to real progress in neurological surgery:

> To successfully cope with the many operative problems offered by the various disorders of the nervous system, a man, after a thorough training in neurology and medicine (in its broadest sense) must study, not only in the neurological clinic but also in the laboratory, the pathology of these afflictions in their histological and—*what is still more important* [my italics]—in their experimental aspects. Anyone, who like myself, has passed from general

surgery into this special branch without this preliminary training finds himself but ill prepared for his new work. . . .[4(p78)]

Since Cushing had trained at Johns Hopkins and was still working there with his mentor William Halsted, his emphasis on laboratory-based, experimental science might not seem remarkable. But it is worthy of remark, because he was prescribing this American version of the German scientific model for *all* neurological surgeons. Only through this rigorous requirement could neurological surgery simultaneously become a truly independent specialty and also produce the kind of advances that would justify its independence.

Nine decades later, with our contributions and our independence well assured, this ideal is still alive and well in neurosurgery. In 1994, the Residency Review Committee for Neurosurgery issued expanded regulations, including a formal requirement that residents must be engaged in ongoing scholarly activities. Although the exact wording of this requirement does not specify scholarship in experimental neuroscience, most residency directors have required such experience for their trainees all along. This is exactly as Cushing would have wanted it, because he was not simply proposing a scientific orientation for his new specialty. He meant very specifically to impose upon neurosurgery a *neuro*scientific ideal. It is by comparison to this standard that we can look at the contributions of other pioneers to the ideals of neurosurgery.

The Neuroscientific Ideal and the Other Early Pioneers

The European pioneers that I have discussed, von Bergmann, Krause, Macewen, and Horsley, were all significantly older than Cushing. The youngest among them, Horsley, was still 12 years Cushing's senior. They had no American counterparts, so any of them could have preceded Cushing as the originator of neurosurgery's goals and ideals. But for one reason or another, none of them rose to the occasion. In his paper on "The special field of neurological surgery," Cushing[4] mentioned only von Bergmann's pessimism about brain tumors; however, in retrospect, it is easy enough to summarize the situation as of 1904.

Von Bergmann and Krause enjoyed both the advantages and the disadvantages of the German university system. They and their scientific work were well supported, but the system itself was not easily changed. Thus, the creation of new specialties was inhibited by a combination of institutional and economic factors.[1] Since von Bergmann and Krause were apparently comfortable within the system, they may have seen little reason to want to change it. In any case, they remained general surgeons with neurological interests. They never became neurosurgeons in the sense of devoting themselves, and their trainees, entirely to this special field. In Britain, Macewen was in a somewhat similar but worse situation. The university system did not support laboratory research, and he remained in a provincial medical center while the British system of medical education and practice had a central focus in London. For these reasons and probably others as well, Macewen too remained a general surgeon throughout his career.

Horsley was potentially in the best position to set neurosurgery's agenda by imposing his own goals and ideals upon it, but in the end he became sidetracked and so left the field to Cushing. Although Horsley's most famous appointment was as Surgeon to the National Hospital, Queen Square, in 1886, he actually lived most of his academic life at University College Hospital and Medical School in London.[21] This reformist institution had welcomed the new experimental physiology, even before it made its more formal appearance at Cambridge in 1873, because Michael Foster had worked there first, in the late 1860s.[12(pp68-73)] By the time Horsley began his scientific career in the 1880s, he had adequate support from University College and other institutions. His devotion to neuroscience was legendary to the point of eccentricity.[27] Indeed, it was probably Horsley's eccentricities that deprived him of his full right to claim the fatherhood of neurosurgery, a title sometimes bestowed on him. When he reached the stage in his professional life where he might have created a school of disciples around him, he began to spend more and more of his passion on other interests.[27]

In comparison to Cushing, Horsley had all of the same founder's opportunities, in addition to a head start, but he either lost or never had the same single-mindedness of purpose. Perhaps of equal importance, neither Horsley nor any of his contemporaries seems to have articulated a vision in the way that Cushing did in the "The special field." If we thus conclude that the Europeans forfeited the opportunity to establish neurosurgery's goals and ideals, the question still arises whether Cushing did it largely on his own, and if so, why? The investigation of this question begins with Cushing's American contemporary Charles H. Frazier.

In retrospect, Frazier was the only American who had an opportunity similar to Cushing's. He was born in 1870, just 1 year after Cushing, and he came to maturity in the same kind of cultural and professional milieu:[18,25,29]

American Progressivism—1890–1920

Frazier's MD at the University of
    Pennsylvania—1892
Surgical training in Philadelphia—1892–1895
Training in Europe with von Bergmann and
    Virchow—1895–1896
Instructor to Professor, University of
    Pennsylvania School of Medicine—
    1896–1901
Dean, University of Pennsylvania School of
    Medicine—1903–1909
Decision to devote full time to neurosurgery—
    1918–1919
Professor and Head of Department of Surgery,
    University of Pennsylvania—1922.

The essential difference between Frazier and Cushing is that Frazier made the decision to devote his full efforts to neurosurgery at a much later stage in his life. Cushing struggled with this problem at the beginning of his academic career (1901–1904) and made his decision when he was 35 years of age.[10(pp204,239)] Frazier was 48 or 49 years old when he reached the same point.[18,29]

Both before and after that decision, Frazier's most important contributions to neuroscience and neurosurgery were in various aspects of pain. This work was done in fruitful collaboration with his neurological colleagues Charles K. Mills and William G. Spiller. Some of Frazier's younger contemporaries felt that he was quite dependent on the neurologists for research inspiration and in clinical practice,[2(p365)] although that was not his later reputation.[29] In a manner that strikingly par-

allels Cushing's "Special field" lecture of 1904, Frazier[9] gave a general address on "The achievements and limitations of neurologic surgery" in 1921, soon after he too had taken his full-time vows. In that paper, his view of Horsley is quite telling:

> . . . I have always pictured the era of surgical neurology as beginning with the work of Sir Victor Horsley. How fortunate it was that the pioneer in this field should have embodied all qualifications that even now we conceive as ideal: he was the experimentalist, the neurologist, the surgeon, all in one. . . . His fundamental knowledge of neurology, his enthusiastic pursuits in the experimental laboratory, especially in cerebral localization, his ingenuity in matters of surgical technique were the foundation stones of his brilliant career.[9(p543)]

In this passage, Frazier was clearly accepting the neuroscientific ideal as it has been discussed here, but this was 17 years after Cushing's "Special field" lecture. Exactly when Frazier came to the conclusion that neurosurgeons need to be independent of neurologists is not so clear. The earliest of the many distinguished neurosurgeons who trained with Frazier were with him in the late 1910s. By 1935, the year before his death, Frazier was praised as a "neurosurgeon who combines neurological conceptions with surgical solutions."[29] In sum, Frazier functioned on the European model until at least a decade after Cushing had articulated his distinctly personal and American ideal.

In addition to Frazier, we must briefly consider two other early American pioneers, Ernest Sachs and Walter Dandy. They were contemporaries of Cushing but just enough younger so that they did not share his window of opportunity.

Sachs was 10 years younger than Cushing and earned his medical degree at Johns Hopkins in 1904. Cushing was his much admired instructor in surgery, but Osler made a larger impression at the time.[26(pp25-26)] Sachs interned at Mt. Sinai Hospital in New York, where his uncle, Bernard Sachs, was a prominent neurologist. The uncle convinced the young graduate to take up neurosurgery, because the results of brain tumor surgery had been uniformly poor in the hands of the general surgeons. Since the world's only prominent practicing neurosurgeon at the time was Horsley, Sachs set out to work with him. But first he planned to go to Berlin for some preliminary training. On the way, Sachs wrote:[26(p32)]

> . . . I wanted to stop in London to meet Sir Victor and be sure I should be welcome in his laboratory. The instant I met him all misgivings vanished. A more informal and delightful person I have never known. . . . Apparently my decision to prepare myself for this work pleased him, for as he told me later . . . I was the first one to do this.

More to the point, Sachs was the *only* person who trained with Horsley for the specific purpose of becoming a neurological surgeon. He worked with Horsley from 1907 to 1909. During that time, he turned down an offer to work with Cushing so that he could finish the work on the thalamus that he had undertaken in Horsley's laboratory.[26(pp47-49)] After a brief return to New York, he went to the recently reorganized medical school at Washington University in St. Louis in 1911, "with the special purpose of developing neurological surgery in the Middle West."[26(p55)] After World War I, the university gave Sachs the first formally titled Professorship of Neurological Surgery in the history of the world. Both the professorship and the new departmental laboratory were financed from the professor's earnings! Shortly thereafter, in 1921, he began to train the large number of fellows who brought prominence to the neurosurgical program in St. Louis.[11,26(pp89-92)]

One of the major elements in the success of the Washington University program has been its collaboration with experimental neuroscientists of Nobel Prize quality. Joseph Erlanger was chairman of physiology when Sachs arrived at Washington University, and Herbert Gasser came in 1916. They revolutionized neurophysiology in 1922, when they demonstrated the existence of the single-neuron action potential with the then new "cathode ray oscillograph."[16] Since Sachs had worked with Horsley, one cannot attribute his fulfillment of the neuroscientific ideal directly to Cushing. But neither can one claim that Sachs led the way in North America. Cushing articulated the ideal and practiced it first, and the same conclusion applies even more clearly to Dandy.

Walter Dandy was born in 1886, 17 years after Cushing. He received his medical degree from Johns Hopkins in 1910. After 1 year of work in Cushing's laboratory, Dandy entered the regular Surgical Service at Johns Hopkins as one of Cushing's assistant residents. A year later, in 1912, Cushing went to Harvard without Dandy, thus leaving the younger man in the lurch since Dandy did not have another position in the Johns Hopkins residency system. Eventually, Halsted made a place for him, and Dandy went on to a brilliant career in the laboratory and the operating room. He founded neurosurgery as an independent entity at Johns Hopkins, but he trained only a small number of neurosurgeons in his own program.[8]

Dandy certainly exemplified the neuroscientific ideal and, in so doing, advanced it enormously. But that is as much as can be said. In addition to his chronological disadvantage vis-à-vis Cushing, Dandy remained a self-imposed outsider with respect to the inner circles among the early pioneers, so he did not have the same self-made bully pulpit that Cushing achieved. Perhaps more to the point, he probably did not have the larger vision that Cushing expressed so forcefully.

Penfield and the Furtherance of the Neuroscientific Ideal

In the generation that followed the early pioneers, it was Wilder Penfield (1891–1976) who had a vision of similar breadth and the equally remarkable ability to instill it in others.[2(pp142-144)] Although he reached his professional maturity and did his major work after the First World War, he was educated and had part of his medical training when American progressivism was still very much alive.

Penfield was born in the sprawling frontier town of Spokane, Washington. From the age of 8 years until he left for college, he lived in Hudson, Wisconsin. Despite its underlying Midwestern conservatism, Wisconsin was a major center of progressivism. One of the movement's most prominent advocates, Robert M. La Follette (1855–1925), was Governor of Wisconsin from 1901 to 1906 and Senator from 1906 to 1925. How much Penfield was influenced by that regional tradition is hard to say, but there is no doubt that he set out to conquer the world from

Hudson, Wisconsin, and he succeeded.[19(pp22-28)] For the earlier part of that success, the relevant dates are:[19,24]

American Progressivism—1890–1920
Penfield's BLitt at Princeton—1913
Rhodes Scholar at Oxford—1915–1916
MD at Johns Hopkins—1918
Intern with Cushing at Brigham Hospital—
    1918–1919
Neurology and neurophysiology training in
    England—1919–1921
Surgical faculty (self-training in neurosurgery) at
    Columbia—1921–1928
Move to McGill—1928
Opening of the Montreal Neurological
    Institute—1934.

Penfield brought two new elements to the neuroscientific ideal: 1) the proposition that neurosurgeons have an obligation to contribute to science and human welfare because they enjoy the unique privilege of operating on the living human brain; and 2) the idea that all of the neurosciences can best be pursued in mutual coordination with each other, preferably within the corporate structure of institutes devoted to that purpose. In neither of these contributions was he completely original, but for both he created the paradigms that were emulated by the rest of the world.

With regard to deliberate experimentation on the human nervous system, Cushing published a paper in 1909 on stimulation of the postcentral gyrus.[5] In it, he mentioned that Krause and Frazier had already done likewise for the precentral cortex. However, Cushing did not make any philosophic statements about scientific obligation in his paper. The person who did make such statements and followed them to their logical conclusion was Otfrid Foerster (1873–1941) of Breslau.[36,37] Foerster had started out as a neurologist with an interest in rehabilitation, especially for tabetics. He thought of dorsal root section as a way of trying to alleviate tabetic spasticity and convinced a surgeon to carry out the operation. Eventually, he simply started doing neurosurgery himself, without any formal surgical training, out of frustration with the general surgeons' poor results. Throughout his long and productive career, Foerster insisted on the need to make careful neurologic and physiologic observations on any patient who had a deliberate surgical lesion or intraoperative testing. Among his many contributions, we owe our basic knowledge of human dermatomal patterns to Foerster's monumental efforts.[33,36,37]

Foerster began publishing papers on dorsal root section in 1908, but his interests and his contributions ranged from the cerebral cortex to the peripheral nerves. Penfield spent 6 months with Foerster in 1928, just before moving to Montreal. It was this experience that convinced Penfield of the feasibility and importance of excising epileptogenic cortical scars in large numbers of patients.[23,24] And no doubt he imbibed much of Foerster's passion about human experimentation. So the question arises whether it was Foerster or Penfield who brought this element into our neuroscientific ideal. The only reasonable answer, of course, is that they both did. However, according to the selection criteria that I proposed at the outset, Penfield's importance looms larger because he promulgated his own version of the idea to large numbers of other neurosurgeons.

Foerster trained only one neurosurgeon, Ludwig Guttmann, who emigrated to England to escape the Nazi threat and later founded the important spinal cord rehabilitation center at Stokes Mandeville. In fact, Foerster was something of a pariah in his own country until late in his life or even after his death, and the last part of his life was spent in the shadow of the Nazi menace.[2(p136)] For all of these reasons and probably others, Foerster was not in a position to create a large school of disciples. Penfield, on the other hand, trained more prominent neurosurgeons than any other person in history. He did it through the mechanism of the Montreal Neurological Institute, which he envisioned and founded.

Penfield's idea of a neurological institute had important predecessors, but he ultimately fashioned his own conception and made it real. Just before he left Germany in 1928, he visited the large and productive laboratory of the Vogts in Berlin. Many years later, Penfield recalled his reaction:[23(pp173-174)]

There was much to learn in this splendid laboratory complex, dominated by the Vogts and dedicated to the broad field of neurological science. But it seemed to me dangerously isolated, too far removed from patients and from general medicine and surgery. The New York Neurological Institute, I reflected, suffered from the opposite form of isolation and the National Hospital at Queen Square, London, likewise. They were concerned with neurological patients but were too far removed from basic science and the other disciplines of medicine, too far away in space and in awareness. . . .

I wanted to see neurology and neurosurgery united in one academic department. I had struggled to make myself a little of everything—surgeon, neurologist, laboratory man. In the end I had learned that I could not master it all well enough to trust myself to be a lonely dictator, as Vogt was, or Foerster for that matter. It seemed to me that there was only one way to give the neurological patient the best in every aspect of diagnosis and treatment and one way to plan research through the years. That was by means of a working fellowship arrangement, the establishment of a team that could work near the bedside of the patient.

Thus, the basic idea of a research institute was derived from the German model, but an important part of Penfield's conception was American. Although he was sometimes amused by the foibles of the German professorial system, he had a strong distaste for its unquestioning authoritarianism.[23(p179)] Penfield's cultural roots were in the frontier openness of Spokane and especially in the egalitarian progressivism of Wisconsin. Those influences are discernible in this passage. Historically, I think it is not too metaphorical to say that Penfield's concept of a neurological institute, a place for all of the neurosciences, can be viewed as a broadened expression of Cushing's neuroscientific ideal.

Conclusions

Given Harvey Cushing's legendary status in the history of neurosurgery, it may seem tautological to conclude that his ideals formed the essential core of the developing profession's view of its own mission. But legends may or may not hold up under close scrutiny. Therefore, it is in-

deed interesting and important to see that Cushing's centrality has been borne out even more than I had thought it would be. He was simply the right person in the right place at the right time. Cushing would have been an outstanding figure in any era, but his role in the history of neurosurgery would have been decidedly different if he had started out a decade sooner or a decade later.

Cushing's window of opportunity was a matter of historical happenstance, but the void that he filled was not formless. It was, in fact, a very specific time in the history of medicine and in American history, and the same statement obviously applies to the other early pioneers of American neurosurgery. It is always a rather tricky business to ascribe the motivations of individuals to the general culture in which they lived, and yet it is sometimes inescapable. Our early pioneers lived in the era of American progressivism.

The leaders of progressivism were not physicians, and medicine is not usually thought of as one of the professions that attracted them. But the mainstream Progressives did look to science as a model of rationality, and they were very concerned with public health, so there was a connection to the new scientific medicine.[34(pp113-116)] In addition, there are some striking parallels between the biographical characteristics of the typical Progressives and many of neurosurgery's early pioneers:

. . . From its birth in the Middle West, a generation of intelligent youth . . . channeled their urges to help people into professions that had not existed for their mothers and fathers . . . settlement work, higher education, law and journalism all offered possibilities for preaching without pulpits. Over the long term, their goal was an educated democracy that would create laws that would, in turn, produce a moral democracy. The place for Christianity was in this world.[3(p15)]

In sum, most Progressives grew up in Midwestern Protestant homes, where education and service to others was emphasized and discipline was enforced. As they matured, they moved away from their parents' formal religious practices but not from their moral implications. These biographical characterizations are fulfilled by Cushing, Dandy, and Penfield—the three most prominent figures in the American pantheon of five that I have been discussing. In his address on "The special field of neurological surgery," Cushing was arguing for the recognition of a new specialty in medicine, but historically we can view the process as leading to the establishment of a new profession. And surely all these men were driven to make the human world a better place through their work in the here and now.

Perhaps the most important characteristic that the early pioneers shared with the Progressives was their conviction that any difficulty can be surmounted if it is approached with enough intelligence and focused tenacity. Cushing and the others pushed themselves and their associates to the limits of their technical/manual and scientific abilities. That is why they were often thought to be so excessively demanding, and that is also why they succeeded. The obstacle that they faced would yield to nothing less because it was the nervous system, the most complex system in the body. That is why I have emphasized the *neuro*scientific nature of Cushing's scientific ideal. To use a Darwinian metaphor, one could say that the nervous system selected its opponents by virtue of its complexity.

It follows, then, that the ideals of the early neurosurgical pioneers were formed in some measure by the very nature of the difficulties that they were trying to overcome. But the difficulties were more than just technical and scientific. They were conceptual.

There is a great mystique about the brain. Since it is acknowledged to be the source of human intelligence and action, it is intimately connected with a wide array of beliefs and practices. In order to investigate the organ that drives these beliefs, and especially to invade it physically, a person must grapple with his or her personal conceptions of these beliefs. It is this necessity, I believe, that forces most clinical and experimental neuroscientists to a deeper level of self-reflection than they might otherwise achieve. It happens to us, and it happened to our early pioneers even more forcefully, precisely because they were the pioneers on a new frontier. Their ideals are the legacy that they have left to us from their struggles to understand and heal the nervous system.

References

1. Bonner TN. The German model of training physicians in the United States, 1870–1914: how closely was it followed? *Bull Hist Med.* 1990;64:18-34.
2. Bucy PC, ed. *Neurosurgical Giants: Feet of Clay and Iron.* New York, NY: Elsevier; 1985.
3. Crunden RM. *Ministers of Reform. The Progressives' Achievement in American Civilization, 1889–1920.* Urbana, Ill: University of Illinois; 1984.
4. Cushing H. The special field of neurological surgery. *Bull Johns Hopkins Hosp.* 1905;16:77-87.
5. Cushing H. A note upon the faradic stimulation of the postcentral gyrus in conscious patients. *Brain.* 1909; 32:44-53.
6. Donald DH. Foreword. In: Wiebe RH. *The Search for Order 1877–1920.* New York, NY: Hill & Wang; 1967:vii-ix.
7. Flexner A. *Universities, American, English, German.* New York, NY: Oxford University Press; 1930.
8. Fox WL. *Dandy of Johns Hopkins.* Baltimore, Md: Williams & Wilkins; 1984.
9. Frazier CH. The achievements and limitations of neurologic surgery. *Arch Surg.* 1921;3:543-559.
10. Fulton JF. *Harvey Cushing. A Biography.* Springfield, Ill: Charles C Thomas; 1946.
11. Furlow LT. Ernest Sachs 1879–1958. In: Bucy PC, ed. *Neurosurgical Giants: Feet of Clay and Iron.* New York, NY: Elsevier; 1985:367-372. (Reprinted from *Surg Neurol.* 1975;3:173-175.)
12. Geison GL. *Michael Foster and the Cambridge School of Physiology. The Scientific Enterprise in Late Victorian Society.* Princeton, NJ: Princeton University Press; 1978.
13. Greenblatt SH. Cerebral localization: From theory to practice. Paul Broca and Hughlings Jackson to David Ferrier and William Macewen. In: Greenblatt SH, Dagi TF, Epstein MH, eds. *A History of Neurosurgery.* Park Ridge, Ill: American Association of Neurological Surgeons. In press.
14. Greenblatt SH. The historiography of neurosurgery: organizing themes and methodological issues. In: Greenblatt SH, Dagi TF, Epstein MH, eds. *A History of Neurosurgery.* Park Ridge, Ill: American Association of Neurological Surgeons. In press.
15. Hanigan WC, Ragen W, Ludgera M. Neurological surgery in the nineteenth century: the principles and techniques of Ernst von Bergmann. *Neurosurgery.* 1992; 30:750-757.
16. Hinsey JC. Herbert Gasser (1888–1963). In: Haymaker W, Schiller F, eds. *The Founders of Neurology.* 2nd ed. Springfield, Ill: Charles C Thomas; 1970:213-217.
17. LaFeber W, Polenberg R. *The American Century. A History of the United States Since the 1890's.* New York, NY: John Wiley & Sons; 1975:41-43.
18. Lewey FH. Charles Harrison Frazier (1870–1936). In: Haymaker W, Schiller F, eds. *The Founders of Neurology.* 2nd ed. Springfield, Ill: Charles C Thomas; 1970:559-562.
19. Lewis J. *Something Hidden. A Biography of Wilder Penfield.* Toronto, Canada: Doubleday Canada; 1981.

20. Ludmerer KM. *Learning to Heal. The Development of American Medical Education.* New York, NY: Basic Books; 1985.
21. Paget S. *Sir Victor Horsley. A Study of His Life and Work.* London, England: Constable & Co; 1919.
22. Penfield W. An address on the field of neurosurgery. *Can Med Assoc J.* 1928;19:654-655.
23. Penfield W. *No Man Alone. A Neurosurgeon's Life.* Boston, Mass: Little, Brown & Co; 1977.
24. Preul MC, Feindel W. Origins of Wilder Penfield's surgical technique. The role of the "Cushing ritual" and influences from the European experience. *J Neurosurg.* 1991;75:812-820.
25. Rhoads JE, Langfitt TW. Charles Harrison Frazier 1870–1936. In: Bucy PC, ed. *Neurosurgical Giants: Feet of Clay and Iron.* New York, NY: Elsevier; 1985:361-364. (Reprinted from *Surg Neurol.* 1977;7:253-254).
26. Sachs E. *Fifty Years of Neurosurgery. A Personal Story.* New York, NY: Vantage Press; 1958.
27. Sachs E. Victor Horsley. *J Neurosurg.* 1958;15:240-244.
28. Shucart WA. Fedor Krause 1856–1937. In: Bucy PC, ed. *Neurosurgical Giants: Feet of Clay and Iron.* New York, NY: Elsevier; 1985:121-124. (Reprinted from *Surg Neurol.* 1975;3:115-117).
29. Stengel A. An appreciation [of Charles Harrison Frazier]. *Ann Surg.* 1935;101:vii-viii.
30. Swazey JP. *Reflexes and Motor Integration: Sherrington's Concept of Integrative Action.* Cambridge, Mass: Harvard University Press; 1969.
31. Temkin O. Materialism in French and German physiology of the early nineteenth century. In: Temkin O. *The Double Face of Janus and Other Essays in the History of Medicine.* Baltimore, Md: Johns Hopkins University Press; 1977:340-344. (Reprinted from the *Bull Hist Med.* 1946;20:322-327).
32. Turner FJ. *The Frontier in American History.* New York, NY: H Holt & Co; 1920.
33. Wartenberg R. Otfrid Foerster (1873–1941). In: Haymaker W, Schiller F, eds. *The Founders of Neurology.* 2nd ed. Springfield, Ill: Charles C Thomas; 1970:555-559.
34. Wiebe RH. *The Search for Order 1877–1920.* New York, NY: Hill & Wang; 1967.
35. Young GM. *Victorian England. Portrait of an Age.* 2nd ed. New York, NY: Oxford University Press; 1964.
36. Zülch KJ. *Otfrid Foerster. Physician and Naturalist.* November 9, 1873–June 15, 1941. Berlin: Springer-Verlag; 1969.
37. Zülch KJ. Otfrid Foerster 1873–1941. In: Bucy PC, ed. *Neurosurgical Giants: Feet of Clay and Iron.* New York, NY: Elsevier; 1985:127-132. (Reprinted from *Surg Neurol.* 1973;1:313-316).

CHAPTER 3

Modern Neurosurgical Philosophy

Robert G. Ojemann, MD

Modern neurosurgical philosophy has evolved from the general principles put forth by the medical philosophers who preceded us, and from the principles that neurosurgeons have found important as we deal with the issues of modern medicine, attempting to build a better life for our patients, ourselves, and society.

Sir William Osler was a great physician and also was considered a great medical philosopher. Quest[9] has written that "Osler . . . admonished us to illustrate with our lives the Hippocratic standard of learning, sagacity, humanity and probity." He quoted Osler[7] as follows:

Of learning, that you may apply in your practice the best that is known in our art, and that with the increase in your knowledge there may be an increase in that priceless endowment of sagacity, so that to all, everywhere, skilled succor may come in the hour of need. Of a humanity, that will show, in your daily life, tenderness and consideration to the weak, infinite pity to the suffering, and broad charity to all. Of a probity, that will make you under all circumstances true to yourselves, true to your high calling, and true to your fellow man.

To each one of you the practice of medicine will be very much as you make it—to one a worry, a care, a perpetual annoyance; to another a daily joy and a life of as much happiness and usefulness as can well fall to the lot of man, because it is a life of self-sacrifice and of countless opportunities to comfort and help the weak-hearted and to raise up those that fall. In the student spirit you can best fulfill the high mission of our noble calling—in his humility, conscious of weakness, while seeking strength; in his confidence, knowing the power while recognizing the limitations of his art; in his pride in the glorious heritage from which the greatest gifts to man have been derived; and in his sure and certain hope that the future holds for us still richer blessings than the past.

In considering this topic, I will discuss the philosophic approach to the art of neurosurgery—i.e. how we use the knowledge we have acquired, and the science of neurosurgery as it relates to the acquisition of new knowledge and techniques. The ethics of neurosurgery governing our decisions and choices on a moral and rational basis is referred to, but is the subject of another chapter. Other factors relating to the philosophic considerations include the relationship with medical and paramedical personnel, the influence of factors outside the physician's office and hospital environment, the physician's physical and mental health, and the physician's family. Some aspects of this author's approach to this subject have been presented elsewhere.[3-6]

Basic Principles

To do what is best for our patients is the basic principle underlying all of our professional activities. This should be the over-riding consideration as we try to treat and prevent illness. Sorensen[11] has written:

. . . we should inexhaustibly seek for excellence in our practice of medicine. If we desire less than excellence, we lack personal honesty. It is inconceivable that a neurosurgeon would consciously render mediocre patient care, but in our haste of pursuing less laudable goals and misplaced priorities, we may find our patients receiving substandard treatment. May we have the insight to search ourselves, discover our weaknesses, and resolve to change them for the benefit of our patients.

Quest[9] has stated: "Our most important commitment is to our patients. All of us must continually review our resolve to do our utmost in our patient's behalf." Pellegrino[8] noted:

> Any ethics of the process of clinical decision must begin with a clear notion of the "good of the patient." This is a complex notion, to which it is easy to give superficial assent. All too often, it is little more than a rhetorical device. It is rarely carefully analyzed, yet it is the final criterion of whether a decision is morally sound. It is, therefore, the unifying theme of all medical ethics, and particularly of any ethics of moral choice and decision-making.

Providing optimal patient care requires a continuous quest for new knowledge. King[1] has written: "It is true, of course, that only a master of what we know from science can become a responsible master of this art. Competence does not stem only from a heart of gold; indeed, compassion without science is dangerous. Errors born of ignorance are as lethal as actions that stem from a venomous spirit." For the practicing neurosurgeon, this means a never-ending program of education which is necessary if we are to continue to give our patients the best possible care. We cannot close our minds to the changes that are occurring in the neurosciences. Quest[9] has written: "Each one of us, no matter how great, no matter how humble, can contribute to our specialty's growth by our commitment to increasing our knowledge of the nervous system and its disorders, supporting research, and to improving our judgment and technical abilities."

The acquisition of new knowledge demands the reading of appropriate books and journals, attendance at postgraduate courses and annual meetings of regional and national societies, the use of audio and video tapes and computer searches of the literature, and discussions with informed colleagues. Failure to acquire new information keeps the patient from consideration of the latest techniques and the neurosurgeon from the studies evaluating new ideas in relation to previous treatment programs. It is imperative that we practice both the science of gaining new knowledge and the art of applying what we learn to our patients. Only in this way will we keep our minds sharp and make our own assessment of the importance of proposed new treatment programs.

Application to Patient Management

In making the patient the focus of our professional lives, neurosurgeons need to develop a philosophy to guide us in this encounter. King[1] wrote: "Large portions of every interaction between physician and patient lie outside of science and in the realm of art." As we meet the patient, we need to keep in mind that the individual is deeply concerned as to what he or she is about to hear or will have recommended in the way of an invasive procedure. The neurosurgeon should display a feeling of confidence and not uncertainty, understanding and not disinterest, humility and not arrogance.

Schwartz[10] has written: "In the past, ours [neurosurgery] has been in many ways a favored field of medicine, guarded by its mystique and prestige from many of the assaults directed against the profession at large. . . ." But such is no longer the case, for neurosurgeons are expected to have more compassion and understanding because, after all, we are working with the brain. Too often in the recent past physicians have been characterized in the media as having a tendency to talk down to their patients, of being arrogant, and of lacking an understanding of the patient's needs and wishes. While I believe we have made progress in this area, I still see patients who spontaneously report this type of experience.

These philosophic principles come into focus throughout our management of the patient. The initial encounter between doctor and patient often sets the tone for the future relationship. A patient should be seen as close to the scheduled time as possible. Long waits are difficult for apprehensive and anxious patients. In recording the history of the illness, the neurosurgeon should pay special attention to how the symptoms are affecting the patient's daily life and normal activities. Concern and compassion with a friendly, supportive attitude is shown, but at the same time, the patient is not allowed to wander away from the primary purpose of the conversation. Lack of sensitivity, abrupt adverse comments, showing a lack of interest, and an air of arrogance are to be avoided in our relationships with patients.

In thinking about treatment options, several questions may need to be considered. What is the expected natural history of the lesion being treated? What are the chances of the recommended treatment improving or relieving the patient's symptoms and of preventing future disability? What are the risks of the treatment? Will the recommended treatment likely lead to a better outcome than the natural history? When presenting the recommendation to the patient, adequate time should be taken to explain what is involved in the treatment and to answer the patient's questions. It is important to discuss with the patient what his or her hopes and expectations from the planned treatment are. It is also important to listen to the patient and his or her family and consider their needs, wants, and wishes in relation to neurosurgical recommendations and decisions. Over and over again I hear, "The doctor spent so little time explaining the problem to me." Pellegrino[8] wrote:

> A biomedically good decision is one that is scientifically correct but it is not automatically a good decision from the patient's point of view. It must be placed within the context of the patient's life situation and his value system. It must square with what the patient thinks "worthwhile," given the circumstances and choices illness force upon him.

He went on to say that "it would be hard to deny that one observable feature unique to humans is the capacity to make choices, to set up a life plan, and to pursue one's goals for a satisfactory life among the many possible ways to conduct a human life."

With the development of new therapies and techniques, and increased knowledge about the natural history of some of the problems neurosurgeons treat, the decision whether to observe the patient, to institute some form of medical treatment, or to recommend surgery, radiosurgery, or some combination of therapies may be difficult. Do not hesitate to consult other colleagues when the chosen course is unclear or to seek the help of other specialties if necessary in doing what is best for the patient. A request for a second opinion should be greeted with support and encouragement. The neurosurgeon who has strong philosophic principles and whose knowledge and skills are up-to-date should have no concern about the request.

The physician should speak frankly, as patients generally know when they have a serious illness. It may not be necessary to tell the patient everything initially, but questions should be answered honestly and in a straightforward fashion. The patient will appreciate this and will have confidence in the neurosurgeon's continued care and in future discussions.

In our daily work, neurosurgeons interact with numerous other physicians and paramedical and nonprofessional personnel. The neurosurgeon must pay attention to those with whom he or she comes into contact, be courteous, and instill confidence and understanding. There should be honesty and straightforwardness in any interactions. In the end, no one wins if attempts are made to do otherwise. It should make no difference whether one is talking to a fellow physician, to a secretary, or to the individual who cleans the office.

As the cost of health care escalates and new systems of health care delivery are being considered, the good of society tends to come into conflict with the good of the patient. In 1983, Pelligrino[8] wrote:

> A growing body of criticism takes physicians to task for exalting individual patient good over that of society. Yet, that is the commitment the patient expects. Are we justified in violating that trust without changing the explicit promise we make to help the patient?

Can physicians be agents of social and fiscal good and still serve the . . . patient good . . . ? In the years immediately ahead, this will be perhaps the most vexing dilemma the physician will face.

Clearly, this has become an increasing concern. However, I believe we can continue to focus on what is best for the patient and still respond to the needs of society.

Personal Factors

While the neurosurgeon can experience great satisfaction in restoring a patient to good health, disappointments and frustrations are not uncommon. Many physicians are helped by developing a strong philosophic foundation to help them in their daily lives. Dr. Bruce Sorensen[11] quoted Dr. Morgan Martin[2] as saying:

> The physician needs a belief system, whether he calls it philosophy, faith or their combination known as religion. He needs almost automatic assumptions to sustain him with his patients and preserve him for his family. Faced with life and death, pain and suffering and problems that do not lend themselves to solution, he must fall back on what he is and what he believes.

Osler firmly believed that he needed spiritual support in his daily activities.[11] Sorensen[11] wrote (and I agree):

> More and more, it becomes evident that occurrences transpire in our lives, private, public, and professional, which can only be explained by a power greater than that that can be found on this terrestrial sphere. To establish a relationship with our creator is a maturing experience, not a sign of personal weakness; it is a pearl of great price to be sought after with eager diligence.

An important factor that allows a neurosurgeon to focus on patient care is a stable, happy home environment. This is not always easy to achieve with unexpected emergencies that often come at inopportune times. But with careful planning and understanding by both the neurosurgeon and the spouse or companion, signifi-

cant segments of time can be spent with the family and this goal can be achieved. Harvey Cushing's daughter Betsey said that had it not been for the love, devotion, and understanding of her mother through 10 years of courtship and 37 years of marriage, he would have accomplished but a small fraction of the contributions that he made.[3]

Conclusion

Stern,[12] concerned about the morality of our profession, said:

> Perhaps the physical and worldly rewards warp the perspective and judgment of some. Perhaps arrogance and lack of social conscience are evident in others. Perhaps even deceit or dishonesty, or even cruelty, afflict a few, while the ravages of mental or physical illness consume an added number. I worry about these errors of our ways, but I worry more about the prostitution of the larger number who, captured by the messages of cynicism, turn to self-serving pursuits. Their energies are motivated by self. We all are vulnerable to such temptation. . . . We can raise our sights to those goals the achievement of which can ennoble our efforts. We can consider a nobleness of purpose.

It is never too late to change the focus of life. We should not become so fixed in our ways that we cannot make a change if it will improve the lives of our patients, those with whom we work, and society. The added benefit, of course, is that our own life will be better for having done this. Finally, as Sorenson[11] has stated: "The future always arrives a little before we are ready to give up the present. Is it not now time, regardless of our years, to review, to change, to correct, and to improve all areas of our lives?"

References

1. King RB. Traditions, transition, and the torch: the 1981 AANS presidential address. *J Neurosurg.* 1981; 55:329-336.
2. Martin M. Should the physician gaze eastward? *JAMA.* 1976;236:835-836. Commentary.
3. Ojemann RG. The tradition of Harvey Cushing commemorated by a stamp in the Great American

stamp series: the 1987 AANS presidential address. *J Neurosurg.* 1987;67:631-642.

4. Ojemann RG. Skull-base surgery: a perspective. *J Neurosurg.* 1992;76:569-570. Editorial.

5. Ojemann RG. Clinical decision making in skull base surgery. In: Tindall GT, Cooper PR, Barrow DL, eds. *The Practice of Neurosurgery.* Baltimore, Md: Williams & Wilkins; 1994. In press.

6. Ojemann RG, Black P McL. Difficult decisions in managing patients with benign brain tumors. *Clin Neurosurg.* 1989;35:254-284.

7. Osler W. *Counsels and Ideals and Selected Aphorisms.* Birmingham, Ala: Classics of Medicine Library; 1985.

8. Pellegrino ED. "The common devotion"—Cushing's legacy and medical ethics today: the 1983 Harvey Cushing oration. *J Neurosurg.* 1983;59: 567-573.

9. Quest DO. Presidential address: Commitment and contribution. *Neurosurgery.* 1988;22:981-985.

10. Schwartz HG. Today's needs and neurosurgery's response: the 1968 AANS presidential address. *J Neurosurg.* 1968;29:221-228.

11. Sorensen BF. Presidential address: "Physician, heal thyself." *Clin Neurosurg.* 1978;25:1-8.

12. Stern WE. A nobleness of purpose: the 1980 AANS presidential address. *J Neurosurg.* 1980;53: 136-143.

CHAPTER 4

Patient-Centered Neurosurgery

Robert E. Maxwell, MD, PhD, FACS

*Saying is one thing and doing is another; we are to consider the sermon and
the preacher distinctly and apart.*

—Montaigne

"Patient-centered care" and "patient-focused care" are contemporary buzz words used by health care professionals, administrators, and bureaucrats to promote differing concepts of how health care can be provided and, in some cases, changed to best serve our patients. The constructs for change are usually served up with a dollop of self-interest depending on the perspectives and incentives perceived by the individual or organization promoting the need for a different way of delivering health care.

The social scientist and public health official envision patient-centered care as a comprehensive cradle-to-grave system that will provide preventive health maintenance and delivery of care so that a greater number of citizens will enjoy healthier and more productive lives. The administrator of a hospital or health maintenance organization emphasizes excellence in providing patient services in a cost-effective way. The nurse and other allied health providers see patient-centered care as an opportunity to empower the patient by providing a more collegial, open, warm, and supportive atmosphere. In addition, they want to have more time for professional rather than administrative tasks and to have a sense of real responsibility for the outcome of their work.[6]

Each of these "patient-centered" concepts has exceptional merit and will be studied, debated, reworked, developed, and promoted by their re-spective advocates and constituencies. It is increasingly apparent, however, that change in the focus of patient care is imminent. A few of the many factors influencing the rapid evolution in health care delivery include: technology-driven increases in medical care costs, a patient population with higher expectations for services, an aging population in need of more efficient and effective health care, increasing numbers of uninsured patients, the movement of health care from the in-patient to the out-patient setting, and the shorter hospital stay.

The neurosurgeon striving to achieve the best surgical result for each of his or her patients is going to be expected to take responsibility for how effectively and efficiently an optimum outcome is achieved from both the patient's and the payer's perspectives. The most valued neurosurgeons will be those who provide creative energy to formulating and guiding the process.[9] Implicit in the concept of patient-centered care is the obligation of the physician as a professional, not businessman, to champion the patient's needs for high-quality medical care and good service. It is increasingly apparent, however, that we must work to identify and eliminate waste and increase efficiency so that care is not rationed and services compromised because of real or perceived shortages of resources. Thomas Langfitt,[7] in his honored guest presentation before the Congress of Neurological Surgeons in 1987, said: "Given the richness of our nation and some of the ways in which those rich resources are wasted, I am not sympathetic to the financial cost issues in this case."

The neurosurgeon's concept of patient-centered care is consistent with those of other health care providers, but the emphasis is likely to be at a more intimate and personal level. The neurosurgeon encounters relatively few patients, but the encounter is often in a setting fraught with unsettling physical and emotional trauma for the patient and family. The critical issues come down to the needs of the patient and how these needs are to be met, not with what the neurosurgeon or other care givers have to offer. Patient-centered care is itself centered on a systematic awareness of values and relative value judgments. What is the value of prevention, acute care, surgery, and rehabilitation?

Awareness

Patient-centered care begins with awareness of the emotional as well as the physical stresses the patient and family are experiencing at the time of their first encounter with the neurosurgeon. Any serious injury or illness requiring a neurosurgical consultation is likely to engender emotions ranging from trepidation to terror. Physical and emotional pain may add to the confusion and disorientation that accompanies the sense of ignorance and loss of control that can befuddle even the most competent and prideful of individuals. Fear of loss, loneliness, and financial burden may either numb the senses or trigger a seething anger that makes communication difficult if not nearly impossible.

Fulton Haight,[5] an attorney, helps us look at this traumatic first encounter through the patient's eyes:

> How odd it is that the physician finally chosen to perform the invasive procedure is someone never before met, a person whose professional credentials (if known at all) are known only by recommendation, an individual with whom the patient may hope to spend at most perhaps 20 quick minutes. At this meeting, what is the most pressing issue discussed? Sure, the doctor's and patient's common purpose and joint commitment to

recovery is covered, but the main subject is the signing of a paper upon which the surgeon, this near total stranger, basically disavows responsibility for the consequences of the surgery he or she is about to perform.

In such a setting, the neurosurgeon must not only be aware and faithful to the principle of the primacy of the patient's preference, but also have a self-awareness of the tendency to be uncomfortable telling the patient distressing information. There is also a tendency for the patient and family to hear only what they want to hear. The patient depends on the physician for an open, honest, and informed opinion about the natural history of the disease or condition, a review of the treatment options available, and as accurate an assessment as possible of the risks of any proposed operation or procedure. One of the "arts of medicine" is to provide this information and assessment, including a "worst case scenario," without destroying hope or, on the other hand, creating unreasonable expectations. One approach is to give the patient the "truth" with a positive slant for prognosis and to give the family the "truth" with the most dire implications of the disease, injury, or surgical procedure being considered. The act of weighing the amount of responsibility to give either the patient or the family suggests a familiarity and relationship between the neurosurgeon and the patient that is difficult to achieve in one or two brief meetings. Consultation with other caregivers more familiar with the circumstances and dynamics of the patient and family may be helpful in this regard.

The individual's "health right" is more than one of awareness and respect for quality-of-life considerations. It is the fundamental right of the patient to know and understand the natural history of the disease being considered and the implications of any therapeutic decisions for that particular patient, at that time, in that setting, and yes, by that particular neurosurgeon. Communication gaps between the patient and the neurosurgeon are traps for the inexperienced or unwary, a fact often exploited by attorneys following a maloccurrence or bad outcome. G. K. Chesterton said: "A man does not know what he is saying until he knows what he is not saying."

From this, a patient would do well to infer that one does not know what one is hearing until one knows what one is not hearing.

Patients judge the quality of care by its impact on their lives. They want to know whether a prescribed drug or procedure will relieve their pain or alleviate anxiety, whether it will preserve or restore their ability to climb stairs, dress, feed themselves, or change their appearance, sexuality, or mood.[13] Physicians measure and monitor tumor size, but may not assess whether the patient is comfortable or functional. The patency of a clogged vessel is measured, but the patient's ability to return to work may not be assessed. Are symptoms such as pain and the epileptic condition with devastating functional consequences treated with the promptness and vigor afforded structural lesions? Many patients who present with disabling and intractable epilepsy are still not recognized as potential candidates for surgical treatment and are destined (from youth) to a lifetime of needless morbidity, limited opportunity for normal development, and an inability to realize their full potential. The loss for the person, the family, and the community is devastating, but largely unmonitored and, therefore, not fully comprehended by society.

Often there is no scientific or medically dictated right or wrong answer or decision. Most of us instinctively and intuitively realize that more care is not always better care. But what is the likely outcome of the act? What is the objective? Is it humane and compassionate? Is the evaluation, monitoring, and treatment consistent with the patient's life path? An operation that is appropriate for one patient may be totally inappropriate for another. Treatment decisions involve value judgments that we are not informed enough to make unless we know the patient very well. Symptoms affect patients in different ways and patients attach different values to their relief. The only way to obtain such intimate information is to expect and encourage patients to play an active role in their own care.[13] The neurosurgeon must participate in the effort to find out what patients want and need, and then find a way to give it to them.

The neurosurgeon must be the patient's staunchest advocate and should strive to identify and empower nurses and other staff who have proven themselves competent to also be advocates for the patient. In addition, we need to be aware of how orders and patient management decisions influence the number of times hospital staff are traipsing in and out of patients' rooms to deliver various services, invading their privacy and disturbing their rest. The patient is encouraged to assume a leadership position in patient-centered care, but patients tend to be passive, particularly when they are sick and find themselves in a strange environment, their clothes taken away and replaced with a short, skimpy gown tied in the back.

It is important to patients that all caregivers be introduced or introduce themselves and explain what they are doing. Patients want a high quality of care delivered by caregivers who know them and their individual needs and preferences. They are dissatisfied when exposed to a myriad of people asking redundant questions and remaining perpetually ignorant about the patient under their charge. How insensitive or even cruel to subject the patient with a crushed spine, severed spinal cord, and complete loss of neurologic function to repeated pinching, poking, and requests to "lift your legs" or "wiggle your toes." Patients and families sometimes wonder, "Doesn't anyone talk to each other around here or read the medical record?" Patient-centered care should allow the patient and the family to sense that there is a well thought-out and communicated "grand plan" for their care.

It is helpful to know what prior knowledge a patient brings to the patient-neurosurgeon dialog. What is the patient's background, environment, prior experience, and aspirations? How will all of this affect the way the neurosurgeon's counsel is interpreted? When discussing carotid vascular occlusive disease with a plumber, one may want to use different words and analogies than when talking with a musician. Prior knowledge affects how easily a patient makes connections with new information. One of the keys to learning and memory is the richness of the connections a bit of information has. The more connections, the easier it is to remember and understand.[15] A patient has the potential to bring more to the interpretation of the situation if we take advantage of his or her knowledge and experiences. Unless the patient is asked for his or her understanding of what is being explained, however, the neurosurgeon will never really know what is being learned.

Service

Patient-centered care is based on the tenet that the patient deserves and has the right to expect more than knowledge, good clinical judgment, and technical competency when he or she presents to the neurosurgeon. Patients have a right to expect "service" in its most comprehensive connotation.

Service is so critical because it engenders a self-confidence in the patient and the family that they have made a good choice and are in safe hands. Prompt, attentive service gives the patient confidence that the family doctor or primary care physician referred the patient to the right place and gives them confidence not only in the neurosurgeon, but in the entire health care system or provider network. Service should be perceived as the medium by which we can not only more efficiently cure the disease or excise the pathology, but also heal and transform the individual through the trust engendered by personal commitment.

Service means reasonably prompt access for the patient once the referral is sought. The true emergency, be it a subarachnoid hemorrhage from a ruptured aneurysm or the sudden evolution of signs and symptoms of increased intracranial pressure from an obstructed shunt or intracranial hematoma, is almost always recognized as such and is promptly evaluated and treated. Is it reasonable, however, to expect a patient with severe sciatica or headaches to wait 1 month or 6 weeks to be seen because the neurosurgeon is out of town or "booked solid"? If the neurosurgeon is unavailable, perhaps a colleague could see the patient and relieve the pain and mental anguish immediately. If not, then prompt referral to another neurosurgeon or allied specialist in the community is appropriate. The practice of only referring or recommending another specialist at great distance, inconvenience, and expense to the patient and family is deplorable when comparable, competent expertise is available close to home.

Almost as important to the patient as prompt access is ease of access. This is particularly a problem in large, urban medical centers serving regional areas and rural populations. Well-thought-out and readily available directions, maps, parking, and even valet service go a long way toward instilling confidence that the system and the professionals in it are thoughtful and looking out for the needs of the patient. Friendly, helpful, courteous staff offering and providing some personal amenities while the patient is waiting to see the doctor is important, but few things show more respect for the patient than being punctual and respectful of the patient's time. This includes the provision of ready access to ancillary services, such as the laboratory, electroencephalography, electromyography, and diagnostic imaging.

The neurosurgeon will never get a second chance to make a good first impression, and that impression is critically important to the patient and the family. Surgical scrub attire is not appropriate for patient encounters outside of the operating theater, and patients expect and respect the professionalism conveyed by a suit or clean white coat.

The neurosurgeon who sits down and converses with the patient in a warm, open, and relaxed manner will almost always be perceived as giving the patient adequate time and sharing of one's self. The nurse clinician, physician's assistant, and house officer all contribute and share in patient care and communication, but are not satisfactory surrogates for the neurosurgeon being available and attentive.

The patient and family appreciate immediate feedback of important information, such as the results of diagnostic imaging and pathology reports. It is often helpful and almost always prudent to communicate with the referring physician as early as possible during the decision-making process. The hospitalized patient and particularly the family prefer regularly scheduled rounds so they can be available and prepared to discuss proposed treatments, progress, prognosis, and discharge planning. It is particularly important to schedule in advance any conference where informed consent issues are to be addressed so that friends and family of the patient can be present if the patient so desires.

When are our patients being offered services? Are patients being awakened at 5:00 in the morning to have blood drawn because the laboratory has a 3- to 4-hour turnaround time? Are patients scheduled for surgery on the day of admission to the hospital being asked or told to arrive at 5:00 AM because overnight-stay facilities are not available or because of inefficient registration, laboratory turnaround, anesthesia workup, or inflexible operating room schedules? Yes, it is deplorable that insurance companies and other third-party payers insist that the patient assume the health risk, financial burden, and inconvenience of same-day admission, so that their chief executive officers can pull down high salaries and bonuses with the savings that accrue from this practice. But we, as the patient's physician and advocate, must try whenever possible to schedule admission, tests, and surgery to meet the needs and convenience of the patient.

Adequate time must be available and allotted for the task at hand. Surgery scheduled and performed under the stress of other important and pressing commitments may interfere with intraoperative judgment and execution. The neurosurgical corollary of Murphy's Law must be: "If something can go wrong, it is most likely to do so when there really isn't adequate time allotted to deal with it." The patient has a right to expect personalized postoperative as well as preoperative and intraoperative care. It is generally unwise and certainly unfair to the patient for the neurosurgeon to perform surgery just prior to leaving town.

In recent years, there has been a tendency for some surgeons to delegate the preoperative history and physical examination to the internist, and the patient's postoperative care to the intensivist. Certainly, consultation with other physicians with special expertise is appropriate and commendable to assist in the evaluation and management of complicated medical and surgical problems. But there is no better opportunity for the neurosurgeon to truly get to know the patient and establish rapport than through the medium of obtaining a thorough and comprehensive history and physical examination. The experienced neurosurgeon may, on rare occasion, be comfortable accepting another clinician's findings on physical examination; however, he or she should almost never delegate the delicate art of obtaining an accurate clinical history in any but the most straightforward and obvious cases, and even then with full awareness of the potential perils and pitfalls of this practice.

Neurosurgeons need to stay involved in the care of their patients in the intensive care unit (ICU) and be available thereafter. No one is better quali-

fied to discuss with the family the care and prognosis for a patient with neurologic conditions. Larry Pitts[11] said: "It is the neurosurgeon's obligation to his or her patients to take charge of their neurologic problem, to be available, to be at the bedside often enough to assess change, and to help counsel other physicians and the family about what therapies and diagnostic studies are in order."

The mood and trend in patient-centered care is shifting toward the multiskilled caregiver. In this evolving and restructured health care system, patients and families will interact with fewer people and thereby enhance the concept of "continuity of care." The neurosurgeon must ponder whether this tendency is consistent with asking the physician's assistant, nurse clinician, or internist to take the history and perform the physical examination, the chest surgeon to expose the spine, the orthopedist to perform the fusion, the intensivist to manage the patient in the ICU, and the physiatrist to oversee routine postoperative convalescence.

In the hospital of the 1990s, a typical patient interacts with about 60 different employees during a 4-day stay.[8] Is it any wonder that the patient can't remember the neurosurgeon's name 2 years after a spinal operation? Does the neurosurgeon know the name of the patient's primary nurse? How closely are they working together? Is the neurosurgeon reading the patient's nursing care plan? Is the neurosurgeon talking regularly with the patient's primary care or referring physician?

J. Daniel Beckham,[1] in writing about his son Andrew's critical illness, observed:

> Most doctors are visitors to the world of the patient. The patient's world, particularly for those who are hospitalized for any period of time, comes to consist of a tightening circle to which the physician is often an outsider. The circle consists of concentric rings of relationships that may shift and flux but most often include family members, nurses, and the relatives of other patients. It is a group that quickly develops a deep reservoir of shared experience because of mutual involvement on the same battlefield.

Lest the neurosurgeon object, declaring that the real battlefield is in the operating theater, it must be realized that the surgery was a different battle and that the patient and family only later received a vague briefing on that relatively brief skirmish. But they are left to fight a physically, emotionally, and resource-draining battle that may go on for days and weeks, if not longer. It is, therefore, easy to understand how they, like the foot soldier, may come to lack considerable empathy for the doctor who, like the general absent during much of the shooting, arrives for brief moments in clean uniform "helicoptered in from the rear."

At the core of patient-centered care is the concept that knowledge and technical competence are just half of the story. The other half is excellence in providing service. The neurosurgeon with personal attributes of honesty and integrity, and in command of a large body of cognitive knowledge and manual skills will still be perceived as uncaring and lacking compassion if there is not an ethic of service. Charles Bosk[3] wrote: "The key problem is maintaining in definitions of competence a professional ethic of service for without an ethic of service, competence loses much of its meaning and much of its value."

Competence

J. Daniel Beckham[1] wrote in an article about his son's illness:

> Compassion is no substitute for competence. In superficial, brief medical encounters, a smiling face and a gentle hand impress. In the long run, it is competence that is valued. The patient and family are looking for confidence, born of knowledge, and demonstrated through competence that is too often perceived as being in short supply in an industry increasingly characterized by pool nurses and part-time doctors.

Donald Quest,[12] in his Presidential Address to the Congress of Neurological Surgeons in 1989, said:

> We are not all gifted technically and we are not all skillful and deft surgeons; but we can all commit ourselves to improving our judgment and our operative techniques; we can read and view tapes of those who are superb technical surgeons. Each one of us can

contribute by our commitment to increasing our knowledge of the nervous system and its disorders, to supporting research, and to improving our judgment and technical abilities as surgeons.

The concept of patient-centered care challenges, or at least calls to question, the very definition of clinical competence. What is the standard to which competence and quality of care are to be compared and who will be responsible for quality control? Proliferating technology and changes toward more centrally administered systems for health care delivery will inexorably alter the delicate relationship between patient, neurosurgeon, and the payer for health care services.

Patient-centered care is oriented toward the generalist. Academic centers during the past half century have prepared health care professionals to be specialists rather than generalists, however, and this is increasingly the case in neurosurgery, where subspecialty certification is currently an issue promoted by a small but vocal lobby. The vast majority of neurosurgeons are well trained and do most things very well. The poorly trained individual without the requisite aptitude, skills, and character for neurosurgery does almost nothing well. It must be recognized that subspecialty certification is a guild protection device that will not guarantee competence, but may make specialty care more costly and less accessible to the patient.

It should be obvious and apparent that a particular skill or technique does not make a professional. It is the constellation of knowledge, training, experience, and skills acquired over time through professional education and practice that forms a professional identity. Certain personality characteristics, such as flexibility, adaptability, innovativeness, a positive attitude, and an ability to control stress and ambition, are associated with successful performance within a profession such as neurosurgery.[17]

One standard of competence by which we will almost certainly be judged is how well we assume and exercise responsibility to use technology in a wise and efficient manner and only when it is of proven advantage for our patients. This implies continuing education not only of ourselves, but also of our patients as consumers of valuable health care resources.[16]

Clinical scientists have traditionally measured and monitored the outcomes of medical care through mortality, morbidity, and complication rates. Patient-centered care provides the clinical neuroscientist the impetus for analyzing outcome by how patients feel, how they function, and whether they are able to work and perform the other daily activities important in their lives. How does the treatment proposed or executed compare with the expected natural history of the disease or disorder being treated? Is the natural history of the disorder known? Has the effectiveness of the proposed treatment been scientifically validated?

A very important development in health care is recognition of the centrality of the patient's point of view when monitoring the quality of medical care outcomes.[4] The purpose of medical care for most patients is the achievement or realization of a more effective life and the preservation of function and well-being. The patient and the family are the best sources of information regarding the achievement of these goals, but how often and how systematically is information sought from patients about their experiences and perceptions of disease and treatment? Such information is not a part of the medical record and is, therefore, rarely available for analysis in the current health care database.[18] Patient-completed health status measures have become tools of health services research, however.[14] The neurosurgeon will soon be analyzing this kind of data and be able to consider the patient's point of view regarding his or her functional status and well-being in addition to the traditional biomedical measures used to assess outcome in clinical practice and trials.

Patient-centered care delivery is based on the principle of case management utilizing a "critical pathways model" or protocols of care. The neurosurgeon will be valued who accepts this model as an opportunity to influence and assure an enhanced and more efficient standard of care for patients rather than condemning it as a "cookbook" approach to be rejected without a fair trial or careful analysis. The "critical pathways model," however, should always be considered a dynamic, working prototype in evolution, not a rigid formula for patient care. Adaptations and exceptions to treatment and outcomes algorithms will be necessary and are to be expected as dictated by the

peculiarities of a particular case. There will always be outliers.

Tracking a patient's progress is easier when protocols define the plan of care, responses to therapeutic regimens, and the expected outcomes. The volume of data in the medical record is reduced by the adoption of standard patient care protocols based on expected activities and outcomes for particular diagnostic groups of patients. "Charting by exceptions" has been recommended and implies recording only those instances where a patient's response to care deviates from that expected according to day of stay for a particular diagnosis. This reduces the time the staff must spend documenting activities and, thereby, increases the time available for direct patient care.

In the patient-centered environment, the neurosurgeon needs to be patient, supportive, and flexible while making sure that the focus is on the needs of the patient rather than the needs or wants of the caregivers, discipline, department, or health maintenance or management system. The neurosurgeon has an obligation to educate the individual patient and society about such things as injury prevention and to train the next generation of neurosurgeons. We must have a continuing commitment to research and need to collaborate with physicians, surgeons, and scientists from other disciplines if we are to provide the best possible care for our patients.

A neurosurgeon must accept some personal risk as an obligation inherent in the trust placed by our patients and society. Communicable diseases have always been a threat to physicians. The threat of hepatitis, AIDS, or Creutzfeldt-Jakob disease should be no more a deterrent to our administering to the ill than was smallpox or yellow fever to previous generations of physicians,[2] nor should fear of litigation affect our willingness to accept challenging cases and do what is right and appropriate for our patients. To paraphrase former President Harry S. Truman: If you can't stand the heat in the kitchen, you shouldn't be a cook.

The neurosurgeon must try to be where the action is and be involved with both quality and cost issues. Patient-centered care requires the standardization of care, the development of critical pathways to guide standardization, and more accountability for patient outcomes in a holistic sense. If we do not provide leadership, these issues will be guided by parties who are perhaps less sensitive to the special needs of our patients with disease and injury affecting the nervous system.

Leonard Peikoff[10] has written about the new and deadly pressure on doctors within the United States that continuously threatens the integrity of their medical judgment: "There is mounting pressure to cave in to arbitrary, politically mandated economies, while blanking out the effects on the patient." Directly or indirectly, a doctor who insists on quality patient care, and thereby implicitly drives up cost, is likely to incur the displeasure of hospital, government, or third-party payer administrators.[10] People who go into the health care professions love people and have a sense of calling. But put good people into a bad system and it makes it difficult for them to do good things.

Through the mechanism of politically motivated devices such as the integrated service networks being mandated by the state of Minnesota, the doctor is threatened with exclusion from the system and the patient loses the freedom of selecting a physician. Under the ever-evolving present system, administrators not only have to cut services drastically, but it is in their interests to conceal this fact from the patient. The system is rigged to restrict the quality of medical care in such a way that the patient does not understand what is happening. The patient does not know medicine and does not appreciate what is being taken away, but rather relies on the doctor's integrity to tell him or her what services are available and necessary. The doctor cannot allow the system to compromise that integrity by not telling the patient the full truth and, thereby, be part of the conspiracy of silence. The heart and soul of patient-centered medicine rests on the principle that the doctor will have the moral courage to stand up for what is best for the patient.

References

1. Beckham JD. Andrew's not-so-excellent adventure. *Healthcare Forum J*. May/June 1993:90-98.

2. Black PM. Risky business: is personal risk an obligation in treating patients? *Clin Neurosurg*. 1989;35:487-499.

3. Bosk C. What are the determinants of a competent neurosurgeon? *Clin Neurosurg*. 1989;35:474-486.

4. Geigle R, Jones S. Outcomes measurement: a report from the front. *Inquiry*. 1990;27:7-13.

5. Haight F. Law and medicine: when will the hostage taking cease? *Clin Neurosurg*. 1990;36:92-107.

6. Henderson JL, Williams JB. The shape of things to come. Part 7: the people side of patient care design. *Healthcare Forum J*. July/Aug 1991:44-49.

7. Langfitt TW. Critical care: when is enough enough? *Clin Neurosurg*. 1987;35:15-28.

8. Lathrop JP. The patient-focused hospital. *Healthcare Forum J*. May/June 1992:76-78.

9. Lathrop JP. The do-it-yourself restructuring test. *Healthcare Forum J*. May/June 1993:108-111.

10. Peikoff L. The forgotten man of socialized medicine: the doctor. *Clin Neurosurg*. 1990;36:108-121.

11. Pitts LH. Neurosurgical critical care: who's in charge? *Clin Neurosurg*. 1989;35:55-62.

12. Quest DO. Presidential address: commitment and contribution. *Clin Neurosurg*. 1989;35:3-14.

13. Silberman CE. Providing patient-centered care. *Health Management Q*. 1992;14:12-16.

14. Stewart AL, Ware JE Jr, eds. *Measuring Functioning and Well-Being. The Medical Outcomes Study Approach*. Durham, NC: Duke University Press; 1992.

15. Svinicki M. What they don't know can hurt them: the role of prior knowledge in learning. *POD Network*. 1993-1994;5:4.

16. Tindall SC. Problems imposed by the new technology. *Clin Neurosurg*. 1992;39:533-543.

17. Vaughn DG, Fottler MD, Bamberg R, et al. Utilization and management of multiskilled health practitioners in US hospitals. *Hospital and Health Services Administration*. 1991;36:397-419.

18. Ware JE Jr. Measures for a new era of health assessment. In: Stewart AL, Ware JE Jr, eds. *Measuring Functioning and Well-Being. The Medical Outcomes Study Approach*. Durham, NC: Duke University Press; 1992:4-11.

CHAPTER 5

Ethics and Etiquette in Neurosurgery

William F. Collins, MD

Webster's Third International Dictionary defines ethics as "the discipline dealing with what is good and bad or right and wrong or with moral duty and obligation." Etiquette is defined as ". . . behavior prescribed by . . . rule or custom . . . [or] the rules of conduct, action, or practice binding on members of a profession . . . in their relations with one another."

The Question Of Ethics

Philosophers both religious and secular have tried for centuries to define what is good, moral, and obligatory—that is, to define a theory of morality that could be universally accepted. The enlightenment of the 18th century contains a classical summary of that quest and the multiple concepts considered. Three of the many divergent views are presented in the writings of Hume, Rousseau, and Kant. David Hume did not believe religion had all the answers and enlarged the definition of what was considered to be moral to include not just that which had been said to come from a God, but also those actions and concepts that are utilitarian for society as shown by the approbation of society. The implication was that the more utilitarian an action is for society, the greater the probability that it is moral and good.[2,3] This is in contrast to Jean-Jacques Rousseau's concept that what is moral comes from God. He did not believe that all that society approved was moral, but rather that progress in the arts and sciences—almost always approved by society—often leads persons and society away from morality.[7] Im-

manuel Kant, upset by both the skepticism of Hume's belief that the origin of morality was not from God and Rousseau's limitation of a God-given basis for all morality, proposed that while he believed in the God-given origin of morality, a practical solution to determine what was right and moral was to utilize the categorical imperative.[4,5] Kant's categorical imperative was to test an action with the following: "Act only according to that maxim whereby you can at the same time will that it should become a universal law." He asserted that if the action could fulfill that imperative, the action or concept was moral.

Despite the reflections and abilities of these and other philosophers, it was and is easy to find a portion of everyday activities or of the actions of society that could not be accepted by these concepts as moral, yet remain moral to persons and society. Defining the canons of a religion and presenting them to the faithful has been one of the more successful means of having multitudes accept concepts as moral. Unfortunately, the multitudes often assume that all who are outside the belief in those concepts are immoral, even when a majority of people are outside that fold. If one is an agnostic and does not believe in God or knows nothing of God's laws, are the actions of that person immoral? If a society finds it useful—thereby approving—the killing of humans on the basis of their beliefs, does that make the killing moral? When an action that helps one person but harms another does not fulfill the Kantian categorical imperative because it cannot become a universal law, is it always necessarily immoral? These questions and many more have concerned ethicists for generations. The important aspect of such inquiry is neither the questions nor the answers, but the recognition of the method used to develop both, and the realization that any concepts one has must be considered in light of that process. A bit fanciful but still useful in action and contemplation is the suggestion of Hume that to understand the values and morals of a society or a person, one should read the poetry and the stories of that society or enjoyed by that person.

A Practical Approach to Ethics

Perhaps a more practical question is "Can ethics be useful as a guide or director of a person, a profession, or a society?"[1,8] That question has no encompassing answer, for ethics does not direct what to do but how to do it. That is to say, ethics is not a category of rules or of rights and wrongs. It is, rather, a means to deal with the generalities of what makes actions right or wrong as opposed to whether an act in itself is right or wrong. Ethics is not the list of positive concepts of what is right or of negative concepts of what is wrong, but instead presents a way for one to move toward a more meaningful existence and the pursuit of excellence. It is not the mechanical application of rules and the attempt to force persons into a mold, but rather the effort to encourage creativity in searching for ways to improve responses to situations beyond what may have been considered. To place it on a categorical or scientific basis would require something not obtainable—a moral theory that is acceptable to all, in all circumstances. While it cannot be a list of dos and do nots, it can be a direct means of focusing the human effort to make choices that are more valuable to persons and society. It is not static nor can it be by definition a completed concept, for it must evolve with the changes it confronts either in substance or in concepts, and respond in kind if it is to effect the common good.

What does it take to be ethical? It requires reflection on one's own moral values, for one must realize that moral values learned from the family—the most common donor of ethical behavior—or from other common donors such as re-

ligious experience, societal groups, or formal education, while perhaps acceptable as a basis for one person's actions, are not an absolute morality when applied to others. It insists as well that one has an interest in human values and their meaning, and an interest in making such values real and effective for oneself and others by making choices based on reflection and knowledge. The ethical person must find meaning in life, drawing conclusions about reasons for actions from reflection upon past personal experiences and the reflections of others who have considered the discipline of ethics. The ethical person must desire to lead a meaningful life that contributes to the commonweal, and then train to their best ability so as to make as meaningful a contribution to society as possible. These actions require a personal honesty that allows one to evaluate one's performance without being fooled by false rewards or discouraged by lack of attainment of what were predetermined goals. Educated ethical physicians should be familiar with classical and contemporary philosophers if only so their reflections on past and present experiences can be freed from parochial concepts. In this way, they can better consider others' concepts of morality and the meaning of life. Thus, for the ethical physician, ethics should be pervasive in all actions, as well as in all considerations.

Medical Ethics and Neurosurgery

Changes in the discipline of ethics occur in medicine as in other aspects of society, for society and medicine have become more complex with technical advances. In medicine, these advances have enlarged the areas of ethical concern to include situations not imagined by our forefathers and therefore not covered by many older ethical concepts and oaths. Some of these areas include mechanical and pharmacologic prolongation of life, alteration in concepts of death, use of organs in transplantation and of abortive tissues to treat human disease, handling of incompetent or impaired physicians, and problems of societal and personal costs of medical care, to name just a few of the recent additions. The increased complexity of society continues to increase the complexity of ethics, particularly in the relationships of society to medicine and medicine to society. Professionals with an understanding of the discipline of ethics will have a better chance to interact positively to these changes.

Where medical ethics is different from general ethics is in its greater focus in time and degree with continuation or cessation of life. It can be focused even more sharply in neurosurgery where an added factor in *continuation*-of-life decisions may be that *prolongation* can be obtained only at the cost of permitting or causing loss of neurologic function. The focus is also that decisions must be made with relatively little time and, at times, inadequate information. The latter issue— i.e. the amount of available information—has become in some ways less of a problem with modern imaging techniques, but in the process has made some treatment decisions even more difficult. The time limitation for making a decision is one of the reasons why it is important for the physician to consider in advance not what decision is to be made, but how it is to be reached. It would be easy to decide that all life must be maintained at any cost, or that only that life which the physician believes acceptable should be allowed to continue. Medical ethics demands, however, that all aspects of meaning in life be considered, and not just those within the prejudice of the physician. What may not be a meaningful life to the physician can, to a family or patient, have significance out of the ken of the physician, unless the physician looks at and brings into the decision process all of the interests of the various persons involved. This does not mean that the patient should make the decision alone, but rather that the physician must consider the values of all persons involved when advising a course of action. This can be difficult, for the axiom is that while a disease may be confined to a patient, an illness affects all in the patient's surround.

How do neurosurgeons usually fulfill these requirements to be ethical people? Most define an area of performance that is within legal and professional limits without considering what is truly ethical by the above standards. Some probably do become ethical persons, but I know only those who have made the effort, not those who have succeeded. They, with that effort, have enriched the lives of their patients and themselves.

A Neurosurgeon's Personal Approach to Ethics

How does this author fit into the situation of medical ethics? I am one of those who have tried to consider ethics in my actions since my early exposure to a Jesuit elementary education and to rudimentary college philosophy. Neither philosophies were or are the main basis of my concepts. I was exposed to medical practice as the son of a general practitioner, and I believe the morality of service to patients and medicine that was played over and over in our family became a portion of my values, definitely influencing me. My ideas have evolved from various concepts that I use in general to determine what is the best way to add value and meaning to the life of a patient or a patient's family. I try not to have fixed concepts of morality or immorality, and continue to be amazed at how other persons can look at the same situation I am considering and reach a different conclusion. My basic (but not bound) concepts are that life is precious and should be preserved if it can have any meaning for anyone, and that when I cannot cure or treat a disease, I should attempt to help heal the persons involved with the illness.

The concept of attempting to heal family and patients when cure or treatment is not possible is difficult to define and often very consuming of time and emotion. My gain has been a better understanding of how illness affects patients and families, along with an added variable to my consideration of the best means of adding value to both my life and that of my patients. We shall briefly discuss etiquette before returning to some examples of the application of ethics in clinical neurosurgery.

Etiquette in Neurosurgery

There is no categorical imperative in etiquette, for the rules of etiquette are neither universal nor the same for different ages, societies, or even genders. Etiquette depends on societal rules that concern dress, language, body posture, body movement, spatial relationship to another, and body functions. I remember working hard to learn to speak some Japanese during the time I was stationed by the Army in Japan. On arriving at a party given by one of the medical school professors, I was dismayed at being asked *not* to speak Japanese since I would almost certainly insult someone. Such a request was difficult for the professor, for he was a kind gentleman, but he was even more concerned with the comfort of all his guests. It is not possible to learn in a brief time the nuances of spoken Japanese; later I realized that I would have degraded some important people with my use of the language. Etiquette in the profession of medicine may not be as difficult to learn as using spoken Japanese, but it has rules of conduct that can reflect adversely upon the person who remains unaware of them. It has some traps that can cause difficulties, especially when combined with ethical concerns.

As with any etiquette, medical etiquette requires respect for the person or persons to whom one relates, so as not to cause unnecessary discomfort or embarrassment. Basic social etiquette in any society is the starting point of professional etiquette. While in some social situations there can be marked variation in manners, with some persons able to deviate significantly from the norm in dress or speech, most persons in important situations adhere to the norm—and one should consider most professional situations as important. Professional society is generally important to those using it. Its etiquette is more rigid because much of the manner, speech, and dress of the professional has intrinsic meaning for the persons or the situation involved. Thus, in professional situations, less deviation is tolerated without reflecting poorly on the deviate. Notice how formally dressed most speakers are at a medical meeting and how limited the variations are in dress for participants, even though after the meeting or at informal functions the dress can be varied. Notice the effect of informal dress on patients or on the health care workers on the hospital ward or in the clinic. Another major aspect of professional etiquette that often bothers physicians is the unwritten rule that criticism of the profession or of a professional should be confined to the profession and not be brought to laypersons.

Etiquette in clinical neurosurgery is no different from general professional medical etiquette. Medical etiquette is most easily discussed by dividing situations of usage into doctor-to-patient, patient-to-doctor, doctor-to-doctor, and doctor-to-patient-to-doctor interactions combined with the manipulations patients or doctors can perform within such situations.

Doctor-to-Patient and Patient-to-Doctor Interactions

The physician should convey by dress, body movement, and speech that a doctor is present and concerned with the patient's problem. It is easiest to convey that impression by dressing as the patient believes a doctor should dress. A white coat is a common signal, while short pants without a shirt or shoes requires an explanation to convey the impression. Body movements should include staying at an interpersonal distance, usually the distance it takes to touch by extending an arm, until a contract for care has been agreed upon or unless physical action is necessary for immediate care. Speech should be modulated, nonjudgmental, and should allow ample time for the patient to present concerns and for the physician to answer questions. I do not call patients by their first names, nor encourage patients to use mine. This appears to undermine the authority that I feel is necessary for optimal care. Although I am aware that many physicians believe filling out a preliminary questionnaire helps clarify an initial consultation, I have found that it depersonalizes the consult and interferes with my doctor-patient relationship. Sometimes at a later visit or after the examination, I offer the patient the opportunity to fill out a questionnaire or to write down their complaints or questions, and I believe this does not have the same negative effect since the relationship has already been established. The physician should not be judgmental by expression or speech, and should show no emotion that would inhibit gaining information or confidence. There should be no implication that the information being obtained is anything but private. Undressing for an examination should be private and, if an intimate examination—a term that varies from patient to patient—is considered, the presence of an aide or a member of the family often will prevent unnecessary embarrassment for the patient or the doctor.

Finally, the results of the examination and the problems or questions being asked or arising from diagnostic tests can be discussed with the patient, but a neurosurgeon is typically a consultant. The patient should be informed that, while the neurosurgeon will discuss their situation, the findings of their examination and the final test results along with the neurosurgeon's opinion will be sent to and discussed with their primary physician. I do not discuss in any concrete terms the opinions or recommendation of the referring doctor unless they are the same as mine or can easily be modified by the testing requested. Expanding that etiquette, I do not allow a patient to believe that I accept their criticism of another doctor, but neither do I stop them from presenting it. I try to have my patients respect my recommendations so that they will do what I recommend. This often means answering, within the limits of professional courtesy to the referring doctor, more of their questions than often I would like to answer, and later answering their telephone calls. I do not hesitate to tell a patient when they are interfering with my ability to function by the number and timing of unnecessary calls, for I believe the patient must follow the rules of etiquette in dealing with me. I do not hesitate to inform a patient that he or she is out of line when they are, and I try to put my concern about their actions as part of my general concern for them and my other patients. At the end of an office visit, when I think a patient may have had some difficulty understanding what I have said, I often ask my nurse to talk with the patient on the way out to be certain that there is no confusion or misunderstanding. While this can increase the number of questions and the time necessary to answer them, it has saved me from mistakes and often saves time in the long run. The situation should be controlled so both the patient and the doctor are as satisfied as possible.

Doctor-to-Doctor and Doctor-to-Patient-to-Doctor Interactions

As a neurosurgeon, one is dependent upon referring physicians, and the etiquette of doctor-to-doctor relationships often determines if one will receive consultations from other physicians or neurosurgeons. With any etiquette, and particularly professional etiquette, the correct behavior in doctor-to-doctor relationships begins with respecting the other physician. After a consultation, I convey to the referring doctor my opinion and any additional information I have obtained as soon as is practical. At times this may require a phone call, especially if there is need for emergency treatment or if I strongly disagree with the referring doctor's diagnosis or recommendations. In the latter situation, the conversation can be started by stating that I disagree with their opinion, but I try to soften this by asking to discuss the basis for the referring doctor's diagnosis, inferring or stating that there may be information I did not receive that would change my opinion. In the case of a major difference, I always add the statement that because I was not certain that the difference was justified until I had all the information from the referring doctor and the tests I had ordered, my difference of opinion was not discussed with the patient. This gives the referring physician an opportunity to explain his or her conclusion, and indicates a sensitivity to the problems of professional disagreement. When the call or contact is made early after the consultation, it allows the consulting physician to continue to be a part of the decision-making process, and to hold the respect of the patient by being on the inside of a change in treatment plans or diagnosis if this is required or allowed.

What is more difficult is the patient that plays with physicians by quoting opinions that may or may not be true, and who may attempt to verbally chastise doctors in general. The patient often starts by stating that you are an exception and then particularly insults the referring or treating doctor. Be careful, for you can be certain you are the next to be chastised no matter what such a patient says. The physician should be aware of what the rules of professional etiquette and ethics are for dealing with such patients. These do not allow comments to be made to the patient that either support or deny the accusations. Any conclusions drawn must wait until all aspects of the situation are carefully considered, and no action should be taken based only upon information from the patient. In the process of reflective contemplation, information from the doctor being attacked is necessary, and that physician should be told what is happening. Most times, the entire episode is a figment of someone's imagination, but as a physician one is compelled to consider all alternatives. At times the information obtained may indicate that the problem is incompetence on the part of the referring physician or surgeon (for one or more reasons). I will use this situation to return to the application of ethics to specific cases in clinical neurosurgery.

Situational Applications of Ethics

There are almost endless situations where ethics apply to the practice of medicine. I will discuss three that are frequently encountered: the impaired or incompetent physician, active prolongation or ending of life, and the impact of technical advances and their cost benefits.

The Impaired or Incompetent Physician

Information indicating that the referring or treating doctor may be the problem often is obtained by examining the patient and the records brought to the consultation. These may make it clear not only that the treating physician may have reached the wrong diagnosis, but that a portion of the patient's disability may have resulted from the treatment used or, in part, from a lack of correct treatment. Professional etiquette states that one does not discuss professional problems with laypersons. On the other hand, the American Medical Association in its 1980 code of ethics states: "A physician shall deal honestly with patients and colleagues and strive to expose those physicians deficient in character or competence or who engage in fraud or deception." What should a physician do and how do ethics apply?

The ethical physician tries to make choices that are best first for the patient and second for all others involved or who could be involved. Medical ethics does not dictate what one should do but rather implies how to proceed. Reflection and consideration must continue until as much information as possible is gathered, since a decision to start or not start an action has to be based on that information. Do not start a process that will lead to an action before deciding that the chosen action is the best way to improve the situation. Consideration will include the possibility that this episode is a simple mistake, evidence of a lack of concern for patients, evidence of incompetence, evidence of substance abuse, evidence of fraud, or none or all of the above. Do not jump to conclusions before you have information, since any action may have a negative effect upon you, the patient, or the doctor involved, while you should be acting to improve the situation.

Ethically, deciding whether to take an action and what action to take should not be based on your considerations alone. If at all possible, one should discuss the information with a peer, contact the involved physician, listen to his or her explanation, and decide if the situation indicates that a discussion should take place with an institutional or medical society ethics committee, realizing that even that action can cause problems. If you believe there is a problem, you must first protect the patient from further harm, and then determine if any action you take will bring about the most meaningful result for everyone. The action must include consideration of whether the referring physician needs help in the form of treatment and/or should stop practicing, neither alternative being easy or simple to undertake. A quick idea for some is to support a malpractice action, but a malpractice action may have little value in the situation for the patient, doctor, or society. One of the problems with malpractice suits is that they may prolong the physical symptoms and the adverse emotional effects on the patient, with the patient ending up with little to compensate for the situation. In addition, malpractice actions rarely stop incompetent physicians from practicing, which may be the best goal of the action. The one choice the ethical neurosurgeon cannot make is to ignore the problem. In my career, I have talked three neurosurgeons out of continuing neurosurgical practice by appealing to their basic values to stop doing things they were not competent to do, and to consider how else they might contribute. Two of the three remained my friends.

Prolonging or Ending Life

The second situation where ethics enters into neurosurgical practice is the question of prolonging or ending life in a patient for whom "quality of life" does not appear to be a possibility. This may be a newborn infant with significant congenital defects, a young male with a serious head injury, a middle-aged person with a large dominant cerebral hemorrhage, or an elderly person with dementia or a disease more debilitating than old age. As an ethical physician, it should be clear that one must obtain and reflect upon the concepts and desires of the patient and the patient's family. Since they often do not realize, due to lack of experience, what the life is they are considering prolonging or not prolonging, it is the duty of the physician to instruct them as completely as possible. I believe that it is not the family's or the patient's role to decide what to do, but for the physician, after due consideration, to present a clear recommendation for the family to accept or reject. Realize that if the recommendation is contrary to their ideals and concepts, they may refuse to accept that advice. Do not abandon the patient or family because of their refusal, but continue to assemble information for them and yourself to consider. In these circumstances, having to put decision-making into a courtroom means to me that the physician failed to prepare himself or herself, the family, and/or the medical personnel taking care of the patient for what was the best choice for everyone involved.

In all these situations, decisions are not easy, and there is always the morality of a physician deciding if a patient should live or die. The issue has been discussed under the terms "active" or "passive" euthanasia. Passive euthanasia is not acting to stop a process that the physician can stop, thus allowing a patient to die. Active euthanasia is causing the patient's death by a definite action, such as injection of a lethal dose of a drug. Some persons call this "killing the patient," and in fact the active ending of life is not

legal. This must be considered even when discussing ethics and morals. There are very cogent arguments that there is no difference between the two, and I concede these arguments are persuasive. For instance, if a patient with terminal cancer, who has had and continues to suffer from severe pain, requests an end to life, is it less moral to end it with an injection of barbiturates or morphine than it would be to not treat a condition such as pneumonia that will kill the patient in a few days but would have been easily treated with antibiotics? Is it moral to prolong the suffering when one can give the patient a merciful death? The terms active and passive euthanasia are pejorative to me, for they imply that there is either only death or life in the equation. Consider again the terminal cancer patient. I agree life is not worth much if one must suffer constantly, but I find unacceptable the argument that only death could end the suffering because it may simply reflect ignorance on the part of the physician as to how to control pain. In some patients, control of pain may require drugs that can shorten life, but the intention is to relieve suffering, not to end life. That, to me, is different than ending life because pain cannot be controlled—it means that the basis for the action is ignorance, which is not an acceptable reason.

A more difficult problem is the infant with multiple defects, a number of which would be lethal unless corrected. Is a low IQ (and how low), paraplegia (and what level), or other loss of function (and how much loss) enough to not treat a fatal condition? I cannot answer this in all instances, but I try to discuss the realities of the situation. I have managed patients where the family, for various reasons, could not accept withholding treatment, and on occasion have been pleasantly surprised many years later to see how both the family and the patient have a meaningful life even though the life would not be meaningful to me.

In contrast, there is the case of cerebral hemorrhage with mass effect that will kill the person within hours or days, but the removal of which would leave the patient at best aphasic and hemiplegic. This person had already developed a lifestyle that will no longer be possible, and I cannot recommend to a family to operate. Assuming that my prediction is an absolute certainty, would I do it if they insisted? Fortunately, I have not had to do so, and now I no longer operate. I have thought of the situation and decided I might, if the family has a reason for such a life, although I could not envision it myself. Of course, this assumes an absolute and perfect prediction of outcome, which is not the case in many clinical situations.

Ethics and the Cost of Care

Finally, I would like to discuss the cost of medical care. Many do not consider this a part of ethics but rather just a side issue in terminal care or in the treatment of conditions where there is no chance that the patient will contribute to society following treatment. In the near-terminally ill whose life is extended, the added cost of that period of time and increased intensity of hospitalization often is born by third-party payers or the government, and is not a concern of the family or the doctor. Ethically, it must be a concern because it places an extra financial burden on the clients of the insurer or the taxpayer, and eventually affects all of us even though it may be in any one instance a minor portion of the health care costs to society. It must be a concern because physicians must consider all of the factors that increase costs and consider them in a cost-benefit-outcome evaluation. Resources are limited, even though in the United States most people act as though they do not believe this to be so. It is clear that when medical care uses too high a percentage of the gross national product, the government will intervene, as is happening now. Even if the govenment becomes the main provider, the ethical physician must still consider all aspects of costs because increased cost in a government system will cause caps and rationing to be instituted, and I find that unacceptable. Also, no health care system in any developed country has been so satisfactory that private practice disappears; costs may be the factor allowing or blocking it.

Conclusion

In summary, the ethical physician must, by reflection and consideration, attempt to make decisions that are best for both medicine and society. The ethical physician must recognize his or her morals and how they developed, and particularly not assume they are the absolute morality for everyone. Ethics is not a list of what to do, but rather presents a way to move toward a more meaningful existence and the pursuit of excellence. Etiquette, in contrast, is the behavior prescribed for society and professions. Both ethics and etiquette are necessary for an individual to attain a position in society or a profession, and to maximize creativity and valued responses to situations beyond what may have been considered without them.

References

1. dePender W, Ikeda-Chandler W. *Clinical Ethics: An Invitation to Healing Professionals.* New York, NY: Praeger; 1990.
2. Hume D; Gaskin JCA, ed. *Dialogues and Natural History of Religion.* New York, NY: Oxford University Press; 1993.
3. Hume D; Selgy-Bigge LA, ed. *Enquiry Concerning Human Understanding and Concerning the Principles of Morals.* 3rd ed. Oxford, England: Clarendon Press; 1975.
4. Kant I; Infield L, trans. *Lectures on Ethics.* Indianapolis, Ind: Hackett; 1980.
5. Kant I; Paten HJ, trans. *Grounding for the Metaphysics of Morals.* New York, NY: Harper & Row; 1964.
6. Mappes TA, Zembaty JS. *Biomedical Ethics.* 3rd ed. New York, NY: McGraw-Hill; 1991.
7. Rousseau JJ; Cole GDH, trans. *The Social Contract and Discourses.* Revised and augmented by Brumfitt JH, Hall JC. New York, NY: Random House; Everyman's Library; 1992.
8. Zucker A, Borchert D, Stewart D. *Medical Ethics: A Reader.* Englewood Cliffs, NJ: Prentice Hall; 1992.

CHAPTER 6

Mind, Consciousness, and the Neurosurgeon

William Feindel, MDCM, DPhil, FRCSC, FACS

The Mind: Philosophy's Conundrum

Over many centuries, philosophers and physicians, poets and priests have pondered, debated, and written at great length on how mind may relate to brain. And it is not surprising that neurosurgeons, from their unrivaled vantage point of dealing with the human brain, sometimes in conscious patients (as during epilepsy surgery), should seek answers to this seductive conundrum. The neurosurgical viewpoint is naturally influenced by experiences from the day-to-day diagnosis and treatment of brain-disordered patients; mind and brain are seen to be deranged and to recover in parallel. Being pragmatic artisans, their approach to this ancient riddle usually has taken the form of matching what are recognized as attributes of mind to selected cerebral structures, whose functions, as they became known, seemed to make them possible candidates for subserving mind. Obviously, loss of brain produces loss of mind. But, as Sherrington[80] remarked: "Mind, meaning by that thoughts, memories, feelings, reasoning, and so on, is difficult to bring into the class of physical things."

The first problem, then, and one over which philosophers have always contended, is to define what we mean by mind. The second, and more difficult issue, has been to correlate what we call mind with our inadequate knowledge of the vast anatomic and molecular complexity of the human nervous system.

This review highlights the history of some of the major proposals that have been put forward to explain how the abstraction, mind, may be explained by the action of a material brain. It then will focus on the contributions of Penfield in relating a long series of cerebral localization studies to a centrencephalic system that he postulated as underlying mind. The last part offers a working model of a neural substrate for the expression of mind. It is based on the amygdaloid complex, coupling its rich anatomic connectivity with its demonstrated role in a particular variety of focal seizures, characterized by automatism and amnesia, which transiently ablate mind.

Metaphors for Mind and Memory

From antiquity, philosophers have shown deep concern about the nature of mind and about the closely related question of memory. Plato (428?–348? BC), in one of his dialogues,[73] has Socrates make the imaginative supposition that there exists in our minds a block of wax, bigger in some, smaller in others: "Let us, then, say that this is the gift of Memory, the mother of the Muses, and that whenever we wish to remember anything we see or hear or think of in our own minds, we hold this wax under the perceptions and thoughts and imprint them upon it, just as we make impressions from seal rings; and whatever is imprinted we remember and know as long as its image lasts, but whatever is rubbed out or cannot be imprinted we forget and do not know." This platonic metaphor of the signet ring impressing wax became much quoted.[32] It may be regarded, noted Leddy,[52] as the prototype of all subsequent arguments that offer an exclusively mechanical or materialistic explanation for the operation of memory.

Plato's student, Aristotle (384–322 BC), wisely defined memory as "that faculty whereby we perceive time." But his insight into the mind-brain puzzle was limited by the meager understanding in his time of the brain's anatomy and function. Aristotle[4] made the safe observation: "The brain, whenever there is one, is placed in the front part of the head"—not, perhaps, a major revelation. He went on to describe the brain as fluid, cold, and bloodless (how advantageous for the neurosurgeon!). He regarded the brain as a cooling mechanism to temper the heat and seething of the blood boiling in the heart. The brain, he further maintained, is not responsible for any of the sensations, the seat and source of sensation being in the heart.[3] But he then made the contradictory observation that smell, hearing, and sight are all located in the head. The fact that the brain has no sensation of itself perhaps contributed, Sherrington[78] surmised, to Aristotle being misled about the brain and its correlation with mind. His view of the heart as the center of feelings and emotions still lingers on in our language in expressions such as "hearts and minds," or "heartfelt thanks." And whenever we speak of "learning by heart," we pay homage to Aristotle.

Hippocrates (460?–377? BC), a generation before Aristotle, had observed nature and man in lieu of what he called "unproven hypotheses of the philosophers." In addition to drawing up a moral code for physicians, Hippocrates left an extensive commentary on many aspects of medicine. In the well-known lyrical passage on epilepsy, he wrote:[41] "Some people say that the heart is the organ with which we think and that it feels pain and anxiety. But it is not so. . . . Men ought to know that from the brain and from the brain only, arise our pleasures, joys, laughter, and jests, as well as our sorrows, pains, griefs, and tears. Through it, in particular, we think, see, hear, and distinguish the ugly from the beautiful, the bad from the good, the pleasant from the unpleasant. . . ." And he concluded, "To consciousness the brain is messenger."

Galen's Chambered Brain

This enlightened view of the brain and mind, although taken up by loyal disciples of Hippocrates, did not become as widely accepted in medical teaching as the writings of Galen (AD 131?–202?).[7] Better informed about brain anatomy than Aristotle, Galen dismissed the notion of the heart and body as the seat of sensations. He considered that the brain's fluid-filled hollows served intellectual and mental activity as well as memory. His doctrine and many variations of it became blended with Augustinian and Thomasian theology to permeate the scholasticism of the Middle Ages.

Three chambers, or cells, of the brain usually were postulated. The most anterior, depicted as receiving sensation from the eyes, nose, mouth, and ears, was the seat of *sensus communis;* there, fancy and imagination resided.[7] This communicated through a vermis to the middle cell, the site of reasoning and judgment. The posterior chamber was for memory. This scheme, figured with prolific variety in medieval manuscripts and books, is exemplified by the cartoon from the encyclopedia *Margarita Philosophica* of 1503 by Gregorius Reisch, a Carthusian monk of Freiburg (Figure 1).[75]

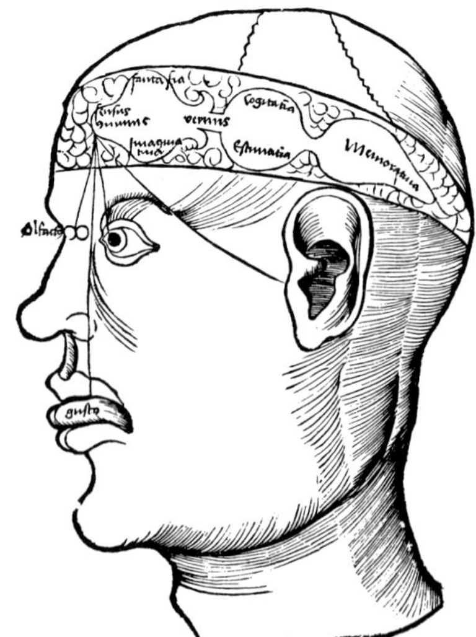

Figure 1. *Cartoon of the medieval cell doctrine showing the three brain cells (ventricles) to which mental faculties were assigned, taken from the encyclopedia* Margarita Philosophica *by Gregorius Reisch (1503).[75] (Illustration kindly provided by the Wellcome Institute Library, London, England.)*

Even Leonardo da Vinci's kaleidoscopic genius was taken in by this dogma. Within a sagittal section of the human head sketched from the centurion, Leonardo (1452–1519) copied faithfully the supposed functions of this three-celled arrangement (Figure 2). Later, when he drew the true shape of the wax-casted ventricles of the ox brain, probably the first anatomic demonstration of its kind, he persisted in tagging them with the same labels they had been assigned by the ancients.[82] In 1543, Vesalius (1514–1564) produced in his fine atlas *De Fabrica* more accurate anatomic figures of the brain and its ventricles, but he sagely refrained from interpreting the uses of the parts.

Descartes' Pineal Machine

A century later, René Descartes (1596–1650), acclaimed for bringing together algebra and geometry, introduced an elaboration of the medieval brain scheme.[8] He proposed the pineal gland as the receptive center of all sensations entering the brain. He depicted the refraction of visual images on passing through the lens of the eye (taken from his detailed study of dioptrics). But he imagined that these images passed by way of nerve tubules to the ventricular lining, thence to the pineal gland, and eventually out again from the brain to activate muscles (Figure 3).

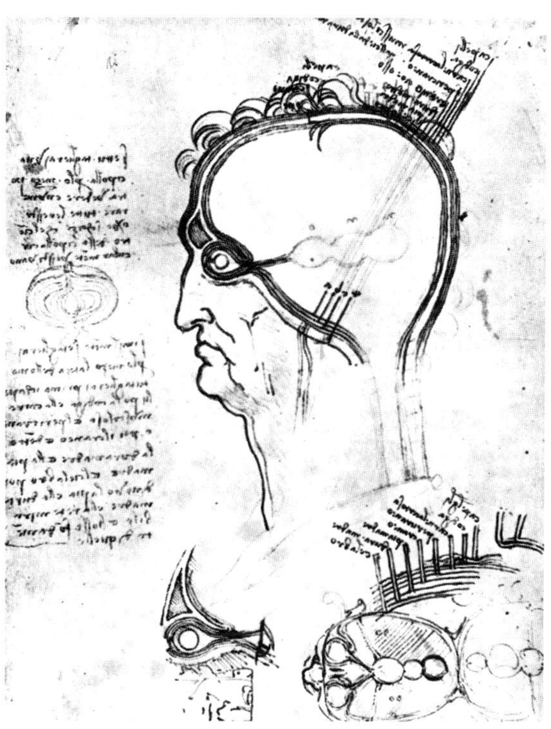

Figure 2. Drawing by Leonardo da Vinci in about 1490 showing the three cells within the head according to the medieval doctrine, with the anatomic layers of the cranium and brain coverings compared to the cut surface of an onion. In other drawings, Leonardo depicted for the first time wax casts of the true shape of the ventricles. (Reproduced by gracious permission of Her Majesty Queen Elizabeth II, from the original in the Windsor Royal Library, England.)

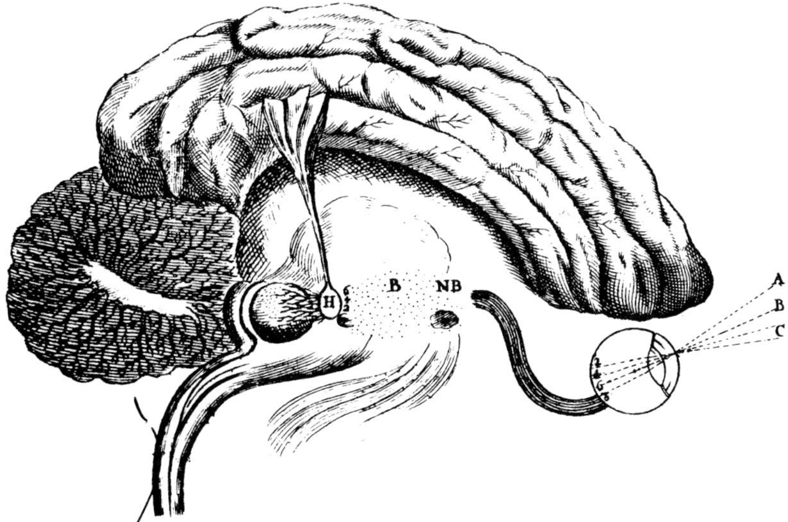

Figure 3. Depiction by Descartes of his notion of how visual impulses pass via nerve tubules from the eye, across the ventricular region, to reach the pineal gland (H) (Figura 35, De Homine, 1662).[9]

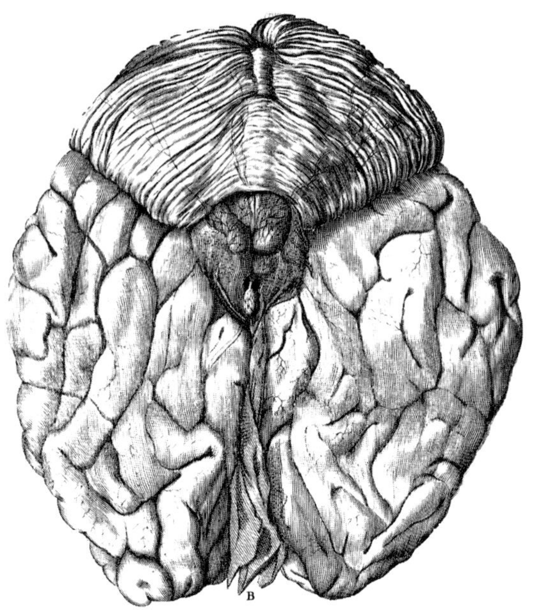

Figure 4. *A dissection from Descartes showing the location of the pineal gland just above the colliculi and lying between the separated cerebral hemispheres. The folia of the cerebellum are finely drawn and the cerebral convolutions moderately well depicted (Figura 53, De Homine, 1662).*[9]

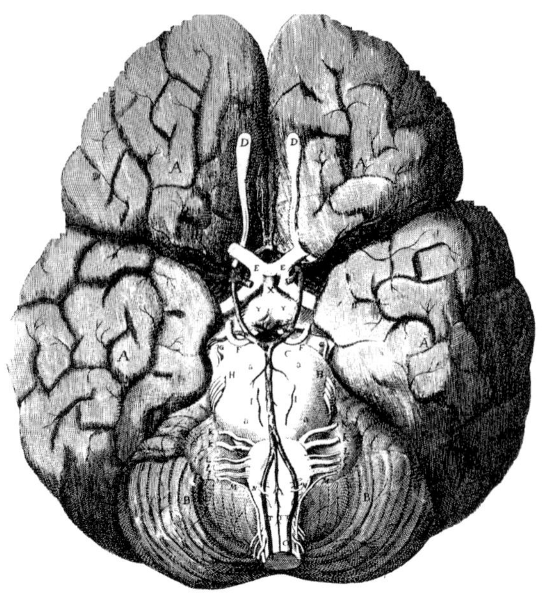

Figure 5. *The famous "Figura prima" drawn by Sir Christopher Wren for* Cerebri Anatome *(1664) by Thomas Willis.*[84] *The details of the arteries, cranial nerves, and the convolutions surpass in accuracy those depicted in any previous anatomic figures.*

"Omnes homines ex anima et corpore sunt compositi," Descartes[9] began in *De Homine* (1662): "All men are composed of a mind and a body." He courageously promoted the concept of the machine model of the body, with many functions taking place automatically, as in the works of a clock. He assigned to the actions of such an automaton not only the autonomic or involuntary visceral functions of the body, but also the reception of sensation, the imprinting of ideas in the organ of common sense and imagination, and the retention of these ideas in the memory. We recognize in this sequence of features the familiar labels of medieval brain localization. Although much engaged in anatomic dissections during his years in Holland,[53] Descartes devised a pineal scheme that was evidently short on neuroanatomy and suffered from the naive state of cerebral physiology in the mid-17th century.

However, his views on the brain and on mathematics had the merit of lending themselves to analysis and argument; they generated an astonishing canon of Cartesiana, running now to more than 3500 items.[77] Taken in that light, Descartes brought to the mind-brain problem a more mod-

ern angle as to how mental action might be based on demonstrated brain structures.[48,49] Mathematically, his proposal seemed plausible: the pineal gland, deep in the geometric center of the brain, was selected to fulfill the role of sensory reception and then transmit this into motor action (Figure 4). It was reminiscent of Galen's idea of the valve-like function of the pineal gland as gatekeeper in controlling the flow of nervous humors. Descartes' obeisance to the still-pervading doctrines of Aristotle flavored his exposition with a certain intellectual ambiguity. But his pineal machine can be viewed as the forerunner of far more sophisticated attempts, vigorously contested in our own time, to explain the mind-brain relationship.

Willis and the Brain's Cortex

The first systematic efforts at correlating the anatomy and physiology of the brain were made in the later part of the 17th century by Thomas Willis (1621–1675) and his circle of Oxford colleagues.[19] Appointed Sedleian Professor of Nat-

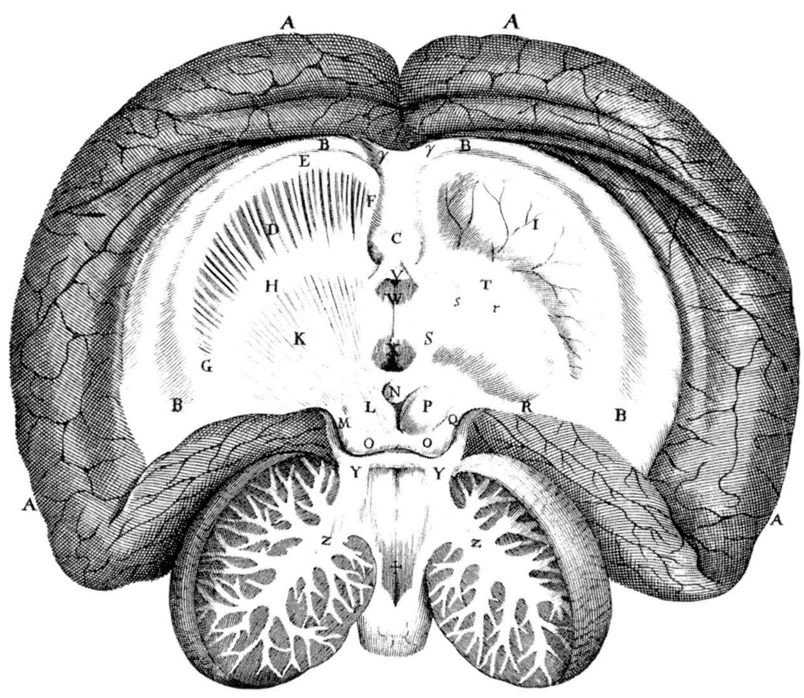

Figure 6. *Dissection of the brain with the cerebral hemisphere reflected forward and the corpus callosum divided to show the corpus striatum (D, H, K), the columns of the fornix (C), the anterior commissure (V), and the pineal gland (N). The style of the figure suggests it also was drawn by Sir Christopher Wren. It appeared in* De Anima Brutorum *(1672) by Thomas Willis.*[85]

ural Philosophy at the University in 1660, Willis was required to lecture weekly on the writings of Aristotle with "Comments on the Offices of the Senses, both external and also internal, and of the Faculties and Affections of the Soul, as also of the Organs and various provisions of all these."[21] Frustrated by the unsatisfactory state of knowledge of the brain in the works of Aristotle, Willis devised an ambitious plan to study the anatomy of the brain and the spinal cord, as well as the cranial and autonomic nerves in man and in many species of animals. He expounded to his readers that he had "resolved to unlock the secret places in Man's Mind," devoting himself "wholly to inquire into the offices and uses of the Brain."[21]

The work of Willis represented the first serious break from the Aristotelian legacy.[42] His enterprising approach resulted in *Cerebri Anatome,* a book that provided the most accurate and detailed description yet published of the anatomy of the nervous system.[84] Furthermore, he added interpretations based on clinical observations, pathologic confirmation, and experimental findings.[85] To help him, he assembled a team of Oxford scholars from medicine, anatomy, chemistry, physics, and pharmacology. Two of them, Christopher Wren (1632–1723), astronomer, geometer, and architect, and Richard Lower (1631–1690), physiologist and pioneer transfuser, etched elegant copper plates of the dissections showing the base of the brain and cranial nerves (Figure 5) and the fornix, anterior commissure, and corpus striatum (Figure 6). This was the first multidisciplinary team (in the history of neurology) that combined brain science and clinical neurology.

Willis also dismissed the Cartesian role of the pineal gland with an irrefutable argument that, ironically, might have been applied by Descartes himself from his experience with dissections of animal brains. Willis wrote: "We can scarce believe this to be the seat of the Soul, or its chief faculties to arise from it because animals, which seem to be almost quite destitute of Imagination, Memory and other superior powers of the Soul, have this Glandula or Kernel large and fair enough."[21] (See Figure 6.) As Sherrington[78] stated, Willis "shifted the seat of the anima from the chambers of the brain to the actual substance of the brain itself. For him, the crust of the brain, grey in contrast to the underlying white matter, was the great seat of the animal spirits." Sherrington continued: "As to the localization of mind, his view was that the higher up toward and into the grey crust of the brain a reflex action occurred, the more did conscious mind attach to it. Willis put the brain and nervous system on their modern footing, so far as that could be then done."

A student of Willis, John Locke (1632–1704) diligently wrote down the professor's lectures in brain anatomy.[21] Later, Locke became a physician and, after a good deal of politicking, devoted his time to the landmark in English philosophy, *An Essay Concerning Human Understanding* (1692). In his introduction, Locke[54] shied away from the mind-brain problem, cautiously stating: "I shall not at present meddle with the physical considerations of the mind; or trouble myself to examine wherein its essence consists. . . ." But among his provocative queries 300 years ago, he asked, "How do we separate imagination and madness?" And his question remains, so far, unanswered.

Phrenology

Introduced in the 1790s by the anatomist Franz Joseph Gall (1758–1828), aided by his pupil Johann Caspar Spurzheim (1776–1832), phrenology postulated that the brain was the organ of the mind with faculties located in specific areas of its surface.[7] These, in turn, were reflected by bumps or indentations of the skull overlying these different areas. It was a partially correct idea of cortical localization based on absurd premises. As ventricular localizations of the mind had pervaded medieval thought, so phrenology, another cerebral fantasy, flourished in the first three decades of the 1800s. It was taken up by enthusiastic and flamboyant followers, some of whom, such as the Fowlers of New York, turned it into a great commercial success.[7]

The numbering of mental faculties and quali-ties went to ridiculous extremes (up to more than 150 in toto). The numbered regions mapped on the skull were made to correspond to areas located directly beneath on the surface of the brain as, for example, depicted by the French phrenologist T. Thoré in 1836.[7] The temporal lobes figure in this numeration using the qualities of *Merveillosité, Secrétivité,* and *Distructivité,* all aligned along the first temporal convolution. They are offset by *Gaité* on the third temporal convolution and *Idealité* on the nearby orbital surface of the frontal lobe. Despite the tenuous scientific basis of phrenology, the drawings of the brain surface published by Gall and his near contemporaries (for example, Gratiolet[38]) compare favorably with modern anatomic illustration (Figure 7). And the phrenologists can be given much credit for popularizing the topic of localization of brain function, which has become such a prominent scientific topic since their time.

Sherrington's Dualism

Sherrington's masterful studies of the physiology and anatomy of the nervous system, beginning with spinal reflexes and ranging through decerebrate preparation to cortical stimulation and ablation, brought an erudite background to his rigorous neurobiologic analysis of the mind-brain problem.[13,79] In his final summary, *Man on His Nature,*[78] he explains at length the origin of the experiential basis of the dualism of "energy" and "mind" that was central to his philosophy. "The brain and the psyche lie together, so to say, on a knife edge," Sherrington suggested—a syzygy, one assumes, quite acceptable to neurosurgeons. In his last word on this topic, Sherrington[80] observed: "The physical basis of mind encroaches more and more on the study of mind, but there remain mental events which seem to lie beyond any physiology of the brain." Eccles[11] provided a valuable commentary on Sherrington's arguments and extended these into his own detailed proposition on the role of the microarchitecture of the cortex as a neural basis for consciousness. Taken together, the writings of Sherrington and Eccles serve as firmly based neurophysiologic contributions essential to any modern consideration of mind.

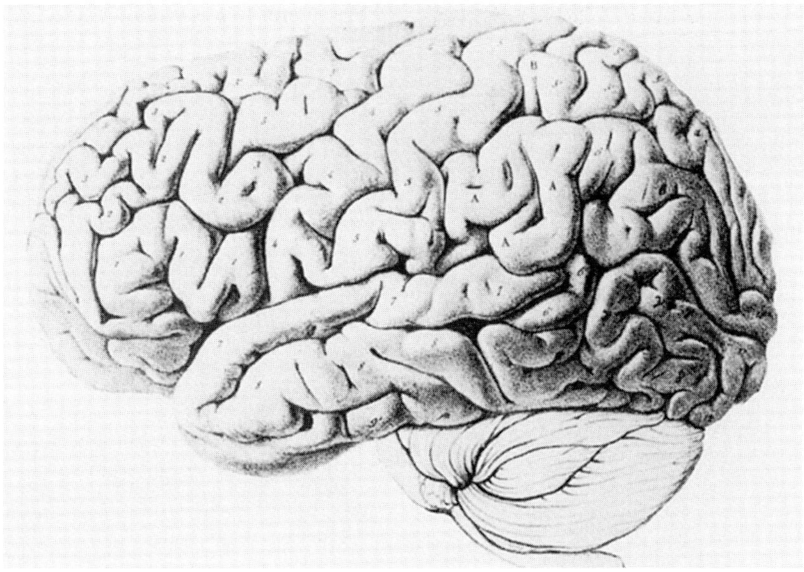

Figure 7. *Illustration from the atlas (1854) of Gratiolet*[38] *depicting the cerebral convolutions before any evidence for localization of cortical function was available.*

Definitions: Mind, Memory, Consciousness

The *Oxford English Dictionary (OED)*[58] gives 21 main definitions of the term "mind," and more than 30 additional variations of meaning. Anciently derived, the word goes back through Middle English to the old Teutonic *mynd*, which, in turn, comes from the root *mun*, meaning "to think, remember, or intend." It is related to a Sanskrit root, *man*, and the Latin *mens*, both of which have the meaning of "thought," to the Greek *memona*, meaning "I yearn," and to the Latin *mamini*, meaning "I remember."

From the 14th century, the term "mind" also has been defined as "faculty of memory." Another variation is expressed in the meaning "mental or psychical being or faculty." A submeaning of that again is given as "the seat of a person's consciousness, thoughts, volitions, and feelings; the system of cognitive and emotional phenomena and powers that constitutes the subject being a person; also the incorporeal subject of this psychical faculties, the spiritual part of a human being; the soul as distinguished from the body."

The term "memory," derived from an Indo-Germanic root through the Latin *memoria*, was used in English by Chaucer in 1374 and by Cax-

ton in 1484. The *OED* gives the definition "the faculty by which things are remembered, the capacity for retaining, perpetuating, or reviving the thoughts of things past." But 20 additional shades of meaning are given, ending with an 18th-century usage: "to come to one's memory, to recover from unconsciousness."

Considering the definition of "conscious," we find that it comes from the Latin *con* ("together") and *scio* ("I know"), as in "knowing something with others, knowing in one's self, privy to." In 1651, Hobbes wrote in *Leviathan*:[58] "Where two or more men know of one and the same fact, they are said to be conscious of it one to another. It is used to refer to one's sensations, feelings or thoughts etc."

The term "consciousness" is explained in the *OED* by seven examples, one being "the state or fact of being mentally conscious or aware of anything." The implication appears to be that awareness relates to what passes within one's own mind as well as the body's surrounding environment. A common difficulty arises when the expression "loss of consciousness" is used to mean loss of awareness and not unconsciousness or coma. The vagaries of the meanings of the terms conscious, consciousness, and unconsciousness make it difficult to come to a precise inquiry of how these

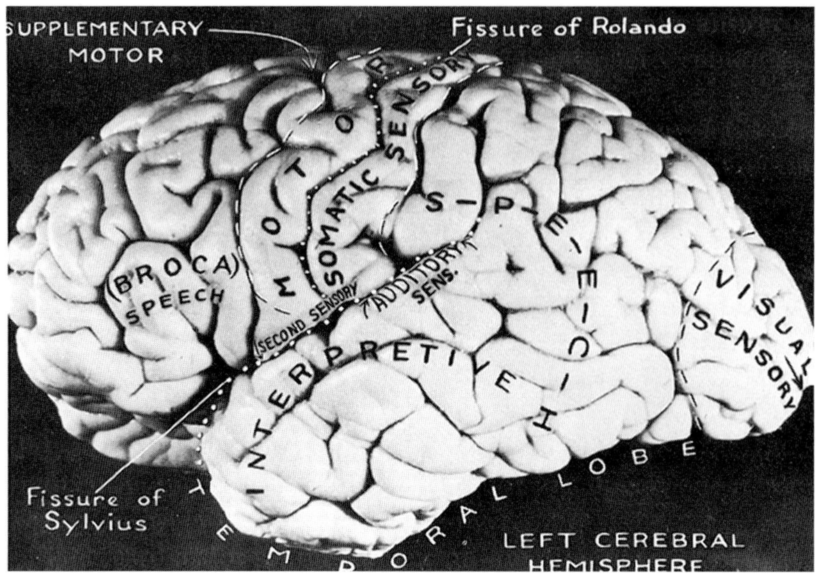

Figure 8. *Areas of cortical localization defined by stimulation studies. (Reproduced from reference 71 with permission.)*

relate in brain action.[81] As MacIntyre[55] notes: "There is no one clear-cut concept of the unconscious, as there is one clear-cut concept of the electron." He pointed out that even Freud, in his early attempt to write an account of psychology for neurologists, tried to explain mental phenomena in terms of the "billiard-ball universe" of Newtonian mechanics.

Thus, the subtle intertwinings of meanings and nuances of meanings for these important terms contrive to make extraordinarily complex any attempt to relate these abstractions to a functional matrix within the central nervous system.

Consideration of the term "soul," often used as a synonym for mind in the spiritual sense, lies far beyond this brief essay; it is best left to those with the philosophic or ecclesiastic stamina to deal with it.

Penfield's Centrencephalic System

In his final monograph, *The Mystery of the Mind* (1975), Wilder Penfield (1891–1976) put together a distillation of his evolving views of functional localization and interaction within the human brain.[65] As a working definition of mind, he quotes *Webster's Dictionary*: "The element in an individual that feels, perceives, thinks, wills, and especially reasons." However, he cautioned that discussion of the subject will make this definition inadequate. He attributed his early curiosity about the mind-brain relationship to his study with Bazett during the 1920s of the decerebrate preparation in Sherrington's Oxford University laboratory.[23] A section of the brain stem at the level of the colliculi eliminated the higher brain stem and cortex to render the animal an automatic reflex preparation,[12] reacting somewhat like the Cartesian model.

Later, in 1940, Penfield's careful study with Hebb[40] and other associates of a series of patients with large surgical resections of frontal lobe tissue provided a landmark in understanding how brain affects mind. In one patient, documented in detail, with injury and scarring of the frontal lobes resulting in uncontrollable epileptic attacks, measured removal of at least one-third of both frontal lobes was followed by striking improvement not only in seizure control but in personality and intellectual capacity. No clinical or psychometric evidence of deterioration was detected. "It becomes evident," wrote Hebb and Penfield, "that human behavior and mental activity may be more greatly impaired by the positive action of an abnormal area than by the negative effect of its complete absence." "Nociceptive brain," it was called, which led to the surgical cliché "bad brain can be worse than no brain."

Penfield recorded his extensive observations from more than 1000 craniotomies carried out with the patient under local anesthesia (Figure 8). He stimulated the cortical surface to evoke epileptic auras and to register, with Jasper, electrical abnormalities in order to localize the region for surgical excision.[66] This catalog of well-documented cases formed the anatomic and physiologic basis for mapping cortical areas relating to sensory, motor, speech, and memory function (Figure 9). The stimulation results were compared with changes in function or sparing of function (as in the case of speech) after precise surgical ablation of circumscribed zones of epileptogenic tissue.[63] Penfield's studies with his associates over the years were reported serially in numerous scientific papers and monographs.[57,66,69–71] The surgical outcomes in regard to seizure control were carefully tabulated and conclusions were drawn regarding the functional anatomy of the human brain defined in the course of this therapeutic approach.

Penfield reproduced by stimulation of the cortex "flashbacks," or memory recall, a phenomenon

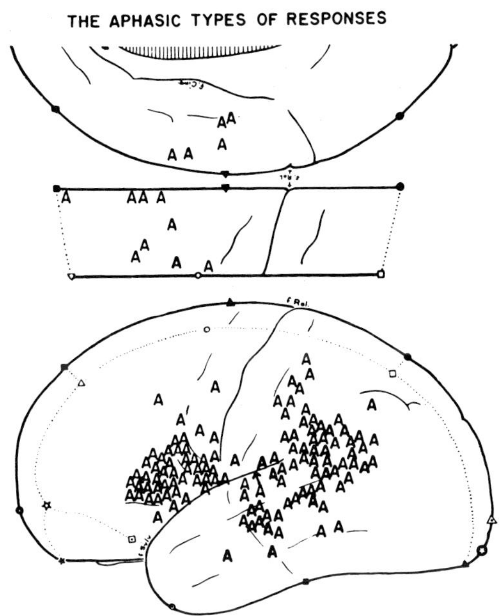

Figure 9. The aphasic types of responses mapped by cortical stimulation. Note the clustering of response sites in the posterior inferior frontal (Broca's) region and in the parietal temporal (Wernicke's) region, extending forward into the midtemporal region. (Reproduced from reference 71 with permission.)

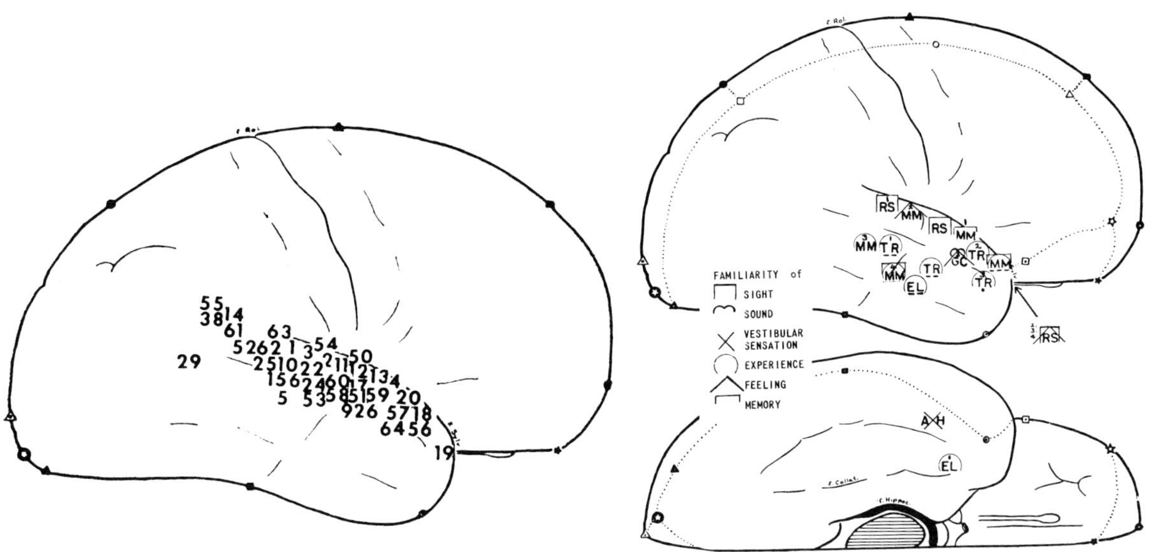

Figure 10. *(Left)* Auditory experiential responses to stimulation that included the sound of familiar voices or music, obtained from the first temporal convolution and extending posteriorly. Responses could be evoked from the left side as well. (Reproduced from reference 69 with permission.) *(Right)* Brain map showing sites where electrical stimulation produced illusions of familiarity, a variety of experiential response. (Reproduced from reference 57 with permission.)

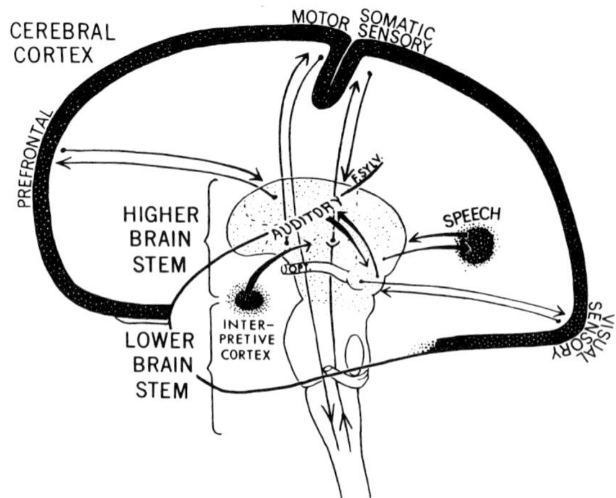

Figure 11. Diagram by Penfield suggesting the reciprocal flow of electrical potentials between the cortex and the higher brain stem. Activation by stimulation of the interpretive cortex of the temporal lobe results in flashbacks from the record of past experienc. (Reproduced from reference 65 with permission.)

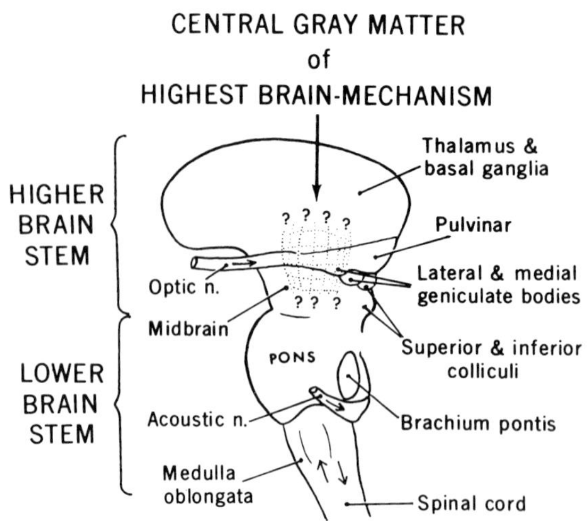

Figure 12. Drawing by Penfield showing the components of the higher and lower brain stem. (Reproduced from reference 65 with permission.)

that he first observed during an operation in 1933. He later interpreted these various experiential responses as the activation of the brain's record of consciousness (Figure 10). In 1952, Penfield presented a paper entitled "Epileptic automatism and the centrencephalic integrating system,"[61] in which he proposed that epileptic discharge passed directly from the anterior frontal cortex and also from the anterior temporal cortex to the diencephalon, where the interfering discharge inactivated the highest brain mechanism most closely related to consciousness (Figure 11). He further suggested an automatic sensorimotor mechanism in the diencephalon and the highest brain mechanism, with the afferent stream of sensory information leading from the former to the latter. He argued that the epileptic discharge, by acting selectively, can deactivate the mechanisms in the higher brain stem whose action is indispensable to the very existence of consciousness (Figure 12).

Some difficulty arises from Penfield's use of the term "unconscious," as when he writes: "In an attack of automatism a patient becomes suddenly unconscious; since other mechanisms in the brain continue to function, he changes into an automaton."[64] He then goes on to describe the features of automatism as evidenced by a patient having a temporal lobe seizure. He notes that the patient "may continue to carry out whatever purpose his

mind was in the act of handing on to his automatic sensory motor mechanism when the highest brain mechanism went out of action. Or he follows a stereotyped, habitual pattern of behavior. In every case, however, the automaton can make few, if any, decisions for which there has been no precedent. He makes no record of a stream of consciousness. Thus, he will have complete amnesia for the period of epileptic discharge and during the period of cellular exhaustion that follows." Penfield continued: "In general, if new decisions are to be made, the automaton cannot make them. In such a circumstance, he may become completely unreasonable and uncontrollable and even dangerous." It is clear that what Penfield is describing as unconsciousness is impairment of awareness, certainly not implying a state of coma, which is the more commonly applied neurosurgical usage. A thoughtful discussion of the condition of consciousness in epileptology is offered by Gloor.[33] But he, too, uses loss of consciousness to describe impairment of awareness.[36]

The notion of a subcortical region accessible from both hemispheres of the brain was proposed by Penfield in an attempt to understand the mechanism of consciousness, its sudden impairment during epileptic seizures (especially, as in petit mal, with little in the way of motor or sensory manifestations), and in connection also with the cortical activation of memory storage.[62,64,65] Jasper[46] has referred to this concept as "one of Penfield's most stimulating legacies to neurology and the neurological sciences" and added: "The centrencephalic system served as a framework on which was woven Penfield's continued search for the highest level of neuronal integration, in the sense of Herbert Spencer [1820–1903] and Hughlings Jackson [1835–1911], the search for brain mechanisms underlying conscious perceptual awareness and purposeful behaviour."

Penfield coined the word "centrencephalic" in 1950, but he already had suggested[59] that Hughlings Jackson's "highest level" should be sought "not in the new brain but in the old," meaning the diencephalon as opposed to the cerebral cortex. He agreed with Jackson that sensory and motor cortical areas were at the middle, not the highest, level of neuronal integration, and he drew upon studies by Hess on diencephalic centers for sleep and waking.[60,62]

His proposal preceded the work of Moruzzi and Magoun[56] (1949) and others on the ascending reticular activating system of the brain stem, but that work added further evidence to support Penfield's definition of the centrencephalic system simply as "that central system within the brain stem which has been, or may be in the future, demonstrated as responsible for integration of the function of the two hemispheres."[62]

The concept of the centrencephalic system was abnegated vigorously by Walshe[83] because it failed to define an anatomic basis. Penfield[62] replied:

We are not discussing a new or separate block of brain. There is no centrencephalon as distinct to diencephalon . . . to suppose that centrencephalic integration is possible without utilization of the cortex would be to return to the thinking of Descartes and to enthrone again a spiritual homunculus in some area such as the pineal gland. It would be equally absurd to consider that the reticular formation is functionally separate from cortex. . . . Consciousness exists only in association with the passages of impulses through ever-changing circuits of the brain stem and cortex. One cannot say that consciousness is here or there. But certainly without centrencephalic integration it is nonexistent.

"Penfield's lifelong search," Jasper[46] concluded, "for a better understanding of the functional organization of the brain and its disorders during epileptic seizures is symbolized in a way by his hypothesis of the central integrating system. It is a sort of conceptual bridge he has built between the brain and the mind. He concluded that we shall probably never be able to cross that bridge. Perhaps he is right, but many have been inspired by his efforts." In his summary of 1975, Penfield[65] stated: "The behavior of the automaton during an attack of epileptic automatism reveals what the brain without the mind and without the mind-mechanism can still do. It reveals what the moment-to-moment function of the normally active mind must be. If, as I have said, an attack of automatism falls upon a patient while he is in the act of planning a project, the automaton (which he becomes) may discharge that purpose in remarkable detail." But Penfield continued: "The human automaton, which replaces the man when the highest brain-mechanism is inactivated, is a thing without the capacity to make completely new decisions. It is a thing without the capacity to form new memory records and a thing without that indefinable attribute, sense of humor. The automaton is incapable of thrilling to the beauty of a sunset or of experiencing contentment, happiness, love, compassion. These, like all awarenesses, are functions of the mind."

After these arguments and a description of the two portions of the brain that relate to higher brain action as compared to automatic action, Penfield was reluctant to assign any neuronal structure or system to mind. He adopted a dualist hypothesis echoing this statement by Sherrington:[79] "That our being should consist of two fundamental elements offers, I suppose, no greater inherent improbability then that it should rest on one only."

Penfield's presentation added significantly to earlier studies by physiologists who argued from experimental animal findings or to those by neurologists, psychologists, and psychiatrists, whose views interpreted the external motor and emotional behavior of patients with brain disorders. Whatever qualifications the reader might have in accepting Penfield's final proposition that there is something that characterizes mind as distinct from physical brain, this summary of his research indicates how fundamental his findings are to our present understanding of memory, learning, language, and behavior. It represented for Penfield a final statement on his own work. In it he brought together his views on cerebral localization and his re-interpretation of the significance of the centrencephalic system. While his philosophic interpretations of the observations could well be challenged, it is evident that any serious approach to the analysis of the brain-mind question must inevitably take into account Penfield's body of contributions on what he referred to as the mind and the highest brain mechanism.[12]

It is a well-established observation that unconsciousness results when there is inactivation of a rather large and ill-defined zone of the diencephalon, the thalamic nuclei, and adjacent structures. Such inactivation may be brought about by pressure, trauma, hemorrhage, and local epileptic discharge; it occurs normally in sleep. Penfield noted, as did Jefferson,[47] Cairns,[5] and others (see Jones[50]), that injury or interference with such areas of the higher brain stem could impair or abolish consciousness. Penfield[65] reasonably concluded from these results that "the indispensable substratum of consciousness lies outside the cerebral cortex, probably in the diencephalon (the higher brain stem)." He postulated, therefore, that the central diencephalic region of the brain (the centrencephalic system) is involved in giving conscious experiences to the subject, in fact that it is the "seat of consciousness."

In concluding, Penfield[65] argued that the activity of the highest brain mechanism seems to correspond with that of mind, switching it off and on. It might do this by supplying and taking away energy that could come to mind from the brain. Penfield added: "But to expect the highest mechanism or any set of reflexes, however complicated, to carry out what the mind does, and thus perform all the functions of the mind, is quite absurd." He thus seemed to interpret the mind as something separate from what he termed the highest brain mechanism and presumed that it also must remember by making use of the brain's recording mechanisms. This part of his treatise is more difficult to understand; he appears to choose a proposition "that our being is to be explained on the basis of two fundamental elements."

Penfield queried, "What form does this mind-energy take?" He suggested that a special form of energy activates the mind during waking hours; this must be derived somehow from neuronal energy. Penfield did not dismiss the idea, as stated by others before him, that energy from without can reach a man's mind. His view in this respect resembles that of Sherrington. It also recalls the presentation by William James,[45] who took the ground that "The mother sea and fountainhead of religions lie in the mystical experiences of the individual, taking the word mystical in a very wide sense." James attached the "mystical or religious consciousness to the procession of an extended subliminal self. . . ."

It became evident that Penfield[65] ultimately related mind to spirit as we use these two terms "in ordinary conversation." He asked, "What becomes of the mind after death?" He posed the question and then attempted a thoughtful, although incomplete, answer. He concluded that there is no good evidence "that the brain alone can carry out the work the mind does." And he suitably ended with the quotation, suggested by his philosopher friend Charles Hendel, from Einstein (1879–1955), who surmised "The mystery of the world is its comprehensibility."

The Amygdala: Mindless Automatism and Amnesia

As Penfield emphasized, seizures that begin with local epileptic discharge in the sensorimotor, visual, auditory, or speech areas do not manifest automatism during the evolution of the attacks. But automatism is characteristic of seizures beginning in the temporal and, to a lesser extent, the frontal lobes. To understand more clearly the neuronal substrate of automatism, a study was carried out in 1951 on a series of 150 patients with well-defined temporal lobe seizures.[28,29] Three-quarters of these patients were found to manifest features of automatism, often at the early stage of their seizures, and to show postictal amnesia for the automatic acts that occurred during the time of the seizures. It was further observed that stimulation deep in the temporal lobe during therapeutic surgery produced certain aspects of automatism.[28] The patient would become unaware, mouth inappropriate maundering com-

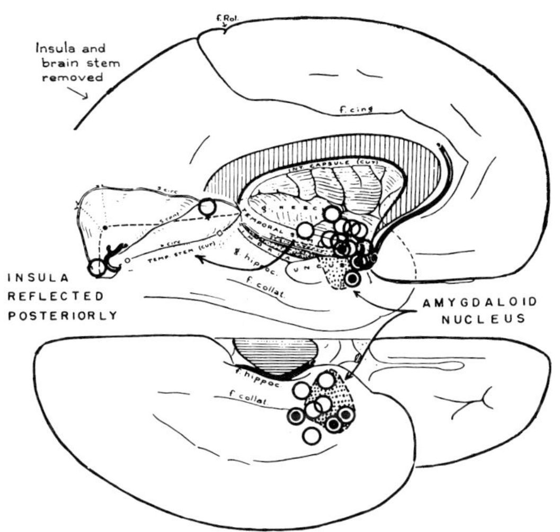

Figure 13. Sites in the amygdala and anterior insular cortex where stimulation produced features of automatism with amnesia and suppression of electrical activity of the cortex. (Reproduced from reference 28 with permission.)

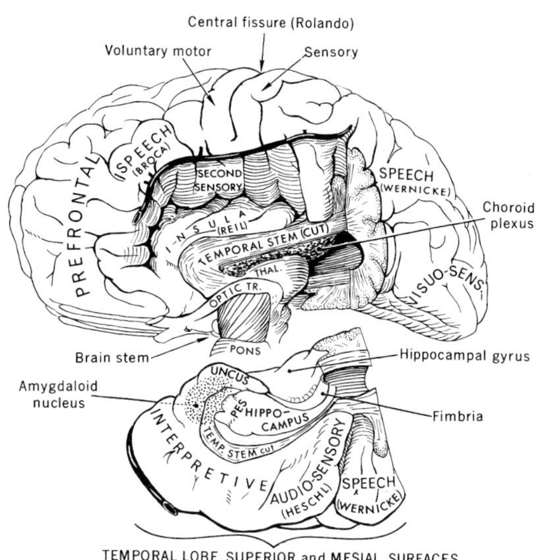

Figure 14. Anatomic dissection, with the entire temporal lobe laid aside, showing the relationship of the amygdaloid nucleus, the uncus, the hippocampal complex, and the anterior insular cortex. (Modified from reference 28.).

ments—one patient said, "Time and space seem occupied"—or make semipurposeful movements, plucking at the surgical drapes but being unresponsive to verbal commands. Or stimulation would evoke in the patients such phrases as "all mixed up," "could not get my thoughts straight," or "I can't remember anymore." Later, they would have no memory of the episodes or the comments. Most of the positive stimulation points were clustered in and about the amygdala and the juxtaposed anterior insular cortex (Figure 13). It was concluded that the neuronal discharge set off by the stimulations produced a train of complex events in the brain that seemed to disengage the patients' awareness, memory recording, and rational speech from their motor and sensory activities. It was apparent that the patients had "lost their minds," in the sense of temporary functional ablation of memory input and conscious awareness. The results indicated that the amygdala acted as a generator of these particular types of attacks and thus should be removed during the temporal lobe resection.[28]

During the 40 years since this hypothesis was proposed, it has been vindicated by similar but more extensive stimulation responses using ana-tomically placed depth electrodes,[36,37,39] by identification of amygdala abnormality on magnetic resonance imaging (MRI),[25] and by the beneficial surgical outcome after temporal lobe resections that include the pathologic amygdala.[18,23,25,30] These results enlarged on the concept of the separation of conscious mental activity from automatic involuntary action, so well described by Hughlings Jackson in his extensive writing on uncinate attacks.[43,44] These were well categorized by the ictal and postictal behavior of Jackson's patient "Z," a physician who kept detailed accounts of his sometimes elaborate attacks of automatism and amnesia.[25,28]

In the 1950s, when the periamygdaloid region was identified as the site where seizures could be provoked, little was known of the amygdala and its connections. It seemed evident that the amygdaloid region might provide an anatomic structure of significance in the mechanism of memory recording as well as being a generator of the epileptic discharge.[17,22] This region included the uncus, the amygdala-claustrum complex, and the anterior insular cortex deep in the sylvian fissure (Figure 14), all of which are susceptible to damage by tentorial herniation.[10,18] Experimental

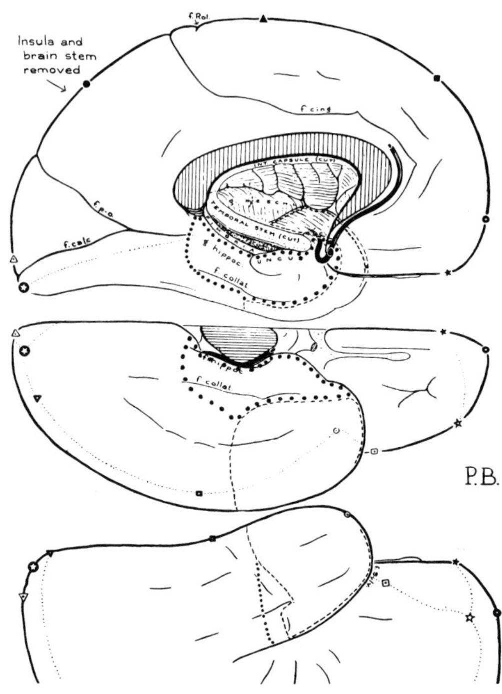

Figure 15. Patient P. B. (1951) The first surgical excision is outlined by the broken line and the second excision, which included the uncus and hippocampus, by the dotted line. Stimulation in the anterior mesial temporal region produced confusion and amnesia. (Reproduced from reference 28 with permission.) After the second operation, the patient exhibited severe disturbance of recent memory.[66,68]

studies also had demonstrated that this suppression of cortical activity could be reproduced by stimulation of the amygdala in the cat brain to mimic closely in character and distribution the response from stimulation of the reticular formation.[27] On the basis of these behavioral changes, together with the widespread suppression of the electrical activity of the cortex produced by periamygdaloid stimulation, this region was proposed along with the diffuse projection systems of the thalamus and brain stem as capable of exerting diffuse regulatory effects on other parts of the brain. Feindel and Penfield[28] concluded: "Evidence, in particular from these studies in man, indicates that the periamygdaloid region is also concerned in the process of memory recording and the maintenance of the normal conscious state, both of which are clearly essential factors in the mechanism of behavior." The severe and unexpected disturbance in recent memory in a few

patients after resection of the amygdala and hippocampus also targeted these structures as critical for memory function (Figure 15). Further study elucidated that this devastating memory disturbance depends upon the presence of bilateral abnormality of the mesial temporal region.[67,68,76]

These findings have been confirmed in thousands of patients where surgical cure or marked reduction of seizures have also been shown to bring significant improvement in verbal memory and behavioral performance.[22,34,35] The early detailed examinations of patients before and after surgical treatment developed into a long, fruitful collaboration of surgeons and psychologists that threw light on many aspects of brain function, such as speech, cerebral dominance, and the role of the temporal lobe, particularly the amygdala and hippocampus, in automatism and amnesia.[18,20,25,26,28,29,68]

In the past two decades, extensive anatomic research on the amygdala at the human and primate level has identified its wide reciprocal connections with the hemispheral cortex, the deep forebrain and midbrain, and certain brain stem nuclei.[1,2,16] Juxtaposed between the rhinal cortex and the hippocampus, the amygdala also has distinct reciprocal connections with each. Moreover, it is endowed with receptor sites for most of the major chemical neurotransmitters, including dopamine, opiate, serotonin, somatostatin, noradrenaline, acetylcholine, and a range of other neuropeptides.[1] In some ways, its position within the temporal lobe, interposed between the cortical mantle of the hemisphere and the deep subcortical structures, is reminiscent of the thalamus and striatum. But its close connection to entorhinal cortex and the hippocampal complex endows it with a particular potential in memory function.

During what we may call "amygdaloid seizures," the ictal obliteration of memory recording and of the mind-brain mechanism results in the patient behaving like a mindless automaton without memory input. Thus, the complex partial seizure dissects, as it were, by this disengaging epileptic discharge, a semiseparable neural system, of which the amygdala and its reciprocally connected network represent crucial components.[25] Arguably, then, this system must be closely identified with structural substrates for the functional expression of mind.

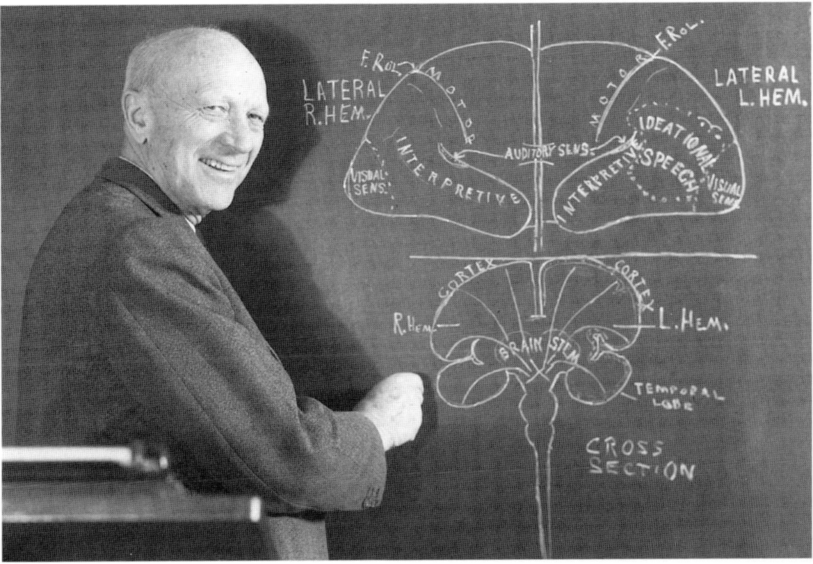

Figure 16. Photograph of Wilder Penfield lecturing on cerebral localization (1963)—mind examining brain.

The Ultimate Problem

This brief overview of the problem of correlating mind and brain indicates how thoughtful philosophers and brain scientists have struggled to clarify their views on this topic.[17,51,52] Much of the discussion has focused on the work of Wilder Penfield, who, more than any neurosurgeon, brooded over this question of how brain action can explain mind (Figure 16). And as the debate and the search go on, neurosurgeons will continue to make their unique contributions to this intriguing conundrum. We can readily agree with William James' statement[45] that the task of explaining the connection between the mind and brain presents "the ultimate of ultimate problems."

What of the future studies of mind? One promising avenue of research on the human brain has been the exciting developments over the past two decades in brain imaging technology.[24] In the early 1970s, computed axial tomography broke a certain barrier in reconstruction of images from a mass of digital information produced by an x-ray beam scanning through the head. This provided remarkable advantages in the speed and precision of localization, and even the nature of cerebral lesions, via a harmless noninvasive method. Matching of the site and size of a lesion with the clinical symptoms and signs and behav-ioral features gave an improved understanding of the influence of localized brain damage on brain function, as, for example, in studies of speech, sensory, and motor function.

But the most revolutionary approach to a detailed study of localized brain function has been the rapid development in the technology and scientific application of positron emission tomography (PET),[24] where functional aspects of human brain disorders can be examined for the first time in their natural state. The most common scanning techniques, utilizing radiolabeled glucose kinetics or radiolabeled oxygen that enables the display of local changes in blood flow activated by selected tasks, have allowed the investigation of a wide range of neurologic and psychiatric conditions not possible before.[74] Indeed, the use of PET seems to be limited only by the degree of ingenuity of the researchers in preparing the appropriate radiochemicals and posing the correct probing questions to examine many aspects of brain function. For the first time, it can be shown how multiple brain regions, cortical as well as subcortical, come into play during the testing of brain responses to carefully chosen tasks involving language.[6] Moreover, research into the 50 or more messenger chemicals in the human brain already has shown promise in defining both normal and abnormal cerebral function using PET. It seems quite probable that, in time, the vast amount of data on neurotransmitters derived from experimental studies at the cellular levels will be replicated at the human neural level.[31]

With the advent of MRI, it is possible to register accurately the anatomic location of the molecular changes in the brain by matching MRI and PET images, thus greatly enhancing the value of both methods for the study of functional localization in the brain. And, recently, the rapid anatomic mapping of focal cerebral blood changes using MRI alone offers a significant advantage in the simplicity, repetition, and precision of such activation research.

Over the next few years, we can expect to experience impressive advances in our understanding of how the brain works during mental activity as sampled by cognitive challenges using these remarkable imaging methods. As we look over the past half century, the productivity of neuroscience research has increased in exponential fashion. As I wrote a decade ago:[65]

> Perhaps at no previous time in the history of science has there been such widespread interest, as is evident, in the brain and its function, and how that function relates to human behavior. For compelling and obvious reasons, this topic has always been foremost in the attention of neurologists, neurosurgeons, and psychiatrists. Over many years, as well, the study of the brain has attracted the talents of scientists trained in anatomy, physiology, pathology, and other biological disciplines. Increasing numbers of intellectual emigrés coming from such fields as mathematics, physics, chemistry, electronics, and computer sciences have recently added fresh impetus to our exciting researches in the neurosciences.

These comments apply even more to the rapid current pace of major inroads into brain research.[31] The activity in this immensely productive field is exemplified by several recent lively publications. Edelman,[14,15] with a persuasive, brilliant fire-and-brimstone approach, brings Darwinian selectivity to bear on the problem of consciousness. Penrose,[72] on the other hand, applies his expert background in quantum mechanics and black holes to neurobiology to explain

with charming Cartesian directness his thinking about the "imperial" mind. Like many others, they bring to contemporary neuroscience the advantage of a fresh look at mind and consciousness, which serves as a stimulus to those using more traditional avenues of research.[31]

In this respect, they bring to mind the first multidisciplinary brain research team gathered around Thomas Willis at Oxford more than three centuries ago. His lectures and writings enunciated with remarkable prescience the problems of mind and brain that will continue to daunt neuroscientists for years to come. Willis[84] put it well in "The Preface to the Reader" of *Cerebri Anatome*: "Wherefore, to explicate the uses of the Brain seems as difficult a task as to paint the Soul of which it is commonly said, That it understands all things but itself." And Penfield echoed Willis when he commented in the Foreword to the tercentenary edition of *The Anatomy of the Brain and Nerves*:[21] "If it seems to neurologists today that our present understanding of the brain and mind of man is hardly more than a beginning of science, it may be reassuring to recall that our task is the ultimate one. The problem of neurology is to understand man himself. We must analyze the means by which man, the creator of science, has done what he has done. This may well be the most difficult, and surely it is the most important, task of all."

References

1. Aggleton JP, ed. *The Amygdala*. New York, NY: Wiley-Liss; 1992.
2. Amaral DG, Price JL, Pitkänen A, et al. Anatomical organization of the primate amygdaloid complex. In: Aggleton JP, ed. *The Amygdala*. New York, NY: Wiley-Liss; 1992:1-66.
3. Aristotle; Lawson-Tancred H, trans. *De Anima (On the Soul)*. New York, NY: Penguin Books; 1986.
4. Aristotle; Peck AL, trans. *Parts of Animals*. London, England: William Heinemann; 1961.
5. Cairns H. Disturbances of consciousness with lesions of the brain-stem and diencephalon. *Brain*. 1952; 75:109-146.
6. Chertkow H, Bub D, Meyer E, et al. Dissociation of brain regions for semantic memory and imagery demonstrated with positron emission tomography. *Nature*. In press.
7. Clarke E, Dewhurst K. *An Illustrated History of Brain Function*. Berkeley, Calif: University of California Press; 1972.
8. Descartes R. *Principia Philosophiae*. Amstelodami:

Apud Ludovicum Elzevirium; 1644.

9. Descartes R. *De Homine*. Lugduni Batavorum: Francisum Moyardum et Petrum Leffen; 1662.

10. Earle KM, Baldwin M, Penfield W. Incisural sclerosis and temporal lobe seizures produced by hippocampal herniation at birth. *Arch Neurol Psychiatry*. 1953;69:27-42.

11. Eccles JC. *The Human Mystery*. New York, NY: Springer-Verlag; 1979.

12. Eccles JC, Feindel W. Wilder Graves Penfield (1891–1976). *Biographical Memoirs of Fellows of the Royal Society*. London, England: Royal Society of London; 1978;24:472-513.

13. Eccles JC, Gibson W. *Sherrington: His Life and Thought*. New York, NY: Springer-Verlag; 1979.

14. Edelman GM. *The Remembered Present: A Biological Theory of Consciousness*. New York, NY: Basic Books; 1989.

15. Edelman GM. *Bright Air, Brilliant Fire: On the Matter of the Mind*. New York, NY: Basic Books; 1992.

16. Eleftheriou BE, ed. *The Neurobiology of the Amygdala*. New York, NY: Plenum Press; 1972.

17. Feindel W. The brain considered as a thinking machine. In: Feindel W, ed. *Memory, Learning and Language: The Physical Basis of Mind*. Toronto, Canada: University of Toronto Press; 1960:11-23.

18. Feindel W. Response patterns elicited from the amygdala and deep temporoinsular cortex. In: Sheer DE, ed. *Electrical Stimulation of the Brain*. Austin, Tex: University of Texas Press; 1961:519-532.

19. Feindel W. Thomas Willis (1621–1675): the founder of neurology. *Can Med Assoc J*. 1962; 87:289-296.

20. Feindel W. Memory and speech function in the temporal lobe in man. In: Brazier MA, ed. *Brain Function II*. Berkeley, Calif: University of California Press; 1964:276-298.

21. Feindel W. *Thomas Willis: The Anatomy of the Brain and Nerves*. Montreal, Canada: McGill University Press; 1965.

22. Feindel W. Temporal lobe seizures. In: Vinken PJ, Bruyn GW, eds. *Handbook of Clinical Neurology*. Amsterdam: North Holland Publishing; 1974; 15:87-106.

23. Feindel W. Wilder Penfield (1891–1976): the man and his work. *Neurosurgery*. 1977;1:93-100.

24. Feindel W. Historical background of PET. In: Diksic S, Reba RC, eds. *Radiopharmaceuticals and Brain Physiology Studied with PET and SPECT*. Boca Raton, Fla: CRC Press; 1990:1-10.

25. Feindel W. Recall, amnesia and experiential responses from stimulation of the human amygdala. In: Squire LR, Mishkin M, Shimamura A, eds. *Learning and Memory: Discussions in Neuroscience*. Geneva, Switzerland: Elsevier; 1990:72-80.

26. Feindel W. Toward a surgical cure for epilepsy: the work of Wilder Penfield and his school at the Montreal Neurological Institute. In: Engel J Jr, ed. *Surgical Treatment of the Epilepsies*. 2nd ed. New York, NY: Raven Press; 1993:1-9.

27. Feindel W, Gloor P. Comparison of electrographic effects of stimulation of the amygdala and brain stem reticular formation in cats. *Electroencephalogr Clin Neurophysiol*. 1954;6:389-402.

28. Feindel W, Penfield W. Localization of discharge in temporal lobe automatism. *Arch Neurol Psychiatry*. 1954;72:605-630.

29. Feindel W, Penfield W, Jasper H. Localization of epileptic discharge in temporal lobe automatism. *Trans Am Neurol Assoc*. 1952;77:14-17.

30. Feindel W, Rasmussen T. Temporal lobectomy with amygdalectomy and minimal hippocampal resection: review of 100 cases. *Can J Neurol Sci*. 1991; 18:603-605.

31. Fischbach GD. Mind and brain. *Sci Am*. 1992; 267:48-57.

32. Fox A. *Plato for Pleasure*. London, England: John Murray; 1962.

33. Gloor P. Consciousness as a neurological concept in epileptology: a critical review. *Epilepsia*. 1986;27 (suppl 2):S14-S26.

34. Gloor P. The role of the amygdala in temporal lobe seizures. In: Aggleton JP, ed. *The Amygdala*. New York, NY: Wiley-Liss; 1992:505-538.

35. Gloor P, Feindel W. Affective behavior and temporal lobe. In: Monnier M, ed. *Physiologie und Pathophysiologie des Vegetativen Nervensystems, II: Pathophysiologie*. Stuttgart, Germany: Hippokrates-Verlag; 1963: 685-716.

36. Gloor P, Olivier A, Ives J. Loss of consciousness in temporal lobe seizures: observations obtained with stereotactic depth electrode recordings and stimulations. In: Canger R, Angeleri F, Penry JK, eds. *Advances in Epileptology: XIth Epilepsy International Symposium*. New York, NY: Raven Press; 1980: 349-353.

37. Gloor P, Olivier A, Quesney LF, et al. The role of the limbic system in experiential phenomena of temporal lobe epilepsy. *Ann Neurol*. 1982;12:129-144.

38. Gratiolet LP. *Mémoire Sur Les Plis Cérébraux de l'Homme et des Primates*. Paris, France: A Bertrand; 1854.

39. Halgren E, Walter RD, Cherlow DG, et al. Mental phenomena evoked by electrical stimulation of the human hippocampal formation and amygdala. *Brain*. 1978;101:83-117.

40. Hebb DO, Penfield W. Human behavior after extensive bilateral removal from the frontal lobes. *Arch Neurol Psychiatry*. 1940;44:421-438.

41. Hippocrates; Jones WHS, trans. *Select Works*. New York, NY: GP Putman; 1923-1931; vol. 2.

42. Isler H. *Thomas Willis, 1621–1675: Doctor and Scientist*. New York, NY: Hafner Publishing; 1968.

43. Jackson HJ. On a particular variety of epilepsy ("intellectual aura"): one case with symptoms of organic brain disease. *Brain*. 1888;11:179-207.

44. Jackson HJ, Colman WS. Case of epilepsy with tasting movements and "dreamy state": very small patch of softening in the left uncinate gyrus. *Brain*. 1898;21:580-590.

45. James H. *The Letters of William James*. Boston, Mass: The Atlantic Monthly Press; 1920; I & II.

46. Jasper HH. Wilder Penfield: his legacy to neurology. The centrencephalic system. *Can Med Assoc J*. 1977;116:1371-1372.

47. Jefferson G. Disintegration of consciousness follow-

ing posterior fossa lesions. In: Jefferson G, ed. *Selected Papers*. Springfield, Ill: Charles C Thomas; 1960: 526-537.

48. Jefferson G. The mind of mechanical man. In: Jefferson G, ed. *Selected Papers*. Springfield, Ill: Charles C Thomas; 1960;10-23.

49. Jefferson G. René Descartes on the localization of the soul. In: Jefferson G, ed. *Selected Papers*. Springfield, Ill: Charles C Thomas; 1960:45-69.

50. Jones BE. Basic mechanisms of sleep: wake states. In: Kryger MH, Roth T, Dement WC, eds. *Principles and Practice of Sleep Medicine*. 2nd ed. Philadelphia, Pa: WB Saunders; 1994:145-162.

51. Laslett P, ed. *The Physical Basis of Mind*. New York, NY: Macmillan; 1950.

52. Leddy JF. An historical introduction. In: Feindel W, ed. *Memory, Learning and Language: The Physical Basis of Mind*. Toronto, Canada: University of Toronto Press; 1960:3-10.

53. Lindeboom GA. *Descartes and Medicine*. Amsterdam, The Netherlands: Rodopi; 1979.

54. Locke J. *An Essay Concerning Human Understanding*. Oxford, England: Clarendon Press; 1692.

55. MacIntyre AC. *The Unconscious*. London, England: Routledge & Kegan Paul; 1958.

56. Moruzzi G, Magoun HW. Brain stem reticular formation and activation of the EEG. *Electroencephalogr Clin Neurophysiol*. 1949;1:455-473.

57. Mullan S, Penfield W. Illusions of comparative interpretation and emotion. *Arch Neurol Psychiatry*. 1959;81:269-284.

58. Murray JAH, Bradley H, Craigie WA, eds. *The Oxford English Dictionary*. Oxford, England: Clarendon Press; 1933.

59. Penfield W. The cerebral cortex in man, I: the cerebral cortex and consciousness. *Arch Neurol Psychiatry*. 1938;40:417-442.

60. Penfield W. The cerebral cortex and the mind of man. In: Laslett P, ed. *The Physical Basis of Mind*. New York, NY: Macmillan; 1950:56-64.

61. Penfield W. Epileptic automatism and the centrencephalic integrating system. *Res Publ Assoc Res Ment Dis*. 1952;30:513-528.

62. Penfield W. Centrencephalic integrating system. *Brain*. 1958;81:231-234.

63. Penfield W. The nature of speech. In: Feindel W, ed. *Memory, Learning and Language: The Physical Basis of Mind*. Toronto, Canada: University of Toronto Press; 1960:55-69.

64. Penfield W. A surgeon's chance encounters with mechanisms related to consciousness. *J R Coll Surg Edinburgh*. 1960;5:173-190.

65. Penfield W. *The Mystery of the Mind*. Princeton, NJ: Princeton University Press; 1975.

66. Penfield W, Jasper H. *Epilepsy and the Functional Anatomy of the Human Brain*. Boston, Mass: Little, Brown & Co; 1954.

67. Penfield W, Mathieson G. Memory: autopsy findings and comments on the role of the hippocampus in experiential recall. *Arch Neurol*. 1974;31: 145-154.

68. Penfield W, Milner B. Memory deficit produced by bilateral lesions in the hippocampal zone. *Arch Neurol Psychiatry*. 1958;79:475-497.

69. Penfield W, Perot P. The brain's record of auditory and visual experience: a final summary and discussion. *Brain*. 1963;86:595-696.

70. Penfield W, Rasmussen T. *The Cerebral Cortex of Man*. New York, NY: Macmillan; 1950.

71. Penfield W, Roberts L. *Speech and Brain Mechanisms*. Princeton, NJ: Princeton University Press; 1959.

72. Penrose R. *The Emperor's New Mind: Concerning Computers, Minds, and the Laws of Physics*. New York, NY: Penguin Books; 1991.

73. Plato; Fowler HN, trans. *Theaetetus*. London, England: William Heineman; 1967.

74. Raichle M. Exploring the mind with dynamic imaging. *Semin Neurosci*. 1990;2:307-315.

75. Reisch G. *Margarita Philosophica*. Freiburg im Breisgau: J Shott; 1503.

76. Scoville WB, Milner B. Loss of recent memory after bilateral hippocampal lesions. *J Neurol Neurosurg Psychiatry*. 1957;20:11-21.

77. Sebba G. *Bibliographia Cartesiana*. The Hague, The Netherlands: Martinus Nijhoff; 1964.

78. Sherrington CS. *Man on His Nature*. Cambridge, England: Cambridge University Press; 1946.

79. Sherrington CS. *The Integrative Action of the Nervous System*. New Haven, Conn: Yale University Press; 1947.

80. Sherrington C. Introduction. In: Laslett P, ed. *The Physical Basis of Mind*. New York, NY: Macmillan; 1950:1-4.

81. Skeat WW. *An Etymological Dictionary of the English Language*. Oxford, England: Clarendon Press; 1910.

82. Todd EM. *The Neuroanatomy of Leonardo da Vinci*. Park Ridge, Ill: American Association of Neurological Surgeons; 1991.

83. Walshe FMR. Some reflections upon the opening phase of the physiology of the cerebral cortex, 1850–1900. In: Wellcome Foundation Ltd, sponsor. *The History and Philosophy of Knowledge of the Brain and its Functions: An Anglo-American Symposium*. Springfield, Ill: Charles C Thomas; 1958:223-234.

84. Willis T. *Cerebri Anatome*. Londini: Martin & Allestry; 1664.

85. Willis T. *De Anima Brutorum*. Oxonii, e Theatro Sheldoniano: R Davis; 1672.

CHAPTER 7

Neurosurgical Morbidity and Complications

J. Peter Gruen, MD, Jeffrey Evan Thomas, MD, and Michael L.J. Apuzzo, MD

A Unified Philosophy of Complications

Complications are inevitable in the practice of every neurosurgeon. Patients die, are neurologically devastated, or more often are disappointed by the results of procedures for which they and their surgeon may have had unrealistic expectations.

Complications or lack thereof are one measure of a neurosurgeon's competency. Clinical series on surgical techniques always report associated complications. Techniques, like surgeons, are made or broken based on complications and the frequency with which they occur.

The specter of potential complications hangs over the neurosurgeon from the positioning of the patient until the final closing stitch. It remains not just through the surgical procedure but into the recovery period and sometimes for months thereafter. The avoidance and management of complications is an important topic in the neurosurgical literature, featured as the title of a recently released neurosurgical text.[1]

Much of neurosurgery can be managed based on knowledge derived from textbooks, journals, and scholarly discussions. The management of many aspects of complications (the patient's reaction to them, as well as the family's and the surgeon's own) requires more complex strategies than can be summarized by an algorithm flow diagram or in the chapters on medicolegal and ethical issues, seemingly obligatory in recent neurosurgical texts.

It is from a wealth of personal, social, and emotional experiences, the elements that are the basis of a philosophy toward life and death, that the neurosurgeon must draw to construct an appropriate philosophy toward a particular complication in a particular patient. An appeal to some published authority, some citable entity, is futile in facing a patient whose life has suffered from the surgeon's intervention.

While it is possible to glean from publications and professional meetings a *sense* of the philosophy of neurosurgery toward complications, there is no *single* philosophy. They are as numerous and diversified as the neurosurgeons who create them.

To understand an individual neurosurgeon's philosophy toward complications, it is essential to understand the individual as the product of many factors. Besides those of upbringing such as parents, society, education, economic status, culture, and national politics, important influences on the neurosurgeon's psyche include medical and residency training as well as the state of neurosurgical art, both technologic and scientific. Even after all of these factors have been analyzed, it may be difficult to predict how a neurosurgeon will approach a complication because a philosophy is not an immutable construct, but rather a dynamic, organic system of interrelated ideas and concepts in the light of which an adverse intraoperative event is viewed.

What Is a Complication?

Before developing a philosophy about complications, the neurosurgeon must have a personal concept of what a complication is. Because a complication usually is an event happening to someone else, its definition is observer-dependent. What to the patient may be a complication may be an acceptable epiphenomenon to the neurosurgeon.

The relative importance of adverse events differs as well: to a patient, an extra day in the hospital may be a significant complication whereas to the surgeon it may be a trivial logistic glitch. A simple wound infection readily treatable with a 1-week course of oral antibiotics and of little significance to the neurosurgeon may conjure images of bodily invasion to the patient.

What the neurosurgeon really wrestles with in coming up with a philosophy toward a complication is not so much the complication itself, but rather the implications of that complication for the patient, society, and the neurosurgeon himself or herself. Complications can be viewed broadly according to the aspect of the patient's life they affect. These include:

1. Mortality
2. Identity
3. Independence
4. Cognition and functional intelligence
5. Personality and emotions
6. Pain and comfort
7. Physical appearance and body image
8. Convenience in daily living

Obviously, the complication that results in a patient having to take medication on a daily basis for life is of a different magnitude than one resulting in a vegetative state. The neurosurgeon's ranking of these complication implications may differ from that of the affected patient who may not be grateful for a complication that is less serious than that of the patient in the next bed.

Mortality

Each person has an attitude toward life and death, and his or her own mortality. For some, the former naturally progresses into the latter. From this perspective, death may be seen not as a fearsome outcome, but as just a natural occurrence. If a patient has suffered much during the course of an illness, death may be deliverance into a more peaceful, painless state and thus not really a complication at all.

Identity

In our fiercely individualistic society where independence is vital to a positive self-image, many feel that a permanent vegetative state is worse than death itself. To some neurosurgeons, this is the most feared complication of all. Although the patient probably is not cognizant of being in this state, the family members often are aware of this situation. The neurosurgeon (especially if inclined to identify with the vegetative patient) may appreciate the hopelessness of the situation for which he or she may have been responsible. For aggressive, assertive individuals, hopelessness can be a source of great frustration. Anger and hostility toward the vegetative patient can affect not only the philosophy toward that particular patient but toward all who suffer an adverse outcome.

Independence

Definitions of disability differ. The overall perspective toward a disability is closely linked to its occurrence as a surgical complication. Weakness, blindness, and deafness are three of the more common or at least more readily apparent deficits that can result from neurosurgical procedures. Even a slight decrease in vision can be devastating to the fully-sighted.

Cognition and Functional Intelligence

In addition to overt neurologic disabilities, there are those functions less readily quantitated or even investigated, including cognition, foresight, insight, and functional intelligence. Only relatively recently has neurosurgery reached the point where manipulations that impact aspects of cognition can be safely done while leaving completely intact traditionally tested modalities such as motor strength, cranial nerve function, and the five senses. Subtle deficits not appreciated by the standard neurologic examination may result from new procedures. Patients may feel themselves quite disabled by these problems, which can be denied by a neurosurgeon who does not objectively verify their existence.

Personality and Emotions

Another intangible area where complications can occur and severely impair a patient's functional abilities is that of emotions. Many physicians have problems dealing with the emotional aspects of illness. As an accompaniment of a surgical complication, or perhaps as a result of surgery itself, a patient may manifest emotional behaviors that the neurosurgeon finds annoying or unbearable. Depressed, hostile patients often can be extremely demanding of the frequently inadequate amount of time the neurosurgeon appropriates for patient encounters.

If surgical sequelae include increased emotional lability, the neurosurgeon may be in a quandary as to whether expressed feelings are legitimate and appropriate or are merely the manifestation of neurologic damage.

In medical school and thereafter, the disciplines that deal with patient and physician emotions are sometimes dismissed as "soft." Many physicians' philosophies of emotionality are not particularly well-informed with respect to psychiatric, psychologic, or sociologic principles. Consequently, they are limited in their ability to formulate philosophies toward emotional reactions to surgical complications.

What the neurosurgeon articulates as a philosophy of complications is just an intellectualization of emotional responses to having harmed another human being. Whether deliberate or accidental, whether the patient assigns blame or not, the neurosurgeon must grapple with negative feelings that may include frustration, fear, guilt, and helplessness.

The neurosurgeon may be angry with the patient for not keeping silent about discomfort or disability. Vocal patients have broken some kind of contract whereby they subordinated their opinions, desires, and feelings in exchange for the care of the physician.

It is not the neurosurgeon's fault that this contract exists; often it originates with the patient. But the same patient who subscribes to the contract when all goes well may abrogate it the instant something goes wrong. At this point the neurosurgeon is suddenly transformed from angel to devil and, if caught unawares by this shift in patient sentiment, may respond with defensiveness or hostility.

Preoperative discussions protect against some but not all guilt. No matter how carefully all potential mishaps have been explained to a patient, such an occurrence usually is met with anger and retribution by the individual who, despite a signature on a consent form, assigns to the surgeon responsibility for damages done. The surgeon's philosophy toward complications must accommodate this often irrational aspect of a patient's reactions.

The neurosurgeon cannot separate the patient's emotional reaction to a complication from his or her own. The patient will respond to cues from the neurosurgeon in assessing the gravity and implications of the complication. The neurosurgeon, empathizing to whatever degree possible, will experience some of the patient's disappointment, fear, anger, and sadness.

Pain and Comfort

Pain is subjective in the patient. Unless inquiries are made about pain, the surgeon may assume there is none.

Physical Appearance and Body Image

In a society obsessed with youthfulness and body image, disfigurement can be perceived by the patient seemingly far out of proportion to its consequence in terms of bodily well-being. What to a neurosurgeon may seem a trivial 2 or 3 centimeters of forehead scar, well worth it to achieve better access to a frontal lesion, may represent facial mutilation to the sensitive patient.

Convenience in Daily Living

Changes in routine require behavioral adjustments that may cause considerable inconvenience to the patient. A neurosurgeon may blame a patient who slowly and grudgingly makes life changes to accommodate the consequences of a complication, dismissing the patient as "noncompliant." This defensive philosophy shifts blame from the surgeon to the victim of the complication.

Factors That Contribute to the Neurosurgeon-Philosopher

A neurosurgeon's philosophy toward complications is conditioned to a significant extent by factors such as relationships with siblings and parents. Such factors as parental divorce, physical or emotional abuse, alcoholism, and major family illness all have important effects on the developing neurosurgeon's adult psyche. From this largely subliminal inner world of impressions and emotions emerges a philosophy toward life, self, goals, means, and responsibility. Even proceeding into adulthood, the impact of various life experiences, both happy and sad, will be reflected in the neurosurgeon's philosophy toward complications, which is always as amenable to correction and modification as an ever-evolving personality.

Physical factors such as gender, race, and age on entering the profession influence perspectives toward neurosurgical patients, practice, and complications. Economic, cultural, and religious conditioning results in value systems upon which the neurosurgeon draws for cues as to the appropriate response to adverse outcomes. Historical factors shape the nation, economy, and society in which the future neurosurgeon grows up. Education, from elementary through medical school, is likewise a conditioning process that for the neurosurgeon culminates in residency training. At each step, philosophic tools and methods of analysis are acquired. Once in practice, the community of neurosurgeons, of medicine, and of society at large continue to influence the philosophy toward complications, setting the standards for what is appropriate, fashionable, and medically defensible.

Physical Factors

Gender

Women are entering neurosurgery in increasing numbers. One projection is that, in the next 50 years, one-half of all neurosurgeons will be female. While generalizations are understandably offensive, a "feminine" perspective on complications is probably somewhat different from the "masculine." While many male neurosurgeons are compassionate and nurturing, these attributes generally are perceived as being more strongly manifested by their female counterparts. As women move into positions of leadership, the feminine influence in all aspects of neurosurgical philosophy will broaden and deepen.

Race

In the United States, the legacy of slavery and a century of institutionalized racism have left scars in the psyches of black and white Americans alike. African Americans are even more a minority in the ranks of neurosurgeons than in the population at large. This status, which places them under often excessive and unreasonable scrutiny, may engender a defensive posture with respect to colleagues and patients alike. Faced with an actual or potential complication, a black neurosurgeon cannot but respond in a way reflective of his or her social, economic, and historical background.

Asian Americans, a growing minority in medicine and neurosurgery, have fared better in our racist culture largely because, as voluntary immigrants, they brought with them national values of educational and economic success. While they are able to integrate in many ways, their physical appearance always distinguishes them. This awareness of a non-neutral physical difference between themselves and the majority cannot but influence their attitude toward their work and complications that occur therein.

White Americans carry a heavy racist baggage. Some flaunt prejudiced attitudes as a mark of their own perceived superiority, others accept the challenge of continually monitoring themselves in this respect. Despite this, it seems that an adverse outcome in an African American, Hispanic, or Asian patient may not have the same significance to the self-proclaimed or subverted racist. Society, racist itself, appears to condone this attitude, because the legal and economic consequences of complications are seemingly different for white and nonwhite victims.

Age

The "younger" generation of neurosurgeons is older every year. Medical school class mean ages are rising as applications from "mature" students increase. This is a group of people who have experienced life outside of medicine. A number of them already have families, and are less vulnerable to many of the socialization forces of residency, be they positive or negative. Their more mature attitudes toward life's vicissitudes undoubtedly affect how they view complications both within and outside the operating room.

Appearance

Outlook on life and self is an important factor influencing an approach toward complications. In our present society, youth, physical appearance, and athletic prowess are highly emphasized and determine, to a large extent, an individual's sense of self-confidence. The continued societal reinforcement of good looks and physical prowess imbue their possessor with a sense of strength. Taken intemperately, they contribute to delusions of omnipotence, which then invariably are incorporated into the philosophy of complications.

Economic Factors

Acceptance of complications requires acceptance of the culpability for their causation as well as responsibility for their management. People who grow up "spoiled" and excessively praised may arrive at adulthood feeling they are somehow specially privileged or gifted. When faced with a complication, they may lapse into denial that they could possibly ever do anything "wrong."

Potentially disabling dependency can be engendered by parents who unduly protect their children or meet their every need, thereby depriving them of the opportunity to make mistakes. Once on their own, dependent individuals who have been spoiled may not be able to withstand the stress of scrutiny of a complication.

Many students come to medical school at the often strenuous (sometimes irresistible) urging of parents and families. Some are deprived of the opportunity to make a decision for or against a medical career and thus of the opportunity to make their own decisions about important life issues. They come to accept a reality in which other people "know best." Applied to their eventual neurosurgical practice, this attitude can translate into one of disregard for the patient who presumably cannot know what is "best" for himself or herself and therefore has no legitimate input into assessing the impact of a surgical complication.

Dependency into early adulthood may also deprive the neurosurgeon of the challenge of assuming personal responsibility for actions and responding appropriately. Parental protection can persist psychologically even when the parent is not physically present. Such internalized voices conveniently may absolve the neurosurgeon of culpability before it is possible to think through the situation and determine whether guilt actually exists.

The economic environment in which one grows up affects attitudes toward acquisitiveness and the desire to gain at the expense of others. In times of depression, survival itself may require subordination of humanistic and/or altruistic values. Lessons learned in times of hardship at an impressionable age can be carried into adulthood. A child who grew up in an economic environment where the family's survival was threatened has suffered a psychological trauma, the memories of which may surface with the stimulus of any personal or professional adversity. A different but equally potent trauma results to the psyche of an individual who is well provided for, comfortable, and safe in the midst of poverty and suffering. While in the present there may be material plenty for all, images of past economic injustice can influence the meaning of and therefore the approach to a neurosurgical complication.

National and Cultural Inputs

Cultural values affect the attitude of neurosurgeons toward complications. Some societies are more lenient toward criminals, others punish even minor infractions severely. The response of a neurosurgeon to personal misconduct, even if inadvertent, may reflect more the standards of the society in which he or she grew up than in which he or she currently resides.

In developed countries, there is great concern about individual rights, which are sometimes expendable in the underdeveloped world. While homelessness and hunger cause consternation on the part of most Americans, they may be more tolerated in some parts of the Third World. Neurosurgeons brought up in countries where large masses of people are begging, living, and dying in the streets may not attach the same importance to a minor complication as does an American.

Debate continues to rage over the issue of capital punishment, about which most Third World countries are far less squeamish. While the majority of modern nations at least pay lip service to the sanctity of life, it is clearly not equally sacred everywhere.

In some societies, particularly more traditional societies in the Third World, physicians are perceived as having almost god-like powers. Neurosurgeons may benefit (or suffer, depending on the individual's perspective) from this tendency for deification. In such a role, the neurosurgeon may be above reproach for an operative complication.

Those societies tending to elevate the status of physicians often demonstrate a commensurate demotion of the status of patients. Perceived as ignorant, unwashed masses, their physical suffering is grist for the neurosurgical education mill. Even in the United States, patients are sometimes discussed as "cases" or "consumers." The objectification of patients engenders similar attitudes toward the complications that befall them.

Religious Factors

Rituals and attitudes toward death and dying vary with different societies. The Judeo-Christian moral code underlying much of Western philosophy is not universal. Islam is poorly understood and perhaps therefore feared by many Westerners. Asian belief systems are multifarious and tend to be obscure to many non-Asians. Immigration has brought to the United States large numbers of physicians whose religious values are very different from those with which "native" Americans are comfortable or at least familiar. The philosophy toward complications in this country reflects its "melting pot" character. In their acceptance of certain types of complications, immigrant neurosurgeons might aggressively pursue types of procedures and techniques that their American colleagues would approach with more circumspection for fear of complication.

Historical Roots

Social Attitudes

Social attitudes have been revolutionized in the last 20 to 30 years. In addition to the Civil Rights movement, which dramatically changed the legal and social status (at least on paper) of the 12% of the population that is African American, a sexual revolution has led to dramatic changes in attitudes toward abortion, contraception, promiscuity, marriage, and sexual orientation.

Among the many groups now requiring special rights are patients. While even the most strident advocates of patient rights acknowledge that surgical complications are inevitable, such watchdogs frequently are less sympathetic to extenuating circumstances that may have contributed to their occurrence. The surgeon can no longer assume that he or she has the right to cause complications without justifying them and making some provision that they will not be repeated.

The AIDS epidemic has forced the neurosurgeon to deal with increasing numbers of patients from groups traditionally held in low esteem. Coming to terms with the reality that a surgical complication is no less significant if it occurs in a homosexual or intravenous drug abuser with a soon-to-be-fatal illness has been a challenge to the philosophy of neurosurgeons individually and as a community.

Wars and Violence

Another area of major sociopsychologic upheaval has been in attitudes toward violence. Appalled by its explosive increase as a factor in crime, while at the same time drawn to it as a form of entertainment, America is clearly ambivalent. While the intention of neurosurgery is to help patients, it is ironic how similar are many of the sequelae of surgical misadventures and those of uncontrolled violence.

War is a virtually universal phenomenon, whether viewed on television from the comfort of the living room couch or experienced on the battle front. While Americans are predominantly acquainted with the former, immigrants from many parts of the world have fled either past or current conflicts. Such victims of national violence have different attitudes toward war than those for whom it is no more real than a Hollywood battle scene. The refugee, grateful just to be alive, may wonder about all the fuss over operative mishaps that result in relatively minor degrees of patient disfigurement or discomfort.

Education

Emerging from divergent educational backgrounds, some neurosurgeons are products of state-controlled public education systems, while others have had the benefit of selective private institutions. Inasmuch as there is an aristocratic class in the United States, no other force acts so effectively to maintain its distinctions as the educational system.

Any force engendering in the neurosurgeon the sense of being unlike or better than patients from different educational backgrounds interferes with the ability to accept a complication. The degree to which the neurosurgeon can identify with the patient rather than seeing him or her as "other" is affected by the nature of educational experiences. When such projection occurs, injury to the patient is tantamount to injury to the surgeon. The care taken by a white middle-class neurosurgeon to avoid a complication to a patient of similar socio-economic background may be greater than that for someone poorer or with darker skin. There also may be different philosophies in an individual neurosurgeon depending on whether identification with the patient is possible.

Medical Training

While a personal philosophy toward complications is devised by each neurosurgeon, most are influenced by real or perceived attitudes toward complications gleaned from authoritative sources within the neurosurgical community.

Training programs have a profound impact on the philosophy of neurosurgical residents. From the attending staff at academic neurosurgical centers, trainees learn what they are supposed to think and feel when faced with an adverse outcome. They may be made to feel ashamed for being oversensitive, or embarrassed at their natural fear of harming another human being. While

not frankly "brainwashed," residents throughout the unnatural and grueling process of training are vulnerable to suggestion from professors whom they admire and desperately want to emulate. While some are strong enough to resist it, there is undeniably a large group of neurosurgical residents who take what their teachers tell them as gospel. Not only do they assimilate the values of authority figures, but they incorporate them into the process of "hazing" their juniors. Many of the lessons and impressions of early training follow the neurosurgeon long after training is complete; indeed, for most these endure for their entire career and lifetime.

All neurosurgeons are students throughout their careers in the sense that the learning in neurosurgery never stops. Their philosophy toward complications reflects "where they are" with respect to training and practice. Surgical experience is attended by complications. The philosophy of a junior neurosurgical resident to an intraoperative mishap is and should be very different from that of the attending neurosurgeon. However, the younger perspective on complications is no less valid than the older, but may reflect lesser experience.

The neurosurgical literature is full of explicit and subliminal statements of philosophy toward complications. Reading the literature, one has the sense that complications are the cornerstones of advancement in neurosurgery. In the white light of "science," complications lose their emotional coloration. The larger the series, the more complications. In a published series, a case is no less a trophy because it is marred by a major complication.

Sensitivity to complications and their management seldom is discussed in neurosurgical texts. Such chapters, when they appear at all, are likely buried among the chapters on legal and ethical aspects of neurosurgery. Schooled on these books, many neurosurgeons formulate their philosophies of complications accordingly. The agenda in texts and the literature is weighted heavily toward technical and scientific advances in neurosurgery. But none of these advances eliminates complications—and some have added new ones.

The major neurosurgical organizations are influenced heavily by academic neurosurgeons. These are the same people, with the same philosophies, who edit and contribute most heavily to the neurosurgical literature. Membership in neurosurgical organizations does not necessarily impose allegiance to any philosophy, but the prevailing attitudes of the top officials in these organizations are extremely influential in how neurosurgeons and society as a whole view neurosurgical complications.

Societal and Governmental Influences

The recent controversies over health care reform have been instructive to those interested in the philosophy of physicians toward their patients. Their loud protests of interest in patient well-being and rights have fallen on the hostile ears of a government and society convinced that what doctors really are after is maintenance of their privileged financial and social status. Physicians see bureaucrats, voters, and patients as potential adversaries. The Clinton Administration's efforts may have made this more acute, but the relationship has been one of conflict. All medical students are told that they will be sued at least once during their medical careers.

The conflictive relationship of neurosurgeon to potential patients has an enormous impact on the physician's philosophy toward complications. A complication carries with it not just the threat of a lifetime of guilt for injury done to another human being, but also of severe financial and professional pain.

A seeming army of adversarial overseers pesters the most conscientious, well-intentioned neurosurgeon. In addition to Quality Assurance personnel, ostensibly hired to watch out for the interests of the hospital, patient, and neurosurgeon alike, are Utilization Reviewers and, increasingly, third-party payer representatives who want an accounting of every move made toward a patient. Complications take on a surrealistic quality when interpreted and replayed by often poorly informed watchdogs serving as advocates of a position but rarely of the truth. Not only does the neurosurgeon have to deal with overt surgical complications, but some are defined for him by non-neurosurgeons based on medically and surgically untenable criteria.

Consumer advocates abound. Proposals have been put forth to make complications public record for review by any citizen, prospective pa-

tient or not. Our society, obsessed with youth and vigor, fascinated with medicine, grows more sophisticated. The patient increasingly determines what will or will not be a complication. The boundary line between "acceptable" and "unacceptable" complications more frequently is decided by consumerism or in court Complication signifies the physician's vulnerability and as such demands a self-reckoning of limitations.

Historical Perspective

Social and historical changes have dramatically altered attitudes toward most aspects of life and death. These changes affect attitudes toward surgical complications as well. Neurosurgical techniques have evolved considerably, as have the complications resulting from their implementation.

The Roots

Neurosurgery has gone through several distinct phases. The pioneers at the turn of the century were experimenting with the application of general surgical techniques on nervous system tissue, with varying degrees of success. Informed consents were neither required nor rigorously obtained. Had they been, perhaps few patients would have submitted to procedures seldom attempted and having dubious outcomes.

Those were the days when neurosurgeons were real "cowboys." The club of colleagues scrutinizing a neurosurgeon's performance was small, with shared cultural and social values. The bold, sometimes reckless (at least from the standpoint of complications) group of pioneer neurosurgeons worked hard to minimize the damage done to patients. Over several decades, they brought the rate of adverse events down to an acceptable range, legitimizing the field of neurosurgery.

Under these circumstances, expectations for outcome were low. Mere survival of the early operations was a good outcome. The threshold for what constituted a complication was high. Neurosurgeons at that time could afford to be bold. They operated without a pack of hospital, government, and third-party payer watchdogs constantly at their heels.

Patients usually were unsophisticated about medicine and unlikely to bring lawyers into their relationships with physicians, who were often viewed as unapproachable, all-knowing figures.

In this context, a complication was an unfortunate but acceptable event whose occurrence represented an opportunity for technical advancement and benefit to subsequent patients.

The Present Generation

Successors to the early pioneers, the current ascendant generations of middle-aged and elderly neurosurgeons have benefited immeasurably from the groundbreaking work of neurosurgery's founding fathers. By and large, they have a philosophy toward neurosurgery that is pragmatically grounded in accepted practice and tradition. Their inherent conservatism is tempered by the fact that neurosurgery is the specialty par excellence of technical innovation.

The next wave of neurosurgeons developed and improved upon the basic techniques of their predecessors. This generation faced increased scrutiny from society and medical regulatory forces and was able to force the complication rate down further. However, the pressure to minimize complications became so great in the litigious, regulated climate that new techniques and approaches sometimes were avoided or only timidly applied in an effort to avoid consequences.

Many neurosurgeons in current practice have benefited from pre-"health care reform" economics. The more entrepreneurial have achieved affluent (some would say opulent) lifestyles. Some perceive that this is their due after years of sacrifice through medical school and residency training. Others, even while reaping great material benefits from their practices, have retained a more humble and grateful attitude. Both perspectives on material success are reflected clearly in the philosophies toward complications of these two broadly characterized groups of neurosurgeons.

Future Outlook

The next generation of neurosurgeons will not likely have the same earning potential and will find themselves closer to the middle class, from which most of their patients will come.

The philosophy of complications for this older, increasingly female and nonwhite generation will be the outcome of the interplay between two conflicting forces. On the one hand are humanizing forces, including the various rights movements and forces for social change. Societal attitudes toward medicine, neurosurgery, and neurosurgeons are changing and forcing neurosurgeons to at least acknowledge the perspectives of many of their patients who have different lifestyles, belief systems, and views toward surgical complications.

Paramount among the dehumanizing forces at work is an obsessive and all too often unquestioning fascination with technology. Technology is expanding the neurosurgeon's operative field of vision and extending his reach while at the same time creating a new world of previously unimagined complications.

When all that is technical and scientific is exhausted, the technician rests. The physician remains, his humanity, his compassion, his courage—his own participation in the human condition.

Redefinition of Success and Failure

Many of the social, economic, and political factors mentioned above are changing the landscape in which neurosurgery is practiced in North America. For many neurosurgeons currently in practice, emerging and threatened changes are distasteful or even unacceptable. While neurosurgeons were previously allowed virtually unlimited leeway in decision-making, they are now increasingly called upon to justify surgeries that carry even minimal risk to patients. And in the event of a complication, the scrutiny can be intense.

Definition of a complication is difficult due to the rapid evolution of the field, which tends to render ambiguous, and therefore jeopardizes, the philosophic assessment of a complication.

Poised to assume leadership in neurosurgery is a generation of neurosurgeons trained during a time of shrinking resources in a society that ever less respectfully examines every word the doctor says. This new generation is used to being considered human. As they graduate from medical school, the fiercest competition is not for the most difficult residencies but rather those that optimize "lifestyle." It is no longer anathema to put family first and career second. There is perhaps a tendency to accept the status quo in order to avoid provoking a complication by trying something new. Fear of innovation could lead to a period of stagnation in neurosurgery unless society can come up with a formula defining complications specifically and allowing for a certain frequency of these along the advancing frontier of the field.

Neurosurgeons also must increase their awareness of complications that have hitherto been unseen because they were not looked for. Application of improved and more sophisticated preoperative cognitive and psychologic testing is essential to permit recognition of subtle deficits resulting from more precise surgical lesion and graft placement.

The assessment of outcome for any given patient is subject to some degree of leveling by the neurologic surgeon. Due to the constraints of time, we tend to be satisfied with visible normal function, and are in danger of overlooking the complexities of the individual. Detailed neuropsychologic and speech testing usually are not an important part of our armamentarium and are unlikely to change fundamental surgical practice. They are important, however, for more individual consideration of the patient and more realistic assessment of the consequences of neurosurgery. The neurosurgeon must be able to anticipate complications and to explain them accurately to patients in order to avoid being held responsible for those that may be imaginary or contrived. Better monitoring and objective testing are necessary for optimal documentation.

Conclusion

The philosophy of neurosurgical complications is a reflection of the very specific "types" of people who tend to be selected to enter the field. The "typical" neurosurgeon is far from typical by societal standards. Neurosurgeons are notoriously hard-driving, overachieving perfectionists, classic "type A" personalities. Despite the stresses in neurosurgery, most who complete their residency stay

in the field. The ability to tolerate tragedy in the lives of others may be due to personal strength and character but also may result from callousness and distance. A cultivated apathy toward the problems of others can lead to the attitude that a complication is of no great consequence.

The same basic aggressiveness and decisiveness that mark the personality of a neurosurgeon also tend to color the judgment and appraisal of the chance to benefit the patient. The neurosurgeon likes to operate. Neurosurgical operations for control of pain, neural transplantation, and psychologic manipulation are among the more dramatic examples of the neurological surgeon's confident but sometimes premature expectation of effective intervention.

While most neurosurgeons, being overachievers, probably wonder at some time if they have the "right stuff" for neurosurgery, a subpopulation exists who are truly incompetent. They may be sheltered by postgraduate education credits and the lack of viable peer review mechanisms at the institutions where they work. Such neurosurgeons will have an increased incidence of complications and must come to terms with the reality that, by virtue of their sheer lack of ability, patients are being harmed. A healthy, well-founded philosophy of complications affords the best protection against instincts that urge incompetent neurosurgeons to persist in a field for which they are unsuited. The resultant philosophic conflicts engendered also can protect the patient.

Social and personal factors affect the neurosurgeon's sense of personal responsibility. Is it a responsibility to society? To the neurosurgical community? To the patient? Or to the neurosurgeon himself or herself? The answer to the question is not based on ethics but rather on philosophy. In Western cultures, with heavy legal and social pressures, the patient may not necessarily be paramount in the neurosurgeon's reckoning of personal responsibility.

Who is the perpetrator of a complication that occurs to a patient who pressured a reluctant neurosurgeon to operate? As the roles of patients and physicians, their interrelationship, and the ultimate participation of third-party payers and government in the relationship evolve, so too will the concept of the surgical complication and, necessarily, the philosophy of the surgeon toward it.

While managed care may alter some of the specifics, the American health care system undoubtedly will remain fee-for-service, with economic factors figuring prominently in the physician-patient relationship. The litigious tendency of our society only further reinforces an attitude that the cost of complications should be borne more by the neurosurgeon's wallet than the patient's suffering.

Some neurosurgeons view what they do as supremely important, while others are more modest in their self-appraisal. Once the endeavor itself competes with the patient's well-being as the object of the neurosurgeon's attention, a complication becomes a blemish on a surgical record rather than a personal tragedy.

Not all neurosurgeons are in the field for altruistic or humanitarian reasons. Some may think of their hands, skills, and judgment not as instruments for betterment of the human condition but more as vehicles for their own personal, financial, or social advancement. Most neurosurgeons have, to some degree, some or all of these nonhumanitarian motivations. The degree to which these are important affects the ability to see complications as tragic or annoying.

To the majority of neurosurgeons, the first question asked when faced with a complication is "Did I do the best operation I could?" Usually, this leads to reflection about the event precipitating the complication. The neurosurgeon learns from this, thereby improving in technique and becoming better prepared for subsequent surgery. A similar questioning surrounds important judgments and decisions.

The instructional utility of complications is certainly not a reason to pursue them deliberately. But it mitigates somewhat the sense of tragedy accompanying their occurrence. The complication signifies the physician's vulnerability, and as such demands a reckoning of personal limitations. If a "neurosurgical personality" exists, it is probably one unaccustomed to failure. The field comprises high-functioning, high-achieving, competitive individuals who are drawn not only to the frontier of modern medical knowledge but also to the mysteries of the brain. The philosophic implications of the ability to manipulate (and potentially harm) the source of the essence of humanity are staggering. The time spent agonizing about culpability, asking forgiveness, and resolving to do better is, for each and every neurosurgeon, the most important in his or her professional life.

Reference

1. Apuzzo MLJ, ed. *Brain Surgery: Complication Avoidance and Management.* New York, NY: Churchill Livingstone; 1992.

CHAPTER 8

The Philosophy of Dying and Death

Howard H. Kaufman, MD

Men fear death as children fear to go in the dark, and as the natural fear of children is increased with tales, so is the other.
—Francis Bacon (1561–1624)

The life of a single human organism commands respect and protection, then, no matter in what form or shape, because of the complex creative investment it represents and because of our wonder at the divine or evolutionary processes that produce new lives from old ones, at the processes of nation and community and language through which a human being will come to absorb and continue hundreds of generations of cultures and forms of life and value, and, finally, when mental life has begun and flourishes, at the process of internal personal creation and judgment by which a person will make and remake himself, a mysterious, inescapable process in which we each participate, and which is therefore the most powerful and inevitable source of empathy and communion we have with every other creature who faces the same frightening challenge. The horror we feel in the willful destruction of a human life reflects our shared inarticulate sense of the intrinsic importance of each of these dimensions of investment.
—Ronald Dworkin, 1993

We hold these truths to be self-evident, that all men are created equal, that they are endowed by their Creator with certain unalienable Rights, that among these are Life, Liberty and the pursuit of Happiness. That to secure these rights, Governments are instituted among Men, deriving their just powers from the consent of the governed. . . .
—Declaration of Independence, 1776

We the people of the United States, in Order to form a more perfect Union, establish Justice, insure domestic Tranquility, provide for the common defense, promote the general Welfare, and secure the Blessings of Liberty to ourselves and our Posterity, do ordain and establish this Constitution for the United States of America.
—Constitution of the United States, 1787

We the peoples of the United Nations determined . . . to reaffirm faith in fundamental human rights, in the dignity and worth of the human person, in the equal rights of men and women and of nations large and small, and . . . to promote social progress and better standards of life in larger freedom . . . and for these ends to practice tolerance and live together in peace with one another as good neighbors. . . .
—Charter of the United Nations and
Statute of the International Court of Justice

Dying and death are an inevitable part of living and must therefore be accepted. However, they are also a defeat of life and so are dreaded and resisted. One's approach to death and dying may be based on values derived from this world or from another. Whether death can be transcended and whether there are planes of existence, and therefore systems of meaning, beyond the temporal realm are questions that have fascinated and occupied the attention of humans since the awareness of death began over 70,000 years ago. Because we live in a heterogeneous society, we need to be aware of multiple secular and religious beliefs about dying, and to understand— and attempt to resolve—the issues and conflicts between them.

The neurosurgeon, as all practicing physicians, treats or gives advice about dying in many circumstances. Such encounters involve the ultimate crisis, the extinction of the individual who has lost control of his fate and is often in physical and mental anguish. Our professional role has been greatly expanded in the last several decades by the development of technologies for prolonging life. But prolonging life may only be temporary, causing physical and mental suffering to the patient, as well as expending scarce resources. Under such circumstances, it is important to determine one's appropriate role and to act according to sound philosophic principles.

Philosophy means literally "love of wisdom" and is most generally used today to mean "that department of knowledge which deals with ultimate reality, or with the most general causes and principles of things."[94] It encompasses many disciplines. For the purposes of this discussion, bioethics, theology, and the law will be particularly considered since the concepts of these disciplines and their interplay are used to guide actions that lead to living or dying, and in fact have taken these issues out of the exclusive domain of the physician.

It is also important to keep in mind that the United States is a heterogeneous culture where different philosophic systems may be in conflict. However, its unique history with an emphasis on freedom and tolerance provides the political processes, and its tradition of the rule of law provides a framework for resolving controversial issues.

After a review of bioethics as well as the legal situation in the United States, a description of its demography, and recent historical developments, this chapter will consider a number of specific subjects including abortion, the infant, the adolescent, personhood, refusal and demand of care, suicide, assisted death, aging, and conditions dangerous to the physician.

Background

Bioethics

The modern consideration of death began with Herman Feifel's *The Meaning of Death* (1959) and Elizabeth Kubler-Ross's *On Death and Dying* (1969). The seminal works on modern medical ethics have been said to be the Episcopal Joseph Fletcher's *Morals and Medicine* (1954) about patient autonomy, and the Methodist Paul Ramsey's *The Patient as Person* (1970) about the relationship between the patient and the physician. The discipline is called "bioethics," a term coined by Van Rensselear Potter: "I chose 'bio-' to represent biological knowledge, the science of living systems, and I chose 'ethics' to represent knowledge of human value systems."[49] Bioethics is "a minor form of moral philosophy practiced within medicine"[49] which may have begun in Seattle in the 1960s in the applied ethics utilized in deciding who would be given dialysis. It expanded in response to the technologic developments that extended the natural life span of human beings but at the same time led to many conundrums in initiating and withdrawing care. Landmarks in this movement include the founding of the Hastings Center in 1969 and the Kennedy Institute of Ethics in 1970, as well as the establishment of several government bodies to consider ethical issues.[104] It has involved philosophers, theologians, social scientists, and lawyers. The importance of this movement has been emphasized:

> By facilitating open discussion and examination of the ethical premises underlying life and death decisions, bioethics has expanded medicine's reflective horizons. In fact, encouraging health practitioners to become self-reflective is the major contribution of bioethics to American health care.[3]

Heifitz[44] has discussed the origin and nature of moral behavior. He describes ethics as a philosophic discipline that develops principles by which to judge right and wrong, and morality as the application of these principles. He feels these principles should be universal, should be in harmony with human nature, and should benefit the individual and society. He cites three sources of ethics—religion, biologic data, and pure reason. Religion gives rise to dogma and religious philosophy, the latter being more flexible. The concepts of religion cannot be verified and therefore should not be forced on others. On the other hand, they should be heard and considered. Biologic data from lower animals are discounted as being too restricted to use for analyzing human behavior. Pure reason is problematic because it depends on the validity of primary assumptions and is based on the quality of reasoning. Heifitz suggests that ethics must be based on two assumptions: 1) the need to avoid harm to ourselves, our families, and our community; and 2) the need to live in social groups. He cites the primary moral principles in order as nonmaleficence and freedom, qualified by the absence of harm (which are required for a free society), followed by action for the common good (which could cause risks to freedom if given too high a priority), and beneficence. He includes as secondary principles justice, or the equal treatment of all, and privacy, or the freedom to make a choice of what is not wanted. Heifitz recommends using these primary and secondary principles to decide how to resolve moral issues, and states:

> Moral behavior is the product of human reason and emotion, modified by our physical and cultural environment and possibly by our genetic imprint. The degree of importance each factor is given in the final pattern is variable.

Decision-making requires balancing and flexibility. In terms of individual decision-making, refusal of care or seeking of death can harm others such as family or community. In the case of someone who is incompetent, substituted judgment of best interests requires intelligence and rational thinking.

An excellent overview of medical ethics can be found in the classic text of Beauchamp and Childress,[4] who also utilize a hierarchic system of organization. They describe the two theories, utilitarian and deontologic, that govern choices in cases of conflict. The utilitarian theory seeks to determine which choice maximizes benefits and minimizes evil. The deontologic theory uses criteria of right and wrong based on particular political, religious, and other beliefs. The beliefs of the major cultures and religions of the world relative to the issues discussed here have been reviewed in detail elsewhere.[6,8,45,64] Next in the hierarchy are four principles that are general and fundamental, namely, autonomy, nonmaleficence, beneficence, and justice, in that order of importance. These are followed by rules, specific to contexts and restricted in scope, including veracity, privacy, confidentiality, and fidelity. Lastly are specific decisions and actions. In addition, the authors note that all decisions and actions should be founded in moral ideals, which are to be desired even if not required, and virtuous character traits, which are morally valued. The major problem arises at the level of theory, where a deontologic theory may prevent the compromise required to resolve conflicts. But again, this is where both respect for the freedom of others and tolerance must be invoked.

The decision-making process requires gathering facts, developing options, and making decisions based on ranking values and principles.[28] Physicians should guide patients through these issues but not decide for them. Patients have a right to be told the truth and to be made aware of the prognosis in order to make spiritual and temporal preparations.[7] Physicians must be trustworthy, and patients must believe physicians to be advocates of their best interests.[7] It is appropriate for such decisions to be difficult and hard fought. It would be best if they were kept from the political arena and freed from the spectres of malpractice, litigation, and administrative cost containment.

Legal Situation

The intellectual climate in the United States involves a liberal political philosophy in which personal freedom and privacy are honored and protected, at least if these do not harm others. This concept leads to a way to resolve conflicts:[29]

Does a state protect a contestable value best by encouraging people to accept it as contestable, understanding that they are responsible for deciding for themselves what it means? Or does the state protect a contestable value best by itself deciding, through the political process, which interpretation is the right one, and then forcing everyone to conform? The goal of responsibility justifies the first choice, the goal of conformity the second. A state cannot pursue both goals at the same time.

Dworkin's conclusion is obviously that the former goal is the proper one. For a pluralistic society to function, it is necessary to recognize the individual's right to make decisions for and about himself above all other principles, and this tolerance is the price required for our "adventure in liberty."

The political embodiment of the social contract of our country is the Constitution, including its amendments, specifically the first, third, fourth, fifth, and fourteenth.[44] In a superb treatment of the Constitution as it relates to life and death decisions, it was pointed out that the Constitution should be interpreted in terms of its broad principles, which is what its framers intended to achieve in terms of liberty and equal concern for its citizens, even if they seem to conflict with apparent details. Dworkin[29] concludes of the Bill of Rights:

> Read in the most natural way, the words of the Bill of Rights do seem to create a breathtakingly abstract, principled constitution. Taken at face value, they command nothing less than that government treat everyone subject to its dominion with equal concern and respect, and that it not infringe their most basic freedoms, those liberties essential, as one prominent jurist put it, to the very idea of "ordered liberty" [Cardoza, 1937]. The system of principle this striking language mandates is comprehensive because it commands both equal concern and basic liberty, which in our political culture are the two major sources of claims of individual rights. Since liberty and equality overlap in large part, each of the two major abstract clauses of the Bill of Rights—the due process and the equal protection clauses—is itself comprehensive in that same way.

Our society is regulated by the rule of law. In the words of Joseph Campbell, "Lawyers and law are what hold us together. There is no ethos."[2] And it is the Supreme Court's interpretation of the intent of the Constitution that ultimately determines how an issue will be resolved. Consideration of end-of-life decisions in the public arena, and government activity involving the judicial, legislative, and executive branches began with the Quinlan case (1976), and there have been many important court cases since.[2,6,8,40,102] Growing legal interest and action, particularly at the state level, has been detailed.[40]

A recent guide for physicians reviews the relevant court cases. It emphasizes the importance of *Quinlan* (1976), in which a state supreme court allowed the withdrawal of a respirator on the judgment by a physician of lack of recoverability, and *Cruzan* (1990), in which the United States Supreme Court allowed stoppage of artificial feeding and hydration based on the patient's prior expressed wishes.[7] Many issues have been argued and case law developed, particularly regarding self-determination and quality of life.[8] Legislative activity is now more widespread through the states than court cases, ranging from brain death to living wills and designation of surrogates. But the Supreme Court and the Congress have not provided national standards.

It has been argued that court and legislative action is too easily swayed by political pressure, that the participants are often not well versed on the issues, that the process is slow and costly, that the venue is too far removed from the actual situation, and that family privacy is violated. In addition, actions may vary from state to state, and cases and laws need to be reconsidered as innovations occur.[40] Some also have argued that in the case of moral choices it is better to keep discussions private, but court involvement indicates the current failure of private decision-making.[8]

By today's ethical and legal standards, patients have a right to determine what will happen to them based on their own values, while physicians must educate them and act as their advocates.[14] This is embodied in the concept of informed consent, which requires that patients be informed of diagnosis, prognosis, and options, but also requires competence and the ability to understand and make reasonable judgments, and must be voluntary. Exceptions to this occur when a patient waives this right and therapeutic privilege, and when disclosure is judged to be harmful to the patient.[102] This right persists even after competence is lost, as embodied by advance directives which include living wills and appointment of a proxy (details vary from state to state).[17] In their absence, substituted judgment, namely what the patient would have wanted, can be employed. Barring such indications, decisions should be made on best interests, namely what most reasonable people would want. In fact, the public favors the right of individuals to control their own fates. Surveys show 80% of those responding favor permitting people to refuse care, 55% favor allowing patients to end their own lives, 60% favor allowing physicians to assist dying, and 70% favor mercy killing.[28] The Federal Patient Self Determination Act of 1991 mandates that funded facilities provide information about and facilitate advanced directives.

Demographics

The demographics of the United States[95,103] demonstrate not only how heterogeneous a population we have, but also the resultant need to try to accommodate each other in order to have a functioning society. Statistics from 1990 and 1991 indicate that there were almost 249 million citizens. The growth rate was less than 1%, the birth rate 1.5%, the death rate 0.9%, and the immigration rate 0.6%. There were large numbers in each 5-year age segment until a gradual tapering in those over 45 years old (Table 1). There were slightly more females (129 million vs. 123 million males). Nine percent (22 million) were foreign-born, including 31% from Central and South America, 25% from Asia, and 22% from Europe. In terms of all citizens, 23% were of German descent, 16% of Irish descent, 13% of English descent, 6% of Italian descent, and 5% Native American; all other countries had fewer descendants. Racial breakdown included 80% white, 12% black, 3% Asian or Pacific Islander, and 0.8% Native American; 9% were considered

TABLE 1
Population by Age, United States, 1991

Age	Population (in 1000s)
Under 5 years	19,222
5 to 9 years	18,237
10 to 14 years	17,671
15 to 19 years	17,242
20 to 24 years	19,372
25 to 29 years	20,844
30 to 34 years	22,242
35 to 39 years	20,573
40 to 44 years	18,779
45 to 49 years	14,101
50 to 54 years	11,646
55 to 59 years	10,423
60 to 64 years	10,582
65 to 69 years	10,037
70 to 74 years	8,242
75 to 79 years	6,279
80 to 84 years	4,035
85 years and older	3,160

TABLE 2
Family Income, United States, 1990

Income Level	No. (in 1000s)
Less than $5,000	2,239
$5,000 to $9,999	3,882
$10,000 to $14,999	5,065
$15,000 to $24,999	10,473
$25,000 to $34,999	10,521
$35,000 to $49,999	13,018
$50,000 or more	20,892

Hispanic but could be of any race. In terms of religious preference, 56% were Protestant, 25% Catholic, 2% Jewish, and 6% of other persuasions, while 11% had no preferences. In terms of income, for 66 million families, 21% were considered under the poverty level (Table 2). Schooling of those over 25 years old included 11% with a grade school education, 11% with some high school, 38% who graduated high school, 18% with less than 4 years of college, and 22% with 4 or more years of college. These figures, all of which are factors associated with different life views, emphasize the great diversity of beliefs that can be expected.

Two million people in the United States die each year, and health care costs almost one trillion dollars a year and is 13% to 14% of the gross national product. Medicare and Medicaid arose in the 1960s and 1970s to fund care of the elderly and the indigent. Various government programs pay 42% of health care costs, and new initiatives may increase this considerably. Unfortunately, one-fifth to one-fourth of these funds is spent on administrative costs. A large proportion is expended in the last year of life, and only 10% of people treated in intensive care units (ICUs) live and leave the hospital.[8]

In response to rising costs, health policy in the United States is undergoing a revolution, with a focus on cost containment and rationing. Since those over 65 years old constitute 11% of the population but consume 30% of health care expenditures, their care, especially at the end of life, is receiving particular consideration. However, only 10% to 12% is spent on patients who die, and at most, 27% of this (or 3% of total costs) might be saved by eliminating unwanted and futile care.[30] Unfortunately, it appears that new systems are being devised that create disincentives to treatment without adequate safeguards.

The Fetus

The neurosurgeon may be involved with a fetus in several circumstances, including counseling the mother, abortion, surgery on the fetus, and research on and use of the fetus.

Once a mother decides to carry a pregnancy to birth, she accepts a moral obligation to the fetus. She should maintain a healthy life style and have regular prenatal care, lack of which is the greatest risk factor in fetal damage. This is of interest to the neurosurgeon in that it may prevent premature labor and diminish the risk of intraventricular hemorrhage. There have been extensive discussions of these obligations.[29,46]

The absolute sanctity of fetal life, regardless of other considerations, has been contested. If human life is inherently sacred, the fetus would need to be protected except to save the life of the mother. If, on the other hand, its rights had to be balanced against the rights of the mother, other

relatives, and society, its rights might be altered, especially depending on its age. It has been argued that a mother has rights of privacy and self-determination, that she should not be forced to assume risk for another person, that her rights supersede the rights of a fetus even to the point of aborting it, and that she is in the best position to choose when abortion is appropriate.[2]

A middle-of-the-road approach may involve trying to determine a point at which the fetus does have rights that can compete with the mother's—the point at which the potential to become a human being is realized sufficiently to warrant protection. Several stages in development might be considered significant besides the conceptus (which is a new genotype with the potential for life). Other stages that have been mentioned include implantation (6–14 days); sufficient development of the nervous system so there is limited (reflex) response to stimuli and the possibility of a personal identity (8 weeks); recognizability as a human (12–16 weeks); development of a neocortex and an integrated nervous system, a patterned electroencephalogram (EEG), the presumed ability to react to painful stimuli, the possibility of self-consciousness, and viability (the ability to survive *ex utero* [live birth]), all of which occur at about 23 to 24 weeks; and finally, birth with breathing.

Some even feel that what is important is the development of such characteristics as consciousness, language, abstract reasoning, and self-awareness,[1,46,54,98] which occur well after birth. In many cultures, even a young infant does not have human status. For example, Australian aborigines do not consider a child a human being until after the age of 1 year, and infanticide is practiced until that time. This subject will be discussed in the next section.

Different parties often have competing interests for or against abortion. The child has an interest in living if it is healthy and may expect a socially satisfying life, the mother has an interest in controlling her life as she feels is most appropriate, and society has a need to protect the mother's rights and to avoid the burden of an impaired child or one without parental support. On the other hand, the child has an interest in existing, the mother may need to be protected from making a poor decision, and society needs to protect the vulnerable. Resolution of these interests is at times difficult and must be individualized to some extent.

Abortion remains a problematic issue and a subject of great controversy in our society, with opinions ranging from total opposition to abortion to allowing any abortion on demand. Because of the moral stance of each faction involved, it is hard to imagine a true compromise. The current liberal legal approach is based on a constitutional rights argument and was embodied by the Supreme Court decision *Roe v Wade* (1973), in which it was decided that a fetus was not a legal person with rights until viability in the third trimester.[2,29,44] It has been argued that the issue of sanctity of life lies in the religious sphere, and that decisions about abortion therefore are protected by the freedom of religion amendments.[29] In a review of 100 public opinion surveys done from 1962 through 1993, it was found that a large majority feel abortion is morally wrong but want it to be legal. They think that it is the mother's right to decide—within limits involving spousal or parental (for minors) notification, that it is acceptable in order to protect a mother's health, in cases of rape, and for a severely impaired fetus, but that it should be funded by government programs only when "medically necessary." Activists on both sides of the issue have played vigorous roles in partisan politics and violent confrontations, and can be expected to continue to do so.[12]

In terms of neurosurgical advice, with modern diagnostic techniques fetal abnormalities such as hydrocephalus and myelomeningocele can be detected *in utero*.[33] The neurosurgeon can inform the mother of the expected neurologic problems and give her some idea of the expected functional and social disabilities. At that point, she would need to decide if a premature death was preferable to severely impaired life. But decisions about the quality of life are based on value judgments and may include consideration of intellect, physical impairment, independence, and productivity, which may differ from person to person. If the neurosurgeon cannot accept the mother's decision, another consultant should be suggested.

A novel area is fetal surgery, which does carry risk to fetus and mother and is in its early stages of development. This usually has been left to the discretion of the mother.

There are several other issues the neurosurgeon may face involving research on and use of an aborted fetus.[101] It should always be remembered that the fetus is a symbol of human life and should be treated with respect. However, living human beings have a vital interest in use of the fetus in research and treatment. The first question is whether using fetal tissue implies sanction of and collusion in abortion. It has been stated that the decision to abort should be separated from the informed consent to donate fetal tissue. Some feel even this does not really separate the two, while on the other hand, some have gone so far as to suggest that conception in order to provide life-saving fetal tissue for a loved one should be permitted.[46,100] Transplantation of fetal tissue has received great interest. There is growing evidence that fetal tissue transplantation may be helpful for Parkinson's disease as well as other diseases.[98,100] More research in these and other applications is needed, but must be done thoughtfully and with sufficient oversight to avoid any suggestion of impropriety. Research of the fetus *in utero* has been useful, but here protection similar to that in any living human must be observed. Research on the living fetus *ex utero* is useful, but must be done with sensitivity.[54,98] The moratorium on federal funding for fetal research established during the Bush administration was eliminated by President Clinton when he took office.[46] New guidelines for the use of fetal tissue have been issued (National Institutes of Health [NIH] Revitalization Act of 1993 [P.L. 103-43]), and the first new NIH grant for human implantation of fetal tissue has been awarded.

The Infant

If an infant cannot participate in ethical and moral debates and decisions, the question arises as to how to treat infants who are terminally ill or expected to survive with severe disabilities. This is a significant problem. About 200,000 or 6% of infants born annually require intensive care due to prematurity, congenital anomalies of various organs, gastrointestinal problems, infections, or problems from diseases of the mother such as diabetes mellitus, drug abuse, or AIDS. Many will not survive, and over 10% of such patients may not now be treated,[3] although there is some variation depending in part on the type of hospital, and no societal norms have been established.

Death may not be the ultimate harm to befall such an infant; rather a life of suffering may be worse. Using substituted judgment or "best interest" criteria as defined by the parents, it may be decided that it is not proper to treat.[2,44,102] However, difficult questions may be raised such as the certainty of the prognosis, the possibility that there may be some new treatment discovered to correct the problem, or whether the mental or physical deficit is severe enough to truly make life not worthwhile. The formula developed by Shaw to help this evaluation is:

> Quality of life = natural endowment ×
> (home and societal support).[3,102]

This reflects the problem that, in many cases, children who are saved have inadequate services later in life. Decision-making should be done by informed and wise parents in the child's best interest. Federal regulations published in the *Federal Register* in 1985 do not require treatment if the patient is comatose, if care would prolong dying, or if care would be futile and inhumane.[8,102]

In a sociologic study,[3] the various roles of physicians, nurses, and parents, and decision-making/effecting were analyzed. Problems were identified, and a plea was made to empower parents, to develop more consistent policies, to prevent these problems on the one hand, and to provide comprehensive services on the other.

The problem of parents insisting on futile treatment for a mentally or physically devastated infant will be discussed later. On the other hand, the parents may not agree to useful treatment, particularly in a handicapped child, or they may abandon the child. Here the state has an interest in preserving life and protecting the vulnerable. In such cases, the physician may need to have a guardian appointed for the child.[28]

The Child and Adolescent

The older child presents many similar issues. On the one hand, the parents presumably know the child's best interests and should have the right to rear the child. On the other hand, the child, being vulnerable, deserves the protection of the state. The secular orientation of our society is obvious when one considers how the courts have acted to promote medical care ahead of religious concerns.[28]

Another issue is how to weigh a child's wishes against the parents' wishes. The question is when do children have the perspective, experience, and judgment—and therefore the right—to make their own decisions. There is also the practical issue of maintaining privacy and confidentiality if one is to win the trust of a child. The issue has been confused by a variety of laws granting rights and obligations at different ages: voting at age 18 years, army service at age 18 years, drinking at age 21 years, and age of majority at 13 to 19 years depending on the state. In addition, marriage, childbearing, and living alone can lead to emancipation. A complicating factor arises when parents are paying the medical bills. The trend now is to work with the child, particularly if the problem is straightforward, and to let him or her know if one plans to discuss the problem with the parents.

Brain Death and Permanent Vegetative State

> . . . the death of persons—of human persons—is of profound moral importance and . . . therefore people generally are very concerned that the criteria of death reflect this importance and provide reliably accurate methods for determining the death of persons.[39]

The questions of what is life and when is it lost must be considered first in philosophic and then in physiologic terms. In philosophic terms, there is perceived to be something unique about a human being separate from organic or somatic functioning. This is embodied in the dualist concept of body and soul which dates from the teachings of Plato and Aristotle. It is therefore necessary to define what is essential to humanity or personhood and to determine what must be lost in order to define death.

From ancient times, it was felt that the locus of this unique quality resided in the brain.[25,77] The mind is identified more specifically with the neocortex, where self-awareness and reasoning are thought to be located. Following this concept, it is not until neocortical functioning occurs that a true human being exists, and once this is lost, human life is over.

However, it is now possible to support vegetative functions in patients whose brains have irreversibly ceased all function (and even more easily in those who have lost only neocortical function).[9,34,70,74] This situation has resulted in a need "to define death by criteria that did not depend primarily on the cardiorespiratory function that life support systems artificially preserved."[25]

Brain Death

A physician has been required to declare death since 1903 in the United States.[6] The modern scientific concept of brain death was first developed from research into the neuropathology of respirator brain at the Massachusetts General Hospital (C Miller Fischer, personal communication) and by EEG studies of similar patients in France, where the term *coma dépassé* (beyond coma) was used to describe irreversible brain damage.[35,65,72] There are several detailed reviews about the clinical determination of brain death.[11,27,72] The first widely recognized criteria on how to define brain death were evolved by the Harvard ad hoc Committee on Brain Death in 1968,[5,35] and the concept also was discussed in the Declaration of Sydney of the 22nd Congress of the World Medical Assembly.[8] Various groups in the United States and throughout the world formulated other criteria.[72] The NIH funded the Collaborative Study which developed additional recommendations.[107,108] A group of consultants to the President's Commission for the Study of Ethical Problems in Medicine and Biomedical Research and Behavioral Research further refined the criteria.[59,61,78] Important exchanges of information occurred during symposia sponsored by the New York Academy of Sciences (1978)[56] and by the Massachusetts Neurological Association (1981). The current standard, the guidelines of the President's Commission, has several advantages:

This societal resolution has relied upon the perceived clarity of medical criteria for neurological death (as opposed to the obvious uncertainties and delays with most forms of higher brain death), the pressure to achieve permission to save other lives with transplantation, and the political acceptability of incremental change.[59]

These criteria have proven to be reliable, although theoretically they may not be proven mathematically.[23,59,92] Further, they fulfill the requirement stated by Shewmon,[92] which is that they are "self-evident on a priori grounds." Since no adult has been reported to have survived when the diagnosis of brain death was made using the criteria of the President's Commission, the criteria can be employed with confidence. However, it has been pointed out that even when the criteria are met, there may be EEG, evoked potential, or neurohumoral function.[41]

The criteria of the consultants to the President's Commission (1981) advocated that laws should define brain death as "irreversible cessation of all functions of the entire brain."[52,61,78] The criteria involve clinical evidence of loss of brain function and a period of observation which can be shortened by confirmatory tests, particularly cerebral blood flow studies. In cases falling outside these guidelines, consultation with physicians with particular expertise may be helpful, and other criteria and tests can be used. The difference between these criteria and older sets lies mainly in the rapidity with which brain death can be declared. Since cardiovascular collapse is increasingly likely during observation of a brain-dead body, many transplantable organs may be lost if older standards are used.

Many physicians have the expertise and experience to declare brain death. General medical curricula and testing of physician qualifications should encompass brain death. Some criteria (and state laws) suggest that two physicians must agree on the diagnosis of brain death, particularly when organ retrieval is being considered. If an EEG is obtained, the electroencephalographer may be the second physician. However, if the diagnosis is straightforward and clear, and if the physician involved is well-trained and experienced, it would seem reasonable for a single physician to certify brain death.

Once a patient is declared brain dead, ventilator support legally can be terminated. Some believe that the physician has the authority and responsibility to stop life-sustaining treatment when a patient is brain dead and that the option to continue care should not be given to the family. Others feel the families should be asked for permission to stop care and turn off the respirator. In any case, when managing distraught or otherwise difficult families, it is prudent to listen for and consider objections. Many families may benefit from a short period of time to adjust to the sudden tragedy and hopelessness of the situation. They may need this opportunity to develop trust in the physician and the diagnosis. If the family objects to discontinuation of the respirator, particularly because of family stress or religious reasons, it may be wisest to delay until these feelings are addressed. A consultant, a chaplain or minister, or an ethics consult may be helpful. When brain death has been caused by criminal assault, thoughtful legal advice becomes essential.

Criteria for the declaration of brain death in children less than 5 years old has been considered problematic. The advisors to the President's Commission suggested that there might be significant, although not well-defined, differences in the brains of those under 5 years of age that allow some functions of the brain to recover from clinical states that would be accepted as indicative of complete and irreversible loss of brain function in adults.[61] Additionally, the distress of brain death is compounded by the emotions generated by the death of a child, one whose vulnerability and unfilled promise magnify the tragedy of any death. But in the last few years, reliable guidelines for this age group have also been developed.[51,55]

Judeo-Christian thinking generally supports the concept of brain death.[20,73,99] The concept that brain death is equivalent to death as diagnosed by the criteria of loss of respiratory and cardiac function is also accepted by medicine and the law in the United States. A model brain death law, the Uniform Determination of Death Act, was approved in 1980 by the President's Commission, the American Medical Association (AMA), the American Bar Association, and the National Conference of Commissioners on Uniform State Laws. This states that brain death is equivalent to death recognized by cardiopulmonary standards. However, it reserves actual criteria and determination to the medical profession. At least 39 states now have brain death laws, and a few others have formally accepted brain death as death in rulings of the states' supreme courts. Precedents are now so overwhelming that brain death standards probably can be applied anywhere in the United States, although practitioners should know the status of their local laws. Still, there can be problems:

> . . . brain death criteria, used in cases where a human being is maintained on artificial ventilation, are far less detectable or even understandable by the ordinary non-medical person, and therefore subject to far greater suspicion.[25]

There is an imperative to define death when it occurs. Humanism, the dominant secular philosophy of our time, emphasizes the value of the life of each individual.[25] Thus, it follows that the determination of the ending of a life has tremendous importance. On the one hand, a living person should not be treated as dead. On the other hand, a dead person also should not be treated as being alive. Preservation of somatic function long after the brain has been destroyed is inappropriate because it ignores the reality of the situation, keeps the family and friends in the limbo of uncertainty and false hope, violates the trust of the family and society that the physician can recognize death, requires health care workers to treat a dead body, expends resources without benefit, and might be perceived as an indignity to and abuse of the body. Exceptions can be made in rare circumstances, for example, in an attempt to salvage a viable fetus.

There is another reason to declare brain death, including brain death in children. Recent advances in transplantation provide the opportunity of using the organs of a brain-dead person to improve or to save the lives of others, and even conserve money because of diminished medical costs and increased productivity.[71,79,86,87] The advances currently being made are reflected in the rising numbers of transplants (now about 20,000/year)[31] and the rising rates of organ and donee survival. However, between 1988 and 1991, when candidates increased 55%, donors only increased by 16%. By March 1993, 30,000 patients were on waiting lists, but six people awaiting a heart or a liver died every day. Cadaver donors remain at about 4,000/year even though more potential donors exist.[26]

A special problem is the need for pediatric organs. The use of cyclosporine for immunosuppression, beginning in 1983, eliminated the devastating side effects of impairment of mental and physical development caused by the high-dose steroid therapy used previously, and thus made transplantation more attractive for children. Some organs for transplantation in children must be size-matched, particularly the heart. In 1990, almost 1000 children aged 1 to 15 years were awaiting organs, and perhaps 1000 children are born each year with congenital heart (or liver) problems who could benefit from a transplant. But 30% to 50% of all children registered for transplants will die while awaiting them. Therefore, when the potential recipients are small children, young donors must be identified and utilized. Anencephalics might become donors, but this would constitute only a small number.

The causes for the problem of too few available transplant organs are numerous. Currently, donation is based on voluntarism and altruism.[19] But although surveys have suggested the public largely understands brain death and generally looks favorably on donation, this is not a universal attitude, particularly among a number of minorities.[18,38,57,84,86,87] Also, many people who would wish to donate do not tell their families, and families who have not been told are more reluctant to donate organs.[38] In addition, organs are lost when patients are not vigorously resuscitated or supported.

The Uniform Anatomical Gift Act (1968) now adopted in all states permits the patient to make a directive in advance. Forty-nine states have rules to encourage this statement on the driver's license. Thirty-eight states have Routine Inquiry/ Required Request laws (1987) mandating inquiry of next of kin, but these have not had much effect.[18,19] National laws to promote transplantation include the National Organ Transplantation Act of 1984 (PL 98–507) and

Amendments in 1988 (PL 100–607) and 1990 (PL 101–616). They established a national organ procurement network and a scientific registry as well as a Task Force, all of which have led to ongoing activities.[31,86,87] The Surgeon General sponsored a workshop in July 1991 whose recommendations include strategies to increase donations.[69,79] There have been many proposals, including improvement in donor identification and care, more effective contact with donor families, universal checking for donor cards, and public education. Other suggested solutions include presumed consent, mandated decision-making, and rewarded gifting.[18,19,86,87,96,105] In several countries, organs are harvested based on "presumed consent" if the deceased had not previously objected. But it has been suggested that "mandated choice" is a better solution.[97] A recent Gallup poll suggested financial rewards would not be helpful.[38]

Because facilitating transplantation can create good, in many cases saving life, it is permissible, virtuous, and, in the eyes of many, obligatory.[54] Professional obligations as well as the ethical and religious imperatives of beneficence, charity, and honesty compel physicians to be proactive and facilitate transplantation by informing the family about this possibility when it exists. The AMA Code of Medical Ethics (1992) declares: "The voluntary donation of organs in appropriate circumstances is to be encouraged," and organized neurosurgery has supported this approach.

Other solutions are being considered. Xenographs are being tried, creating their own ethical issues. Artificial organs are being investigated. Use of live donors is being expanded. And the use of non-heart-beating cadaver donors is again being explored. The University of Pittsburgh has developed a protocol in which terminal patients who elect to have life-sustaining treatment stopped and who wish to donate organs are taken into an operating room, treatment is stopped, and their organs harvested if they do not breathe and their heart stops in a short period. This may increase the donor pool by 20% to 25%. A review of the evolution of this controversial protocol, its status, and the experience with it, as well as critiques about it, have been published.[53,110]

Permanent Vegetative State

Descartes stated the concept of higher brain function with elegant simplicity: "Cogito ergo sum." Consciousness has been defined as "our immediate sense of the present and what amounts to memory (the source of the revisions of reality . . .)."[80] As to the exact location of consciousness in the brain, "On the basis of modern evidence for the massive parallel processing of information within the brain, . . . consciousness is not a unitary phenomenon but rather a continually changing, updated and edited version of the world that derives from many neurological sources."[80] The problem is that there is no consensus about exactly what constitutes consciousness, how to determine whether it is lost, or how to know whether that loss is irreversible.[111]

The concept of a higher brain or neocortical standard of personhood based on consciousness is already being utilized implicitly if not always explicitly. In recent years it has become widely accepted that it is not ethically required to give any support to breathing patients, not even water, if the patient is not sentient or will not suffer discomfort.[23] Although this approach alters the way we deal with the living, we have not treated such patients as dead, which would mean they could be buried or have their organs harvested.[25,77]

It has also been pointed out that: 1) there may be viable cells (and by necessity blood flow) in patients who meet the current definition of brain death; 2) this is accepted under "a gentleman's agreement that cellular functions did not count;" and 3) this qualification opens the argument that the issue remains loss of "key functions" or "higher brain function," which must be defined and agreed upon and then subjected to measurement.[106]

The determination of the permanent vegetative state requires a specific definition together with an evaluation of prognosis. A task force including representatives from the American Academy of Neurology, the American Academy of Pediatrics, the American Neurological Association, the American Association of Neurological Surgeons, and the Child Neurology Society have considered this subject in depth. Their report, which has already been approved by three of the parent organizations, begins with the definition: "The vegetative state is a condition of complete unawareness of the self and the environment accompanied by sleep-wake cycles with either complete or partial preservation of brain stem and hypothalamic autonomic functions." The report includes an extensive literature review of the various causes of the permanent vegetative state, including traumatic and nontraumatic brain injury, degenerative and metabolic disorders, and developmental malformations, the times at which it can be known to be permanent, and the epidemiology. It notes that there are estimated to be 10,000 to 25,000 adults and 4000 to 10,000 children in the permanent vegetative state and that their care costs between 1 and 7 billion dollars/year (R Cranford, personal communication, 1993).

More research needs to be done to facilitate diagnosis and prognosis of this state. Indeed, a recent survey of ethicists has demonstrated tremendous variations in thoughts about such patients,[37] and there is a need for explicit discussion to develop standards for dealing with them.[40] It has also been proposed that people should be allowed to choose their own definition of death and to include a higher brain definition as one option.[106]

A related issue is the status of anencephalics, a group who are clearly not brain dead, and whether they can be organ donors, which would require defining a special legal status for them.[2,21,36,42,43,62,88,93,102]

Direction of Care

Problems arise when patients refuse care that is suggested or may demand care that a physician feels is inappropriate. That patients can legally refuse treatment has long been established in the United States.[7,63] Indeed, in a 1914 Supreme Court decision, Justice Cardoza declared, "Every human being of adult years and sound mind has the right to determine what shall be done with his own body."[64] This statement is the embodiment of the Constitutional right of liberty and privacy and the common-law right of self-determination.

Another landmark came in 1957 when Pope Pius XII, in response to the development of technologies that at times only prolong dying, proclaimed that extraordinary care is not obligatory.[7] This right to refuse treatment has led to the endorsement by the Hastings Center (1981), the AMA (1982), and the President's Commission (1983) of withholding and withdrawing unwanted care.

On the other hand, there are religious considerations that obligate a person to care for the body, the gift of God. This is true in Roman Catholicism and perhaps even more in Judaism.[102] Indeed, in Judaism, there is a mandate for a person to live in a place where there is a physician.

This principle was accepted in California in 1986 in the Bouvia case, in which the patient was given the right to refuse food and water.[7] Its effect can be seen in such situations as the right of a Jehovah's Witness to refuse blood even if this leads to death (although this may be limited when it adversely impacts others, i.e. where a mother's refusal of a transfusion will lead to her death and abandonment of a child). There are many cases in which this right has been affirmed.[2,8,29,44,102]

Public polls have revealed that the majority of citizens are in favor of this concept.[40] Many patients have a preference to not have aggressive care when they are terminal. But physicians have not necessarily perceived these desires and tend to give more aggressive care than patients want.[90] Therefore, physicians and patients should discuss explicitly the patient's wishes. However, in acute disabling conditions, such as a spinal cord injury, patients may initially lack a full perspective of the problem and decision-making should be deferred for some time.[75] In cases of conflict, a second opinion, ethics committee consult, or other help should be sought or, if the problem cannot be resolved, the patient should be transferred.

In the case of a cardiac arrest, an immediate decision is necessary, which requires a prior declaration to prevent resuscitation. A great deal of information has been accumulated about prognosis in such areas as cancer and heart disease and, therefore, about when resuscitation may or may not reasonably be expected to be effective in terms of survival to hospital discharge.[64] Indeed, an uncritical approach to this problem would result in forcing many people to prolong their dying in dismal circumstances. Patients and physicians should discuss the patient's prognosis, and patients should be allowed to elect not to be resuscitated. Reasonable reasons for "Do Not Re-

suscitate" (DNR) orders include poor prognosis, poor quality of life before arrest, or a poor quality of life anticipated after resuscitation. This must be based on probability and is a matter of judgment. In fact, in one study only 22% of elderly patients opted for cardiopulmonary resuscitation (CPR) after being informed of the facts, as opposed to 41% of a control group.[68] The need for such directives has been recognized more over the last decade, as indicated by the increased number of patients in ICUs with DNR orders.[48] State laws on this subject first appeared in the 1980s; in 1988 the Joint Counsel for Accreditation of Hospitals passed regulations about DNR orders, and in 1991 the Patient Self Determination Act mandated them for recipients of Medicare and Medicaid funds.[64]

An interesting issue is whether DNR orders should be suspended when a patient goes to an operating room. As many as 15% of patients with DNR orders undergo surgery. The fact of being operated on implies the desire to be treated and to survive the surgery. In addition, arrest in the operating room is generally due to correctable problems, and resuscitation is usually successful. The issue should be discussed with such a patient and agreement reached regarding circumstances in which resuscitation should or should not be attempted.[28,58,100]

The right to refuse treatment extends into the future in the case of incapacitation. This is embodied in the concept of advanced directives, including the living will and the right to appoint a surrogate.[29] The living will was first suggested by Louis Rutner in 1969 and first enacted in California in 1976.[7] A model law for the living will was offered by the National Council of Commissioners for Uniform State Laws in 1984. The advantage of living wills is that they make wishes explicit. One problem, namely that the best interests may change, will be discussed in the section on dementia. Appointment of a surrogate has the advantage of allowing more flexibility but may not always lead to the care the patient would have wanted. Because surrogate laws need not refer to specifics, they are less politically controversial and therefore easier to pass. Currently, at least 47 states have living will statutes, and 50 allow the appointment of surrogates.[7,17,28,40] However, although up to 75% of patients lack decision-making capacity when such choices are required, only about 1 in 10 patients have created advanced directives, and there is a great need for educational efforts to inform people about their rights and options in this regard.[40,89] To correct this problem, Congress in 1990 passed the Federal Patient Self Determination Act, which mandated policies about advanced directives, education of staff, and documentation for a variety of institutions.[28,64]

In many instances, there are no advanced directives, either because the patient neglected to indicate them or was never able to draft any because of limited mental ability. Other patients may deny the severity of medical problems or refuse to consider their mortality and so have not discussed this issue.[8] In these circumstances, substituted judgment based on the patient's prior expressed preferences is required. This is by convention and law given to someone with power of attorney, a guardian, spouse, adult children, parents, and other relatives (typically in that order).[8] If the wishes of the patient are not known, the decisions should be made in the patient's best interests based on quality of life as judged by others. It is now well-established that in circumstances approved by the physician and society, the surrogate can elect to withhold or withdraw care, including nutrition and water.[7]

The next question is what to do when futile treatment is requested. The Hastings Center Guidelines (1981) suggest that patient well-being, autonomy, the moral integrity of the professional, and justice be considered in decisions to forgo treatment. Useful treatment is indicated, but futile treatment is not. In an era of increasing limitations of resources, the issue of demands for inappropriate care must be resolved.

The definition of what is futile is complex, but in general it means something that is of no ultimate value to the patient because it is unable to achieve its physiologic objective. It involves the quality (consideration of sentience, suffering) and duration of life, as well as the concept of certainty of prognosis. Judgment is in part subjective and may take into account the needs of others, as in the case of allocation of scarce resources. It is also concerned with the rights of individuals and families to request care, and the right of the physician to refuse inappropriate

care. Whereas the patient (or surrogate) generally has the right to refuse care unless this adversely affects others, it is not logical to permit requests for useless and expensive care, particularly if paid for by others. This problem has been made more worrisome by the Wanglie case (1991), in which a court in Minneapolis mandated useless care for a vegetative patient because the husband requested it. Thus, although physicians are said to have the right to stop futile care, there is no standard or consensus or law to protect them in a conflict with a family in such circumstances. It has been suggested that guidelines be developed to guide such decisions, that physicians be empowered more, that outside parties participate in decision-making, and that an effort be made to keep such cases out of the courts.[58,67] The neurosurgeon should provide information to help patients and families make individual decisions and should encourage societal solutions for this problem.

Expensive Care and Scarce Resources

Allocation of resources requires consideration of how much money society wants to devote to medical care and, of the total amount, who is to get what. Many societies clearly have limited the funds for medicine, which in the United States has been done only in a fragmented ad hoc fashion. Similarly, determination of who gets what portions of health care dollars has not been discussed comprehensively. Attempts to do so, such as that in Oregon, have been unsuccessful. On the other hand, many parties including payers, hospital administrators and lawyers, and government watchdogs are intruding into patient-physician decision-making and influencing that decision-making based on considerations of cost as well as perceived benefits and risks. Ethics committees can act as patient advocates and counterbalance inappropriate rulings.[28,60] Recent work of interest involves how to determine the dollar value of medical interventions in terms of years of functional life and satisfaction, how much different members of society are owed and should request, and what they are willing to pay for themselves and for others.[2,14]

Transplants, which are facilitated by neurosurgeons and are therefore an area of interest, are an example of a scarce resource, and trying to decide which needy person will be offered an organ is a great problem. Medical and social issues are considered, and a system for sharing on a national level has been developed under the National Organ Transplantation Act (1984). But the issue is still problematic. ICU beds are a scarce resource we need for our patients. ICUs consume 12 to 20 billion dollars a year, one-fifth of hospital resources, and 1% of the gross national product, and still at times there are insufficient beds. This can lead to conflicts when trying to decide who is given a bed, particularly where care may be futile. If, on the one hand, patients and families may wish to have a bed although its use is not medically or morally appropriate, physicians should discourage this. On the other hand, this is where physicians must act as the patient's advocate if it appears necessary. There are many other technologies in short supply where prioritization takes place. To avoid requiring physicians to compromise the care of their patients, one author suggests that expert arbiters aid in decision-making.[28] But a national discussion about developing criteria for prioritization and mechanisms for doing this is necessary. The neurosurgeon should avoid engaging in such prioritization of resources at the bedside of individual patients, where the physician is first and foremost an advocate for the patient's well-being, and is viewed as such by the patient, family, and administrators.

Suicide

The neurosurgeon may be concerned with suicide in several circumstances: 1) in a patient who may be suicidal, where preventive action is indicated; 2) in a patient who may request help in carrying out suicide, where a response must be made; and 3) in a victim of a suicide attempt, such as a self-inflicted gunshot wound to the head, where care is required; but all require consideration of the appropriateness of the act.

Since suicide occurs 30,000 times a year in the United States and is the eighth cause of death, it is a major issue. Suicide is discouraged in the Judeo-Christian tradition, except in unusual circumstances, and is generally rejected in part because of the fear of death.[44] The state has an interest in preserving life, and therefore it has been agreed that it is traditionally bad policy for society to take a permissive approach. Suicide may be made a criminal act by state law, and this is the case in a number of states, but the law has not to date been fully invoked in the United States.[102] Suicide is often the result of correctable circumstances, and therefore prevention and treatment are generally indicated. Current discussion involves condoning suicide under certain circumstances, although criteria have not been fully discussed or agreed upon. The physician should usually encourage the patient to live, except in such cases as discussed below.

Suicide has been described as self-inflicted, self-intended cessation of life. Suicide is an act carried out to remove oneself from an unbearable situation and is characterized by feelings of helplessness and hopelessness. It is the result of the conjunction of three factors: the individual's personality, the general situation, and the specific problem leading to the act. The demographics of suicide speak to these factors. Suicide is particularly common among white males. The rate increases with age (as does the success rate), and since the population is aging, it is expected that the numbers will increase. Suicide is more common after the loss of a spouse by death or divorce, and is less likely when there are children under the age of 18 years at home. While social isolation and physical decline are obviously significant, underlying mental illness is also an important factor. For example, a major depression has been identified in 40% to 60% of victims, chronic alcoholism in 20%, schizophrenia in 10%, and a personality disorder in 9%. A previous suicide attempt has been noted in 7%.

The problem is that while, in retrospect, 80% of victims gave clues to their intent, only 20% of suicides were recognized in advance, and more research is required to understand who is at risk.[13] Still, if a patient is suspected of being suicidal, the physician should facilitate treatment of depression and improvement in the patient's environment.[13] Often, much also can be done to deal with the cause of stress, for example, aggressive pain control for a cancer victim, an area of interest to neurosurgeons.

However, at times when, as in debilitating or terminal disease, suffering cannot be relieved, suicide then may be considered "rational."[22] The circumstances in which assisted suicide or a request for euthanasia have been thought, at least by some, to be appropriate will be discussed below.

When faced with an attempted suicide (for neurosurgeons, generally a self-inflicted gunshot wound to the head), if we accept that the underlying depression can be treated and if we can hope to benefit a patient by care, we obviously should do so. Therefore the judgment to treat should be based on the prognosis of the injury itself.

Physician-Assisted Death: Assisted Suicide and Euthanasia

As medical technology developed methods to support vegetative functions, there arose circumstances in which treatment only extended an agonizing life and prolonged dying. As mentioned, under such circumstances it is generally accepted that the patient (or a surrogate) can request that care be withheld or withdrawn. A logical extension of this right of self-determination is to permit the patient (or a surrogate) to request help from the physician to hasten dying, and it has been suggested that this might even be part of the physician's duty to the patient.[50] This assistance could range from the giving of medication which in addition to relieving pain and suffering might also hasten death (double effect), to giving information about suicide or even helping at suicide (assisted suicide), to overtly ending the patient's life (euthanasia). But it has been suggested that assisting death is morally different from allowing death to occur by withholding or withdrawing care, and that assisting death would have adverse ethical and legal consequences.[14,50,58,63,76] This controversial subject has been colored by the Nazi excesses in the Holocaust as well as by other attempts at "ethnic cleansing."

The most basic issue involves resolving differences of opinion about the meaning of life. The secular argument is that needless suffering is not in the patient's best interest, that the patient has the right to ask that this be stopped, and that the physician is the person who has the expertise and thus the obligation to carry out the patient's wishes. Legally, if there are conditions under which suicide is acceptable, a second person should not be liable for helping someone exercise that right.[8] Several authors have discussed the idea of a constitutional right to die.[29,91] Dworkin[29] talks about the meaning of life to the individual—when does it become so burdensome as to be intolerable?—and suggests that the individual be permitted to choose death.

In traditional religious terms, life is sacred, a gift of God, and suffering is a part of life and growth.[24,64] Jewish and Roman Catholic teachings generally oppose suicide and assisted death, while Protestant doctrine may be more flexible. Another point is that the patient can use dying to set an example for others. In the words of Petrarch: "A good death does honor a whole life."[45] In secular terms, Callahan[16] states that the premature ending of life deprives the individual of the possibility of growth and understanding, and should not be necessary if a patient is given the proper emotional and physical care. It also has been suggested that in a just society, the dying should not have to be concerned about being a personal and financial burden, which might compel them to ask for help in dying. Most states have laws forbidding assisted suicide. However, this is being reconsidered. Euthanasia is not accepted in any state.

At the present time, assisting death is generally considered beyond the professional and moral rights of the physician. Callahan[16] fears that "private killing," giving one person power over another, could be distorted and too easily extended, for example, to the mentally incompetent or anyone who was depressed. Also, if physicians were to participate in euthanasia, this would be a breach of trust, would desensitize them to the value of human life, and would take them down a "slippery slope" to killing in other circumstances. Even assuming acceptance of physician-assisted death in principle, there are many other problems. Prognosis may be wrong or a new cure may be developed, so treatment may be of benefit. In the case of a debilitating but nonterminal illness, the state may have a special interest in limiting suicide.[91]

Interest in assisted suicide has been increased by the activist approach of Dr. Jack Kevorkian. It has been suggested that Kevorkian has not fully informed his patients of alternatives nor given proper care. However, he has stated that at one point he turned down 57 of 60 applicants.[24] On the other hand, when Dr. Timothy Quill prescribed barbiturates to a terminal patient long known to him so she could commit suicide when her life became unbearable, this action received widespread approval.[15,81-83] Agreeing that depression must be recognized and treated, Dr. Quill has argued that there are times when death is the only way to relieve suffering. He has pointed out that fear of facing an agonizing death with no way of controlling pain can distract the patient from enjoying his remaining good days, and that it is humiliating to a patient to have to beg for help in dying. But assisted suicide is illegal in at least 36 states, there are religious proscriptions against it, it can cause guilt in the family, and it can invalidate insurance policies.

There are some patients who cannot end their own lives because of physical or mental incapacity. Dr. Quill[82] recommended that we reconsider aiding death if requested (voluntary euthanasia) because there may be times when life is unbearable but when a patient cannot act alone.

Then there is the issue of patients who do not have the mental capacity because of youth, retardation, or dementia to make such decisions. They may or may not be aware, and they may or may not be suffering. The criteria for euthanasia and who would make the decision require extensive deliberation.[14,102] A related issue is what to do in the case of a mentally incompetent patient who, when still competent, expressed a wish not to live if dementia developed. This will be discussed later.

At this time, public support favors voluntary active suicide and less so assisted suicide, although physicians have expressed mixed feelings.[24,40,76,82] Indeed, attempts made in Oregon (1991) and California (1992) to pass laws allowing assisted suicide and voluntary euthanasia were defeated due to campaigns by medical groups. However, such laws likely will be passed in the near future.

Much can be learned from the Dutch experience with euthanasia.[7,24,64,82] The issue was addressed seriously after Dr. Schoonheim, who had been convicted for the euthanasia of Mrs. Barendregt, was exonerated by the Dutch Supreme Court in 1976. The Dutch Medical Association drew up guidelines in 1984, there was a report of a State Commission on Euthanasia (1985), and there were a number of court decisions, all of which agreed that euthanasia was appropriate under specific circumstances. Initially, each case had to be reported and investigated. This led to underreporting, so in 1991 the rules were changed so that prosecutors could review the case and elect not to investigate. However, there is no legislation legalizing euthanasia, and the situation is still ambiguous in theory. The Dutch rules approve euthanasia for an incurable disease with unbearable mental or physical suffering, no other solution, a voluntary and persistent request, and concurrence of a second physician. The patient need not be terminal. By 1988, 81% of Dutch citizens favored the practice.

A recent Dutch survey suggested that of 129,000 deaths a year, 2300 involved active euthanasia and 400 were assisted suicides. One-thousand of these lives were terminated without request, but 50% of the patients had discussed this previously, and in all but two cases another professional or the family was consulted. Seventy percent of euthanasia patients were expected to die within 1 week, and only 10% in more than 3 months. The underlying disease was most often cancer (83%), severe neurologic disease such as multiple sclerosis or amyotrophic lateral sclerosis (10%), or AIDS. The reasons for the request were most commonly weakness and exhaustion, physical dependence, loss of dignity, and disfigurement. Severe pain was a less common factor, although it also has been suggested that sophistication in pain control and other aspects of terminal care is limited.[24] Eighty-eight percent of physicians reported willingness to carry out euthanasia, but 50% of those had not done so. Morphine was the most common drug used for euthanasia, although barbiturates and curare were recommended, so in many cases the primary goal may have been to kill pain. Interestingly, 50% of requests were not honored. Only 2% of deaths were assisted, and only in very circumscribed situations. Failure to consult with a colleague, lack of reporting, and killing patients without their consent is problematic.

One of the strongest arguments against a liberal policy on assisted death involves the possibility of improving care of terminal patients who suffer from feelings of helplessness and hopelessness, and, particularly, from lack of pain control. The importance of this problem is apparent since 50% of all deaths are the result of a chronic disease with a terminal phase, and 80% of all deaths occur in a hospital. Since people are afraid of suffering, their psychological and physical needs must be attended to. Additionally, they wish to die at home. One of the major chronic diseases is cancer, causing over 500,000 deaths a year, one-half in those over 65 years of age.

One possible solution is hospice care, which costs one-fourth as much as hospital care and is much more appropriate. The modern hospice movement, initiated by Dr. Cicely Saunders in England in the 1960s, provides comprehensive services to the patient and family including emotional support and pain control mainly at home, with short stays in nursing homes and hospitals. Of those receiving hospice care, 90% die at home, the average time after entry into a hospice program being about 2 months. In 1983, Medicare and in 1987, Medicaid funds were approved for hospice care, but funding is low and services are not well-developed. Although hospice care is a better and cheaper alternative to current terminal care, only about 200,000 people in the United States received hospice care in 1992.[24,32] More research and training in this area are required, as well as the expansion of the current system, and this could obviate the need to consider assisted suicide and euthanasia by providing a period of life during its terminal phase that is tolerable and useful.

More specifically, studies of cancer patients have shown that pain control is often inadequate. On the other hand, recent guidelines such as those from the Agency for Health Care Policy and Research can be used to optimize pain control.[47] In England, only 1% of patients in hospice care have poorly controlled pain.[24]

One comprehensive approach was proposed by Heifitz,[44] who categorized patients and suggested the following: 1) competent patients who are physically able should be allowed to commit suicide (and not ask someone to assume any burden for them); 2) competent patients unable physically to commit suicide should be able to request euthanasia; 3) patients in a permanent vegetative state, since they would not suffer from lack of food or water, should have care withdrawn; 4) retarded handicapped newborns should have euthanasia since withdrawing care would cause suffering; 5) retarded children and adults who are unaware of relationships have no interest in living and are a burden on others and could have euthanasia; and 6) retarded children and adults who are aware of relationships should have care. A knowledgeable second party should evaluate all patients. Physicians should not be required to perform euthanasia if they do not want to. He acknowledges that euthanasia has been abused in situations where it was widely permitted.

Dworkin[29] concludes that the issue of controlling one's fate ". . . involves decisions not just about the rights and interests of particular people, but about the intrinsic, cosmic importance of human life itself. In each case, opinions divide not because some people have contempt for values that others cherish, but, on the contrary, because the values in question are at the center of everyone's lives, and no one can treat them as trivial enough to accept other people's orders about what they mean. Making someone die in a way that others approve, but he believes a horrifying contradiction of his life, is a devastating, odious form of tyranny."

Dementia

The conquest of many medical problems has led to the emergence of others as major societal problems. Dementia, particularly Alzheimer's disease, is an example.[10] Although there are over 50 recognized causes of dementia, Alzheimer's disease is responsible for the overwhelming number of cases, now estimated as high as 4 million, with one-third to one-half requiring continuous or nursing home care and accounting for one-half to two-thirds of those in nursing homes. Aggregate costs for these patients have been estimated at over $80 billion.

The disease occurs with increased incidence

TABLE 3
**Estimate of Increased Occurrence of
Alzheimer's With Age**

Age	Percent of Cases
< 65 years	< 1%
65 to 74 years	1%
75 to 85 years	7% to 16%
> 85 years	25% to 48%

with age, with estimates in the ranges noted in Table 3. Since those over 85 years of age constitute the fastest growing segment of our population, it has been further estimated that in less than 50 years, there possibly will be over 12 million Alzheimer's victims whose care costs will total about 150 billion dollars. The issue of how to provide for the current and future victims of dementia is obviously a crucial problem.

To make such determinations requires considerations of the nature of dementia; the rights (and perhaps obligations) of its victims, their families, and our entire society; how to streamline appropriate care; and how to mobilize resources for that care.[10]

Dementia involves deterioration of cognitive and behavioral function to the point where patients are unaware of their plight and even surroundings, and are unable to care for themselves. The disease is insidious in onset, and slow and variable in course. Depending on the patient and the realization of the problem, it may or may not include great fear and suffering, but this is sometimes difficult to determine. In fact, for a long period, the patient may be able to experience considerable pleasure in many aspects of life and thus deserves aggressive medical treatment. During further decline, the patient has certain rights, and the person always has value. The patient always deserves care, relief of suffering, and to be treated with respect and dignity. On the other hand, when there is no benefit from the medical treatment, either because the dementia has proceeded to the point where the mind is completely destroyed or there is a disease in which the burdens of treatment outweigh possible benefits, the patient has the right not to be treated. Indeed, intergenerational jus-

tice mandates that resources not be wasted on such treatment. But determination of that state remains a problem.[10,14]

Society must concentrate on how the disease can be prevented and treated, what services a patient will require, how these services can be provided most efficiently, and how to pay for them. In 1990, a total of only 140 million dollars was devoted to research into Alzheimer's disease, and this needs to be increased. There is a current lack of coverage for the care of such patients in both private and government programs, which needs to be increased, perhaps even by increased taxation specifically for this purpose. While families currently provide a large portion of care, the money and personnel to do this will decline. Better understanding and acceptance by the populace of the value and reward of such care must be emphasized. And it must be decided if use of the patient's own funds is indicated.[10]

One interesting argument revolves around advance directives. Either before or after learning of the disease, the patient may set limits on care, and because of the right of autonomy, should be able to do so. However, it has been argued that since treatment in the early stages of dementia can be in the patient's best interest and lead to improved quality of life (which is a benefit), there should be limits to this autonomy and it should be reconsidered and renegotiated with the patient and/or family periodically. This care must be individualized based on each patient's previous wishes, those of their families and other surrogates who know them well, and the burdens and benefits of treatments required as different medical problems arise.[10]

Last is the issue of what to do at the point when the decision is made that no treatment is indicated. Certainly, withholding and withdrawing treatment, including food and water, is currently accepted as appropriate. But the effect of this and how it can be done most aesthetically needs to be discussed.[10,40] This also raises the possibility of euthanasia, which is currently not ethically or legally acceptable. For it to be accepted, both criteria of a level of dementia and a process for determining that level would have to be evolved, as well as a method for euthanasia that is acceptable to society and particularly to those who would need to practice it.[10]

Aging

The demographics of the country are changing with regard to the number and percentage of people over 65 years of age. This group has been growing steadily, now numbering 30 million people who are 12% of the population. Their number may double in the next 40 years, especially the very old (aged 85 years or older), the number of whom will increase from 3 million to over 20 million. More than one-half of the elderly are females, of whom one-half are widows. While in general the elderly are gaining in affluence, the women are less affluent.

Many older people, because of mental or physical deterioration, have lives of limited quality. Of those over 65 years of age, 2 million are in nursing facilities, and 7 million will spend some time in these. Eighty percent of nursing home inhabitants have mental impairment, 50% of those due to Alzheimer's disease. While in a nursing home they are constrained by rules, and 50% by physical or chemical restraints.[28]

In the United States today, one-third of the federal budget goes to aid older people, essentially creating a welfare state for the elderly. The older 12% of the population accounts for 50% of deaths and consumes 30% of all health care expenditures, especially as they age, particularly in the last year and especially in the last month of life. If current trends continue, the cost of their medical care will continue to rise, and this will be further increased by the ongoing development of new technologies.[40,109]

The growing number of elderly individuals, both vigorous and impaired, in a time of limited resources is forcing them to consider what they want and society to consider what is their due.[14] There are many societal needs, including food, housing, and education, as well as health care, and within medicine, a variety of needs by generations, such as immunizations for children, maternal and trauma care for young adults, and cancer and geriatric care for older individuals. As medical advances have increased life expectancy, there is now the question of how to make these lives meaningful, both to the individual and to society. It has been suggested that more research should be done on the disabling diseases of the elderly, namely Alzheimer's, os-

teoarthritis, osteoporosis, hearing and vision problems, Parkinson's disease, and adult onset diabetes.[109] It should be remembered that the mental dysfunction often seen with various ailments is reversible.[28] Another issue is how to determine the effectiveness of such treatments as CPR, enteral feeding, and dialysis.[109]

Each generation has its own interests, rights, and obligations. The elderly have an interest in living as long as they are sentient, and indeed may continue to grow mentally and spiritually: ". . . the intrinsic capacity for the human being to set new goals, to reconceive the self and what its integrity might mean. This is . . . a matter of meaning, and meaning is at the heart of the ideal of integrity."[66] Also, as members of the human community, they have a right to expect respect, humane treatment, and repayment for their contributions in working and raising families. On the other hand, it is in their best interests to learn to meet death with equanimity. In the words of a Middle Eastern proverb, "The beginning of wisdom comes when a person plants a tree, the shade under which he knows he will never sit." And, having had the opportunity for a full life, they should not make unreasonable demands that compromise the welfare of other generations. Thus, there must be an "ethics of responsibility" with a limit on expectations. Indeed, many elderly do not wish aggressive care with discomfort and little chance of success.[109]

One suggestion, on the basis of intergenerational justice, is to ration care purely on the basis of age. This could be economically quite effective. As stated in the Woody Allen film *Love and Death:* "Death's a great way to cut down on expenses." However, even as the originators of this concept have pointed out, the obvious need to make frequent exceptions to such a rule makes it too simplistic. Another suggestion is to develop a system for allocation of resources rather than rationing. This would require cost/benefit analysis so that reasonable treatment would be given as opposed to very expensive care that only helped a little or treatment that did not lead to high-quality life.[66,109] Discussion of such options must be done publicly in order to set fair guidelines based on trust and solidarity so that all generations will buy into the system.[66] Considerations may include place in the queue, potential quality of life, and, to a lesser extent, value to society, and will have to include allocation decisions for all generations.[44] Extensive societal and political debate is currently underway regarding these controversial issues.

Dangerous Patients

Patients may be dangerous to treat for a variety of reasons. They may be violent or have a communicable disease. Traditionally, no citizen must put himself or herself at risk for another, but physicians are clearly different. They voluntarily choose their profession, and thereby accept its ethical and legal obligations. By law, a physician must treat in an emergency and must not abandon a patient.[2]

The most common dangerous patient today is one with AIDS. Risk of contracting this disease, although less than 1% per exposure, can be minimized by universal precautions, but cannot be totally eliminated, and infection is a death sentence. The question arises as to what the obligations of the physician are when faced with an AIDS patient who will die soon no matter what is done. The arguments for allowing a physician not to treat an AIDS patient involve the physician's autonomy, the question of risk of a disease that will destroy one's life as well as that of one's family, and the fact that most patients with AIDS have contracted it because of self-destructive behavior and therefore physicians should not have to take a risk for such people. The argument for assuming this risk is one's personal commitment to service, the right of people to health care and therefore an obligation of physicians to provide this, the trust of society which must be fulfilled, and one's collegial responsibility to share risks so that they are not concentrated in a few physicians.[85] The issue of responsibility to such patients has never been fully resolved, but professional responsibility was enunciated by the Council on Ethical and Judicial Affairs of the AMA in 1987, which stated that physicians cannot refuse to treat patients because they are seropositive. This was codified in the Disabilities Act of 1990.

Conclusion

Callahan[16] points out that while death is a natural event, it is unique, irrevocable, and complete—a threat to our desire to live and to our social lives. He advocates "trying to understand how we should live with our mortality and how medicine should help us do so." He urges us to accept pain and suffering if necessary, although to minimize this in order to have a "tame death." Indeed, he notes that death in circumstances where there is suffering and in which one no longer has the ability mentally or physically to function is a lesser evil than living. On the other hand, he notes that we can experience and grow to the very end, and that we have obligations to others to set an example in the way we die as they have an obligation to care for us. Thus, we should not give up life easily, but on the other hand should meet death with "self-possession" when it comes. He states that we should "leave open the possibility that we can live in such a way that death has an appropriate, and therefore meaningful, place in our being." He concludes: ". . . death is a part of life, to be accepted, and the grief that goes with it, to be endured." He states that the goals of medicine should be to ensure a good life and a peaceful death.

Since there are many conflicts in our society about dying and death, it is necessary to continue to try to reason out the issues and to try to reach accommodations. The argument that any revision of current policy starts one down a slippery slope is questionable since it would prevent change. Conflicts must be addressed to fulfill our needs and to prevent extreme reactions such as the violence that has been seen in the abortion controversy.

Callahan[16] put the current status of bioethics in perspective:

> How was the acceptance of bioethics in fact gained? I would say that the first thing those in bioethics had to do . . . was to push religion aside. It was clear that the physician as sole decision maker would have to give way to a more complex picture of what moral life is all about. What we began to see was the movement . . . toward a different kind of moral language in the mainstream of public

policy, toward a language of rights, worries about questions of pluralism, efforts to find moral consensus and moral strategies in the face of a diverse cultural situation. . . . Bioethics chose a kind of middle course. That middle course is regulation, regulation being the way we in the United States typically deal with controversial issues. On the one hand you avoid the extreme of simple prohibition of things, while on the other hand you show you are serious and willing to be cautious. What we began to see increasingly was the creation of oversight bodies. . . . The final factor of great importance I would mention was the emergence ideologically of a form of bioethics that dovetailed very nicely with the reigning political liberalism of the educated classes in America.

In recognition of the current absence of a national forum for analyzing ethical issues in medicine, the Congressional Office of Technology Assessment, at the request of Senators Hatfield, Kennedy, and DeConcini, prepared a background paper entitled "Biomedical Ethics in U.S. Public Policy" (1993). They noted the helpfulness of prior federal bodies and the advantages of a well-funded centralized national forum, and made specific suggestions about the factors to be considered in developing one.[104] If properly established, such a forum could be useful in facilitating accommodations on the controversies over dying and death.[2] The neurosurgeon who has always faced these issues at the bedside of individual patients and who possesses a unique philosophic perspective and the command of a vast body of relevant scientific knowledge on death and dying, should aim to play a central and shaping role in the complex and evolving climate of societal consensus and public policy on this subject, which is fundamental to life and to humanity.

References

1. Allen MC, Donohue PK, Dusman AE. The limit of viability: neonatal outcome of infants born at 22 to 25 weeks' gestation. *N Engl J Med.* 1993;329: 1597-1601.
2. Annas GJ. *Standard of Care: The Law of American Bioethics.* New York, NY: Oxford University Press; 1993.
3. Anspach RR. *Deciding Who Lives: Fateful Choices in the Intensive-Care Nursery.* Berkeley, Calif: University of California Press; 1993.
4. Beauchamp TL, Childress JF. *Principles of Biomedical Ethics.* 3rd ed. New York, NY: Oxford University Press; 1989.
5. Beecher HK, Chair. A definition of irreversible coma: report of the Ad Hoc Committee of the Harvard Medical School to examine the definition of brain death. *JAMA.* 1968;205:337-340.
6. Berger A, Badham RP, Kutscher AH, et al, eds. *Perspectives on Death and Dying: Cross-Cultural and Multi-Disciplinary Views.* Philadelphia, Pa: Charles Press; 1989.
7. Berger AS. *Dying & Death in Law & Medicine: A Forensic Primer for Health and Legal Professionals.* Westport, Conn: Praeger; 1993.
8. Berger AS, Berger J, eds. *To Die or Not to Die? Cross-disciplinary, Cultural, and Legal Perspectives on the Right to Choose Death.* New York, NY: Praeger; 1990.
9. Bernstein IM, Watson M, Simmons GM, et al. Maternal brain death and prolonged fetal survival. *Obstet Gynecol.* 1989;74:434-437.
10. Binstock RH, Post SG, Whitehouse PJ, eds. *Dementia and Aging. Ethics, Values, and Policy Choices.* Baltimore, Md: Johns Hopkins University Press; 1992.
11. Black PM. Conceptual and practical issues in the declaration of death by brain criteria. *Neurosurg Clin North Am.* 1991;2:493-501.
12. Blendon RJ, Benson JM, Donelan K. The public and the controversy over abortion. *JAMA.* 1993; 270:2871-2875.
13. Bongar B, ed. *Suicide. Guidelines for Assessment, Management & Treatment.* New York, NY: Oxford University Press; 1992.
14. Brock DW. *Life and Death.* Cambridge, England: Cambridge University Press; 1993.
15. Caine ED, Conwell YC. Self-determined death, the physician, and medical priorities: is there time to talk? *JAMA.* 1993;270:875-876. Editorial.
16. Callahan D. *The Troubled Dream of Life. Living With Mortality.* New York, NY: Simon & Schuster; 1993.
17. Cantor NL. *Advance Directives and the Pursuit of Death with Dignity.* Bloomington, Ind: Indiana University Press; 1993.
18. Caplan A, Siminoff L, Arnold R, et al. Increasing organ and tissue donation: what are the obstacles, what are our options? In: *The Surgeon General's Workshop on Increasing Organ Donation. Background Papers.* Washington, DC: US Department of Health and Human Services; 1991:199-232.
19. Caplan AL, Virnig B. Is altruism enough? Required request and the donation of cadaver organs and tissues in the United States. *Crit Care Clin.* 1990; 6:1007-1018.
20. Childress JF. Protestant perspectives on organ donation. In: Kaufman HH, ed. *Pediatric Brain Death and Organ/Tissue Retrieval.* New York, NY: Plenum Press; 1989:45-53.
21. Churchill LR, Pinkus RLB. The use of anencephalic organs: historical and ethical dimensions. *Milbank Q.* 1990;68:147-169.
22. Cotton P. Rational suicide: no longer "crazy"?

JAMA. 1993;270:797. Medical news and perspectives.

23. Council on Scientific Affairs and Council on Ethical and Judicial Affairs. Persistent vegetative state and the decision to withdraw or withhold life support. *JAMA*. 1990;263:426-430.

24. Cundiff D. *Euthanasia is Not the Answer. A Hospice Physician's View*. Clifton, NJ: Humana Press; 1992.

25. Dagi TF. Death-defining acts: historical and cultural observations on the end of life. In: Kaufman HH, ed. *Pediatric Brain Death and Organ/Tissue Retrieval*. New York, NY: Plenum Press; 1989:1-30.

26. Darby JM, Stein K, Grenvik A, et al. Approach to management of the heartbeating "brain dead" organ donor. *JAMA*. 1989;261:2222-2228.

27. de Villiers JC. Pitfalls and problems in the diagnosis of cerebral death. *Prog Neurol Surg*. 1990;13:180-202.

28. Dubler N, Nimmons D. Ethics on Call. *Taking Charge of Life-and-Death Choices in Today's Health Care System*. New York, NY: Vintage Books; 1993.

29. Dworkin R. *Life's Dominion. An Argument About Abortion, Euthanasia, and Individual Freedom*. New York, NY: Alfred A Knopf; 1993.

30. Emanuel EJ, Emanuel LL. The economics of dying: the illusion of cost savings at the end of life. *N Engl J Med*. 1994;330:540-544.

31. Evans RW, Orians CE, Ascher NL. The potential supply of organ donors: an assessment of the efficiency of organ procurement efforts in the United States. *JAMA*. 1992;267:239-246.

32. Everson LK, Irick N, Iseminger K. Terminal care of the patient with advanced cancer. *Curr Therapy Hematol Oncol*. 1991;4:457-463.

33. Ewigman BG, Crane JP, Frigoletto FD, et al. Effect of prenatal ultrasound screening on perinatal outcome. *N Engl J Med*. 1993;329:821-827.

34. Field DR, Gates EA, Creasy RK, et al. Maternal brain death during pregnancy: medical and ethical issues. *JAMA*. 1988;260:816-822.

35. Fisher CM. Brain death: a review of the concept. *J Neurosci Nurs*. 1991;23:330-333.

36. Fost N. Removing organs from anencephalic infants: ethical and legal considerations. *Clin Perinatol*. 1989;16:331-337.

37. Fox E, Stocking C. Ethics consultants' recommendations for life-prolonging treatment of patients in a persistent vegetative state. *JAMA*. 1993;270:2578-2582.

38. The Gallup Organization, Inc. *The American Public's Attitudes Toward Organ Donation and Transplantation*. Boston, Mass: The Partnership for Organ Donation; February 1993.

39. Gillon R. Death. *J Med Ethics*. 1990;16:3-4. Editorial.

40. Glick HR. *The Right to Die. Policy Innovation and Its Consequences*. New York, NY: Columbia University Press; 1992.

41. Halevy A, Brody B. Brain death: reconciling definitions, criteria, and tests. *Ann Intern Med*. 1993;119:519-525.

42. Hastings Center. *Guidelines on the Termination of Life-Sustaining Treatment and the Care of the Dying*. Briar-

cliff, NY: The Hastings Center; 1987.

43. Hastings Center. Anencephalic infants: a source of controversy. *Hastings Cent Rep*. October/November 1988;18:5-33.

44. Heifitz MD. *Easier Said Than Done: Moral Decisions in Medical Uncertainty*. Buffalo, NY: Prometheus Books; 1992.

45. Hill TP, Shirley D. *A Good Death. Taking More Control at the End of Your Life*. Reading, Mass: Addison-Wesley; 1992.

46. Humber JM, Almeder RF, eds. *Bioethics and the Fetus. Medical, Moral and Legal Issues*. Clifton, NJ: Humana Press; 1991.

47. Jacox A, Carr DB, Payne R. New clinical-practice guidelines for the management of pain in patients with cancer. *N Engl J Med*. 1994;330:651-655.

48. Jayes RL, Zimmerman JE, Wagner DP, et al. Do-not-resuscitate orders in intensive care units: current practices and recent changes. *JAMA*. 1993;270:2213-2217.

49. Jonsen AR. The birth of bioethics. *Hastings Cent Rep*. November/December 1993;23(suppl):S1-S4.

50. Kamisar Y. Are laws against assisted suicide unconstitutional? *Hastings Cent Rep*. May/June 1993;23:32-41.

51. Kaufman HH, ed. *Pediatric Brain Death and Organ/Tissue Retrieval: Medical, Ethical, and Legal Aspects*. New York, NY: Plenum Press; 1989.

52. Kaufman HH, Lynn J. Brain death. *Neurosurgery*. 1986;19:850-856.

53. Kennedy Institute of Ethics. *Kennedy Inst of Ethics J*. 1993;3:103-278.

54. Keyes CD, Wiest WE, eds. *New Harvest. Transplanting Body Parts and Reaping the Benefits*. Clifton, NJ: Humana Press; 1991.

55. Kohrman MH, Spivak BS. Brain death in infants: sensitivity and specificity of current criteria. *Pediatr Neurol*. 1990;6:47-50.

56. Korein J. The diagnosis of brain death. *Semin Neurol*. 1984;4:52-72.

57. Lange SS. Psychosocial, legal, ethical, and cultural aspects of organ donation and transplantation. *Crit Care Nurs Clin North Am*. 1992;4:25-42.

58. Law, Medicine & Health Care. Medical futility. *J Law Med Health Care*. 1992;20:307-339.

59. Lynn J. Brain death: historical perspectives and current concerns. In: Kaufman HH, ed. *Pediatric Brain Death and Organ/Tissue Retrieval. Medical, Ethical, and Legal Aspects*. New York, NY: Plenum Press; 1989:65-72.

60. Macklin R. *Enemies of Patients*. New York, NY: Oxford University Press; 1993.

61. Medical Consultants on the Diagnosis of Death. Guidelines for the determination of death: report of the Medical Consultants on the Diagnosis of Death to the President's Commission for the Study of Ethical Problems in Medicine and Biomedical and Behavioral Research. *JAMA*. 1981;246:2184-2186.

62. Medical Task Force on Anencephaly. The infant with anencephaly. *N Engl J Med*. 1990;322:669-674.

63. Meisel A. The legal consensus about forgoing life-sustaining treatment: its status and its prospects. *Kennedy Inst Ethics J.* 1993;2:309-345.

64. Misbin RI, ed. Euthanasia. *The Good of the Patient—The Good of Society.* Frederick, Md: University Publishing Group; 1992.

65. Mollaret P, Goulon M. Le coma dépassé. *Rev Neurol (Paris).* 1959;101:3-15.

66. Moody HR. *Ethics in an Aging Society.* Baltimore, Md: Johns Hopkins University Press; 1992.

67. Morreim EH. Profoundly diminished life. The casualties of coercion. *Hastings Cent Rep.* 1994;24:33-42.

68. Murphy DJ, Burrows D, Santilli S, et al. The influence of the probability of survival on patients' preferences regarding cardiopulmonary resuscitation. *N Engl J Med.* 1994;330:545-549.

69. Novello AC. From the surgeon general, US Public Health Service: increasing organ donation. *JAMA.* 1992;267:213.

70. Nuutinen LS, Alahuhta SM, Heikkinen JE. Nutrition during ten-week life support with successful fetal outcome in a case with fatal maternal brain damage. *JPEN J Parenter Enteral Nutr.* 1989;13:432-435.

71. Olson CM, ed. Diagnostic and therapeutic technology assessment (DATTA): lung transplantation. *JAMA.* 1993;269:931-936.

72. Pallis C. Brainstem death: the evolution of a concept. *Semin Thorac Cardiovasc Surg.* 1990;2:135-152.

73. Paris JJ. Catholic considerations of brain death and organ retrieval. In: Kaufman HH, ed. *Pediatric Brain Death and Organ/Tissue Retrieval: Medical, Ethical and Legal Aspects.* New York, NY: Plenum Press; 1989:35-43.

74. Parisi JE, Kim RC, Collins GH, et al. Brain death with prolonged somatic survival. *N Engl J Med.* 1982;306:14-16.

75. Patterson DR, Miller-Perrin C, McCormick TR, et al. When life support is questioned early in the care of patients with cervical-level quadriplegia. *N Engl J Med* 1993;328:506-509. Sounding board.

76. Pellegrino ED. Compassion needs reason too. *JAMA.* 1993;270:874-875. Commentary.

77. Pernick MS. Back from the grave: recurring controversies over defining and diagnosing death in history. In: Zaner RM, ed. *Death: Beyond Whole-Brain Criteria.* Boston, Mass: Kluwer Academic; 1988:17-74.

78. President's Commission for the Study of Ethical Problems in Medicine and Biomedical and Behavioral Research, ed. *Defining Death: A Report on the Medical, Legal, and Ethical issues in the Determination of Death.* Washington, DC: US Government Printing Office; 1981.

79. Public Health Service. *The Surgeon General's Workshop on Increasing Organ Donation: Proceedings.* Washington, DC: US Department of Health and Human Services; 1991.

80. Purves D. Book review of Dennett DC, *Consciousness Explained,* 1991. *Science.* 1992;257:1291-1292.

81. Quill TE. The ambiguity of clinical intentions. *N Engl J Med.* 1993;329:1039-1040. Occasional notes.

82. Quill TE. *Death and Dignity. Making Choices and Taking Charge.* New York, NY: WW Norton & Co; 1993.

83. Quill TE. Doctor, I want to die. Will you help me? *JAMA.* 1993;270:870-873. Special communications.

84. Randall T. Too few human organs for transplantation, too many in need . . . and the gap widens. *JAMA.* 1991;265:1223,1227. Medical news and perspectives.

85. Reamer FG, ed. *AIDS and Ethics.* New York, NY: Columbia University Press; 1991.

86. Rivers EP, Buse SM, Bivins BA, et al. Organ and tissue procurement in the acute care setting, I: principles and practice. *Ann Emerg Med.* 1990;19:78-85.

87. Rivers EP, Buse SM, Bivins BA, et al. Organ and tissue procurement in the acute care setting, II: principles and practice. *Ann Emerg Med.* 1990;19:193-200.

88. Rothenberg LS. The anencephalic neonate and brain death: an international review of medical, ethical, and legal issues. *Transplant Proc.* 1990;22:1037-1039.

89. Rubin SM, Strull WM, Fialkow MF, et al. Increasing the completion of the durable power of attorney for health care: a randomized, controlled trial. *JAMA.* 1994;271:209-212.

90. Schneiderman LJ, Kaplan RM, Pearlman RA, et al. Do physicians' own preferences for life-sustaining treatment influence their perceptions of patients' preferences? *J Clin Ethics.* 1993;4:28-33.

91. Sedler RA. The Constitution and hastening inevitable death. *Hastings Cent Rep.* September/October 1993;23:20-25.

92. Shewmon DA. The probability of inevitability: the inherent impossibility of validating criteria for brain death or "irreversibility" through clinical studies. *Stat Med.* 1987;6:535-553.

93. Shewmon DA, Capron AM, Peacock WJ, et al. The use of anencephalic infants as organ sources; a critique. *JAMA.* 1989;261:1773-1781.

94. Simpson JA, Weiner ESC, eds. *The Oxford English Dictionary.* 2nd ed. New York, NY: Oxford University Press; 1989:11

95. Smith-Morris M, ed. *The Economist. Book of Vital World Statistics. A Complete Guide to the World in Figures.* London, England: Hutchinson; 1990.

96. Spital A. The shortage of organs for transplantation: where do we go from here? *N Engl J Med.* 1991;325:1243-1246. Sounding board.

97. Spital A. Mandated choice: the preferred solution to the organ shortage? *Arch Intern Med.* 1992;152:2421-2424.

98. Steinbock B. *Life Before Birth: The Moral and Legal Status of Embryos and Fetuses.* New York, NY: Oxford University Press; 1992.

99. Tendler M. A Jewish approach to ethical issues in brain death and organ transplantation. In: Kaufman HH, ed. *Pediatric Brain Death and Organ/Tissue Retrieval: Medical, Ethical and Legal Aspects.* New

York, NY: Plenum Press; 1989:31-34.

100. Truog RD. Do-not-resuscitate orders during anesthesia and surgery. *Anesthesiology.* 1991;74:606-608.

101. Turner DA, Kearney W. Scientific and ethical concerns in neural fetal tissue transplantation. *Neurosurgery.* 1993;33:1031-1037.

102. Urofsky MI. *Letting Go: Death, Dying & the Law.* New York, NY: Macmillan; 1993.

103. US Bureau of the Census, ed. *Statistical Abstract of the United States: 1992.* 112th ed. Washington, DC: US Bureau of the Census; 1992.

104. US Congress, Office of Technology Assessment. *Biomedical Ethics in U.S. Public Policy—Background Paper.* Washington, DC: US Government Printing Office; 1993: OTA-BP-BBS-105.

105. Veatch RM. Routine inquiry about organ donation: an alternative to presumed consent. *N Engl J Med.* 1991;325:1246-1249. Sounding board.

106. Veatch RM. The impending collapse of the whole-brain definition of death. *Hastings Cent Rep.* July/August 1993;23:18-24.

107. Walker AE, coordinator. An appraisal of the criteria of cerebral death: a summary statement. A collaborative study. *JAMA.* 1977;237:982-986.

108. Walker AE, ed. *Cerebral Death.* 3rd ed. Baltimore, Md: Urban & Schwarzenberg; 1985.

109. Winslow GR, Walters JW, eds. *Facing Limits: Ethics and Health Care for the Elderly.* Boulder, Colo: Westview Press; 1993.

110. Youngner SJ, Arnold RM. Ethical, psychosocial, and public policy implications of procuring organs from non-heart-beating cadaver donors. *JAMA.* 1993;269:2769-2774.

111. Zaner RM. Introduction. In: Zaner RM, ed. *Death: Beyond Whole-Brain Criteria.* Boston, Mass: Kluwer Academic; 1988:1-14.

CHAPTER 9

Neurological Surgery and Biologic Science

Dennis D. Spencer, MD

Discovery: a seeing or learning of something for the first time (*The World Book Dictionary*); a phenomenon at the core of that part of the human spirit that strives continuously to unravel the unknown and so improve the lot of humans.[13] *Creativity:* a bringing forth of something original; may involve expressing new literature, art, music, or a scientific theorem as a private expression of a universal experience. The individuality of creativity and the theme of relentless search resulting in discovery are linked by similar definitions. In Kant's terms, creativity is imagination and the expression of that imagination.[10] In science, imagination leading to discovery may be the best metaphor for developing a hypothesis: "Imagine if injury to a neuron caused. . . ." Imagination, creativity, discovery: the forces that make us uniquely human and allow, or perhaps drive, us to create our own world in nature's universe. Where does medicine and our own neurosurgical cosmos fit in this philosophic stream?

Introduction

As neurosurgeons, we are faced daily with the stimuli for discovery—neurologic disorders that we treat with limited tools, often with an uncertain outcome and an incomplete understanding of underlying normal functions or of disease pathogenesis. This insecurity whets the normal human insatiable curiosity, implores us to disrupt inertia, and gnaws at us to fill the continuously revised promise to improve the human condition. As Theobald Smith said: "Research is fundamentally a state of mind involving continual reexamination of the doctrines and axioms upon which current thought and action are based. It is therefore critical of existing practices."[8]

The United States has been a fertile garden for creativity and discovery in the arts and sciences. In the sciences, academic medicine has particularly blossomed, perhaps because it stretches from the laboratory into society and is, therefore, sewn into our political fabric. Medicine has benefited in America because we have had the freedom to promote creativity and discovery, not from observations defined by societal or political pressures but rather multifaceted investigations of many phenomena that simply pique man's curiosity. We pick away at the status quo with systematic observation and experimental studies.

We have, in fact, come to expect that the physicians and scientists making up American medical science should be the world leaders in research. Educators and practitioners of medicine and surgery are *expected* to actively participate in discovery. Neurosurgery emerges as a product in the evolution of these expectations. In fact, our sense of who we are and what we do comes from the rich heritage of basic neuroscience as midwife to neurosurgery's birth. To understand the neurosurgeon as a neuroscientist, therefore, we must review this history, critique our contribution to modern neuroscience, define the form of research for which most of us are best suited, envision our role in future discoveries, and address the practical question of how to sustain this vision in a country poised to amend its health care delivery system.

One hundred years ago in this country, medical research in all fields began a rapid rise in large part because medical schools developed clinical departments that accepted the tenets of basic science to study diseases in man. The university accepted the responsibility for the medical schools, which automatically strengthened research and teaching in the associated hospitals. Patients benefited directly from investigative treatment and sophisticated technology for special diseases and indirectly from private practitioners who trained in this environment, which challenged them to constantly search for better ways to solve their patients' problems.

As I discuss the importance of research to neurosurgical growth, I will emphasize the role of *integrated research*. Integrated research occupies the threshold between the laboratory and the bedside, and stimulates the linkage of a basic discovery to human disease. This concept has been buried under the generic rubric of medical, particularly clinical, research. But when properly defined, it explains much of our developmental history and potential contributions in discovery; it should be emphasized as our unique role as we attempt to academically survive.

Integrated transitional, translational research has always bridged the gap between the laboratory and the clinical trial. It entails the application of basic science tools directly to the study of human disease, involving the patient in the process, but precedes the study design of a clinical trial that is critical for the establishment of clinical efficacy of any treatment. Examples range from the first use of cortical stimulation in man adopted from Ferrier's animal stimulation studies, to the recording of the first human electroencephalogram, to experimental imaging studies of the brain that are evolving into a reciprocal loop between the physician and the physicist. The physician-scientist's role is critical and evident. He or she must select the right disease and ask a question that can potentially be answered via proper scientific methodology. In some cases, the physician-scientist is active in both laboratory investigation and clinical care but, at the minimum, he or she requires a fundamental understanding of laboratory language, deft communication with the basic scientist, and an in-depth knowledge of the disease being studied. The neurosurgeon properly schooled in and absolutely respectful of the po-

tential of the laboratory is, therefore, uniquely poised to recognize discovery.

The Origins of Observation and Research in Medicine Prior to the 19th Century

The role of the academic physician and neurosurgeon began with the observational school of medicine championed by Hippocrates. This evolved to our present experimental forms through such notables as Galen, who some think was the first to conceive of medicine as a science. He demanded function, not just structure, and pathogenesis, not just symptoms. Galen's philosophy was challenged and amended by Paracelsus, who extended the four humors through his research in chemistry and pharmacology. But it was the physical sciences, in this case astronomy with Copernicus, Kepler, and Galileo, that stimulated development of the instruments of measuring. This critical moment in history has not been sufficiently recognized in the biologic sciences. It was, however, at this point that medicine was irrevocably restructured and tied to this day to the innovation of measuring tools. The pulsilogum of Galileo was followed by Sanctorius' development of the thermometer contemporaneously with Harvey's measurement of the circulation of the blood. René Descartes first verbalized the importance of tools for new observations and stressed the application of mechanics and physics to the study of the human body.[8]

There is a subtle yet critical philosophic turn of events here that molded discovery in biology and medicine through the turn of the century. It began with Marcello Malpighi (1628-1694), who exemplified the investigator identified not by his master nor subject but by his instrument of measuring.[2] Malpighi called himself a "microscopist," using that designation for the first time, and envisioned himself the Galileo of biology. He examined tissues with his "flea glass" microscope and described for the first time the capillary rete that connected the arterial and venous circulation in the lung of the frog, thus answering Harvey's frustrating question about how the circulation was connected in the tissues. Malpighi was greatly influenced by Giovanni Alfonso Borelli, an

Italian physicist who founded "iatrophysics," the application of physics to medicine. These two individuals revolutionized the way man was to be viewed (both literally and figuratively) and established a never-to-be-abandoned quest for instruments with which we can image the mysteries of the human body.

The Birth of Modern Medical Investigation in Europe

The conjunction of observation and instrumentation is well illustrated in the late 1800s by the two different forms the study of disease took: the school of observation in France and the school of laboratory experimentation in Germany. The classification of diseases by scientific observational measurement was still in its infancy when Louis, during the period of 1820 to 1860 in Paris, contributed the first detailed approach to disease description, forming the basis of information gathering that is fundamental to diagnosis.[8] Louis founded "observational" clinical methods and quantified these observations to describe disease from the history-taking and physical examination to the autopsy. He made statistics the basis of clinical research, and Osler felt that Louis created the American school of clinical medicine by exerting profound influence on his American students, such as Oliver Wendell Holmes, Henry Bowditch, George Shattuck, and numerous others. This marked the period of hospital-based medicine, whose growing competition was the school of laboratory medicine advanced by Francois Magendie. Claude Bernard added the experimental approach to problems of medical science while in Germany, where decentralized universities were introduced into the separate city states, fostering competition in research.

Medical research, then, began as clinical observation in France and moved to laboratory investigation in Germany. Germany became the seat of applied medicine, and it became possible within this system to support careers in research. The clinical chairs in medicine were given to individuals with backgrounds and interest in research stressing physiologic medicine. German research was influenced by the French to concentrate on human disease, but the competitive and well-or-ganized laboratories in Germany gave birth to the riches of true experimental medicine from Liebig and Purkinge to Van Goethe and Muller.

The Emergence of the American Medical System as the Coalescence of European Diversity

In the United States, scientific observation of human disease was performed as early as 1833, when Beaumont reported careful studies on digestion in his patient Alexis St. Martin. American medicine, however, was not prepared to integrate science, and Beaumont's work was largely ignored by universities and medical schools. At the end of the Civil War, there were no clinical research laboratories in this country and no training in research methods. Therefore, our first requirement was for individuals trained in basic science. This initial step was taken with the introduction of preparatory studies at Yale in 1869 and subsequently at Johns Hopkins and at Harvard in 1871.[8]

One of the earliest signs that basic laboratory science was important in medicine came when the Yale Sheffield Scientific School offered a course entitled "Studies Preparatory to Medical Science" to undergraduates preparing to study medicine. The first American laboratory of physiologic chemistry was established at the Sheffield School in 1874, and Russell H. Chittenden was appointed the first chair in 1882. The Sheffield Laboratory was a direct extension of similar facilities directed by Professor Kühne of Heidelberg, emphasizing the impact of the German laboratory on American medicine. This oversubscribed course was a resounding success and the Sheffield Laboratory was moved to the Sterling Hall of Medicine in 1923, following Yale's reorganization into departments in 1919, with physiologic chemistry being one of those departments. Germany's laboratories, particularly those of Carl Ludwig, the Leipzig physiologist, became the training ground for American medical scientists. The German system was adopted, first and foremost at Johns Hopkins, and the milieu in the United States followed Germany's lead and became a similar decentralized system with competition and specialized research roles and facilities. Henry Bowditch, after studying physiology in Ludwig's laboratory in Germany, developed the first university facility in America for experimental physiology at Harvard in 1871. However, funding, appreciation, and demand for his work came with difficulty. The Germans often wondered what happened to all the fine American scientists who had been trained in their country and sent back to America, never to be heard from again. The answer was simple: in the United States, there was no demand for them, nor facilities for their experiments. American medicine was concerned with survival, and practicing was based on Benjamin Rush's theory that all diseases were an "excessive action" in the walls of blood vessels that could be relieved by bleeding and purging.

Franklin Paine Mall, reflecting in the 1890s upon this philosophy of practice, felt that clinical medicine was static in the United States at this time and that providing a basic science background would make the student arriving at the Johns Hopkins clinic intolerant of the state of medicine. Osler during the same period emphasized observation and pathology, stressing the Paris school of Louis, but felt that laboratory methods should be brought to the bedside.[14] He did not, however, emphasize investigating the etiology of disease. Lewellys Franklin Barker succeeded Osler at Johns Hopkins in 1905 and was a strong advocate for university-based medicine and the application of science to clinical medicine. He expressed these views best during an address entitled "Medicine and the Universities,"[1] which proposed that clinical departments should rank with basic science departments in emphasizing research and human disease. While at Johns Hopkins, Barker was the first to organize full-time research divisions in a clinical department, believing that there was a great need to apply fundamental sciences to the solution of diagnosis and therapy. Thus, whereas Osler taught careful observation of disease, Barker began asking fundamental questions about disease.[7] The assimilation of basic laboratory technology and research by clinical departments in selected medical schools signaled the dissolution of the propriety schools in which private practitioners

taught apprenticeship-type medicine of quite variable quality. The ranks of the great clinical teachers steeped in French observational medical tradition continued to include private practitioners; those institutions involved in investigation did not. At the turn of the century, it was not clear whether the medical schools would adopt to education and research a uniform approach that either was observational or also involved investigation.

The Flexner Report: Boosting Medicine as Science

If the influence of the German laboratory was not in itself sufficient to sway the tide, that of Abraham Flexner was. In his report on medical education prepared for the Carnegie Institute,[6] he advocated a uniform scientific medical education format. It was clear to Flexner that medicine had entered the scientific era when physics, chemistry, and biology were to be an intellectual foundation, despite the gap separating simple physical laws and the complex machine of the human body.[11] He believed that the scientific method should be extended from research to practice, so that every diagnosis is approached with the thoroughness of a hypothesis. His caustic muckraking of the nation's medical schools forced a disassembly of commercial proprietary medical education between 1910 and 1930, and led to the maturation of academic medicine as we know it today.

By 1924, the position of basic investigative research in American medical schools was solid, and Abraham Flexner addressed this progress at a 1924 medical education symposium in Chicago, comparing the state of medical education in Europe and the United States between 1909 to 1912 and 1924. He found that no fundamental change had taken place in Europe, except that the new University of Strasbourg was attempting to combine the strengths of the French clinical and German investigation programs. In regard to the United States, Flexner went to the heart of the matter in pointing out that, despite great advances in introducing basic science to American medical education, science was not well integrated into the clinic: "The medical school is, as a matter of fact, an organic thing, laboratories and clinics requiring intimate interaction."[15] Ernest Burton, President of the University of Chicago, also spoke at the symposium and pointed out that the word "research" as a descriptor of the process of discovery was only 50 years old in the literature and 30 years old in medicine but, nevertheless, had exerted a profound effect on how medical education was perceived. He believed that the incorporation of discovery into education, which has a natural dogmatism to repress it, must be reorganized and consciously supported, particularly in medicine and surgery.[15]

Basic Medical Science and the Spawning of Neurosurgery

As the preceding brief history demonstrates, the discipline that developed surgical principles for the nervous system and spine did not, of course, emerge suddenly at the turn of this century. A rich neurosurgical heritage preceded this era, and a more detailed description of this is available elsewhere.[3,4,16,17] The conjunction of classical observation, experimental electrophysiology, and neurosurgical advances is perhaps best illustrated by the first brain tumors that were localized using Ferrier's principles of electrical localization of the motor cortex in animals. From these observations, Charcot, Pitres, and John Hughlings Jackson deduced cerebral motor cortex localization following focal motor seizures in man. In parallel, Bennett, Godlee, Macewen, and Horsley used this electrical localization technique for early tumor excisions.[18]

In the United States, we return to Johns Hopkins for the early growth of basic research in neurosurgery and Harvey Cushing's contribution to Halsted's Hunterian Laboratory for Experimental Surgery and Medicine. Cushing, in fact, decided upon a career in medicine primarily because of his experience in the newly established course of physiologic chemistry offered by Russell H. Chittenden during Cushing's college years at Yale. Basic research applications that Cushing creatively adapted to surgery and neurosurgery, beginning while a medical student at Harvard and extending through his research years at the Hunterian Laboratory, included the clinical use of x-rays, continuous intraoperative recording of the patient's pulse and respirations, the use of the sphygmomanometer, and physiologic saline.

Aside from his work on the pituitary, however, many of Cushing's contributions to the field of neurosurgery were technical. Dandy, on the other hand, who began his training under Cushing, applied himself directly to the laboratory in the study of cerebrospinal fluid, translating his conclusions successfully to the human. Osler and his tradition also influenced Ernest Sachs, while a medical student at Johns Hopkins, to contemplate an academic career that he initiated by studying with Sir Victor Horsley in London, where he researched and described the "optic thalamus." Shortly after World War I, Sachs became the nation's first Professor of Neurological Surgery at Washington University in St. Louis.

The 20th Century's First Epoch of Neurosurgery: Extending Basic Science into the Operating Room

The epoch that made up the first third of this century saw a rising tide of characters who marked our emerging specialty—a variety of talents, surgical skills, and creative minds. Despite the mercurial personalities of Wilder Penfield, Charles Elsberg, Charles Frazier, and Max Peet, to mention just a few, they maintained a common compulsion: to carry fundamental laboratory observations into the operating room. This represented a leap of faith that a basic observation was not to be wasted without trial upon the debilitating neurologic diseases affecting their patients who suffered, by and large, without pharmacologic relief. The conjunction of investigation and the clinical instinctiveness of early neurosurgeons is most amply reported by E. A. Kohn's description of Max Peet in Paul Bucy's *Neurosurgical Giants: Feet of Clay and Iron*.[3] Peet was visiting Wilder Penfield at Presbyterian Hospital in New York City where Penfield, based on his previous 6 years of experimental studies on brain wounds in dogs, was about to excise a right frontal traumatic scar from a young patient. Penfield apparently asked Peet what he would do with this patient in Ann Arbor. Peet quickly replied: "I would take the whole damn thing out." Penfield concurred with Peet's advice and performed what was probably the first prefrontal lobectomy for epilepsy in the United States.[3] It was extrapolation from basic physiologic observations to bedside care that also led Peet to perform sympathectomies for essential hypertension. This group of pioneer neurosurgeons spent most of their professional careers espousing the philosophy and attitude of a basic scientist but, in a practical sense, more clearly defining techniques and confirming neurosurgery's rightful role as a clinical specialty.

In an article published in 1991 entitled "The neurosciences and neurosurgery," Robert King emphasized that during this early 20th century era neurosurgeons were enthusiastically and creatively applying basic neuroscience principles directly to patient care, and contrasted this with the midcentury epoch when neurosurgery turned inward, more concerned with the clinical growth of the specialty and the honing of techniques for a proscribed number of diseases uniquely suited to neurosurgical treatment. This clinical emphasis, he points out, was occurring simultaneously with the tremendous growth of an increasingly complex neuroscientific world. Basic research opened the door for innovative operative treatment of nervous system diseases, such as pain and epilepsy. This clear relationship between understanding anatomy and correlating function with pathology was to be maintained, but it took many different forms as the tradition of research became a formal part of resident education. A common form was and continues to be a traditional anatomy or physiology laboratory operated by the neurosurgical service and designed to solve the surgical problems of the day. Some programs, such as that of A. E. Walker at Johns Hopkins, maintained a strong interdisciplinary research effort. Dr. Walker recalls that in 1947 the training program consisted of only 3 years since most trainees were seasoned general surgeons from the war. The trainees spent 1 year as assistant residents, 1 year with their own service, and 1 year in the laboratory, often studying with either Dr. Walker in neuropathology or physiology, Curtis Marshall in electroencephalography, or Vernon Mountcastle in neuroanatomy (AE Walker, personal communication, 1994). When Henry Schwartz, MD, returned from World War II to assume the

chairmanship of neurosurgery at Washington University, he brought a clear vision that substantial basic research belonged in residency training. He quickly developed a liaison with basic scientist and neurologist Jim O'Leary and the neurophysiologist George Bishop. The neurosurgery residents spent a specified amount of time in the laboratory and were exposed more to fundamental research than to surgical problem solving. Financial support for this training came from a variety of sources. For instance, Drs. Roulac and King were awarded Rockefeller grants for their research time in the late 1940s (H Schwartz, personal communication, 1994). Although some neurosurgery chairmen at the time, such as A. E. Walker and A. Ward, did seek National Institutes of Health (NIH) support and used it to build successful laboratories, in general many neurosurgical leaders rejected government training support just as NIH was beginning to provide substantial dollars for basic science training.

As is well known, despite his resistance to government support, Dr. Schwartz's program turned out more successful academic neurosurgeons and eventual chiefs than any other single program of that era. Many of these former students emphasized basic research in their own programs, and there was a clear relationship of their goals to their taste of discovery in Jim O'Leary's laboratory.

The Second Epoch: Technical Developments, a Clinical Specialty Developing Autonomy

The self-imposed autonomy of neurosurgery, its relative boycott of NIH support, and its emphasis on focused problem solving in research have left an imprint on the field. These aided technical development and clinical expertise such that, during the 20 years between 1960 and 1980, a generation of neurologists were convinced to reverse a traditional mindset that preached conservative management for most neurologic conditions. During this era, technical developments in neurosurgical tools, the microscope, imaging, anesthesia, and specialized neurosurgical care teams brought tumors and vascular and spine disease squarely into the surgical paradigm.

Although the word "paradigm" risks a comparison to its faddish use today, T. S. Kuhn established this as an important philosophic concept in science in 1962, pointing out that most scientists solve puzzles within a relatively rigid "framework" of a scientific paradigm or, in our case, a surgical paradigm.[8] The paradigm defines our known limits in, for example, physics or medicine. As Jack Oliver points out: "The natural pace of science is long intervals of puzzle solving interspersed with brief intervals of upheaval and paradigm discovery."[13] This leads to a new paradigm where there is a framework with a new set of rules for problem solving. For example, for years air studies and arteriography were used as the major diagnostic imaging tools; computerized imaging is then discovered and the rules changed.

To return to the midcentury epoch of neurosurgery, the surgical paradigm, as pointed out previously, consisted of rapid advances specific to the discipline and technique. Much of the trainees' research time during residency was spent honing these skills. There was little cross-fertilization with basic neuroscience. The latter was expanding too rapidly for brief training exposures to provide the skills and credentials for a neurosurgeon to perform independent investigations that could compete successfully for resources.

The Third Epoch: Integrated Research, Back to the Basics

The last 20 years of this century are destined to be marked as the third distinct epoch for neurosurgery. Many of the generation that has just finished or will soon finish training have come seeking to use the advanced techniques and technology of surgery as tools to address new disease processes and to further understand the central nervous system (CNS).

It is less necessary to spend all our research effort on clinical details of the specialty and increasingly possible to use our tools and our unique perspective to explore new areas of human disease. The time is right for neurosurgical scientists to no longer focus solely on the surgical paradigm and to look, for example, at restorative measures such as gene therapy or transplantation in degenerative diseases, CNS trauma, and developmental abnormalities; to put effort into CNS immunology combined with molecular genetics for advancing neuro-oncology; to explore the mechanisms of vascular biology to predict, explain, and modify behavior of cerebrovascular pathology; or to define the substrates underlying the pathogenesis of epilepsy and pain.

In this third epoch, reductionism in the study of the brain takes on new dimensions when you can analyze the energy state and amino acid composition of the brain and its lesions preoperatively using nuclear magnetic resonance spectroscopy, intraoperatively using optical imaging and microdialysis, and postoperatively submitting the resected tissue to the very same measuring tools for in vitro testing of an in vivo hypothesis. Much better animal or in vitro models might then be created for any particular disease once the proper observations have been performed in the human.

Where is the evidence that the young neurosurgeon is vying for a seat in the neuroscience rocket? Robert King, Director of the Research Foundation of the American Association of Neurological Surgeons, provided me with a list of research fellowship proposals and Young Clinician Investigator Awards submitted between 1983 and 1994. The number of well-thought-out and well-mentored proposals have increased from 12 in 1983 to 27 in 1994, and comprise the range of today's cutting-edge investigations in basic neuroscience, including 9 molecular genetics proposals in 1994.[9]

It is the surgical neuroscientist who is in the best position to integrate this application of basic tools to human disease. There are no other members of the neuroscience team in the position to understand the disease and what must be accomplished for control, to manage an invasive interaction and treatment plan, and to balance the ethical consideration of a new treatment and understand what is most appropriate to be extracted from the laboratory to bring to a clinical trial. The surgical neuroscientist may indeed be involved, in small or large part, in a laboratory investigation, but that does not change his or her obligation to integrate the laboratory with the clinic; in fact, it enhances it. Integrated research thus defines this concept of how neurosurgeons can be involved in the process of discovery, particularly if they take seriously Jack Oliver's admonition to keep the big picture in mind.

We must use a long-term perspective to look at neurosurgical science. Discovery will then come from this perspective using new ways of observing and organizing. The neurosurgical scientist should choose a nontrivial question and use his or her special talents and intuition to create relevant hypotheses and not get bogged down in the minutiae of solving secondary puzzles that are distracting. The key suggestion that Oliver makes is that we should cross-fertilize our field with another one. For example, since measuring and the instruments of measuring are so critical to scientific advancement, bring powerful ones from another field to yours. If microdialysis is possible in the animal, then we ought to adapt it to the human and ask an important question that is feasible to answer. I believe that the best way to change our paradigms is to consciously effect cross-fertilization, and to blend the disciplines together in interdepartmental disease-related programs that (and this is *most* critical) *share the same space.*

Integrated research automatically provides the fertile ground for discovery and interdisciplinary investigation. The critical transition into the third neurosurgical epoch harkens back to the first epoch and our early 20th-century vision of the proper medical school where basic laboratory problems are solved in clinical departments and there is less risk of losing sight of the principle goal—the disease question. Although there are many other examples, a neurosurgery change at Yale can be used to illustrate one aspect of this transition from the second to the third epoch of the surgical neuroscientist. When W. F. Collins, MD, assumed the leadership of Yale's neurosurgery section, traditional anatomy and physiology were the mainstay of research activities and training, with emphasis on neuropathology. Dr. Collins succeeded in procuring a grant for a spinal cord injury center that provided resources for much-needed clinical improvements in patient care and a laboratory that over the subsequent 10 years explored spinal cord injury animal models. The goals of the investigations were to describe the pathophysiology of spinal cord injury and to address treatment modalities that would reduce secondary injury. It became clear that the paradigm of pharmacologic manipulation in spinal cord injury was a problem-solving endeavor with

a finite endpoint. Going from the laboratory to the bedside, a large multicenter cooperative study statistically revealed just how much could be accomplished by medical treatment in the human. Although some statistical benefits have occurred, it subsequently became obvious that this paradigm was limited. Because the neurosurgery laboratory at Yale was home to a number of independent PhD investigators in CNS plasticity and development, it was decided to shift the paradigm to involve scientists from other clinical and laboratory departments. Dr. Collins and the director of the neurosurgical laboratories, Charles Greer, PhD, then redirected the spinal cord grant toward the more distant but open-ended goal of regeneration and CNS plasticity. Changing the question but using the same available techniques, such as immunohistochemistry and confocal microscopy, adding sophisticated electrophysiology and biochemistry scientists, and using human tissue, symptomatic epilepsy substrates and neuro-oncology were added to integrated research programs in the 1980s.

The Education of the Surgical Neuroscientist

This example of integrated research emphasizes a major point. If basic science skills are to be important for independent investigation or as tools for communication with laboratory colleagues, mentoring for the neurosurgical resident is necessarily performed in a basic laboratory directed by someone (usually a PhD) who is devoted full-time to fundamental investigation but who is in a clinical department because he or she seeks to have an impact on disease. To provide the tools for discovery to our next neurosurgical generation, we must find a way to maintain laboratory investigations in clinical departments despite the economic stresses. This new era of remodeling and re-integrating basic science into our field must be recognized as critical to our patients' care and not a luxury of academics. If we accept that basic science training is important for all our residents, not just those staying in the university setting but also those who will use critical thinking and problem solving in the practice of neurosurgery, then we must decide what form this training should best take.

The philosophic construct of the surgeon as a neuroscientist should begin with training that provides an integrated format in basic laboratory investigation, biostatistics, and clinical study design. Should we continue to place our research time in the formal training program or adopt training programs similar to our medical and neurology colleagues, where the clinical training stands alone and research is usually part of a subspecialty fellowship that follows? The latter obviously limits the research experience to those who continue in subspecialties, and the subspecialty fellowships will be, by and large, clinical fellowships, unless the individual has laboratory experience or a PhD prior to clinical training. Alternatively, one might provide an expanded postgraduate fellowship in neurosurgery where both laboratory and clinical experience are gained in a well-designed 2-year block following formal clinical training. This format would compensate for the possible paring down of trainees and of formal training time proposed in health care reform. It would select for research training only those individuals who were serious about academic medicine, and put the onus of fiscal responsibility on government training programs. Less of the responsibility would be borne by clinical income, through either the hospital or faculty practice income.

This scenario, however, detracts from providing an integrated research format throughout the training period. Figure 1 outlines the possible relationships of the surgical neuroscientist to research. This integrated research paradigm allows for our field to accommodate and encourage those whose talents lie in the technical realms of surgical care delivery (i.e. instrumentation, intraoperative computer-assisted devices, etc.). It also

The Integrated Research Paradigm in the Interdisciplinary Center

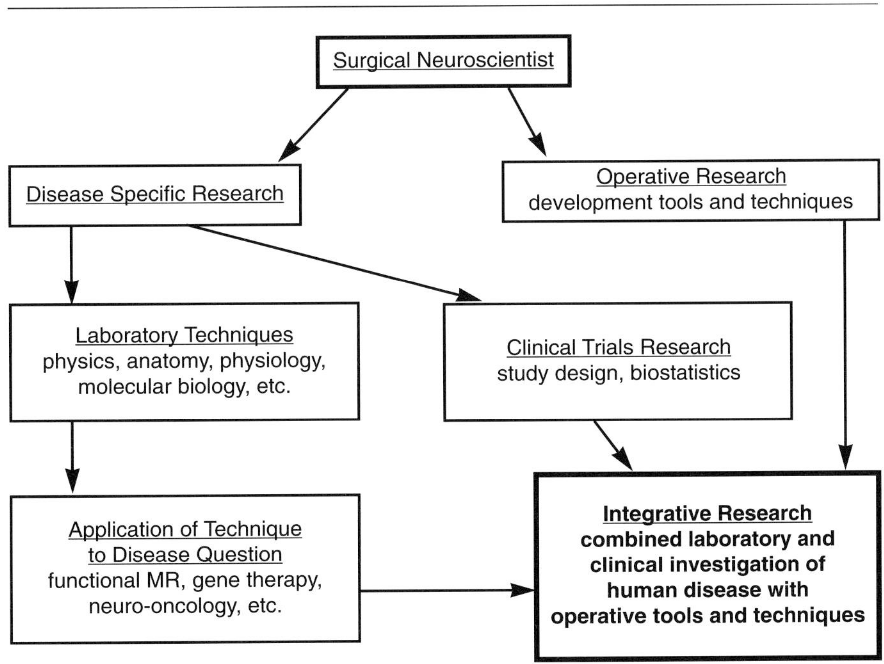

Figure 1. Outline of the various paths academic neurosurgeons may take to finally effect an integrated investigation of human disease. A given individual will require exposure to each of these routes in his or her higher graduate education. Interest and talent will lead the young investigator to emphasize either laboratory investigation, clinical studies, or technical development. Regardless of this emphasis, the neurosurgical scientist needs training in all areas so that proper translation from one realm to another is effected. This investigative endeavor is best performed in the setting of an interdisciplinary center designed for disease-specific research.

allows for the growth of integrated research that is disease-specific and interdisciplinary program-oriented, where surgical techniques are not only developed for patient care but are unique tools in research. Both patient care and research benefit from this programmatic approach, which would bring together neurologists, neurosurgeons, psychiatrists, and basic scientists. We already see these organ- or disease-specific groups forming in our medical centers. Comprehensive epilepsy centers, neurovascular programs, and neuro-oncology programs are just three examples. In some instances, it might make sense to reorganize our departments in this vein rather than keep the medical and surgical substrates that presently exist.

Figure 1 illustrates one concept of academic neurosurgery. The variable role that the neurosur-

geon may take as neuroscientist or technical innovator is emphasized. It should be apparent that graduate education for this individual in a rapidly changing scientific world demands flexibility and a large multifaceted research menu from which the trainee can choose according to his or her educational goals and individual talents. Figure 2 illustrates the training program at Yale, in which research is emphasized relatively early and an attempt is made to maintain the thread throughout clinical training.

Whether you believe that this form of training is necessary for everyone in postgraduate neurosurgery, it seems clear that fewer innovations and discoveries will be associated with neurosurgery as an island unto itself. Under very few circumstances is one person capable of both quality basic research and quality surgical practice. A rich relationship with laboratory scientists and epidemiologists, preferably in a center where they may work together on programmatic themes, seems ideal. The training program is where that mindset begins.

Unfortunately, our own squabbling about who controls medical education may push our academic goals away as we develop plans for health care reform and as the emphasis on primary care drives education outside the university control. The Millis report[12] prepared for the American Medical Association in 1963, entitled "The Graduate Education of Physicians," recommended a national body to develop and maintain graduate medical education that was not divided among hospitals, universities, and specialty boards. Although this governing body was initially fractionalized, leading to many stalemates in specialty growth, eventually the Accreditation Council on Graduate Medical Education was formed, and many rules for change were agreed upon and solidified. However, the educational process remained uneven as long as the universities did not control the continuum of medical education from medical school through fellowships, and as long as education remained mired in the finances of patient care. Up until now, surgery has not been concerned with this since the number of specialists trained has been high and the medical marketplace has defied Adam Smith (i.e. the more surgeons there are, the more surgery is performed) and the unit cost with increasing technical sophistication is dri-

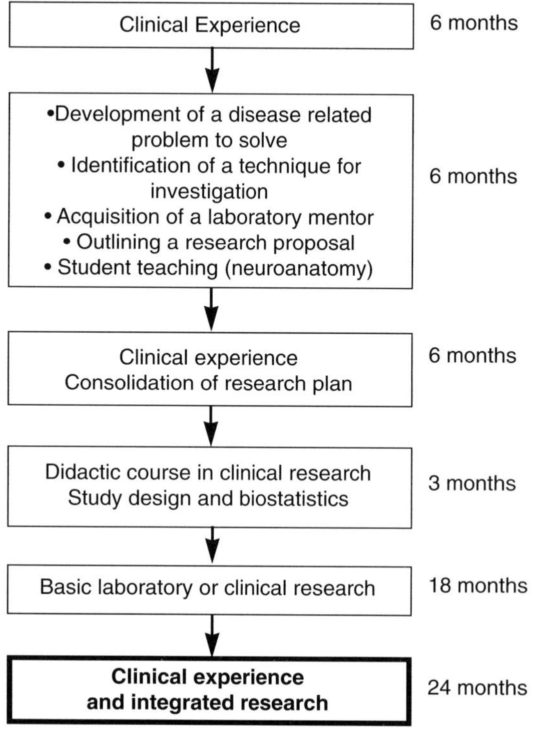

Post Graduate Neurosurgical Training

Preparing for an integrated research environment

Figure 2. *Outline of one possible training format, which emphasizes integrated research on human disease and provides exposure to both clinical and laboratory investigation.*

ven higher. This has allowed academic surgeons to care for fewer patients with a relatively high return per patient. This, in turn, has supported time for research, allowed for reasonable salaries, and given sufficient training time for neurosurgical residents. Postgraduate education is then clearly bound to patient care dollars. When the number of neurosurgeons is decreased and the money tightened, research time will disappear. Education costs must be separated and clearly identified if we are going to maintain the strides we have made in integrating our field with other neuroscience arenas.

Summary

We have come full-circle after a century of progress in medical research. In this third epoch of neurosurgery and neuroscience, we confront a crisis in which our progress is again inextricably tied to basic laboratory discoveries. We should take to heart Rene Dubos' maxim: "Think globally, act locally."[5] In my conversation with Dr. Schwartz as I prepared this manuscript, he reminded me of the wanderlust attitude for research training of the pioneer neurosurgeons. Reaffirmation of basic science in our specialty begins with the concept of an interdisciplinary center that cross-fertilizes our outmoded department paradigm and should include international scholars and training programs. Physicians and scientists from many disciplines and nations should be placed side by side using overlapping techniques, driven by different problems to solve, but together providing a greater chance that some one member will view the whole picture and synthesize a new paradigm. The interdisciplinary center within the university may provide the best compromise between the free-standing institute and traditional, relatively rigid academic structures. By being program- and disease-specific but not department-specific, there will be fertile ground for discovery, allowing diversity, embracing new ideas, and entertaining a range of paradigms as probable or as improbable as their proponents. This center should grow in a medical school where it lies within the invisible walls surrounding patient care. Early but rigorous clinical application of new basic laboratory constructs will be possible under the academic scrutiny of the university and the ethical oversight of both university and hospital. The research and clinical application equilibrium among the center, university, and hospital, with parallel international input, will both maintain the leadership of American medical research and provide a model for discovery as we enter the third millennium.

References

1. Barker LF. Medicine and the Universities. *Am Med.* 1902;4:143.
2. Boorstin DJ. *The Discoverers.* New York, NY: Random House; 1983.
3. Bucy PC. *Neurosurgical Giants: Feet of Clay and Iron.* New York, NY: Elsevier; 1985.
4. Bucy PC. *Modern Neurosurgical Giants.* New York, NY: Elsevier; 1986.
5. Dubos R , Escande JP. *Quest: Reflections on Medicine, Science, and Humanity.* New York, NY: Harcourt Brace Jovanovich; 1980.
6. Flexner A. *Medical Education in the United States and Canada.* New York, NY: Carnegie Foundation for the Advancement of Teaching; 1910.
7. Harvey AM. *Adventures in Medical Research—A Century of Discovery at Johns Hopkins.* Baltimore, Md: Johns Hopkins University Press; 1976.
8. Harvey AM. *Science at the Bedside: Clinical Research in American Medicine 1905-1945.* Baltimore, Md: Johns Hopkins University Press; 1981.
9. King RB. The neurosciences and neurosurgery. *Surg Neurol.* 1991;35:424-428.
10. Klausner NW, Kuntz PG. *Philosophy: The Study of Alternative Beliefs.* New York, NY: Macmillan; 1961.
11. Ludmerer KM. *Learning to Heal—The Development of American Medical Education.* New York, NY: Basic Books; 1985.
12. Millis JS. *The Graduate Education of Physicians: Report of the Citizens' Commission on Graduate Medical Education.* Chicago, Ill: American Medical Association; 1966.
13. Oliver JE. *The Incomplete Guide to the Art of Discovery.* New York, NY: Columbia University Press; 1991.
14. Osler W. The evolution of the idea of experiment in medicine. *Trans Cong Am Phys Surg.* 1907;7:1.
15. *Proceedings of the Annual Congress on Medical Education, Medical Licensure, Public Health and Hospitals.* Chicago, Ill: American Medical Association;1924.
16. Sachs E. *The History and Development of Neurological Surgery.* New York, NY: Paul B Hoeber; 1952.
17. Walker AE. *A History of Neurological Surgery.* Baltimore, Md: Williams & Wilkins; 1951.
18. Wilkins RH. *Neurosurgical Classics.* New York, NY: Johnson Reprint Corp; 1965;361-377.

Neurological Surgery and Clinical Science

Issam A. Awad, MD, MSc, FACS

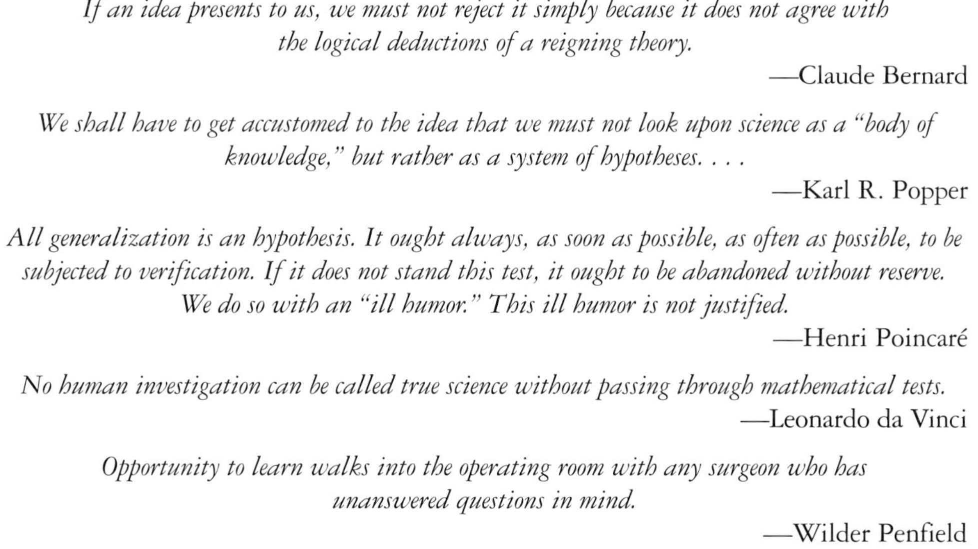

*If an idea presents to us, we must not reject it simply because it does not agree with
the logical deductions of a reigning theory.*

—Claude Bernard

*We shall have to get accustomed to the idea that we must not look upon science as a "body of
knowledge," but rather as a system of hypotheses. . . .*

—Karl R. Popper

*All generalization is an hypothesis. It ought always, as soon as possible, as often as possible, to be
subjected to verification. If it does not stand this test, it ought to be abandoned without reserve.
We do so with an "ill humor." This ill humor is not justified.*

—Henri Poincaré

No human investigation can be called true science without passing through mathematical tests.

—Leonardo da Vinci

*Opportunity to learn walks into the operating room with any surgeon who has
unanswered questions in mind.*

—Wilder Penfield

The Neurosurgical Heritage in Scientific Context

Modern neurological surgery has evolved during a century of extraordinary revolution in medicine and in the sciences. While a close interaction and collaboration among anatomists and surgeons had existed for centuries, the eve of the 20th century witnessed a novel and fruitful cross-fertilization between physiology and clinical medicine. Experimental physiology and pathology became entwined, generating many novel observations regarding the normal and the pathological that evolved into accepted clinical concepts.[4] Claude Bernard's famous animal experiments formed the foundations of modern endocrinology and metabolism;[2] those of Ivan Pavlov were indispensable to relevant foundations of neurology. Work on the spinal roots by Bell and by Magendie, later experimental studies on reflexes by Pavlov and by Sherrington, and the elegant histologic demonstrations by Cajal laid firm foundations for the "neuron doctrine."[10,21,24]

The founders of modern neurological surgery were at the heart of this emerging movement in experimental physiology, and were keen to find its potential applications in their new field.[3] Cushing's pilgrimage to European physiology laboratories during his formative years has been discussed extensively. The association of Horsely with neurologist and physiologist Jackson was a model of clinical neuroscience collaboration emulated in future decades at a number of academic institutions. These early neurosurgical leaders were associated with august institutions of higher learning, where the teaching and practice of medicine were also enjoying an intellectual renaissance. Within this context, they established "schools" of neurosurgery reflecting their own philosophy and vision. Penfield insisted that his pupils spend extensive time in the study of neurophysiology and work closely on clinical problems within a neuroscience team. He firmly believed that the operating room was the surgeon's special laboratory, with opportunity to make unique observations and to advance knowledge.

The extraordinary scientific possibilities of working on the human nervous system in vivo have motivated scores of neurosurgeons who have hence contributed fundamental knowledge to human neuroscience in a way not otherwise possible.[3,10,24] The applicability of phenomena documented in the experimental setting to human function and neurologic disease could not be tested in any other setting. Neurosurgeons became indispensable partners in neuroscience teams interested in human function and disease. They applied this knowledge in creative ways to numerous pathologies, including surgical approaches to the treatment of pain, movement disorders, and epilepsy. Their careful observations and physiologic measurements, in conjunction with radiologic imaging and gross and histopathologic correlations, shaped conceptual advances in cerebrovascular diseases, central nervous system neoplasia, infection, trauma, and spine and peripheral nerve diseases.[3] The current generation of neurosurgeons is breaking new ground, exploring powerful cellular and molecular techniques in deciphering mechanisms of disease and applying innovative treatment strategies.[21]

Experience, Myth, and Bias

Neurosurgeons have always been aware of the tremendous power and privilege associated with their work.[3] Their observations could not be easily verified by nonsurgeons. Their keen sense of

clinical and surgical decision-making could not be matched by anybody not familiar with their domain. A number of pathological entities have become characterized as "neurosurgical diseases," the physiopathology, diagnosis, clinical spectrum, and treatment of which have not been mastered by any other specialist. When these entities were encountered clinically, the neurosurgeon has traditionally been—and to a large extent continues to be—called upon for diagnosis, prognosis, and comprehensive management.

Neurosurgical teachers accumulated and carefully documented and analyzed clinical observations of these neurosurgical diseases. They advanced concepts and strategies based on this experience, which they then taught to their neurosurgical pupils and colleagues. Their opinions carried the commensurate weight of their leadership, innovation, and vast clinical and surgical experience.[3] Their credibility was enhanced by the applicability of their concepts in the clinical practice of other neurosurgeons, and the reproducibility of their results within the limits of reverence to their uniquely superior technical skills.

From the earliest days of modern neurological surgery in this century, controversies arose about different perspectives of disease and its management.[3,9,28] These have traditionally been highlighted by comparing and contrasting results of treatment as presented to and published for neurosurgical peers, and, less commonly, other clinicians. Some controversies were resolved by the collection of convincing data, and others by the accumulated experience of a generation of neurosurgeons. Still others remain to this day, surrounding the whole spectrum of daily neurosurgical practice and more complicated and specialized problems. Some controversial practices are carried on by pupils of various neurosurgical "schools"—at times in ritualistic obedience or in emulation of workable approaches associated with satisfactory individual outcomes. These practices include perioperative adjuvant medical management, procedures of surgical field, minor and major technical steps, and even indications for surgery and the strategic stance toward a disease entity.[9,16]

Neurosurgeons recognized, albeit reluctantly at times, the potential for myth and bias. Cushing humorously admitted, late in his career, that his memory of surgical outcome was tainted by his successes—and that he was humbly reminded of his true results by the famous notebook maintained by a long-term associate and colleague who kept track of the morbidity and/or mortality for every tumor case.[8] The tendency of a surgeon to forget or rationalize bad outcomes, and the role of the nonsurgeon adjudicator are surely not unique to this master teacher!

Most sources of clinical bias are not unique to neurosurgery.[9,14–17,28] The critical difference between association and causation is a fundamental scientific principle. In clinical medicine, it underlies numerous fallacies and misinterpretations, including the mistaken attribution of epiphenomena as causative mechanisms. This could lead to false generalization and to the potentially dangerous approach of modifying epiphenomena in an effort to treat disease. In surgical disciplines, including neurosurgery, surgical outcome could be attributed to a particular factor in the course of treatment, leading the surgeon to falsely invoke an epiphenomenon as the cause of success or failure. Selection bias is another form of this treacherous trap, where inadvertent characteristics of the patient or population, rather than the treatment, account for a given outcome. Unjustified generalization is another common pitfall related to the attribution of a narrow association to causation.[14] This also has commonly resulted in the attribution of an effect to treatment when it was perhaps due to placebo or even to chance alone. Conversely, the absence of a measurable difference between two groups has often been attributed to a true lack of any difference, despite an insufficient number of observations.[14]

Neurosurgeons are particularly vulnerable to observational bias,[9,14] because they cannot objectively divorce themselves from the intense experience of surgery. They tend to document observations in surgical cohorts that they ignore in nonsurgical patients, and to attribute the observed differences to the effect of surgery. This can be further compounded by selection bias, as in selecting surgical candidates based on consciously articulated and inadvertent criteria, and observing and even treating these cases differently from nonsurgical cohorts, yet attributing a

difference in outcome to an effect of treatment. Rationalization of untoward surgical outcome is another common pitfall, including placing the blame for surgical complications on the patient's disease or a serendipitous occurrence, while a similar outcome in nonoperated patients is attributed to omission of surgery. Surgeons are particularly vulnerable to overestimating unverified surgical objectives, such as the extent of resection, and to attributing outcome to having accomplished the said objectives.

Many of these biases are integrated innocently and inadvertently into neurosurgical practice. Every clinician is vulnerable to one or more of them in every treatment decision or intervention, and when making subjective judgments about management value and outcome. The neurosurgeon's biases are more difficult to circumvent, as few neutral (uninvolved) observers are qualified to validate the observational basis of the judgments and opinions. Neurosurgical peers may themselves be subject to the same biases. When such a biased opinion is held by a respected neurosurgical leader or teacher, it may be adopted as fact by the neurosurgical community or by pupils—and becomes a myth.[3,9] Such myths are difficult to refute in view of reverence and respect toward their generator.

Epidemiologists have warned clinicians repeatedly about these prevalent biases. Methodologic strategies of defining populations, cohorts and subjects, standardized observation, control, randomization, stratification, and the statistical analysis of results have been well articulated.[4,9,12,14–17,20,23,25,28] Neurosurgeons have acknowledged more recently their vulnerability to these pitfalls and have proposed specific means of avoiding them in the setting of neurosurgical diseases. The scientific standard in scrutinizing against such bias and in insisting on sound methodology in neurosurgical peer-reviewed publications has become far more stringent in recent years. Multidisciplinary academic teams have integrated non-neurosurgical peers into the arena of evaluation and treatment of many neurosurgical diseases, and hence an inherent protection against some forms of bias. The prevalent practice of research training in neurosurgical residency programs, and credibly proctored conferences and journal clubs are instilling this awareness in future generations of neurosurgical clinicians.

The Science and Art of Clinical Decisions

The Process of Clinical Decision-Making

Clinical decision-making is a complex process integrating concepts about mechanisms of disease, observational information (controlled and uncontrolled) from one's experiences and those of others (published and unpublished), and the results of relevant or possibly relevant research studies. Clinicians acknowledge that this represents a mixture of science and art, through a process reflecting individual style, education, and ethic.[4,16,28]

The science of clinical decisions is based on controlled observations in well-defined cohorts, aimed at testing a specific question of clinical relevance.[12,15–17,25] Such is the hypothesis-driven approach underlying the scientific method. The clinical scientist encounters relevant problems in diagnosis, prognosis, or therapy. He or she formulates these into testable hypotheses and designs studies to prove or disprove them. Testing hypotheses involves statistical analysis aimed at showing whether an observation is due to chance alone, which would deem it insignificant. The lack of observed differences can also be statistically validated using sufficient observations (power) to ensure significance by minimizing the likelihood of chance alone. The role of hypothesis, the reliability of hypothesis-driven research, and the philosophic implications of chance and causation in clinical neurosurgery are discussed later in this chapter.

Methodology of Clinical Science

The methodology of scientific investigation should aim at defining the hypothesis and the cohort to be studied, and articulating the variables to be monitored and the statistical methods to be used in data analysis and hypothesis testing.[15–17] Typically, a null hypothesis is artic-

ulated and a level of significance is chosen, below which the observation could be attributed to chance alone. The size of the cohort and the number of observations are determined so as to ensure sufficient statistical power to prove or disprove the hypothesis.[14,20] The methodology includes specific safeguards against intentional and inadvertent bias. These include prospective data gathering, randomization and concurrent control (preferably placebo), and double-blinding. A study is typically designed to test a specific hypothesis, and care is taken not to extrapolate information to other hypotheses. The cohort studied must be reflective, in an unbiased fashion, of the population with the disease so as to avoid the pitfall of false generalization.[1,15,17,20] Stratification is used to ensure balance in cohort representation of known factors that might influence the outcome.

Such studies are tedious to perform, expensive, and difficult in the setting of surgical disease.[1,15,20] Blinding, and even bias-free randomization, are impossible to achieve in surgical studies. There is also the ethical concern of denying potentially life-saving therapy to patients randomly assigned to receive placebo or nontreatment.[20] Yet, the alternative methods of uncontrolled clinical conclusions can potentially be more harmful and more expensive, especially when doubt is raised about the validity of a surgical treatment from observations alone.[15,16] Neurosurgeons have recognized these considerations in the last two decades and were among the first surgical specialists to experiment with the controlled methodology of clinical trials. Powerful lessons were learned about the potential impact of such trials on clinical practice, and the potential for false generalization and other bias in trial design and execution and in extrapolation of results.[1,15,20] These lessons have assisted in the subsequent design of studies less vulnerable to such pitfalls. For example, concern was raised following the extracranial-intracranial bypass study about the weighting of the cohort with low-risk patients, about preselection bias, and about false generalization of conclusions.[1,20] These factors were more tightly controlled in subsequent carotid endarterectomy trials, with better stratification, selection criteria, and monitoring of potentially eligible non-enrolled cases (preselection bias).

Yet, prospective controlled trials can only answer a single cardinal question with strict reliability,[1,15,20,28] and cannot be used for other secondary observations with the same reliability. They apply to the selected cohort, which cannot reflect—despite stratification—all possible relevant variations in the disease or treatment. The cardinal question is formulated based on a fixed understanding of the disease and treatment, and is inflexible (by strict methodology) to changes in knowledge that invariably alter the question, the treatment, or the population of interest. The results of a clinical trial can become obsolete through changes in knowledge or technology before a trial is completed. A technical innovation of a surgical procedure may lower surgical morbidity to an extent that a procedure may become more effective; similarly, a selection criterion may improve the effectiveness of treatment by restricting it to patients most likely to benefit from it. These factors cannot be anticipated during the design phase of a clinical trial and would invalidate the methodology if they were considered thereafter.

Hence, clinical trials are useful for focused questions regarding a disease and a technology with sufficient maturity and stability. Such questions can be answered with high reliability. Other equally fundamental clinical questions cannot be tackled through clinical trials. Trials cannot give answers to the myriad of subtle questions that could not be lumped into the single cardinal question, but that could have a strong bearing on outcome. For example, while a clinical trial has shown carotid endarterectomy to be effective in symptomatic severe carotid artery stenosis, it did not address with any certainty issues such as timing of surgery following moderate infarction, patient factors that might increase or decrease surgical risk, the myriad of variations in adjuvant surgical technology and medical therapies, patient age, or lesions that are near but not quite at the level of stenosis where benefit was demonstrated. These issues are real and shape clinical decisions in individual patients.

Clinical observations can be validated scientifically through other methodology, which may be more useful albeit less rigorous.[1,5,12,17,20,23,28]

Registries can provide longitudinal databases for documenting disease epidemiology, natural history, and the impact of treatment.[23] Vulnerability to bias can be minimized by documenting as many variables as possible, and using statistical multivariate analysis to examine the individual and additive impact of these variables. Hypothesis-driven strategies, including stratification and prospective monitoring, can increase statistical reliability and minimize bias. Other methodologies include case control studies, population- or experience-based, which allow statistically sound conclusions relevant to the specific population or experience.[17] It may be possible to generalize these conclusions without significant bias as long as all consecutive cases are included in the study and known or suspected relevant disease variables are documented. Again, open articulation of a specific hypothesis and sufficient numbers of observations in relevant cases are essential for the validity of conclusions in these types of studies.[23,28]

Meta-Analysis and the Art of Consensus

Rigorous scientific studies cannot guide all clinical decisions, and every study—even the most rigorous—cannot be generalized to all relevant clinical scenarios.[16,28] Meta-analysis or integration of numerous studies can add certainty to a clinical concept through concurrence and convergence, or can introduce meaningful doubt through contradiction or divergence. Statistical methods have been introduced to assist in such meta-analysis, although the element of consensus may not always be quantifiable.[29] The art of clinical decisions, the sense of good clinicians, is shaped by such consensus—controlled by doubt when there is no consensus and constantly reshaped by the flux of information and individual clinical peculiarities. The clinical conscience consists of such honest reappraisal and self-doubt, a constant reintegration of all relevant information. Such information does and should include one's own experience while at the same time being cognizant of its potential biases. Individual experience is one's personal laboratory, where doubt is generated and hypotheses are formulated. The answers should constantly be sought in the experience of others and in applicable reported scientific studies.[28]

Philosophy of Neurosurgical Science

Hypothesis and Doubt

In his recent thesis on the logic of scientific discovery, science philosopher Karl R. Popper[26] states that a scientific discipline should not be defined through a body of knowledge, but rather as a system of hypotheses. These cannot be justified in principle, but are rather working hypotheses that can never be considered "true" or "more or less certain," or even "probable." This thesis takes into consideration notions about the unity of nature and the importance of hypothesis as advanced by Poincaré, including the concept of generalization as hypothesis.[6,25] It emphasizes doubt as the generator of relevant questions, a concept espoused by many ancient and modern philosophers.[6,22,27] It also reflects the philosophic implications of the theories of modern physics, including Einstein's "space-time" interchangeability in the special theory of relativity[11] and Heisenberg's uncertainty principle,[19] applying statistical probabilities to the very structure of matter.[14] In apparent order there is fundamental uncertainty,[6,25,26,27,30] and from chaos there seems to emerge a predictable order.[6,13]

These notions indicate that hypotheses must arise from our doubts,[25] and should drive our queries. A set of hypotheses must shape our way of thinking, rather than a body of knowledge. A hypothesis is never certain nor permanent. Hypotheses themselves arise from our experience, which is necessarily limited. The "empirical uniformities" sought by Plato and the certainty of scientific knowledge evoked by Comte and the positivists and applied to practical value by the physiologists are themselves subject to uncertainty and doubt.[2,4,6,7,29,30] A system of hypotheses allows the advancement of knowledge and its practical application, as long as these hypotheses themselves do not raise any doubt and hence generate new knowledge through new hypotheses.[25–27]

As neurosurgeons, our scientific positions should reflect this mature climate of thinking. We are certain of our knowledge as long as it stands up to the repeated challenges of our doubts. We recognize the certainty of our knowledge through practical value; yet, we recognize its narrow experiential scope and view it as a "choice of means, not choice of ends."[4,7,22,25] The mature neurosurgical scientist therefore becomes the true master of knowledge rather than its slave, the shaper of an evolving field—a system of hypotheses.[25–27]

Defining Neurosurgical Disease

In a narrow sense, neurosurgical disease can be defined as a set of clinical entities where the opinion or action of a neurosurgeon contributes to advanced knowledge, better prognosis, or more effective treatment than in the absence of such an opinion or action. This is a definition in the tradition of Heidegger's existential philosophy, the meaning of being.[18] It is itself subject to doubt, generating a set of hypotheses about our role, the purpose of our being. Such a definition is practical, self-evident, but also subject to challenge, urging us to constantly justify and re-examine our role. It is perhaps less secure than more arbitrary territorial definitions, but it is on firmer scientific, ideologic, and philosophic grounds.

Perhaps as important as defining neurosurgical disease is to articulate the normal and the pathological in these clinical entities.[4] We must differentiate between the normal state and that which does not require surgical intervention. The lack of need for surgery does not imply normalcy and does not exclude the entity from the category of neurosurgical disease. Our input into an entity can reflect special knowledge, ability to diagnose and to prognosticate, and also to determine the role and timing of possible neurosurgical treatment. In this context, intervertebral disc disease is a neurosurgical disease, and not just when it requires disc excision. Cerebrovascular occlusive disease is a neurosurgical disease, with one of its narrow features the option of vascular neurosurgical intervention. The option of surgery and the body of associated hypotheses cannot be divorced from other aspects of the disease.

The difference between normal and pathological in neurosurgical disease transcends the role of surgical intervention, as important and fundamental as the latter is. It should include a hypothesis-driven definition of the entity based on current diagnostic criteria, itself subject to future revision. There should be an epidemiologic perspective of prevalence and incidence, and a clinical perspective of the spectrum of clinical manifestations—the natural history. This should be articulated in statistical formulas, models of likelihood of clinical behavior.[4,6,27]

Predicting vs. Explaining

Neurosurgical disease cannot be defined solely in statistical and epidemiologic terms. Statistics and epidemiology are used to predict clinical behavior, but not to explain it.[4,6,27] This difference is critical, for prediction is inherently a statistical chance occurrence of limited application to any particular patient. Conversely, explaining reflects on individual cases and uncovers mechanistic host and external factors that influence statistical clinical behavior. Mechanistic explanations allow more individualized predictions of clinical behavior and thus a rational manipulation of this behavior. For example, understanding and explaining why an aneurysm bleeds allow more accurate prediction of when and how often it bleeds. Of equal importance, they allow more rational timing of treatment and perhaps innovative strategies toward treatment.

Georges Canguilhem[4] defines health as an equilibrium that man redeems on inceptive ruptures; the menace of disease is one of the components of health. The science of neurosurgical disease should encompass the deterministic principles of disease behavior, as well as its mechanistic vectors. The neurosurgeon must uncover statistical formulas governing the natural history of disease, but equally importantly the factors that govern lesion behavior in the individual patient—the very factors that cause deviation from the average natural course.[6,30] These factors allow more rational disease prevention and treatment, and more individualized strategies of management. Hence, the neurosurgeon generates hypotheses about when to treat and how best to treat.

From Natural History to Molecules: Dimensions of Neurosurgical Science

Based on the philosophic elements articulated previously, we can propose current dimensions of neurosurgical science. A system of hypotheses would govern the very definition of neurosurgical disease and the diagnostic criteria for the specific clinical entities. The epidemiology of the disease must be studied, defining prevalence and the full spectrum of clinical manifestations, and statistical formulas must be derived to predict the likelihood of clinical behavior.[8]

Further clinical observations should generate hypotheses about factors that determine clinical behavior, including host and external factors. These would include cardinal questions about the impact of therapy on the natural course of the disease at various stages and a comparative examination of different therapeutic approaches, including expectant, nonsurgical, and operative. The role of technology is articulated into "question-driven technology assessment" aimed at sensitivity, validity, and usefulness of technology in diagnosis and treatment, and also cost-effectiveness and generalizability.[5] Experiential observations, a surgeon's traditional tool, are integrated into information from methodologically controlled scientific studies, with consensus sustaining a hypothesis and doubt and controversy inciting its challenge.

These statistically driven clinical experiential elements are further focused toward more individualized predictors, also explaining, through mechanistic hypotheses, the course of the disease. These are formulated within system or cell biology principles and eventually in molecular terms,[10,21,23] starting at the level of the genome, elucidating inherent imbalances, errors, or deterministic combinations predisposing to disease, and factors modulating disease progression and regression. The role of neurosurgical intervention is re-examined within this context with an eye toward refining indications, optimizing timing and patient selection, and articulating the surgical rationale, objectives, and techniques based on these mechanistic concepts.

The above elements are necessarily temporary, to be abandoned without reserve through doubt and the constant test of experiential observations.[25] Bias is minimized through scientific methodology, meta-analysis, and the integration of observations so as to sustain old hypotheses, or generate new ones, shaping and advancing neurosurgical science.[26]

References

1. Awad IA, Spetzler RF. Extracranial-intracranial bypass surgery: a critical analysis in light of the International Cooperative Study. *Neurosurgery.* 1986;19: 655-664.
2. Bernard C. *Lecons de Physiologie Experimentale Applique a la Medicine.* Paris, France: JB Bailliere; 1855-1856.
3. Bucy PC. *Neurosurgical Giants: Feet of Clay and Iron.* New York, NY: Elsevier; 1985.
4. Canguilhem G. *On the Normal and the Pathological.* New York, NY: Zone Books; 1991.
5. Caplan LR. Question-driven technology assessment: SPECT as an example. *Neurology.* 1991;41:187-191.
6. Casti JL. *Searching for Certainty: What Scientists Can Know About the Future.* New York, NY: William Morrow; 1990.
7. Comte A. Considerations philosophiques sur l'ensemble de la science biologique (1838). Fortieth Lecture of *The Cours de Philosophie Positive, III.* Paris, France: Schleicher; 1908.
8. Cushing H, Eisenhardt LM. *Meningiomas, Their Classification, Regional Behavior, Life History and Surgical End Results.* Springfield, Ill: Charles C Thomas; 1938.
9. DeVilliers JC. Some pitfalls and problems in neurosurgery. *Prog Neurol Surg.* 13:1990.
10. Dowling JE. *Neurons and Networks: An Introduction to Neuroscience.* Boston, Mass: Belknap Press; 1992.
11. Einstein A. *The Meaning of Relativity.* Princeton, NJ: Princeton University Press; 1945.
12. Fredrickson DS. Biomedical research in the 1980's. *N Engl J Med.* 1981;304:509-517.
13. Gleick J. *Chaos: Making a New Science.* New York, NY: Viking; 1987.
14. Haines SJ. Six statistical suggestions for surgeons. *Neurosurgery.* 1981;9:414-418.
15. Haines SJ. Randomized clinical trials in neurosurgery. *Neurosurgery.* 1983;12:259-264.
16. Haines SJ. The art and science of evaluating neurosurgical treatment. *Clin Neurosurg.* 1989;35: 451-458.
17. Hawkins C, Sorgi M, eds. *Research: How to Plan, Speak and Write About It.* New York, NY: Springer-Verlag; 1985.
18. Heidegger M. *Identity and Difference.* New York, NY: Harper & Row; 1969.
19. Heisenberg W. *Physics and Philosophy: The Revolution in Modern Science.* New York, NY: Harper & Row; 1958.
20. Langfitt TW. Are randomized clinical trials of surgical procedures feasible? *Clin Neurosurg.* 1989;33: 43-52.
21. Levitan IB, Kaszmarek LK. *The Neuron: Cell and Molecular Biology.* London, England: Oxford University Press; 1991.
22. Marias N. *History of Philosophy.* New York, NY: Dover Publications; 1967.
23. Moses LE. The series of consecutive cases as a device for assessing outcomes of intervention. *N Engl J Med.* 1984;311:705-710.
24. Newell A. *Unified Theories of Cognition.* Cambridge, Mass: Harvard University Press; 1990.
25. Poincaré H. *La Science et L'Hypothese.* Paris, France: Flammarion; 1906.
26. Popper KR. *The Logic of Scientific Discovery.* New York, NY: Basic Books; 1959.
27. Salmon WC. *Scientific Explanation and the Causal Structure of the World.* Princeton, NJ: Princeton University Press; 1984.
28. Schwartz HG, Enthoven AC, Black PM, et al. Symposium on medical decision making. *Clin Neurosurg.* 1986;33:73-113.
29. Scopperud RJ. *American Usage and Style: The Consensus.* New York, NY: Van Nostrand Rheinhold; 1979.
30. Vendryes P. *Vie et Probabilite.* Paris, France: A Michel; 1942.

CHAPTER 11

Neurosurgery and the Surgical Art

Michael Salcman, MD

In what sense is neurosurgery or its practice an art? Why is there any need to formulate an answer to this question so late in our century? Isn't the answer obvious? After all, skill and its display or application, or skill in doing anything as a result of knowledge and practice, is the first definition of *art* encountered in the *Oxford English Dictionary (OED)*. However, the specific use of art as a term to mean "skill in applying the principles of a special science; [a] technical or professional skill" is now considered an obsolete or archaic use of the term. Indeed, such a definition is so general and nonspecific that almost any learned activity might be considered an art. Are medicine and surgery—disciplines uniquely dependent on knowledge of both the arts and the sciences—nothing more than mere technical exercises? Since the old notion of art as a professional skill implies that medicine is simply the practical application of a science, it may unnaturally separate the latter from the former. A utilitarian concept of the arts probably led Jeremy Bentham[1] to declare that each art had a corresponding science. As discussed elsewhere, such compartmentalization between the arts and the sciences is demonstrably artificial and potentially dangerous.[19] Neurosurgery obviously represents the application of an acquired skill, but it cannot be considered an art simply on this basis.

The secondary definition of *art* in the *OED,* usually employed in the plural, refers to subjects or activities wherein skill may be attained or displayed, and it is in this sense that the Arts have been used to denote certain branches of learning. The term was first applied in the Middle Ages to the trivium (grammar, logic, rhetoric) and the quadrivium (arithmetic, geometry, music, astronomy), seven subjects that comprised a course of study introduced as early as the sixth century; our concept of the free or liberal arts derives from this scholastic program. However, these "arts" also were thought to be sciences because they were considered basic to all other areas of study in which further research and refinement were still possible. Obviously, medicine and its subdisciplines, eternally perfectible, are not arts in this meaning of the term. In the alternative sense of art as the "practical application of any science, a body or system of rules serving to facilitate the carrying out of certain principles," medicine may at least claim status as an applied art, a situation no more desirable than considering medicine an applied science. In any case, none of the original subjects of the trivium are today considered to be sciences, and almost none of the subjects in the quadrivium are thought to be arts.

Although the most traditional concepts of art, either as an individual skill or "Art" as a category of learning, are not incompatible with the status of medicine as an art, they are but imperfect and incomplete descriptions. Nevertheless, both medical practitioners and the public at large would be comfortable with the notion of medicine as an art if profound changes in the definition and practice of these two disciplines had not occurred in the 19th and 20th centuries. Confusion in regard to the status of medicine as an art arises chiefly by virtue of two developments: first, a new definition of art that did not even appear in any English dictionary prior to 1880; and second, the contemporary orientation of medicine toward technology and away from humanism.

Medicine as an Art

The modern definition of art is now the one that is almost exclusively employed as the basis for our usual sense of the term when the word (art) is used without qualification. This meaning of the term is given by the *OED* as: "The application of skill to the arts of imitation and design . . . the skillful production of the beautiful in visible forms." This usage began with the artists and critics of the 19th century and continues to the present day. It is based on a Romantic notion of the artist as an intuitive creator of beautiful objects. These artifacts were thought to reflect the artist's mind and hand, even as the purpose of the Creator was reflected in the wonders of the natural world. This conjunction was most obvious in the landscapes of the French Romantic painters, the seascapes of the English master J. M. Turner, the evocation of light by the French impressionists, and the depiction of cataracts, rainbows, and canyons by the painters of the American Hudson River School. In this view, artists are the creators of artifacts, which are in themselves subject to some theoretical standard of beauty or creative significance.

Superficially, the role of the caring physician and the creative surgeon would appear incompatible with such a concept of the nature of art. Nevertheless, John Ruskin,[14] one of the first proponents of the modern view and the foremost art critic of the 19th century, stated: "Fine art is that in which the hand, the head, and the heart of man go together." In the contemporary art world, Ruskin's observation might be considered to apply as much to the process of art as it does to the artistic product. In this sense, certainly, neurosurgery is an art and the neurosurgeon an artist.

Furthermore, artists, scientists, and physicians selectively filter reality, emphasizing features that are of interest to them and ignoring others. In this way, they are capable of forming a world view based on a type of looking. The process of intuition is critical to the process of selection and instrumental in the creation of the artist's or scientist's orientation to the world. As I have previously discussed, artists, scientists, and physicians share a number of other characteristics;[19] as listed by Cavell,[2] these include: precision, accuracy, authority, apprenticeship, argument, rhetoric, definition, community, example, experimentation, and stubbornness. Furthermore, the will to create and heal is the moral force and guiding principle of the medical profession, directly related to what Cavell has described as "The wish to make something, to counter destructiveness, to leave the world marginally better than you found it, to mend it, [that] is at the heart of both the arts and the sciences." This belief in the healing power of art must be very close to what Matisse felt when he expressed his desire that his works should provide the weary businessman with a respite from the quotidian, from the everyday cares of the world:[20]

> What I dream of is an art of balance, of purity and serenity, devoid of troubling or depressing subject matter, an art which could be for every mental worker, for the business man as well as the man of letters, for example, a soothing, calming influence on the mind, something like a good armchair which provides relaxation from physical fatigue.

Of course, Matisse had much more than a simple anodyne for our everyday problems in mind, wishing for his art to have the power to return us to a primitive Golden Age where the spiritual would reign supreme. On the other hand, this view taken to dangerous extremes has sometimes led to confusing the quality of a painting with its ability to provide moral uplift. The excellence of an object has virtually nothing to do with the political beliefs of the artist or the moral lessons implicitly or overtly contained within the object itself. Unfortunately, much of contemporary art is concerned with issues of race, sex, and gender, or the supposed disjunction between man and the natural world brought about by technology (Figures 1 and 2[6]). Attempts by dictatorships of both the left and the right to enlist the artist in the moral education of the populace have always failed to produce significant works of art.[7]

The primary tools of the artist are the same as those of the neurosurgeon. As Vogel[24] has stated: "The eyes and the hands are the most important instruments for a neurosurgeon." These tools are critical to microsurgery, the apex of contemporary practice in our field, a discipline in which the eyes and the hands are still considered more important than conceptual visualization or advanced technology. However, the mere repetition of such handiwork, no matter how difficult or elegant, without exercise of judgment and creative insight is simply a type of craft; the daily practice of microsurgical procedures carried out by rote can hardly be considered art. On rare occasions, however, apparently intuitive and nonreflective behavior can raise itself to the standards of art. This not only occurs at the operating table but also may take place at the artist's easel. When Cézanne said of Monet that "he was only an eye, but what an eye!" he did not mean to disparage him.[15] The color of Monet's haystacks and cathedrals was purposefully laid down in individual small strokes of equal hue or maximum intensity so as to paint the insensible atmosphere of light that stood between the viewer and the object. Furthermore, his haystacks and cathedrals were painted in series so as to illustrate changes in the materiality of his objects and their colors with changes in the seasons and the time of day. Monet knew that the structure of the world (i.e. vision) was a temporal phenomenon. Because he made this knowledge visible, we know that Monet was much more than an eye, or even a hand and an eye—he was a brain intuiting the universe.

The Pterional Craniotomy

In the same way that Monet appears to encapsulate the history of French impressionism, the pterional craniotomy can be said to symbolize the 30-year period of neurosurgery now drawing to a close. In the early 1960s, pioneering applications of the operating microscope in the posterior fossa by Kurze and Rand and in the treatment of cerebral aneurysms by J. Lawrence Pool were succeeded by Yasargil's elaboration of a complete microsurgical technique and philosophy.[11,12,27] The pterional craniotomy became the cornerstone procedure, an approach that largely replaced the more extensive bone removal and brain exposure of former techniques in the treatment of a wide variety of tumors and vascular lesions.[28] Although the operating microscope made exposure of deep structures safe and feasible, it placed a premium on the ability of the surgeon to manipulate specially-designed instruments with small and precise movements. Not all neurosurgeons

caught in midcareer with this advance were able to adapt, and not all new trainees were intuitively able to grasp the subtleties of the technique. It became necessary, therefore, to develop methods for the acquisition of a new way of thinking as well as a novel means of doing.

As one minor example, it is possible to teach the microsurgery of a pterional craniotomy as a series of "cookbook" steps, an approach that I have often found safe and useful with junior residents. After completion of the bone flap and removal of the lateral edge of the sphenoid wing (the pterion) down to the skull base, the dura is opened in a lunate fashion, with the apex of the incision directed into the sylvian fissure. Since much of the logic and rationale of the procedure is based on the purposeful limitation of potentially harmful retraction delivered to the frontal and temporal lobes, the student is taught to think of the initial exposure of the circle of Willis and the pituitary as a series of balletic steps involving a single retractor blade. This retractor is advanced perpendicular to the long axis of the frontal lobe until the olfactory nerve is exposed (first position). The tip is kept perpendicular to the first nerve throughout gradual movement of the retractor posteriorly along the olfactory tract until the optic nerve is discovered. Retraction is now carried out in the long axis of the second nerve (second position), and the arachnoidal adhesions to the frontal lobe are dissected until the carotid artery becomes visible lateral to the optic nerve. At this point, the angle of retraction is once again changed, since it must be carried out in the long axis of the carotid artery (third position) while dissection is gradually advanced distally along this structure. This sequence of steps is virtually foolproof and well serves the student in the majority of situations. However, the experienced and artful operator knows that an almost infinite number of variations can be filigreed upon this basic sequence.

I give a few examples to make it clear that the strategic consequences of each variation in the basic pterional approach are as meaningful as the fugal play of Bach's music. The analogy is not as distant as it might first appear; for example, the physical embodiment of Bach's musical lines is quite visible in the choreography of George Balanchine. As a first point, since the A_1 segment of the anterior cerebral artery is the only major structure to cross the dorsal surface of the optic nerve, exposure of an anterior communicating artery aneurysm may require little or no dissection over the dorsal surface of the carotid artery (position three) and, therefore, little or no retraction of the temporal lobe. In fact, in the majority of cases, the treatment of aneurysms of the proximal carotid artery requires only the placement of a "bookmark" retractor on the temporal lobe. An exception is an aneurysm in the vicinity of the ophthalmic artery, where even gentle retraction of the frontal lobe (position one) may result in premature rupture of a lesion dorsal to the anterior clinoid process. Retraction of the frontal lobe can be minimized through more extensive bone removal at the skull base, early dissection in the sylvian fissure, and packing of the most anterior and deep portion of the field with cottonoid strips.

Aneurysms of the carotid bifurcation and middle cerebral artery always require distal dissection in the sylvian fissure and some retraction of the temporal lobe. The latter maneuver can be dangerous in the treatment of so-called simple aneurysms of the posterior communicating artery. When the dome is judged to lie below the tentorial edge, temporal retraction is relatively safe; when the aneurysm points above this line, a single retractor approach based on the frontal lobe is wise. In each of these situations, the selective application of "pressure" or the intensity of movement felt in certain directions or upon particular structures is a matter of the operator's judgment. Such judgment is a type of wisdom gained from experience in the application of the visual and kinesthetic senses at critical moments in the life of the patient and the life of the surgeon. Profound examples of such learning are to be found in the descriptions given by Drake[3] in regard to his highly intuitive and individualized approach to the treatment of giant aneurysms. The application of such wisdom is a type of art.

Art and Technology

In the evolution of the microsurgical approach to aneurysms in general and the pterional craniotomy in particular, Pool, Yasargil, Drake, and others served as form-givers and artists. The implications of their accomplishments were as evident to their successors as the lessons of van Gogh and Cézanne were for Matisse and Picasso. However, the artists of the early 20th century were already caught up in a zeitgeist and mindset that only now are beginning to affect the daily practice of neurosurgery. In their prescient way, artists often anticipate the elaboration of a new world view before general dissemination of knowledge about recent advances in physics and biology occurs; conversely, developments in the sciences strongly affect the philosophic orientation of the artist, sometimes providing him or her with new subjects and materials from which a contemporary reality can be created.[19] The apparent cultural estrangement of art and science, so eloquently decried by C. P. Snow, is not substantiated by the many historical parallels so evident in the development of both fields.[19,21,22]

From a philosophic point of view, the most profound development in the 20th century has been the elaboration of the Einsteinian universe, one in which the speed of light becomes the only reliable invariant and all events are relativistically contingent upon the speed of the observer and the nature of his frame of reference.[21] The simultaneity of views in a cubist landscape or portrait, the dilation of time visible in a de Chirico, the melting of clocks in a Dali—all are symptoms of this cultural influence. Twentieth-century artists (and the rest of us) have struggled with the apparent absurdities imposed by a world view in which traditional causality and dimensional relationships are thrown out. As a consequence, no prior century has expended so much energy on the measurement of time and the contemplation of space. It is not surprising, therefore, that a contemporary artist like David Wojnarowicz would implant clocks in his soft sculptures of the human brain (Figure 3[26]). This improbable conjunction of seemingly incompatible objects and events is familiar to us from the dream world of psychoanalysis and surrealism, but its origins can be traced to earlier literary experiments in which medical metaphors played a prominent role. In 1868, in *Les Chants de Maldoror*, the Comte de Lautreamont describes a young boy as being "as beautiful as the chance meeting on a dissecting table of a sewing machine and an umbrella."[15] Like the simultaneity of views present in cubism, the strange conjunctions and distortions of time and space in surrealistic painting were remarkably congruent with the predictions of modern physics and neuroscience.

Stereotactic Surgery

The recent emergence of stereotactic surgery, therefore, is the tardy acknowledgment of a relativistic method of looking that was already familiar to artists and scientists at the dawn of this century. Like them, the stereotactic surgeon must feel comfortable with the integration of multiple frames of reference. Naturally, neurosurgeons are happiest when dealing with anatomic space, a frame of reference in which all intracranial structures are related to superficial landmarks. Inferences are drawn in three dimensions and the consequences of one's decisions are directly visible. Throughout the development of our specialty, neurosurgeons have had to learn how to transpose information from two-dimensional radiographic images to the three-dimensional reality of the operative field. Of late, we have become familiar with the x-y coordinate system that orients anatomic structures within single computed tomography (CT) or magnetic resonance imaging (MRI) slices, the scan space of the machine.

Prior to the development of image-based stereotaxy, however, it was relatively difficult to translate or map the location of structures seen in scan space onto the anatomic space arrayed before the surgeon at the operating table. Paradoxically, the CT- or MRI-compatible stereotactic frame does not directly perform such a translation since all points contained within the frame are referenced only to the boundaries of the volume that it contains (i.e. stereotactic space) and not to the actual dimensions of either the patient's head or the scanner. It is for this reason that simple mathematical rules or portable computers are required to translate radiographic (scan space) coordinates into stereotactic coordinates for use in the operating room. Of course, the CT scan or MR image of the frame in place on the patient's head contains all the information required for determining the stereotactic coordinates of imaged targets within the real brain. Therefore, the sequence of a stereotactic procedure flows from an image through a mental abstraction to the reality of anatomic space.

Not only must the contemporary stereotactic neurosurgeon learn to work within multiple frames of reference, he or she usually directs probes or beams of energy at anatomic structures that are shielded from sight. Therefore, the surgeon carries out his or her efforts "on faith" and at a distance, without the reassurance of direct visual inspection, much as the modern physicist must believe in particles that can barely be detected or measured. In this sense, stereotactic neurosurgery is almost a purely mental activity, the essential nature of which is to free the surgeon from the need for coordinated use of the eye and hand. In a similar vein, this century has witnessed numerous scientific and artistic movements in which an idea or concept has taken the place of an actual object, especially when its physical embodiment has become a near impossibility. It was in this spirit that Einstein carried out his "thought" experiments, and that some artists came to believe in the superiority of their concepts to any physical realization of their ideas. The written instructions for a Sol LeWitt wall drawing completely specify the reality of his "sculpture" and only these instructions can be purchased in the gallery. LeWitt's assistants must be hired to carry out a realization of his concept on an actual wall and, if the collector moves, the drawing must be recreated in the new space and painted over in the old.

The Issue of Quality in Art and Medicine

It is easy to scoff at the emergence of a new reality, to treat novel ways of seeing as just further examples of the emperor's new clothes. In our everyday world, acts and objects are usually more important than ideas alone. In the parlance of football, it is necessary to walk the walk as well as to talk the talk. Results count. In Gabor Peterdi's master printmaking class at Yale, where the purpose of the course was to physically create an etching or an engraving, a student enthralled by conceptual art was once offered a "conceptual" diploma as a fitting reward for his nonexistent print. In the everyday world, expectations must be met and ideas used in appropriate circum-

__Figure 1.__ Deborah Kass (b.1952). "One Gold Barbra," acrylic on canvas, 1992. The conceptual basis of much contemporary art is nicely illustrated by this painting, in which the issues of gender politics and technology converge. The portrait of Barbra is not painted but utilizes a 1960s photograph that is silk-screened and centered on a canvas of the appropriate size, color, and format so as to appear to be a genuine work by Andy Warhol, almost identical to his gold portrait of Marilyn Monroe in the Museum of Modern Art in New York. Kass is a radical feminist who has appropriated Warhol's technology and point of view to do to him, a prominent male artist, what he so often did to others—i.e. "steal" their signs and symbols so as to change their meaning by placing them in another context (c.f. his Brillo soap boxes and paintings of Campbell soup cans). Kass chose Streisand as a subject because she was the only major performer of the 1960s not used as a subject by Warhol; Kass feels that Streisand's exclusion was based on her strength and independence as a woman. As evidenced by Kass, Warhol's art, born in the era of television and mass communication, with its explicit questioning of the meaning of authenticity and spirituality in a post-Freudian technological age, has been profoundly influential. (Reproduced courtesy of a private collection.)

__Figure 2.__ Robert Longo (b.1953). "Walk," lead, wood, oil, and plastic paint on aluminum, 1986; Broad Collection, Los Angeles. Longo is an American member of the postmodern or neoexpressionist generation of painters that came to prominence in the 1980s. He has always worked in multimedia with major portions of his oeuvre fabricated by assistants. Many of his best works are commentaries on modern urban life. Here, the "walk" of the mindless cutout figures occurs in a subterranean space beneath the three-dimensional recession of buildings on a major avenue. The city takes the place of the corpus callosum, but instead of binding the right and left sides of the brain, the urban environment acts to split the soul. Although often critical of technology, Longo's art could not have been physically realized in any previous era.[6] (Courtesy of the artist and Metro Pictures.)

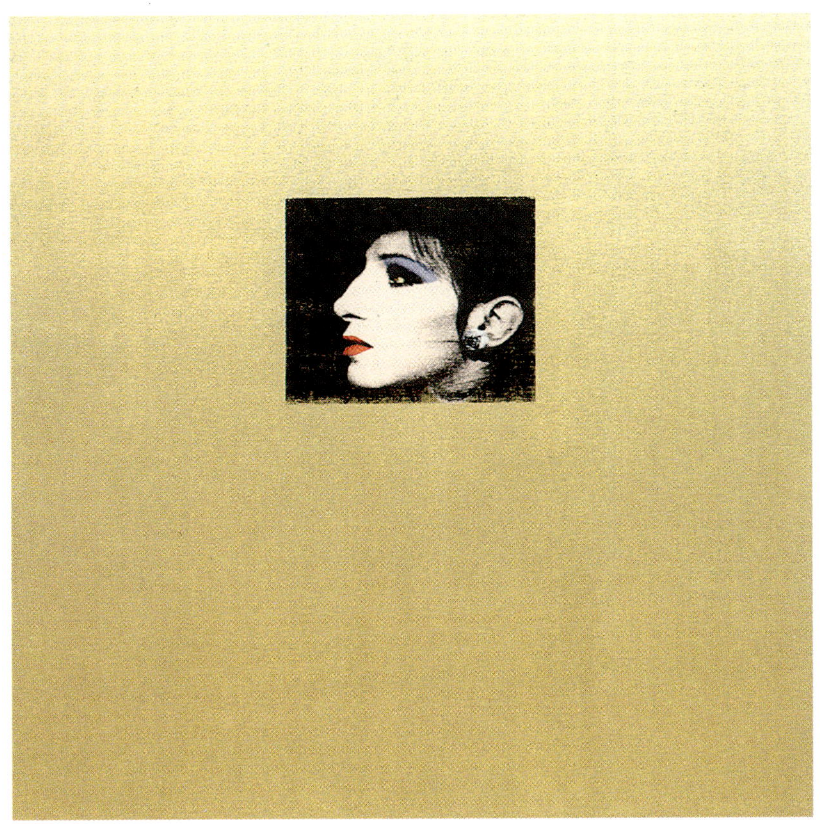

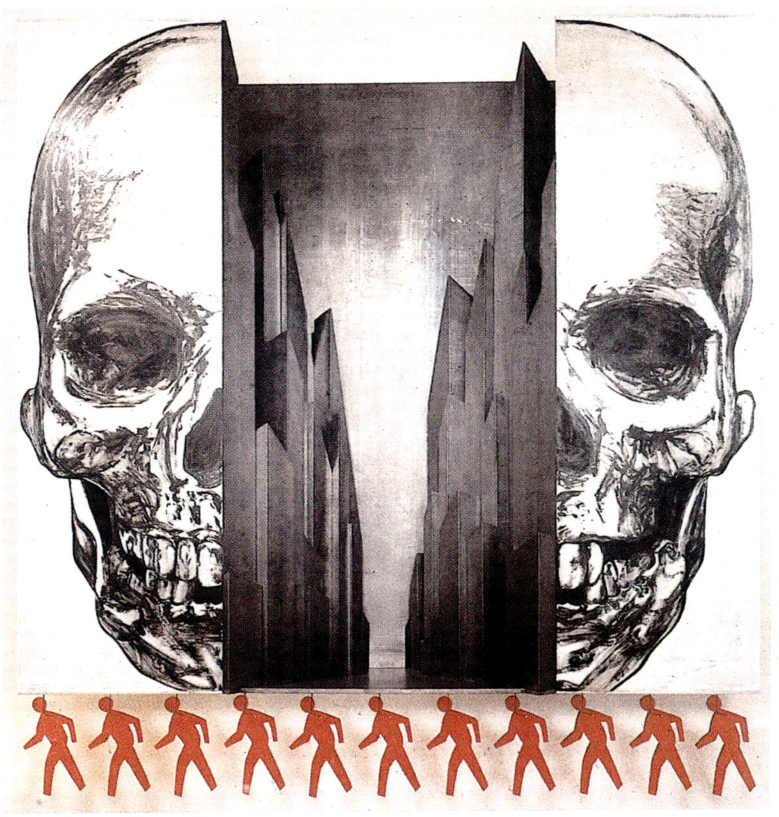

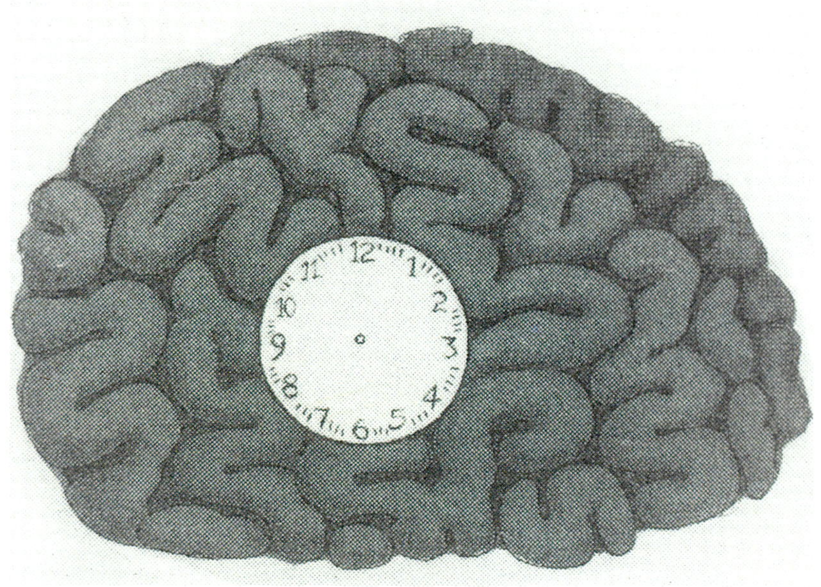

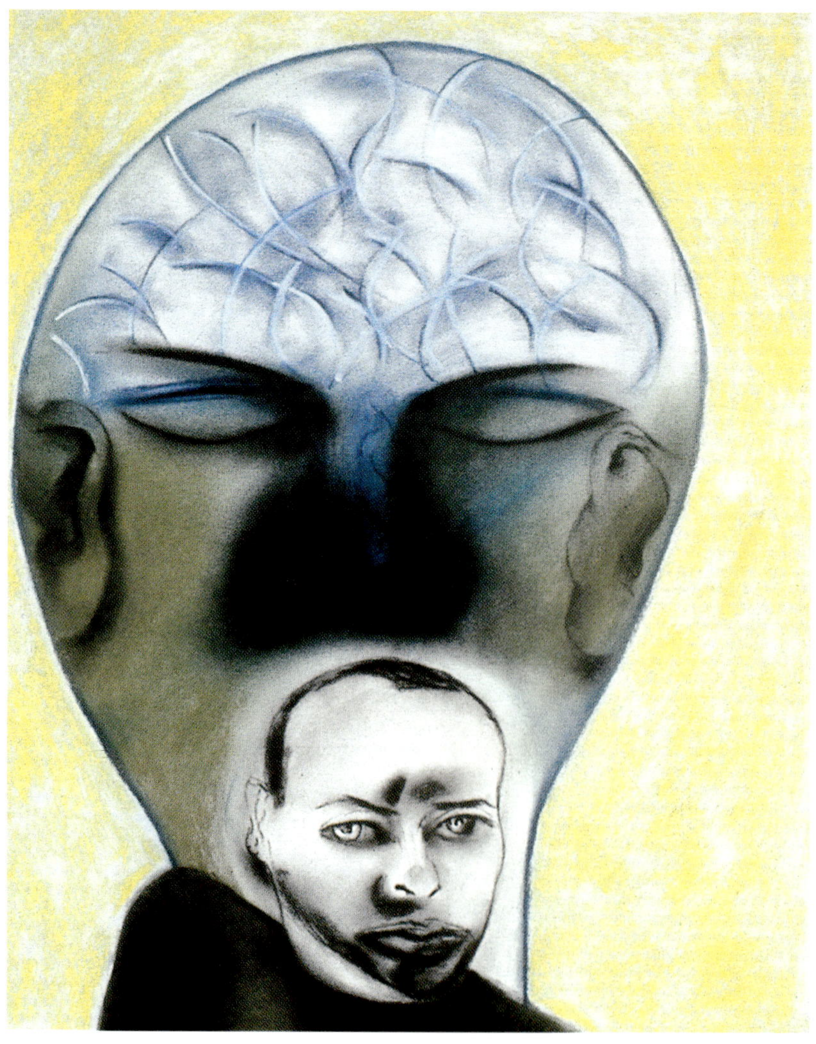

Figure 3. David Wojnarowicz (1954–1992). "Brain-Time," etching, 1988–1989. One of the leaders of the New York East Village scene in the 1980s, Wojnarowicz was a multimedia artist who wrote books, made films, did photography, and worked in painting and collage. His career is exceptional in that he was able to create powerful works of art on political themes. Although his anger and frustration were usually quite visible, the images were always arresting and the subjects complex. Wojnarowicz became an impassioned advocate against the forces that had so brutalized his life on the streets. When he made "Brain-Time" as both an etching and a soft rubber sculpture, he already knew that he was dying of AIDS.[26] (Courtesy of the estate of David Wojnarowicz and PPOW Gallery, New York.)

Figure 4. Francesco Clemente (b.1952). "Smoke in the Room," pastel, 1983. The most important contemporary Italian artist, Clemente is also the most widely traveled and has homes in Rome, Madras, and New York. His works on paper, in pastels, and watercolor are frequently superior to his paintings. His art is closest in feeling to classical surrealism, but he revitalizes this tradition with his color sense and the spirituality and eroticism of his literary and cultural sources: Roman mosaics, Persian miniatures, and Indian legends. (Courtesy of Sperone Westwater, New York.)

stances. On the other hand, received wisdom must not be allowed to constrain innovation.

In his lawsuit against the 19th-century critic Ruskin, James McNeil Whistler countered such narrow-mindedness by claiming sole authority for judging the rightness of his work. As a corollary, some writers adopted the principle that a painting created by an artist should be judged by the degree to which it upheld the aesthetics propounded by that artist. It was but a small step from Whistler's defense of the quality of his art to the position of Marcel Duchamp that anything was to be considered art, even a hat rack or a signed urinal called "Fountain," if the artist said it was art.[25] Of course, the wide-ranging prerogative generally conceded to artists is no longer granted to physicians. The most aesthetically pleasing operation in the world is a failure if the patient is left hemiparetic or dies.

Aesthetics is the slippery slope upon which judgments of quality and importance are made in the arts, and sometimes even in mathematics and science. Except for the underlying anatomy and physiology involved, it is hard to imagine that beauty rather than utility can ever be the standard for the rightness of a surgical procedure. Of course, aesthetic judgments have been applied to ideas and theories as well as to paintings and poetry. In this sense, mathematicians speak of elegant proofs or economic solutions to difficult problems. It is in this spirit that some operations can be described as elegant or beautiful. Although aesthetics change over time and the criteria of a contemporary critic such as Clement Greenberg[5] are unlikely to be those of a Ruskin or Aristotle, beauty is not simply in the eye of the beholder and quality in art goes well beyond the physical embodiment of an idea. In her correspondence with Gustave Flaubert, George Sand[4] wrote that "art, at its greatest, is nothing but the expression of wisdom. Wisdom teaches us to see something outside ourselves that is higher than what is within us, and gradually, through contemplation and admiration, to come to resemble it." Subsequently, many philosophic influences, including French symbolism and Eastern religion, have contributed to the mystic identification of the artist and his work (Figure 4).

In any field of intellectual activity, an appreciation of worth presupposes knowledge. Although considerably more difficult, absolute judgments about and comparative evaluations of paintings and symphonies are hardly more arbitrary than qualitative appraisals of diamonds and houses; a knowledge of the historical record and the eye or ear of a connoisseur are essential. Therefore, aesthetic judgments are inherently elitist and involve an insider's point of view. As a result, the elegance of most mathematical proofs is obvious only to mathematicians, and the heuristic beauty in the structure of DNA is best appreciated by molecular biologists. Similarly, the elegance and economy of movement involved in a neurosurgical procedure are almost certainly irrelevant and possibly quite invisible to our nonsurgical brethren. The perspicacity of the artist is of quite another order. Not only is he often ahead of the zeitgeist, frequently anticipating the discoveries and revelations of his colleagues in other fields, but he is also the most reliable guide to those individuals and things of greatest interest and quality in his own area. If a neurosurgeon seeks to be an artist, then he should follow the precept of McLuhan:[9] "The artist is the man in any field, scientific or humanistic, who grasps the implications of his actions and of new knowledge in his own time. He is the man of integral awareness."

In sorting out aesthetic judgments, history is the great leveler, and the judgment of time is as close to absolute certitude as we are likely to get. From a distance, it is easier to tell how tall the mountains stand and how small the foothills really are. With the advantage of historical perspective, Mendelssohn rediscovers Bach, and Rosenblum[13] can link Turner and Caspar David Friedrich to Pollock and Rothko. As the filmstrip of time speeds up, we also can watch fashions in treatment and diagnosis come and go. The entire saga of medical therapy for subarachnoid hemorrhage and vasospasm takes off from dextran, papaverine, and steroids, progresses through antifibrinolytics and calcium channel blockers, and returns again to volume expanders, a new generation of steroids, and papaverine.[8,10,23] Hence, after more than 50 years in which the survival curves for glioblastoma have not changed appreciably, we can only hope that the arrival of molecular biology truly represents an Einsteinian revolution in our stalled treatment of malignant brain tumors.[17,18] If nothing else, time and history should teach us to be modest in our claims and aspirations. Would the fashionable salon painters of 19th century France ever have dreamed of the anonymity to which history and the impressionist painters have consigned them? Would Newton, so right in so many things, ever have guessed to see his world view overthrown to such a degree that Einstein felt the need to issue him an apology?

It is not only the microscope that evolves but the lens of history. Like the observer and the electron, it is not possible for a new vision to inform art and science without that vision similarly affecting the manner in which criticism and historical judgment are carried out. New methods of seeing, some optical, some mental, have been critical to the development of the arts and sciences in this century and throughout the history of the Western tradition. Even our theoretical views of the manner in which the brain functions have been conditioned by the dominant technologies of our time.[16] Meanwhile, the pace of change has steadily accelerated. The method developed during the Renaissance of using one-point perspective to give a lifelike rendering of objects held sway for more than 400 years until the advent of cubism and its multiplicity of viewpoints in 1907. In rapid succession, however, the recognizable subjects of cubist still lifes were eliminated by the geometric abstractions of Kandinsky, Mondrian, and Malevich; the shallow sense of depth in cubist space was flattened by Pollock, abstract expressionism (1950), and the color field painters (1960s). All that remained was for the reality of paint and canvas to disappear, supplanted as they were (but only for a time) by the pure conception and disembodied ideas of the artist. In physics and cosmology, the Newtonian view of everyday mechanics in a cause-and-effect universe reigned supreme for almost 300 years until it gave way to Einsteinian relativity, multiple frames of reference, an expanding universe, and the study of subatomic particles in a probabilistic world.

The timeline of development in neurosurgery is almost exactly the same. From the time of Ambroise Paré until the pioneering generation of Macewen, Horsley, and Cushing, almost nothing changed in neurosurgery for about 400 years. Cushing's declaration of the specialty occurred in 1905 and progress, although steady, was hardly revolutionary until the 1960s and the arrival of the operating microscope. Since then we have not only witnessed the unaided vision of pioneering surgeons supplanted by microsurgical techniques, but the more rapid development of technologies, such as image-based stereotaxy and frameless surgery, that depend on the computerized acquisition of images, new coordinate systems, and the imminent arrival of virtual reality. Today the neurosurgeon sees his patient with many eyes; he can work with a linear vision that is natural and unaided, with the enhanced single-point perspective of the microscope, in the multiple perspectives of the stereotactic frame, or even without any direct visual or tactile guidance whatsoever. In the molecular surgery of the future, some of the steps in every operation and many of our tools will have become well-nigh invisible, transparent to both the surgeon and the patient. What I have described here as a brief history of neurosurgery is really the progressive refinement of its vision. Is neurosurgery not an art, therefore, so dependent as it is on new ways of seeing?

References

1. Bentham J. The rationale of reward (1825). In: *Oxford English Dictionary*. Compact ed. New York, NY: Oxford Press; 1971:204.
2. Cavell S. Observations on art and science. *Daedalus*. 1986;115:171-177.
3. Drake CG. Giant intracranial aneurysms: experience with surgical treatment in 174 patients. *Clin Neurosurg*. 1979;26:12-95.
4. Flaubert G, Sand G; Steegmuller F, trans. *Flaubert—Sand: The Correspondence*. New York, NY: Knopf; 1993.
5. Greenberg C. *Art and Culture: Critical Essays*. Boston, Mass: Beacon Press; 1961.
6. Honnef K. *Contemporary Art*. Hamburg, Germany: Taschen Verlag; 1988:139.
7. Hughes R. *The Shock of the New*. New York, NY: Knopf; 1981:110-111.
8. Kosnik EJ, Hunt WE. Postoperative hypertension in the management of patients with intracranial arterial aneurysms. *J Neurosurg*. 1976;45:148-154.
9. McLuhan M. *Understanding Media: The Extensions of Man*. New York, NY: New American Library; 1964:71.
10. Pool JL. Cerebral vasospasm. *N Engl J Med*. 1958;259:1259-1264.
11. Pool JL, Colton RP. The dissecting microscope for intracranial vascular surgery. *J Neurosurg*. 1966;25:315-318.

12. Rand RW, Kurze T. Facial nerve preservation by posterior fossa transmeatal microdissection in total removal of acoustic tumors. *J Neurol Neurosurg Psychiatry.* 1965;28:311-316.

13. Rosenblum R. *Modern Painting and the Northern Romantic Tradition. Friedrich to Rothko.* New York, NY: Harper & Row; 1975.

14. Ruskin J. The Two Paths: being lectures on art and its applications to decoration and manufacture (1858–1859). In: *Oxford English Dictionary.* Compact ed. New York, NY: Oxford Press; 1971:ii.

15. Russell J. *The Meanings of Modern Art. The Museum of Modern Art.* New York, NY: Harper & Row; 1981:22.

16. Salcman M. Probability and the brain. *Neurosurgery.* 1979;4:75-82.

17. Salcman M. Epidemiology and factors affecting survival. In: Apuzzo MLJ, ed. *Malignant Cerebral Glioma.* Park Ridge, Ill: American Association of Neurological Surgeons; 1990:95-109.

18. Salcman M, ed. *Neurobiology of Brain Tumors.* Baltimore, Md: Williams & Wilkins; 1991.

19. Salcman M. The education of a neurosurgeon: the Two Cultures revisited. *Neurosurgery.* 1992;31:686-696.

20. Schneider P. *Matisse.* New York, NY: Rizzoli International; 1984:268.

21. Shlain L. *Art and Physics: Parallel Visions in Space, Time and Light.* New York, NY: William Morrow; 1991.

22. Snow CP. *The Two Cultures and a Second Look.* Cambridge, England: Cambridge University Press; 1963.

23. Steinke DE, Weir BKA, Findlay JM, et al. A trial of the 21-aminosteroid U74006F in a primate model of chronic cerebral vasospasm. *Neurosurgery.* 1989;24:179-186.

24. Vogel S. The importance of visual arts in the life of a neurosurgeon. *Acta Neurochir (Wien).* 1993;124:168-171.

25. Wheeler D. *Art Since Mid-Century: 1945 to the Present.* New York, NY: Vendome Press; 1991.

26. Wojnarowicz D. *David Wojnarowicz: Tongues of Flame.* Normal, Ill: Illinois State University; 1990.

27. Yasargil MG. *Microsurgery Applied to Neurosurgery.* Stuttgart: Georg Thieme; 1969.

28. Yasargil MG, Fox JL. The microsurgical approach to intracranial aneurysms. *Surg Neurol.* 1975;3:7-14.

CHAPTER 12

Neurosurgical Education

Julian T. Hoff, MD

Evolution of Neurosurgical Education

Medical education began in antiquity. Surgeons taught their art to apprentices, a practice of the Egyptian, Mesopotamian, Asian, Greek, and Roman civilizations and through the Middle Ages. When surgeons separated from barbers during the Renaissance, education became more formalized. But surgery still depended upon master practitioners assisted by apprentices.[5,12]

Anatomic dissections, particularly by Leonardo da Vinci and John Hunter, marked the beginning of the modernization of surgery as a medical discipline. Schools of surgery emerged in several regions of Europe during the mid-1800s. Billroth, Kocher, Kronicker, von Bergmann, and others became renown for their surgical skills, their innovative procedures, and their willingness to teach others. These masters were general surgeons capable of performing any procedure developed at that time. Included among the generalists were men who later became early pioneers of surgery for brain and spinal cord lesions. Macewen, Horsley, Keen, and Godlee were each practitioners of the surgical specialty to become known as neurosurgery.[2,5]

Because those early neurosurgeons had practices that required surgery for conditions outside the nervous system, they relied heavily upon the diagnostic skills of their colleagues, particularly neurologists and physiologists. Thus, the pioneer neurosurgeon confined his role in patient management principally to the surgical procedure alone. While early neurosurgeons were often accompanied by trainees and observers, they failed to establish a curriculum of study

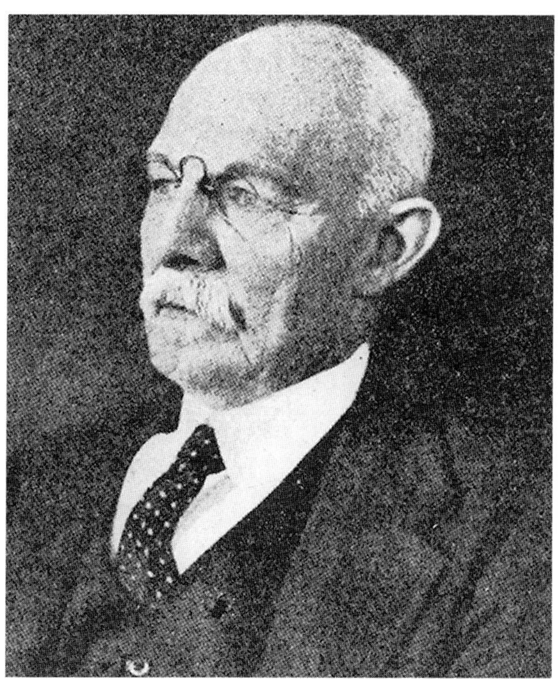

Figure 1. *William S. Halsted, MD (1852–1932)*

and a definition of the new specialty they had initiated, probably because they depended on others for preoperative diagnosis and postoperative care.[2,5]

Surgery education changed dramatically in the late 1800s when William S. Halsted from Johns Hopkins University established a new and exciting method for teaching the surgical discipline (Figure 1).[5] Students were no longer relegated to the observer role, in which they were forbidden to take an active part in patient care. On the contrary, they were expected to immerse themselves in the practicalities of patient care, including preoperative diagnosis, direct participation in surgical procedures, and management of postoperative problems. Halsted emphasized precision in surgical maneuvers, careful approximation of tissues, and practiced anatomic dissections. He, of course, was enabled to do so by the availability of anesthesia for his patients and the aseptic principles provided by Lister and others earlier in the century. Halsted established the innovative concept of resident training in surgery, requiring in-house call, daily rounds, intraoperative participation, and bedside teaching. Halsted's colleague, William Osler, developed similar teaching principles for internal medicine about the same time (1889) at the new Johns Hopkins Hospital in Baltimore.[5,12]

Halsted did not perform neurosurgery himself. He did, however, recognize that desire in Harvey Cushing, one of his medical students. He encouraged Cushing to pursue general surgery at Johns Hopkins first and later encouraged his interest in the surgery of central nervous system disorders.[5]

Harvey Cushing trained in general surgery at Johns Hopkins from 1895 to 1900. He then traveled abroad for 1 year, during which time Horsley and Sherrington in England and Kocher and Kronicker in Switzerland further stimulated his interest in the nervous system. Cushing returned to Baltimore in 1900 to assume a faculty position and devote his practice to patients with neurological problems. He retained the surgical skills and the comprehensive approach to patient problems that he had learned from Halsted and others, and perpetuated the attitude toward training of house officers that he had learned from his master.[4]

Cushing moved to the Peter Bent Brigham Hospital in Boston in 1912 where he became the Mosely Professor at the Harvard Medical School. He brought to the Brigham his rapidly expanding knowledge of nervous system disorders that were amenable to surgery, a profound interest in the education of others in the new discipline he was developing, and a commitment to the best patient care he and his colleagues could provide.[14]

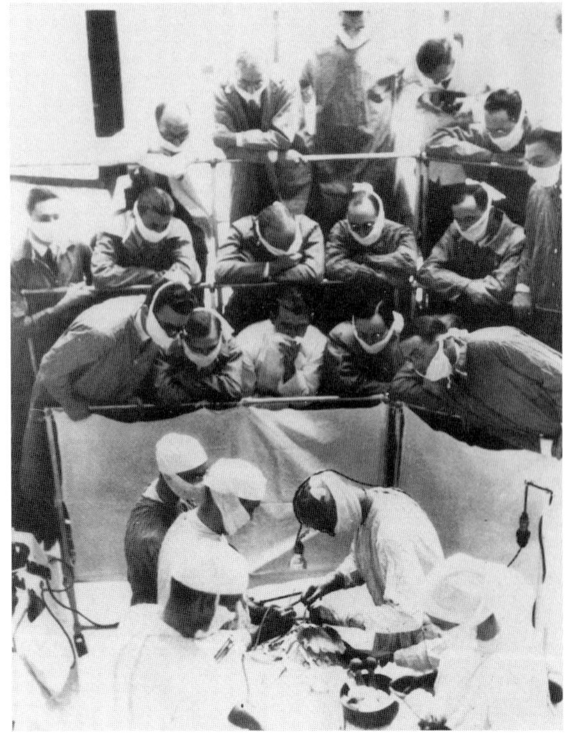

Figure 2. *Harvey Cushing operating (note the headlight). Cushing's colleagues assembled for the first meeting of the Harvey Cushing Society in Boston in 1932, with Dr. Cushing providing a "wet lab" for the members.*

Cushing's residents were "on service" for 1 year, usually toward the end of their general surgery training but sometimes in the midst of it or even at its beginning. He also had many observers from North America and abroad, each of whom stayed for several weeks to months without assigned clinical duties. Cushing had enormous influence on the developing specialty because he was charismatic, a prolific writer, an articulate spokesman, a neuroscientist, an artist, a compulsive and patient surgeon, and a remarkably effective teacher (Figure 2). He was aided throughout his career in Boston by his student and later his colleague Gilbert Horrax and by Louise Eisenhardt, the neuropathologist, both of whom enhanced Cushing's program.[4,8]

Most of Cushing's trainees established training programs of their own throughout the United States, Canada, and Europe. Through his influence on trainees, he established a legacy that differed significantly from the lesser impact on neurosurgery made by Horsley, Macewen, and others in the earliest phases of neurosurgery specialization.[2]

In the 1920s, other schools of neurosurgery emerged in the United States and Canada. Most stemmed from Cushing. Early centers included those developed by Frazier in Philadelphia; Elsberg in New York; Archibald in Montreal; Mackenzie in Toronto; Kanavel and Davis in Chicago; Adson in Rochester, Minnesota; Coleman in Richmond, Virginia; Peet in Michigan; Sachs in St. Louis; Naffziger in San Francisco; and Dandy and Bagley in Baltimore. Most of them were friends and veterans of World War I. They all realized that the development of neurosurgery required the sharing of individual experiences, freely exchanged ideas, and a commitment to teaching the new specialty to the next generation.[2]

Thus, the Society of Neurological Surgeons was formed in 1920, mainly at the instigation of Cushing himself and of Ernest Sachs, his younger colleague from St. Louis. Its principal purpose was to foster a healthy exchange of ideas in patient care, research, and teaching within the framework of good fellowship. There were 20 charter members in this so-called "Senior Society," with an average age of 41 years. They had about 3 years of surgery training each, but only nine members had neurosurgery training that exceeded 6 months. Ten members, including Cushing himself, had no formal training but were exposed to neurosurgery during World War I or in clinics in the United States or abroad before the war. Two of the charter members of the Society were self-taught.[15]

Neurosurgery, thereafter, began to differentiate further from general surgery. Even before then, Cushing recognized that "substantial improvement in neurosurgery would never be achieved until competent men restricted their work to that field alone."[4] Training in 1920, nevertheless, required a full curriculum of general surgery followed by varying degrees of exposure to neurosurgical problems. The first neurosurgeon to be trained exclusively for neurosurgery was Ernest Sachs, later to become the first Professor of Neurosurgery in the world, a position established at Washington University in St. Louis in 1920. Sachs was trained mainly by Horsley in London.[13]

Between 1920 and 1940, the number of neurosurgeons and the number of programs grew. The length of training in neurosurgery increased without progressive responsibility in a defined curriculum. The time spent in general surgery training began to shorten gradually, typically from 4 years to 3 years to 2 years, coupled with a lengthened time in neurosurgery training. By the 1960s, a typical program required 2 years of general surgery followed by 4 years of neurosurgery. During the fourth year of neurosurgery training, the Chief Resident would usually be left alone in the operating room to do his or her work with little supervision, treating patients admitted through resident clinics or the emergency department.[10,11]

The first officially recognized training program was begun in 1933 under the direction of Claude Coleman at the Medical College of Virginia, Richmond. Surprisingly, none of the other training programs that had been established by the 20 charter members of the Society of Neurological Surgeons were acknowledged at that time. One year later, programs in six institutions were identified by the American Medical Association (AMA): the University of California, San Francisco; the New York Neurological Institute; the Boston City Hospital; Strong Memorial Hospital in Rochester, New York; the Medical College of Virginia; and the Presbyterian Hospital in Chicago. By 1940, there were 18 programs officially recognized by the AMA.[10,15]

The American Board of Neurological Surgery

The American Board of Neurological Surgery (ABNS) was established in 1940 at the instigation of the Society of Neurological Surgeons.[9] Its format followed that of the 17 other Boards in existence at that time. The ABNS was comprised of elected members from various societies within the specialty, with a mission to accredit training programs in a systematic way and to certify trainees from those programs. The first Chairman was Howard Naffziger from San Francisco. Fifty neurosurgeons were certified without examination, forming the founding group. The Board continued to accredit programs and certify candidates through an oral examination process until the mid-1950s.[2]

Residency Review Committee

The accreditation of training programs and certification of their trainees by the same group (ABNS) was perceived to be a conflict of interest in the specialty movement. In 1954, both the ABNS and the Council of Medical Education of the AMA agreed that accreditation of programs should become a separate process from certification of trainees. A Residency Review Committee for accreditation of neurosurgical programs was thus created, under the joint sponsorship of the ABNS, the AMA, and the American College of Surgeons. The ABNS thereafter remained a separate and independent body, charged with examining and certifying fully-trained neurosurgeons.[7,9]

In 1981, the Accreditation Council on Graduate Medical Education (ACGME) was formed. It was an agency of five parents (AMA, American Board of Medical Specialties, American Hospital Association, Council on Medical Specialty Societies, and Association of American Medical Colleges) that provided oversight of the Residency Review Committees for all medical specialties. Its charge was to standardize residency training in various disciplines within medicine and to develop general and special requirements for training.

As a result, the proliferation of programs that characterized neurosurgery training in 1965 was sharply curtailed and their growth tightly regulated. The number of training programs fell from 194 in 1965 to 86 in 1969, mostly due to the amalgamation of programs, many of which were in the same locale. The Residency Review Committee for Neurosurgery was given the power through the ACGME to accredit programs based on periodic reviews of the curriculum developed by each program, the availability of its resources, the quality of its faculty, and other sharply defined requirements.[2]

Certification of trainees from programs accredited by the Residency Review Committee was left to the ABNS, where it had originated.

The certification process changed from an all-inclusive oral examination (1941–1970) into staged assessments consisting of a written examination during training, successful completion of an accredited program, 2 years of practice in the specialty, and a final oral examination.[7]

Curriculum Development

The process that evolved from 1940 onward clearly separated the training program as an entity from the trainees within it. The Program Director assumed responsibility for the curriculum and all its elements. General and special requirements were established nationally to provide consistency among programs. Those requirements were periodically revised by the Residency Review Committee, focusing on training essentials including fundamental clinical skills, research opportunity, clinical neurology experience, basic science exposure, the length of training in each segment of training, the quality and quantity of the surgical experience and of the supervising faculty, and the provision for progressive responsibility within the training process. The general aim of each program was to provide an educational experience that would successfully train a medical school graduate to be a safe and competent neurosurgeon within a reasonable period of time. Furthermore, the curriculum was intended to allow the transition of responsibility from a resident neurosurgeon to a fully-trained neurosurgeon without substantial change in the performance of the individual or the expectations of him or her by patients.[10]

Continuing Education

Neurosurgeons require continuing education to keep pace with advancing medical knowledge. To ensure that continuing medical education happens and is not simply an expectation of the professional by the public, organized medicine, including the AMA and the American Association of Neurological Surgeons, established procedures to document time spent by their members in continuing education programs. In addition, continuing education opportunities expanded from the 1960s onward in many insti-

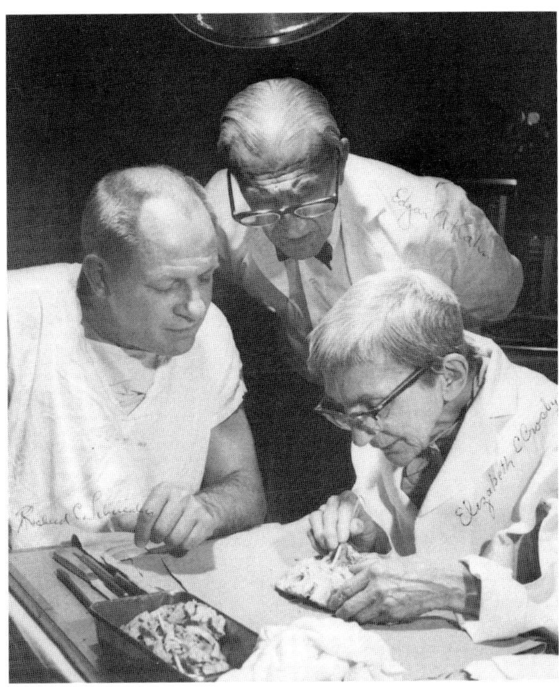

Figure 3. The education of neurosurgeons never ends. This photograph depicts Dr. Elizabeth Crosby, neuroanatomist, teaching two senior students, her colleagues Dr. Edgar Kahn (center) and Dr. Richard Schneider (left), at the University of Michigan in 1978.

tutions. Educational experiences now range from the simple reading of pertinent literature at home to lengthy periods of study in established teaching institutions. Home study courses, practical courses for new diagnostic or therapeutic techniques, annual scientific meetings, and many other formats comprise the available continuing medical education opportunities. That abundant numbers of neurosurgical practitioners participate regularly in many educational events is testimony that neurosurgeons enjoy learning (Figure 3).

Current Teaching Focus

The essentials for neurosurgical education are trainees eager to learn, faculty eager to teach, patients willing to be the subjects of an educational process, optimal facilities, and a curriculum structured for progressive learning.[1] While the essentials for neurosurgical education are clearly defined by the Residency Review Committee, flexibility remains within those requirements. Clinical neurosurgery, neurology, neuroradiology, neuropathology, and the basic neurosciences that support neurosurgery are all obvious necessities. Research is also an essential part of the curriculum, a requirement emphasized decades ago by Horsley, Cushing, Dandy, and Penfield, and more recently by others. The program and curriculum should be well-balanced so that it exposes its trainees to the entire range of the specialty as it is currently practiced in our country. Inevitably, variability exists from program to program. Supervision of the trainee is an obvious requirement, varying individually with each teacher and student depending upon their experience, skill, and knowledge at different levels of training.

Evaluation of and feedback to both the student and the teacher through some objective mechanism is essential for learning. This process allows early identification of individuals not suited for neurosurgery, enabling supervisors to redirect the individual trainee and his or her career goals at an early time. The program itself undergoes peer review periodically by the Residency Review Committee for the quality of its residents and the content of its curriculum, faculty, facilities, and patient material.[1] Assessment of individual residents is currently provided by an in-training examination through the ABNS and by their performance at each step in the training process.

Growth of Neurosurgical Subspecialties

Neurosurgery began as a natural subspecialty of general surgery in the early years of the 20th century. It resulted from focused interests and an expanding knowledge base through an evolutionary process that will continue. Currently, there are several focused groups within neurosurgery itself, including those interested in pediatric neurosurgery, spine and peripheral nerve surgery, stereotactic and functional problems, cerebrovascular disorders, trauma and critical care, neuro-oncology, and the neurosurgery of pain. Pediatric neurosurgery, begun by Frank Ingraham and Donald Matson in the pre-World War II era, was probably the first neurosurgical subspecialty and is the most clearly organized at the present time.

There are many fellowships within neurosurgery, each focused on one or more of the above disciplines.[3] They are currently accredited as fellowships by the institutions where they are offered, but none are recognized by the ABNS or the Residency Review Committee for Neurosurgery and no subspecialty certificates have ever been awarded by the ABNS. The current position of the ABNS holds that subspecialty certification leads to the fragmentation of an already small subspecialty and that certification of smaller and smaller groups will be harmful to the specialty as it matures. However, there is a clear trend toward subspecialty certification within most other specialties recognized by the American Board of Medical Specialties, the parent organization of all the medical specialty boards.[6]

Federal health care reform is presently influencing the specialty and the growth of subspecialties by emphasizing the need for more primary care physicians and fewer specialists and subspecialists. Despite efforts by many to slow the growth of specialization, sophistication in our high-technology society and the inevitable focus of many practitioners will continue. This evolutionary process is predictable, so that further specialty development will, simply, just happen.

Future Teaching Challenges

There are challenges facing neurosurgical education. Resident selection is an ongoing problem. Currently, third-year medical students, with little knowledge of neurosurgery as a life-long occupation, are required to make career decisions based on insufficient information and inadequate exposure to the specialty. Despite that fact, just 15% of those who select neurosurgery as a career fail to complete their training (C Bosk, personal communication, 1994). This failure rate is similar to that found in orthopedic surgery and most other surgical subspecialties.

Resident selection currently depends upon a computer-based matching plan begun in 1983.[10] The matching process, which accounts for the placement of 95% of resident candidates in programs of their choice, is very costly to candidates. The "match" has been successful because of good compliance with the rules by all participants and the high quality of candidates who pursue neurosurgery as a career. A more economical selection process is needed.

Curriculum adjustments must be made periodically. Retention of the basic principles of surgery and the scientific foundations of the specialty will become increasingly difficult to retain as societal pressures demand shorter training periods and more cost-effective delivery of care to patients. Research involvement by neurosurgery residents will be threatened directly by shorter training periods and reduced research funding.

Assuring expertise in the diagnostic techniques we use, coping with a reduced length of hospitalization for patients with neurosurgical problems, dealing effectively with the defensive posture required for our specialty by a litigious society, and teaching students and residents in settings that require ever-increasing efficiency are other challenges neurosurgery educators face.

Funding for resident training remains a problem. How many years are actually needed to produce a neurosurgeon and how many can we afford to train? How many do we really need and of what variety? These and other similar questions are asked of our profession by governmental and private agencies responsible for medical education. While financial concerns and the manpower needs of our country preoccupy policy makers within government, our specialty and its training programs must respond to these concerns by remaining scientifically sound and by requiring a strong and sustained research commitment within every program. Expanding the horizons of our specialty will not happen without new knowledge that benefits patients, and new knowledge about neurosurgical disorders is the direct product of relevant research within the training programs.

Neurosurgical Education Abroad

Neurosurgical education in countries outside North America has followed the same pattern described here. The specialty began within general surgery, then separated at different rates depending upon wars, economic constraints, and other influences in various countries.

The content of neurosurgery as a discipline varies from country to country. Some countries need more neurosurgeons per capita and some need less because the number required for the population depends directly upon the health problems considered appropriate for that specialty in that setting. For example, spine surgery comprises about 60% of the neurosurgical practice in the United States, while it is about 5% in Japan. Most spine surgery in Japan is performed by orthopedic surgeons, implying that that country currently needs fewer neurosurgeons and possibly more orthopedists per capita than their counterparts in the United States in order to provide care for their patient spectrum.

The evolution of neurosurgery internationally, particularly in Europe, mirrored its development in the United States and Canada. Currently, there is an interest in Europe to establish a European Board of Neurosurgery, which aims to standardize the training experience and certify qualified trainees on completion of their training.

Students, Teachers, and Learning Neurosurgery

The style of teachers and the role of students in neurosurgical education have changed over the years. Prior to Halsted, apprentices learned from their masters by watching, duplicating their skills, and sometimes inheriting their judgment. Apprenticeship learning was often successful, although it must have been exceedingly difficult unless the student had natural talent and was a quick learner. When Halsted and Cushing changed training in surgery from the apprenticeship and master format to one of a resident and faculty, substantial gains were made in the ease of learning and the effectiveness of organized study. Despite a better appreciation of structured learning, Cushing continued to do the bulk of his surgery "skin-to-skin," assisted by residents who were primarily observers in the operating room. In fact, Cushing's residents rarely performed an operation as the principal surgeon. Preoperative and postoperative management was also dominated by Cushing with supervised help from residents-in-training.[11]

Hands-on learning and direct experience, often by trial and error, became part of neurosurgical education during the middle part of the 20th century. Often times, charity patients and those admitted to county or veterans' hospitals received most of their care from residents-in-training, some of whom were poorly supervised during their formative years in the specialty.[2] In the 1960s and then onward, increasing supervision came to be expected by residents, faculty, review agencies, including the Residency Review Committee for Neurosurgery, and the public.

Supervised management in outpatient clinics also became important as the need for more accurate diagnosis and efficient workups prior to hospitalization became a necessity in the 1980s and 1990s. Resident participation in the care of all patients, whether private or not, became the standard, with supervision at varying levels of intensity by faculty members.

Interest in improving the education process for neurosurgeons rose steadily after the establishment of the Residency Review Committee, which clearly defined specific and general requirements for resident training. Today, the Residency Review Committee for Neurosurgery is the principal driving force for quality control of neurosurgery educational programs in the United States. It is composed of neurosurgical educators who have long-term commitments to quality training in this country.[1]

Students

Many criteria for the selection of residents have been proposed but none have been universally agreed upon (C Bosk, personal communication, 1994). The following criteria seem obvious. The best candidate for a neurosurgery residency takes great joy in learning and has well-developed study habits. He or she has often been a member of honor societies in undergraduate and medical school. The candidate is emotionally stable and mature for his or her age. He or she has demonstrated a compassionate approach to patients and collegiality toward other health care workers. The candidate has significant outside interests, including sports, music, the arts, etc.

Men and women are equally desirable as resident candidates and equally effective as neurosurgeons. Most physical disabilities, including monocular vision and dyslexia, have not been significant impairments for those entering the specialty. Diversity among residents is enriching not only for the specialty but also for the individual program where they train. Thus, ethnic and racial backgrounds that reflect our society and equal opportunity are sought among the residency applicants.

Teachers

The best teachers of neurosurgery have obvious attributes as well. First, they are excellent mentors with a commitment to teaching and learning. They are eager to constantly improve their own clinical skills and have an abiding interest in research within the discipline. Their moral fiber is beyond reproach, reflecting a stable personal life. Their exemplary behavior is of prime importance because students in most instances emulate their teachers.

Some teachers have an autocratic style; Cushing was such an example.[4,11,14] Others patiently nurture students, taking great care to teach at the bedside, in the operating room, and in clinic. Every teacher must have high expectations of the student and be willing to delegate responsibility in a progressive fashion.

The best teachers are committed to placement of their students in optimal circumstances on completion of their training. Training alone is not enough. Good training and good placement in a practice setting or other appropriate position is a basic responsibility of both the teacher and the student.

Evaluation of residents should be provided regularly so that they have feedback about their progress and their suitability for the profession. Similarly, teachers need feedback from students so that they can adjust their approach and the curriculum that frames the educational program.

Finding the key that unlocks learning enthusiasm in the neurosurgery resident is an ongoing challenge. Each resident is different and each responds differently to teaching methods. The teacher must find the key so that each resident responds optimally and gets the maximal benefit from the training program.

The basic goal of all neurosurgical educators is to equip the trainee with current clinical skills, to stimulate his or her interest in teaching and research, to demonstrate the relevance and fun of continuing education, and to provide the trainee with the opportunity to practice neurosurgery safely and competently.

References

1. American Medical Association. *Graduate Medical Education Directory 1993-94*. Chicago, Ill: American Medical Association; 1993:823.
2. French JD. History of neurological surgery. In: Hoff JT, ed. Neurosurgery volume. In: Goldsmith H, ed. *Goldsmith Practice of Surgery*. Thomaston, Conn: Harper & Row; 1987.
3. Friedman E. *Fellowships for Neurosurgeons 1994*. Park Ridge, Ill: Young Neurosurgeons Committee, American Association of Neurological Surgeons; 1994:76.
4. Fulton JF. *Harvey Cushing*. Springfield, Ill: Charles C Thomas; 1946:754.
5. Garrison FH. *History of Medicine*. 4th ed. Philadelphia, Pa: WB Saunders; 1929:996.
6. Hoff JT. Subspecialty certification. In: Wilkins RH, Rengachary S, eds. *Neurosurgery*. Baltimore, Md: Williams & Wilkins; 1990:414-416.
7. Kline DG. *Fifty Years of Service to American Neurological Surgery: The American Board of Neurological Surgery*. Houston, Tex: Privately published; 1990: 102.
8. Light RU. Cushing's handwriting and remembering Harvey Cushing: the closing years. *Surg Neurol*. 1992;37:147-157.
9. Mahaley JS Jr, Kline DG. The American Board of Neurological Surgery: an historical perspective. In: Kline DG. *Fifty Years of Service to American Neurological Surgery: The American Board of Neurological Surgery*. Houston, Tex: Privately published; 1990: 6-8.
10. Pevehouse BC. Residency training in neurological surgery, 1934–1984: evolution over 50 years of trial and tribulation. The 1984 AANS presidential address. *J Neurosurg*. 1984;61:999-1004.
11. Ray BS. *As I Remember It: An Autobiography*. New York, NY: Privately published; 1990:246.
12. Rutkow IM. *Surgery: An Illustrated History*. St. Louis, Mo: Mosby; 1993:550.
13. Sachs E. *Fifty Years of Neurosurgery; A Personal Story*. New York, NY: Vantage Press; 1958:186.
14. Thomas EH. *Harvey Cushing: Surgeon, Author, Artist*. New York, NY: Henry Schuman; 1950:347.
15. Turnbull F. As it was in the beginning. In: Alexander E, ed. *History of the Society of Neurological Surgeons. 75th Meeting Anniversary*. Winston-Salem, NC: Hunter Publishing; 1984:4-6.

The Neurosurgeon-Patient Relationship as a Framework for Neurosurgical Philosophy

Oliver Woodhouse Grin, MD, FACS

The essential practical application of medical science is to augment patient healing and recovery from illness and disease. This statement and concept places *the patient at the center of the health care process*, since it is the patient who "harbors" the disease or illness, and it is the patient's body and mind that has the potential to heal and recover from the disease—with or without the support of the health care team. How patients develop disease and how they heal from disease then become the two essential features of medical science and thus of the health care system.

As physicians, we have a long history of service to patients, but the methods of that service have obviously changed dramatically over the years. An integral part of this change has been the confusion of roles between patients and physicians to the point that physicians are often called "healers" when, in fact, they are essentially the "helpers" to patient healing. The concept of the physician as healer has led to a physician-centered health care system that is illogical in many ways.

Biology teaches us that the patient has the central role of healing, for it is the patient who is (correctly) at the center of the health care system. This paradigm shift is critical to medical science and our current health care system, as it adapts to new challenges and demands. Neurosurgeons are an integral part of the health care system and are important members of our society, and they should endeavor to understand their role in order to better serve patients, their community, and our nation. In this chapter, I examine the philosophic dimensions of the neurosurgeon-patient relationship and articulate these within the framework of neurosurgical principles, methods, and objectives.

The Doctor-Patient Relationship

A discussion of medical science and the health care system ultimately involves the concept of the doctor-patient relationship. This venerable relationship has a long history dating back to the days of Hippocrates. We are all familiar with the Hippocratic oath which challenges physicians to pledge and commit their actions for the good of the patient. There is the strong caveat to "do no harm." I submit that many of us equate our professional actions with the Hippocratic oath and that it might also mean "do not interfere with healing." This warning makes good sense, particularly when we recognize that as physicians, our role is to augment healing and, if we cannot augment it, we should certainly not stand in the way of patient healing. Hippocrates, in his wisdom, seems to have recognized the fact that it is the patient who is at the center of the healing process.

In the days of Hippocrates and other great physicians of ancient times, a physician directed his efforts to what we call "holistic" medicine, often treating conditions that today we would classify as emotional, spiritual, and psychological. Physicians of those times did not have the extensive knowledge of human anatomy, physiology, and pathology that we have today; they certainly did not possess the medical and physiologic methodology of treating diseases. Consequently, their focus was on the whole patient and not simply the disease.

This model of the holistic physician, attending to all of the patient's needs, has been the model for the doctor-patient relationship for many centuries. In fact, it remains a standard against which most physicians are judged today. This model has been called the "priestly healer" model, which clearly places the physician at the center of the health care process.[5] This holistic approach functioned well as long as our scientific knowledge was limited, an element of trust and faith in physicians was held by patients, and an overall philosophy existed in which patients accept life's events (including disease, trauma, and death) as having a higher meaning. In this milieu, the physician was able to function collaboratively with the patients and families to provide appropriate medical care and service.

The Impact of Technology

In the past century and particularly in the recent decades, medical science has exploded in terms of its knowledge base and technologic capabilities.[3] Neurosurgery itself has arisen out of this technologic revolution and owes its origin to pioneers such as Harvey Cushing and Walter Dandy, and to innovations such as x-rays and electrocautery. The progress in neurological surgery has been so rapid that neurosurgeons of the 1960s hardly recognize the diagnostic and therapeutic capabilities of today's neurosurgeon.

Neurosurgery itself, being a product of this technologic revolution, is a prime example of shifting the physician's primary concern from patient to disease. This shift has tended to focus our thoughts on diagnostic methodology and treatment, rather than on the central role of healing in the patient. Unfortunately, this has also resulted in the health care system focusing on physicians and placing them (instead of the patient) at the center of the health care process.

If we look back in our neurosurgical history, two names that quickly surface are Harvey Cushing and Walter Dandy. Their diagnostic methodology was limited to neurologic exami-

nation, electroencephalography, air encephalography, and primitive angiography. They were delighted to identify and localize a mass or tumor, and arrived quite easily at the decision to "take it out." In the presence of limited information and newly evolving neurosurgical techniques, this seemed very reasonable. The focus, however, was on the disease and not necessarily on the patient.

The doctor-patient relationship in neurosurgery at that time was one of a very empowered neurosurgeon and a very passive patient. Physicians outside the field of neurosurgery had difficulty understanding the complexity of neurologic illness, and had even more difficulty in understanding how the techniques of surgery could be applied to treating such illnesses. This left the neurosurgeon as omnipotent and clearly at the pinnacle of the doctor-centered health care system. Many neurosurgeons clearly enjoyed this position, including Dr. Cushing, who often instructed his residents to "take the patient's problem as your own."[12] This approach was carried so far as to limit the patients' knowledge about their illnesses and the implications of those illnesses. (Several years ago, a disciple of Dr. Cushing's challenged me on the issue of patient education; he told me that in emphasizing patient knowledge about a disease and treatment, I was violating what he perceived as the teachings of Harvey Cushing.)

Technology has continued to support our focus on disease and treatment rather than on patients. Through the eyes of modern imaging, we can now see what was often overlooked 20 years ago, even at postmortem examination. Imagine the delight of Harvey Cushing today if he were looking through today's operating microscopes, having a clear vision of an acoustic neuroma and then being able to remove it with microinstruments and lasers, along with electrical potentials monitoring equipment to help the neurosurgeon preserve the facial nerve. Today's navigation to brain lesions is dramatically different from that of 20 years ago. Our technology allows us to more directly—and safely—approach neurosurgical lesions. We can also better determine if there would be more harm done in surgically treating them.

Imagine the delight of a John Hughlings

Jackson gazing at the magnetic resonance images of a complex skull base tumor that was producing minimal neurologic symptoms and was difficult to localize with certainty. Modern skull base surgery itself has been a focus of bringing all these technologies together and stressing concomitantly the relationships between diagnostic and operative capabilities, and what may best serve the overall health of the patient. Most facets of neurosurgery, including skull base surgery, now require a team of affiliated neuroscientists rather than the solo neurosurgeon with his neurosurgical assistant, as in the days of the neurosurgical pioneers.

All this marvelous technology, however, has not changed the central fact that the disease is a product of the patient and his environment[2] and that healing and recovery are functions of the patient—and augmented by the health care team. Despite our technologic advances, we continue to ignore the central role of healing, possibly because we have no clear way to measure a patient's healing index. More and more, however, as we look at increased surgical capabilities and the demands placed on us by patients who have more complicated medical problems and who are more advanced in years, a measure of the healing capabilities becomes an important aspect in patient care. This requires a return to the holistic approach and patient-centered focus of ancient physicians, and a move away from the current focus on disease and treatment. The latter places the physician at the center of the health care process, whereas the former correctly places the patient at the center.

Principles of Biology and Patient-Centered Care

It has been said that biology teaches us how things work in the living organism. Clearly, if we accept this tenet, the shift from physician-centered care to patient-centered care is mandated. This is based upon the biologic fact that it is the patient who heals and recovers, and that physicians and other members of the health care team augment—but do not control—the healing and recovery potential.

Basic science has also helped us to understand the relationship between mind, body, and healing, again pointing to the central fact that healing is a function of the patient.[10] A new field of study called "psycho-neuroimmunology" deals with the extensive relationships between mind, body, and healing, focusing on the interrelationships between the brain and the immune system. In their most basic functions, both the brain and the immune system are organs that allow an organism to find and protect itself from the environment. In a recent study of apes following an earthquake,[4] those that survived on the lush garden-like side of the fault remained almost unaffected by the event. The apes that found themselves on the rocky, barren side of the fault, where the environment challenged their survival, were forced to transcend their previous instincts and habits, having to find new ways to adapt to their uncomfortable surroundings. This is an example of the premise that through challenge comes opportunity, and meeting a challenge can promote growth—be it physical, emotional, or spiritual.

The Role of the Neurosurgeon

At a recent (1994) meeting of the American Association of Neurological Surgeons (AANS), the organization was compared to a three-legged stool by Dr. Julian T. Hoff in his Presidential Address. He stated that the activities of the AANS were founded upon: 1) patient care, 2) neuroscience research, and 3) teaching. He then suggested that the addition of a fourth leg, socioeconomic concerns, be added.

I believe that neurosurgery may be better viewed as a pedestal stool. The highest pedestal is patient healing and recovery. This is supported by a single post representing clinical neurosurgical care (augmentation of neurologic healing and recovery, led by a neurosurgeon). The post is supported by a base with three legs: 1) research, 2) teaching, and 3) economic issues. To me, the pedestal stool model focuses on augmentation of patient healing and recovery by the neurosurgeon-led neuroscience team.

Traditionally, neurosurgeons have understood the important roles of teaching and research. Teaching is necessary to train neurosurgeons so that they may provide neurosurgical care to patients. The excellence of that care is supported by research, both at the basic and clinical levels. Economic factors have always been essential to neurosurgery, but only in recent years have they become more openly discussed. Clearly, without a sound economic/management structure, be it in individual practices, in universities or large medical centers, or in research foundations or national organizations, neurosurgery would not reach its highest potential.

The Importance of Patient Education

In order to achieve patient-centered care, a system of patient education must be an integral part of the therapeutic plan.[8] If patients are to be at the center of the health care process and if they are to maximize their healing and recovery potentials, they must certainly understand the basics and the risks of their disease, as well as the alternative treatments and associated risks, weighing the benefits of treatment against non-treatment.[6] In this day of health care reform, this educational process also allows patients to understand their own individual illnesses in the context of broader social issues, taking into consideration the position of the government, insurance carriers, managed-care entities, and clergy. All of these entities have a direct impact on the patient and his or her family, and all play a role in this system—one that I feel should be collaborative and not adversarial.

The doctor-patient relationship, in its simplest form, is a process whereby the patient presents himself or herself to the physician for advice and treatment in a patient-centered care system. The patient carries with him or her the disease, the risks of the disease, and his or her own inherent healing and recovery potential, which is often difficult to measure. The physician considers diagnostic possibilities based on clinical experience and laboratory studies (scientific knowledge) and arrives at a working diagnosis based on statistical probability. He or she then makes recommendations for treatment and, again, attempts to tailor it to the patient's needs and healing and recovery potential. The physician must rely on statistics and probability. All of this, in a sense, is risk management, for if there were no risk, there would be no need for management. Given the influence of our judicial system on health care, we have lost sight of some of these basic concepts.

It is important for physicians and their colleagues to help patients understand how this process works and define the true meaning of risk management for them. This will give patients insight into the fact that all management of disease is based on statistical outcomes. If a less than perfect outcome results, it may be a matter of statistics and the patient's own inherent healing and recovery potential rather than a fault of the health care system.

Economics and Neurosurgery

Economics has always been a part of neurosurgical practice, although it is not a subject that is openly discussed. Simply stated, were it not for economics and good business practices, teaching programs and medical schools could not exist to teach neurosurgeons. Certainly, research could not be carried out at a very efficient and useful level. Neurosurgical treatment could not be delivered to patients without the economic and business support for neurosurgeons and other neuroscientists. We have often been hesitant to talk about socioeconomic issues. However, we must continue to recognize that without good economics and good management, there would not be good research, good teaching, good neurosurgeons, or quality neurosurgical care. Additionally, the central role of neurosurgery in augmenting patient healing and recovery would be unfulfilled.

One of the great misunderstandings in current concepts of health care reform is the importance of the impact on patient care derived from the socioeconomic issues. In America, business wants to take a very business-like outlook on health care in terms of applying cost controls and capitation.[9] Alternatively, it does not want to recognize the importance of incentives, workplace environment, and optimizing professional function. I recently asked a bank president (who serves on a hospital board) what would happen if he went to his bank the following day and suggested that everyone take a 20% pay cut, be on-call every third night, be exposed to AIDS daily, and be scrutinized and second-guessed by the judicial system on a regular basis. We need to ask society this same question.

As we enter the era of managed-care contracts and capitation of medical care funds, economics also begins to play a very important role in the medical decision-making process. It is my personal view that, clearly, the patient must be at the center of this process, not only in individual situations but also in society as a whole. Basing health care decisions purely on economics, through a national board or body, and without having the patient at the center would represent fundamental loss of freedom. We hear politicians talking about "freedom of choice" in choosing doctors, but an even more fundamental choice by patients is whether they have the choice of treatment—and if not, on what rules are those choices (or lack thereof) to be based? This issue of freedom in health care—which is a neurosurgical issue, as well—goes to the core of the foundations upon which the United States is based.[1]

As we look at the aforementioned facts, evolution and development of a philosophy of patient-centered care becomes not only logical but necessary. This is based foremost on the strong biologic concepts that: 1) it is the patient who develops the disease as the result of the interaction between his or her genetic inheritance and environment; and 2) it is the patient, based on these two factors, who possesses the powers of healing and recovery. Therefore, it is only logical that the patient must weigh the relative risks of living with the disease or accepting treatment in the hopes of controlling or removing the threat to his or her well-being (or life).[7] This patient-centered approach is augmented through patient education and input by the professional medical team, including the neurosurgeon. The weighing of risks versus treatment involves quality-of-life issues that can be answered only by the patient. Additionally, it should be recognized that as in any major decision in life, the individual making the decision has innate, intuitive insights and capabilities that are not possessed by his professional advisors.

The Enhanced Role of the Neurosurgeon in Patient-Centered Care

Patient-centered care enhances the role and importance of the neurosurgeon by focusing and differentiating the respective roles of the patient and the neurosurgeon. In patient-centered care, neurosurgeons are able to focus their energies and skills on those elements with which they are most comfortable, i.e. neurologic diagnosis and surgical treatment. This facilitates a well-defined responsibility in patient management, incorporating the patient at the center of the process.

It must be pointed out that in this role of augmenting healing and recovery, a neurosurgeon's direct relationship with the patient is extremely important. This relationship not only aids in patients' healing and recovery but also allows patients to inspire us in reciprocal fashion through their direct support and encouragement of the neurosurgeon. It can be argued that patient-centered care makes great theoretic sense, but how is it practically applied? The following are some practical applications:

1) Diagnostic decisions can be made through clinical judgment and the use of appropriate diagnostic tools. This is different from today's current mode where clinical judgment, by virtue of our judicial system, is out of vogue and costly tests are often ordered to prepare for a legal defense ("defensive medicine") rather than for patient benefit. If a patient requests an expensive diagnostic test that the physician believes will yield little or no pertinent information (based on his scientific knowledge, experience, and statistical probability), they can collaborate and come to a mutual decision. If the patient proceeds with the testing, the patient is aware that he or she was empowered to make an informed choice and is responsible for that choice. This collaborative approach enables both the patient and the neurosurgeon to benefit from a doctor-patient relationship based on education and collaboration.

2) We must accept our supportive role in heal-

ing and recovery and the supportive role of our treatments, no matter how elegant they might seem. This places poor outcomes in proper perspective and does not leave surgical treatment as the sole bearer of this onus.

3) We must help patients understand their central role in healing and recovery through a systematic approach to patient education. This includes relating to the patients information about their diseases, their own healing and recovery, diagnosis and various forms of treatment, and the concept of risks of the disease versus the treatment. We can help patients understand that a so-called "cure" may be impossible and that if it does occur, it is from a combination of an appropriate diagnosis of the disease, appropriate treatment, and an appropriate healing and recovery potential. All of this is based on statistical methodology and helping patients understand the concepts of probability and statistical risks.

4) Patients must accept illness as a systems problems for which neurosurgeons are only one of the many team members called upon to help. This team also includes the patient, family members, other neuroscience specialists, nurses, therapists, clergy, and friends.

5) Patient-centered care mandates that we continue to use the scientific method, along with practicing the art of medicine.

As we define and differentiate ourselves as neurosurgeons, while adhering to the tenets of the Hippocratic oath, the tenets of patient-centered care, and the scientific method, we will be called upon to voice our position regarding many current medical/social issues. For example, such things as euthanasia, health care rationing, freedom of choice of physician, and the impact of economics on medical practice can be realistically discussed openly and frankly—within the framework of a patient-centered philosophy.

The Impact of the Judicial System

A major social issue facing the health care system in particular and society in general is our judicial system. The judicial system endeavors to defend the rights of victims, extracting monetary rewards from other segments of society to repair alleged wrongdoings (some say that it creates victims). As we have previously discussed using the biologic model, in most cases the judicial model does not fit, for we have learned that one of the essential principles of biology is that growth and development come only through challenge, which often may be painful. The medical sciences try to help people heal by encouraging them to go forward with their lives and through untoward events and illnesses. The judicial model often hinders patients' healing by focusing on the problem/event and supporting their victimization. University of Pennsylvania Professor Lani Guinier was recently interviewed on C-Span and stated that we need to de-emphasize victimization and talk "the language of healing." How wonderful it would be if physicians, and in particular neurosurgeons, could lead this social change.

Specifically, with respect to our judicial system, the problem of medical malpractice suits has come to the fore.[8] It is puzzling to me that in medical malpractice cases, the science of statistics and probability are never recognized. However, this is not only a problem of our legal brethren but also of our neurosurgical colleagues. I am alarmed that neurosurgeons who purport to believe in the scientific method (including statistics) and to be ethical and honest physicians can testify against another neurosurgeon or physician without gathering all the data available and, most importantly, speaking directly with the physician whom he or she is challenging, thereby completing the database. A complete picture is important, for even when we are involved in medical malpractice cases, we must remain dedicated to the healing of the patient and help determine whether our "legal" testimony will contribute to healing or to continued victimization. If the law prohibits us from following our logic and ethics (i.e. refusing to let us communicate directly with those involved in an honest and forthright manner), then we should refuse to participate at all, for this reflects back to our Hippocratic oath to "do no harm." As we neurosurgeons become more differentiated and adhere to our principles of patient-centered care and scientific method, these shortcomings will no longer be prudent or acceptable.

Spirituality and Healing

During my 25 years in neurosurgery, I have been impressed by the importance of spiritual issues in the lives of many patients. Spiritual issues should not be confused with religious issues, although both may be important to most patients. In a doctor-centered system, these issues are often left at the periphery and not used as a management tool for the patient's illness. In fact, they are not used at all as a therapeutic tool. Nonetheless, many patients and families rely upon spiritual and religious issues as important therapeutic tools. With the patient at the center of the health care process, we can better integrate spiritual and religious concepts with more concrete biologic issues which we physicians are more comfortable and familiar with from experience. In many ways, neurosurgeons have come full circle, for despite our special interest in neurologic diseases, we are being asked to participate in a holistic approach to illness and disease utilizing today's technology.

Partners in Healing

Patient-centered care requires that we not treat patients as victims of disease but rather as *partners in healing*. Furthermore, we must view professionals within the medical profession (along with patients) as a community sharing a common goal of maximizing patient healing and recovery. This requires us to understand our specific roles and functions, to adhere to those roles and functions, and to conduct our relationships within the health care system in a civil and ethical manner.

It is time for neurosurgeons to apply the teachings of biology to society as a whole. By this I mean that a fundamental principle of biology (and the immune system is a splendid example of this) dictates that growth and development are stimulated by challenge. While disease and pain are often unwelcome and uncomfortable, they are also mechanisms for growth and enhancement of the human being.

Just as the immune system combats disease and preserves the organism, we should discourage our patients from becoming victims of it and at the same time "arm" them for their correct role as partners in healing. This is a fundamentally different way of viewing today's society. Neurosurgeons are important, influential members of the medical community, a group that adheres to biologic principles. We can begin to talk about the principles of healing and encourage patients to be partners in healing rather than victims. (We may think that we are already doing this, but I made an interesting discovery at the 1994 AANS meeting. A CD-ROM disk was prepared, containing every word from the abstracts of all the papers and posters presented. *Out of 2.5 million words, the word "healing" appeared just three times.*)

Conclusion

A patient-centered philosophy enhances the role of the physician as well as patient healing and recovery. It allows the neurosurgeon to differentiate each role in a very specific manner and frees him or her from "feeling responsible" for the patient's disease—or for the patient's healing and recovery from the disease. It allows the neurosurgeon to focus his skills on neurosurgical diagnosis and its implication(s). Additionally, it allows the neurosurgeon to focus on the proposed neurosurgical treatment, the relative risks of the treatment, and helping the patient make an educated decision. Lastly, it enables the patient to accept the disease and his or her role in healing and recovery, which in turn helps the neurosurgeon and medical team.

By differentiating the specific roles, the neurosurgeon can act as a coach to patients in healing and recovery, being an enthusiastic supporter. In many ways, this is a return to the holistic, "priestly healer" role of treating the patient rather than the disease. As part of such a system, the neurosurgeon can contribute to the patient's well-being by being a part of a patient education system, thus helping patients understand certain biologic truths (such as disease) and the process of ongoing healing, recovery, and health—and eventually death.[10] This results in neurosurgeons helping patients and their families to accept inevitable events and unplanned outcomes, for patients will recognize that they are part of the biologic and spiritual forces that shape human beings—and all living things.

References

1. Brody H. *The Healer's Power*. New Haven, Conn: Yale University Press; 1992.
2. Cartwright FF. *Disease and History*. New York, NY: Dorset Press; 1972.
3. Charman RC. *At Risk: Can the Doctor-Patient Relationship Survive in a High-Tech World?* Dublin, NH: William L. Bauhan; 1992.
4. Coppens Y. East Side Story: The Origin of Humankind. *Sci Am*. 1994;270:88-95.
5. Detmer DE, Finney MD. Health care issues. In: Bell RM, Dayton MT, eds. *Essentials of General Surgery*. Baltimore, Md: Williams & Wilkins; 1992:8-16.
6. Gerteis M, Edgman-Levitan S, Daley J, et al, eds. *Through the Patient's Eyes: Understanding and Promoting Patient-Centered Care*. San Francisco, Cal: Jossey-Bass Publishers; 1993.
7. Goodman JC, Musgrave GL. *Patient Power*. Washington, DC: Cato Institute; 1992.
8. Grin ODW. Patient education: Protecting the surgeon-patient relationship through the strategy of patient education. In: Benzel EC, ed. *Spinal Instrumentation*. Park Ridge, Ill: American Association of Neurological Surgeons; 1994:275-279.
9. Huber PW. *Liability—The Legal Revolution and Its Consequences*. New York, NY: Basic Books; 1988.
10. Moyers BD. *Healing and The Mind*. New York, NY: Doubleday; 1993.
11. Nuland SB. *How We Die: Reflections on Life's Final Chapter*. New York, NY: Alfred A Knopf; 1994.
12. Thomson EH. *Harvey Cushing*. New York, NY: Neale Watson Academic Publications; 1981.

CHAPTER 14

The Neurosurgeon and Academia

Robert H. Wilkins, MD

'Mongst all these stirs of discontented strife,
O, let me lead an academic life
—Joseph Hall (1574–1656)[3]

And seek for truth in the groves of Academe
—Horace (65–8 BC)[4]

Academic life is viewed by many as an idyllic, unhurried, scholarly search for truth. And in the ideal sense, it is. Yet there are numerous practicalities that intrude on a daily basis. The academic neurosurgeon does not live and work in an ivory tower.

Ideal Academic Life

The ideal academic life is fueled by the excitement of learning and discovery. All who take part are students; most are also teachers. With the acquisition of knowledge and experience, the person who is learning becomes a resource to others not as advanced. The desire to learn and discover must arise within and be satisfying to the individual student, but scholarship is usually stimulated and enhanced by intercommunication with other students who have similar or related interests.

The student who is contributing to knowledge has an obligation to find out what is already known by reading or listening to organized summaries of the topic. Eventually, the student should trace the reference tree back to the original sources. This not only provides a sound foundation for the student's own efforts, but also prevents the unnecessary repetition of work already done. Key to this type of basic information gathering is an extensive library that also can tap into resources of other libraries if necessary. Experienced teachers and one or more mentors likewise are important to this process, primarily to advise the student about how efforts can best be focused so that the pertinent knowledge can be obtained with the least waste of time and energy.

In the next step, that of discovery, the experienced teacher becomes more important than the library, with facilities and equipment assuming importance as well. Concerning research, the teacher can guide the student in formulating hypotheses to be tested, acquiring the skills and materials necessary to perform such testing, planning the experimental work and data gathering, executing the study, analyzing the results, and organizing the information so that it is suitable for presentation and publication.

In the ideal medical academic setting, the student (e.g. premedical student, medical student, resident, fully-trained physician, and faculty member) has free access to an excellent library or libraries, to extensive laboratory facilities, to large and varied patient populations, and—most importantly—to teachers and students at all levels. The student must have adequate time to take advantage of these resources, and should be free from distracting influences such as making a living.

For the academic neurosurgeon, the challenge is how best to achieve these goals within the framework of real life. How best can the neurosurgeon in an academic environment contribute as a scholar and teacher, and how can he or she become a leader and an innovator in medicine?

Regarding scholarship, teaching, and innovation, the academic neurosurgeon must spend considerable time and energy to provide the necessary patient base and grant support to permit both clinical and experimental investigations and instruction. To become a leader in the field calls for an investment of both time and expense in meeting attendance and organizational work related to professional societies. These activities seriously limit the time available for reading, for conducting clinical and laboratory studies, and for trying to advance neurosurgical knowledge. Even so, by collaborating with others, worthwhile and satisfying progress can be made. In the case of the neurosurgeon who collaborates with one or more basic scientists, the neurosurgeon typically provides surgical skill, access to human patients, and an interest in the possible clinical relevance of the study. The basic scientists are more likely to provide the technical expertise, facilities, and equipment for the experiments, and an orientation toward the potential value of the study in advancing basic knowledge. Each participant learns from and is stimulated by the fund of information and the perspective of the others. The sum of such collaboration is frequently greater than its parts.

The neurosurgeon, and especially the neurosurgeon-in-training, can benefit considerably from reading, reflection, and investigative work. Current neurosurgical knowledge is seen in the perspective of its background; neurosurgery is perceived as an evolving discipline that is intimately related to other evolving disciplines. The neurosurgeon who becomes involved in academic life also develops the ability to assess critically scientific and scholarly work, and develops an understanding of how arduous such work can be. For the neurosurgeon who remains in academia, these perspectives continue to mature as basic tenets of daily activity. But even for the neurosur-

geon who leaves academia, these perspectives remain valuable—a strong argument for involving all neurosurgical residents in some form of clinical or experimental research.

How can neurosurgical academic units best achieve their goals, and how can neurosurgical residents best be educated? These important questions have been considered periodically in various forums, including the annual meetings of the Society of Neurological Surgeons. The proceedings of one such workshop were published as a separate issue of the *Journal of Neurosurgery*.[8] In that issue, Dr. W. Eugene Stern[9] summarized his views about ideal residency training in neurological surgery as follows: "A flexible program designed and nurtured by dedicated teachers to provide depth, balance, breadth, and perspective in its offering should graduate an individual worthy of the science and art of surgery, inbred with a thirst for life-long learning, and one whose acceptance of the everchanging character of knowledge will serve him and his patients beyond the finite life-span of technical procedures. . . ."

So much for ideal circumstances . . .

Actual Academic Life

The neurosurgeon in actual academic practice has all of the responsibilities of the neurosurgeon in private practice, and then some, requiring a balance of activity in several areas. Dr. Eben Alexander, Jr.[2] has written about the four-legged stool of academia with the legs representing patient care, teaching, research, and administration.

Patient Care

In the area of patient care, the academic neurosurgeon must be able to attract patients to the institution. Initially, this means that the individual must be adept at some aspect of operative neurosurgery so as to compete successfully with other neurosurgeons. This is, however, only a beginning. The patient and the referring physician must be pleased not only with the outcome of treatment, but also with the neurosurgeon's compassion as well as with the attention and care given by the numerous other individuals at the academic institution who are involved with the patient. The appointment secretary, registration clerk, office or clinic nurse, transporter, laboratory technician, radiologic technologist, neurosurgical resident, and the nurses in the preoperative preparation area, operating room, recovery room, neurosurgical intensive care unit, and neurosurgical floor are just some of the many people who can influence whether a patient is satisfied with his or her care. This is also true for the neurosurgeon in private practice, with minor variations such as the degree of control over the actions of some of the others involved with patient care. For example, the academic neurosurgeon would have direct influence on neurosurgical residents and residents assigned to the neurosurgical service, whereas the neurosurgeon in private practice would have direct control over the secretaries, nurses, physician associates, and others whose salaries and fringe benefits are supplied by the neurosurgeon rather than by a hospital or other medical institution.

In competing with the private practitioner, the academic neurosurgeon has the advantage of 24-hour coverage by the resident staff, and the advantage of easy access to numerous other physicians in a variety of specialties who practice in the same institution. Depending on the quality of the medical center, consultations with such faculty physicians can provide assessment and advice of the very highest caliber.

Involvement of the residents and medical students in patient care is a two-way street, with liabilities as well as advantages. There is no question that residents and medical students stimulate the academic neurosurgeon to stay current and to perform proficiently before this daily audience. The patient also benefits from the increased attention. Yet the additional physical examinations, the discussions on rounds, the multiplicity of the people writing orders in the chart, and the involvement of less-experienced surgeons in the operative procedure add time, inconvenience, and occasional confusion. The patient may get the feeling of being experimented upon. And the sheer complexity and size of a modern academic medical center almost inevitably leads to frequent foul-ups. For example, the patient's chart or radiologic studies may be misplaced or studies may be scheduled at conflicting times.

In general, a nonacademic medical center is more "user friendly." The patient tends to feel more like an individual and less like a number. It is not uncommon that a patient and a referring physician will turn to the community or local hospital for routine neurosurgical problems and only consider the academic center for more complicated or riskier situations.

To stay competitive, the academic neurosurgeon can specialize in some of the more difficult neurosurgical conditions—those that the nonacademic neurosurgeon is just as happy to refer. But this brings an increased level of stress and an increased risk of poor results, as well as a concomitant increased likelihood of malpractice litigation. The academic neurosurgeon also needs to compete for the more routine aspects of neurosurgical practice so that the residents are exposed to these basic and important facets of neurosurgery in addition to the more esoteric ones.

In 1992, the Duke University Medical Center retained Professional Research Consultants, Inc., to conduct an in-depth study of physicians in 65 North Carolina counties to determine their referral patterns, perceptions, and needs.[7] This study showed that the most important factors to a physician in deciding about referring a patient to any physician or institution are (in decreasing order of importance): the satisfaction of previously-referred patients with the consulting physician; the referring doctor's previous satisfaction with the consulting physician; prompt appointment scheduling; the satisfaction of previously-referred patients with the facility; and the referring doctor's previous satisfaction with communication from the consulting physician. The assurance that the patient would be returned to the care of the referring doctor was found to be less important. Of least importance among the factors considered were the consulting physician's professional reputation and whether the consulting physician was on the faculty of a medical school. For overall referrals then, the personal touch is most important. Yet when the 609 physicians surveyed were asked about the main reason why they chose to refer patients to a particular neurosurgeon or neurosurgical group in North Carolina, 37% cited the quality and reputation of the neurosurgeon(s), 13% cited previous favorable experience with the neurosurgeon(s), 13% cited the proximity of the institution, and only 8% cited good communication. Therefore, to attract patients, the academic neurosurgeon needs to develop expertise in some area or areas of neurosurgical practice, but must also maintain the interpersonal qualities that lead to the satisfaction of both patients and referring physicians.

However, in addition to these considerations, the academic neurosurgeon has the responsibilities of assessing and reporting the results and complications of his or her clinical work, and of developing new and better neurosurgical techniques. It is not enough to practice in the present, to perform well the procedures of the present. The academic neurosurgeon must honestly evaluate the outcomes of such procedures and must try to better the prognosis of patients with neurologic disorders that are treated surgically by improving current techniques and introducing new ones.

Teaching

The terms "academia" and "academe" refer to the academic environment or community. They also can mean a place of instruction. The academic neurosurgeon is involved with professional teaching at various levels, from premedical students to experienced neurosurgeons. At different medical centers, the opportunities vary and the emphasis is different. But within any setting, the academic neurosurgeon has the responsibility of instructing others about the field.

In general, the access of the academic neurosurgeon to undergraduates and medical students is limited. Only the basic aspects of neurosurgery can be taught. Yet, the way in which these are transmitted, as well as the personality of the neurosurgeon, can be crucial in attracting students to the field. The charisma of the neurosurgeon is crucial; the subject matter is less important.

The most important and time-consuming form of teaching for the academic neurosurgeon is resident education. Considerable time and attention are spent initially in the resident selection process, both by the applicant and by the academic neurosurgical group. The applicant is seeking the institution and teachers that will provide the best neurosurgical education, and the neurosurgical group is seeking the most qualified residents—those most likely to benefit from the instruction, to have a successful career, and to bring honor to the institution. Although the present

matching system in the United States has flaws, it does place residents in an equitable way. Each year, the neurosurgical faculty at an academic institution is supplied with one or more new residents to instruct.

The formats and techniques of neurosurgical education are discussed in another chapter in this book and will not be dealt with in detail here. However, the academic neurosurgeon must recognize that the main way in which neurosurgical residents are taught is by example. Residents-in-training emulate the teachers they admire, and may adopt negative patterns as well as positive ones. This places an added burden on the academic neurosurgeon who, as a role model, must try to have a consistently positive impact and to restrict the negative influences that may arise from stress and fatigue (e.g. cutting corners in diagnosis or treatment, being curt with a patient or family, or putting off to tomorrow what should be attended to today).

Part of the obligation of neurosurgical educators is to make available to the resident a wide variety of neurosurgical and neurologic conditions for first-hand instruction, while maintaining patient volume sufficient for repetitive encounters. Because of the recent shift in emphasis in American medical practice, the neurosurgical residents must receive more outpatient experience. This will enable them to learn how to assess patients referred for neurosurgical consultation, how to select those who should be treated surgically, how to manage those who are not likely to be helped surgically, and how to follow patients postoperatively. Concerning inpatient treatment and outpatient operations, the neurosurgical teacher must assure that the resident receives enough hands-on surgical experience, in a gradually advancing fashion during the residency, to be able to conduct an independent neurosurgical practice at a reasonably high level of quality at the completion of the residency.

Although the instruction of neurosurgical residents is the primary teaching responsibility of the academic neurosurgeon, there is also a responsibility for the education of fully-trained physicians and neurosurgeons. In the former case, this often means providing physicians with oral or written surveys of current methods or recent developments in neurosurgery or one of its component areas. In the latter case, the academic neurosurgeon provides more focused information at a higher level for neurosurgeons who want to stay current or to add to their own repertoire of neurosurgical techniques.

Research

The academic neurosurgeon has the responsibility of improving the field of neurosurgery. As previously mentioned, this can be done clinically by assessing outcomes and improving neurosurgical operative techniques, as well as by educating residents in such a way that they also will contribute to the advancement of neurosurgery. In addition, the academic neurosurgeon can contribute on a more basic level by experimentation in the operating room and in the laboratory.

The neurosurgeon has an advantage over other researchers in neuroscience by having the opportunity to study directly various functions of the exposed human brain, spinal cord, and nerves. This is of particular importance for the study of higher brain functions such as memory and speech. Such clinical research can be conducted in the course of the academic neurosurgeon's daily practice.

Laboratory research, on the other hand, interferes with daily neurosurgical practice. Ordinarily it is conducted in some other area of the institution, often in a separate building removed from the hospital and clinics. Such research frequently involves significant blocks of time, requiring that the neurosurgeon be insulated during those periods from the demands of clinical practice. In addition, the academic neurosurgeon must take the time to learn the techniques necessary for the research, to read the appropriate literature and attend the appropriate meetings, to interrelate with others who are working in the same area, and to prepare periodic reports for oral presentation and for publication.

It is a difficult balance. The neurosurgeon must compete with full-time researchers for grant support and must try to achieve results that will compare favorably with those of full-time researchers. In fiscal 1991, there were 1492 competing applications to the National Institute of Neurological Disorders and Stroke for research grants, of which 460 (31%) were funded.[5] Among these were 32 grant applications submitted by neurosurgeons, 17 (53%) of which were funded. The success rates for neurosurgery grants during the previous 4 years were: 45% in 1987; 33% in 1988; 35% in 1989; and 18% in 1990. In 1991, there was only one neurosurgical application for a Clinical Investigator Award, and it was not funded.

The academic neurosurgeon who is conducting laboratory research also needs to tend to his or her practice and other responsibilities so that these important aspects will not wither from neglect. Few individuals can conduct such a balancing act for a full career; often the laboratory research dwindles after the first few years as the neurosurgeon's practice builds.

One paradigm that permits a longer dual productivity is the limitation of clinical and research interests to the same area within neurosurgery. In this way, the academic neurosurgeon can study the clinical problem in the laboratory and apply the solutions for the benefit of patients. Dr. Blaine S. Nashold, Jr., a member of the neurosurgical faculty at Duke University Medical Center, was able to be productive in this way over many years. As an example, he studied spinal deafferentation pain in animals and developed a technique of treating such pain by making lesions in the dorsal nerve root entry zone of the spinal cord. He tried this technique in human patients and found that it would bring relief to a high percentage of patients with certain types of pain, such as that caused by brachial plexus nerve root avulsion. He and his laboratory associates continued their concurrent animal studies and made further adaptations in the procedure that improved the results when applied to human patients.

The criteria for academic advancement vary from institution to institution, but often the important considerations include the level of grant support and the number of publications in refereed journals, with the individual as the first or main author of a specified percentage. Thus, the neurosurgeon with a heavy clinical load and no grant support, who publishes book chapters and occasional clinical reports, is at a distinct disadvantage compared with basic science faculty members when it comes to academic advancement. The fledgling academic neurosurgeon needs to keep these facts in mind when beginning a career so that appropriate goals and guidelines can be established early.

Administration

Frequently, academic neurosurgeons take on administrative responsibilities in addition to their other duties. This is most often in the form of committee work within the medical center or university, but at times involves becoming the head of a division or department of neurosurgery or surgery, or accepting an administrative position within the medical school or hospital.

Organizational and interpersonal skills are necessary for the smooth performance of patient care, teaching, and research. These qualities are especially important to the academic neurosurgeon who becomes responsible for the administration of an academic neurosurgical department or division. That individual not only has his or her own patient care, teaching, and research to worry about, but also those of all of the other faculty members. The degree of the chairman's or chief's success is based in large part on how well the interests, desires, and necessities of the entire faculty can be coordinated so that the whole program is productive, with the greatest cooperation and the least friction among the individuals involved. Time, facilities, and equipment must be allotted in a fair and consistent manner, and financial compensation must be reflective of individual productivity.

The administrative heads of academic neurosurgical units ordinarily have had years of training and experience in patient care, teaching, and research. But few have had any formal instruction in "running a business," with all that this entails. Some take the trouble to learn the basics in a structured way, such as by attending an intensive short course at a business school. But most learn as they go, depending on frequent feedback from the other faculty members to achieve a balanced program that is beneficial to all.

Among the responsibilities of the unit leader is the nurturing of the faculty. New members must be given encouragement and financial help to get their clinical and experimental work up and running. They also must be given guidance in the early years so that they can direct their energies in the most productive ways. As their experience grows and their productivity increases, they should be supported for academic advancement and perhaps eventually for consideration as a head of a neurosurgical unit. In the concluding years of academic practice, the senior faculty members also should be supported; the unit leader needs to encourage the senior members to maintain their interest in the unit activities and to continue to exert their mature influence on the younger faculty members, residents, and students.

Although the neurosurgical chairman or chief is responsible for coordinating the activities of the faculty and encouraging their development, the main responsibility lies in directing the instruction of the residents. As director of the residency training program, the chairman or chief must assure that the trainees receive their education according to the general and special requirements of the Accreditation Council on Graduate Medical Education for residency training in neurological surgery, and according to the rules and regulations of the American Board of Neurological Surgery and the Residency Review Committee for Neurosurgery. These many requirements include the necessity for a sponsoring institution such as a medical school to demonstrate commitment to the program in terms of financial and academic support. To quote from the Special Requirements for Residency Training in Neurological Surgery:[1]

> The training program in neurological surgery must include a minimum of one year of training in an accredited program in general surgery or at least 1 year of a program accredited for the acquisition of fundamental clinical skills. . . . The neurological surgery training program is 60 months in duration, in addition to the year of acquisition of fundamental clinical skills, 36 months of which must be on the clinical service of neurological surgery. . . . A block of training of 3 months minimum in an accredited neurology training program must be arranged for all trainees. . . . There must be a well coordinated schedule of teaching conferences, rounds, and other educational activities in which both the neurological surgery faculty and the residents participate. . . . Educational experience in neuroradiology and neuropathology must be an integral part of the training program and designed for the education of the neurological surgery resi-

dents. . . . The program must provide opportunities for experience and instruction in the basic neurosciences. . . . The residents should participate either in ongoing clinical and/or basic research projects. . . . There must be resources for the education of neurological surgery residents in anesthesiology, endocrinology, ophthalmology, orthopaedics, otolaryngology, pathology, and psychiatry.

These requirements have been designed to ensure that the focus of each neurosurgical training program is on resident education rather than service to the institution. It is the responsibility of the program director to see that this happens—that the resident is educated rather than simply instructed in current neurosurgical thought and techniques. The resident must be prepared for a career that will be characterized by the steady expansion of medical and neurosurgical knowledge, and by sequential changes in medical and neurosurgical practice.

Three decades ago, Professor Moody E. Prior[6] summarized this view as follows:

> . . . training which is confined solely to mastering a highly specialized activity alone creates the technician and not the man who can innovate or give to his particular science or skill a new and original direction. In the present state of learning and technology, the specialist is our chief hope to advance knowledge and improving practice, but originality is not stimulated by narrowness. The history of learning affords us many instances which suggest that unusual and important developments in the arts and sciences arise often from a stimulus outside the particular art or science itself. The failure to see experience outside the scheme of a limited discipline impoverishes the mind, and so, in the very interests of specialization itself it becomes necessary to provide for breadth in the education of the specialist. . . .

Conclusion

Because an ideal is a conception of something in its perfection, the ideal academic life can be thought of as the ultimate in how the life's work of an academic should be conducted. This ideal existence cannot be realized for numerous reasons. In constantly striving for it, however, the academic neurosurgeon can be sure of contributing as much as is possible to the advancement and dissemination of knowledge. At career's end, the academic neurosurgeon will then have the satisfaction of having achieved something worthwhile despite the obstacles.

References

1. Accreditation Council for Graduate Medical Education. *Essentials and Information Items 1993–1994.* Reprinted from: Graduate Medical Education Directory 1993–1994. Chicago, Ill: American Medical Association; 1993:58-62.
2. Alexander E Jr. Perspectives on neurosurgery: presidential address. *J Neurosurg.* 1967;27:189-206.
3. Hall J. *Discontent of Men With Their Condition.* Cited by: Bartlett J; Beck EM, ed. *Familiar Quotations: A Collection of Passages, Phrases and Proverbs Traced to Their Sources in Ancient and Modern Literature.* 15th ed. Boston, Mass: Little, Brown & Co; 1980:257.
4. Horace (Quintus Horatius Flaccus). *Epistles.* Bk II, 14 BC, epistle ii, line 45. Cited by: Bartlett J; Beck EM, ed. *Familiar Quotations: A Collection of Passages, Phrases and Proverbs Traced to Their Sources in Ancient and Modern Literature.* 15th ed. Boston, Mass: Little, Brown & Co; 1980:109.
5. National Advisory Neurological Disorders and Stroke Council. Minutes of meeting. May 21–22, 1992; Bethesda, Md.
6. Prior ME. Education for our times. *Key Reporter.* 1965;30:2-6.
7. Schleff T. *Duke University Medical Center: 1992 PRC Referring Physician Study Executive Report.* Omaha, Neb: Professional Research Consultants, Inc; 1993.
8. Society of Neurological Surgeons. The education of a neurosurgeon: report of a workshop for neurosurgical training program directors. *J Neurosurg.* 1969; 30:323-364.
9. Stern WE. Men for all seasons: an inquiry into principles, practices, and prejudices governing training of neurosurgeons. *J Neurosurg.* 1969;30:338-341.

CHAPTER 15

Neurosurgery and the Law

W. Ben Blackett, MD, JD

Neurosurgeons, like other specialists, use legal advice and require personal legal representation from time to time throughout their professional lives. This legal assistance may involve professional corporations, partnerships, medical building and other real estate transactions, peer review and hospital credentialing disputes, estate planning, divorce, antitrust problems, Employee Retirement Income Security Act (ERISA) law compliance, office formation or breakup, tax planning or Internal Revenue Service (IRS) disputes, patent and copyright law, and, of course, medical malpractice claims. The need for legal advice and representation seems likely to increase as the federal and state governments involve themselves more in medical rule-making, administration, and enforcement.

Like medicine, law has become increasingly specialized, and the days of the solo lawyer able to handle any matter well and efficiently are gone. And, as in medicine, specialization has contributed to public estrangement. If a number of public opinion polls are to be believed, people like and trust their own lawyers but have a poor opinion of lawyers in general. Much the same sentiment has been expressed in regard to physicians. The relationship between professional groups is influenced by interactions that have been either supportive or damaging. Not surprisingly, the major interaction for neurosurgeons (along with other high-risk specialists) has been with trial attorneys doing plaintiff personal injury litigation. By and large, the medical profession has viewed these contacts negatively, and that has at times colored the entire physician-bar relationship. In the area of medical malpractice disputes, physicians and plaintiff trial attorneys not only square off frequently in court but also in almost yearly legislative battles in which the medical societies support and the bar opposes various tort reforms. The negative perception of the bar is influenced not just by the ever-present concern about being second-guessed in medical malpractice lawsuits, but about frivolous claims, exaggerated claims, and the whole adversarial process with its time demands, interruptions, continuances, and inefficiencies. Particularly offensive to most physicians (and here they have lots of company) is the aggressive advertising of some personal injury attorneys in the telephone yellow pages, on road signs, and on television. There is a growing feeling that equity, fairness, and even good taste are often missing from the system.

But, we are a society of laws, and the universe of law and of lawyers is large. It cannot be realistically appreciated if viewed too narrowly. The following are some selected topics of medicine, neurosurgery, and the law. They are presented with the hope of providing a philosophic perspective on this very important facet of neurosurgical thinking and practice.

Law and Equity: A Historical Note

Certain legal remedies, such as restraining orders, contempt citations, injunctions, cease and desist orders, specific performance, and rescission, are called equitable remedies. These hail from the equity jurisdiction of the English Chancery courts. Although the terms "law" and "equity" now sound roughly synonymous to our ears, this was not always the case. Law and equity were derived from different institutions, and there was a significant period during which they were at war with each other. Our legal system evolved from that of England's, and that system was derived from royal decrees. Early kings freely exercised the power to intercede in all matters within their realm (which was anywhere they could enforce their authority). The modern vestige of that power is the authority of governors and presidents to issue pardons to persons accused or convicted of crimes.

The common law courts of England were established by royal decree. Also established by royal practice, if not decree, was the king's privy counsel. The privy counsel represented the king and eventually delegated much of its day-to-day authority (including its judicial function) to the chancellor. The chancellor presided over what came to be known as the "courts of equity." These exercised the inherent authority of the king to intercede in any dispute, but since legal disputes also were heard and decided by the courts of common law, there was a split judiciary. The common law courts evolved a rather rigid structure and, because of this, could not exercise the freedom of action available in the courts of equity. For a considerable period of time and despite these differences, the two systems complemented or at least did not seriously interfere with each other.

Toward the mid-15th century, however, the common law courts became progressively more rigid and formalized, greatly limiting their effectiveness in many situations. Suits at common law were categorized into particular "forms of action." These forms of action had names that are only vaguely recognizable today, such as trover, assumpsit, replevin, trespass, and trespass on the case. These forms or writs were both precise and exclusive. A complaint, however meritorious by generally accepted standards of fairness or morality but which did not fit a particular writ, would not be heard by the court and therefore had no remedy at common law. Although the solicitor or barrister of the day tried his best to fit the facts of his case into one of these forms of action, if the common law judge decided the facts did not fit

the chosen writ, the case would be dismissed and could not be brought again—even under another writ. The slightest oversight or failure to correctly predict the court's determination could be fatal to the case.

The chancellor, on the other hand, presiding over the equity court and exercising the king's overriding authority, could fashion remedies and hear cases not cognizable at law. The chancellor's theme became: "for every wrong a remedy." While the common law courts for the most part decided property rights and were said to operate *in rem,* the courts of equity enforced their decisions against the litigants themselves and were said to operate *in personum.* The equity courts developed rather ill-defined and not entirely consistent operational principles called the "maxims of equity." The equitable maxims included:

1. Equity regards as done which ought to be done.
2. Equity looks to the intent rather than to the form.
3. He who seeks equity must do equity.
4. He who comes into equity must come with clean hands.
5. Equality is equity.
6. Where there are equal equities, the first in time shall prevail.
7. Where there is equal equity, the law must prevail.
8. Equity aids the vigilant, not those who slumber on their rights.
9. Equity imputes an intention to fulfill an obligation.
10. Equity will not suffer a wrong without a remedy.
11. Equity follows the law.

Certain acts of the equity courts caused great consternation and aroused strong opposition among the common law judges and lawyers of the time and their supporters in Parliament. Equity courts sometimes enjoined enforcement of decrees at common law and even enjoined prosecutions at common law. The common law courts in turn released on habeas corpus writs persons already imprisoned by the chancellor for violation of equitable injunctions. These and other conflicts were part of the climate leading up to the so-called "Long Parliament" of 1641 (which, among other things, ended the court of Star Chamber and tried to limit equity jurisdiction) and the overthrow and eventual execution of Charles I.

The double-court system survived King Charles I to become particularly contentious during the rein of King James I. The major combatants at that time were Chief Justice Coke and Chancellor Ellesmere, whose verbal and procedural confrontations finally pushed the king to intervene. Kings James I ordered a commission to study and resolve the conflict. Based on this commission (and perhaps his desire to maintain the power of the royal court system), James I ordered the courts of equity to:

> . . . continue to give such relief as shall stand with the merit and justness of the cause and with the former ancient and continued practice and (precedent) of our chancery.[43]

The common law champions, unwilling to push the king too far, drew in their horns somewhat and an uneasy truce replaced the open fighting.

The dual system was transplanted to the American colonies, where running conflicts continued between the colonial governors appointed by the crown and the courts that were heavily influenced by local legislatures. The United States Constitution gave the U.S. courts jurisdiction over both law and equity[39] and, of course, abolished the powers of the English throne. In 1934, the U.S. Supreme Court was given authority to combine the still separate functions of law and equity and, in 1938, adopted the first set of Federal Rules of Civil Procedure. (These were amended in 1975 and are currently undergoing further amendment.) Although now blended into one court system and with a modern judge acting as both common law judge and equitable chancellor, the requirements for giving so-called "equitable relief" have not entirely lost their origins or rationale. The equitable remedies attempt to fill in the gaps where strict application of the older common law principles would result in an incomplete or unjust result.

Due Process

Due process is an ephemeral concept present throughout the law, yet nowhere comprehensively defined. It underlies all of our Western notions of equal protection, judicial impartiality, and protections against arbitrary and capricious decisions. Daniel Webster in *Dartmouth v Woodward*[10] defined "due process" as: "The law which hears before it condemns; which proceeds upon inquiry and renders judgment only after trial." The concept of due process was contained within the charter of King Henry I in 1100, the Magna Carta of 1215 (King John), and the Magna Carta of 1225 (King Henry III), which states that:

> No free man shall be seized or imprisoned or stripped of his rights or possessions or outlawed or exiled or deprived of his standing in any other way, nor will he proceed with force against him, or send others to do so, except by the lawful judgment of his equals or by the law of the land. To no one will we sell, to no one will we deny right or justice.

The due process ideal was valued at least by the English middle and upper classes by the 13th and 14th centuries. Its greatest challenge came from the "other face" of the chancellor. The same system that gave birth to the courts of equity fathered the courts of Star Chamber (so named for a star decoration in the court chamber). The courts of Star Chamber, which existed between the 1400s and 1641, had both civil and criminal jurisdiction. They were secret tribunals conferred by the king, with the authority to compel answers under oath and mete out punishments including fines, brandings, the pillory, and mutilation, but not the death penalty. They used no juries and dispensed with the procedural safeguards of the common law courts. The courts of Star Chamber were used with increasing frequency and oppressive results during the reign of Charles I to enforce unpopular policies. They became a symbol of the attempt by Charles I to govern without consulting Parliament and were abolished by Parliament in 1641. They remain perhaps the leading example of an arbitrary and capricious tribunal within the English legal system, and a historical reminder of the need for due process protection.

Due process is expressly mentioned in the Fifth and Fourteenth Amendments of the U.S. Constitution, yet the concept is embodied throughout the constitution, in each of its amendments, and in the rules of criminal and civil procedure. In a procedural sense, it means "no short cuts." Everyone properly before the court or any other adjudicative body or tribunal is entitled to all of the protections afforded by law, and if not properly before the court, no binding determination of rights or duties can be made. Central to the concept of due process are the requirements of jurisdiction and notice. Theologic considerations aside, there are no courts of unlimited jurisdiction. Jurisdiction means that the subject of litigation is before a court or other body that has the authority to hear and decide the matter. A bankruptcy court is without power to decide a personal injury dispute. A tax court cannot rule on a municipal code violation. A case brought in a court with no jurisdiction must be dismissed by the judge *sui sponte* or on motion for dismissal for lack of jurisdiction. The requirement of notice means that one's rights may not be affected without notice within a proper jurisdiction and an opportunity to appear and contest any disputed claims.[30]

Courts of law are highly experienced with the requirements of due process. Judges and attorneys in a courtroom are alert to any procedural failure of due process. The same cannot be said for many quasi-judicial tribunals that handle matters on a less formal administrative basis. Due process issues are not uncommon in proceedings such as government administrative hearings, professional disciplinary hearings, zoning board hearings, tax board of equalization hearings, and hospital or medical society membership disputes. Hospital bylaws, under prodding by the Joint Counsel for Accreditation of Hospitals, now have extensive written procedures for hearings and appeals designed to avoid due process legal challenges.

Most courts do not consider disputes "ripe" for adjudication until all avenues of administrative appeal have been exhausted. At that point, a lawsuit can be brought to court raising the issue of due process failure and asking for judicial remedies.

Punitive Damages: Criminal or Civil?

Criminal and civil law have important distinctions, yet features of these separate systems often are lumped rather casually together. Perhaps nowhere else are the distinctions more confusing than with the subject of punitive damages. A criminal act is an act contrary to a statutory prohibition of some unit of government. The offended party is the government and not the individual (of course, an offended individual also may have a civil cause of action against the perpetrator). A criminal charge is brought by an official prosecutor representing some level of government. Punishment may include a fine and/or imprisonment. Statutes generally give a monetary range of fines or imprisonment for a particular violation. Any fine assessed is paid to government coffers and none of this goes to any private party. There are special rights given to criminal defendants including the right to counsel (free if necessary), speedy trial (civil trials are frequently scheduled years into the future), right against self-incrimination, the right to a jury trial, and others. There are also special rules of court procedure for criminal cases. In federal courts, these are detailed in the Federal Rules of Criminal Procedure. The various states have adopted their own rules of criminal procedure that, in general, closely parallel the federal rules. The burden of proof in a criminal case is "beyond a reasonable doubt." While defying precise mathematic quantification, this is generally considered to be something significantly beyond a 50% likelihood. Eventually, the criminal defendant will be found either guilty or not guilty of some charge. Compromises negotiated by the prosecutor, known as plea bargains, usually result in a guilty plea to some lesser charge. Criminal cases may be major (various classes of felonies) or minor (various classes of misdemeanors), and may be inherently evil *(malum in se)* or the violation of some rule not involving evil motive or moral turpitude *(malum prohibitum)*. Even an offense such as overtime parking (a mere *malum prohibitum* misdemeanor) is a criminal case and distinguishable from a civil case. Civil cases may also be brought by government prosecutors, as in certain IRS or antitrust prosecutions under civil statutes, but most civil cases are between private parties (individuals or corporations). These are processed under the rules of civil procedure, which differ from the rules of criminal procedure. Judgments in civil cases will be made regarding liability, not guilt. The concept of guilty or not guilty is exclusive to criminal law. The burden of proof in a civil case is "the preponderance of the evidence," sometimes also stated as "more likely than not." This definitely is less than the "beyond a reasonable doubt" burden of the criminal prosecutor and usually is defined as anything in excess of 50%. There is no imprisonment in civil cases. The debtors' prisons of Charles Dickens' era are no more. Instead, monetary damages in civil cases are intended to "make whole" the injured party. They include special damages (out-of-pocket calculable damages) plus general or non-economic damages (pain and suffering). In some states, damages may also be allowed for loss of a chance, hedonic damages, emotional damages, and even wrongful life.

Punitive damages, which are recognized in most states, exceed the intent of "making whole" the injured party and are in a highbred class of their own. Damages in civil cases often are much larger than the maximum statutory fines levied against a criminal defendant for seemingly comparable wrongdoing. The disparity between civil damages and criminal fines for behavior that society tries to discourage is nowhere more apparent than with punitive damages. Both criminal fines and civil punitive damages are designed to punish reprehensible behavior, but there the similarity ends. Criminal fines are limited by statute and are paid entirely to the government entity that prosecuted the defendant. Civil punitive damages, in contrast, are paid to the plaintiff, are subject to the attorney's contingency fee (usually 30% to 50%), and have no statutory upper limit. In *Texaco v Penzoil,* punitive damages were set by a jury at $3 billion.[37]

The concept of damages in excess of the amount needed to compensate for loss was recognized as early as 1793.[41] The term "exemplary damages" (a current synonym for punitive damages) was first used in a companion case.[21] In the United States, acceptance of punitive damages has varied from state to state but historically used to be confined to those cases that were particularly egregious, such as intentional torts and flagrant disregard for the consequences of one's actions. Such actions often were described as "wanton and willful" or "malicious behavior." Historically, punitive damages were small and rarely awarded, but over the past 30 years have increased dramatically in both size and frequency.[13,32]

Punitive damages have been a particular concern of manufacturers and a particular delight of plaintiff attorneys. The most frequent battlefield has been in the area of product liability, but punitive damages are also a major financial risk for all business and professional activities. The largest punitive damages award of all time was in a commercial contract interference dispute.[36] Punitive damages awards are "all over the map." They bear no consistent relationship to actual damages or to potential future damages. Since civil punitive damages, like fines in criminal cases, are intended to punish the miscreant individual or corporation, should they be subject to the Eighth Amendment's proscription against "excessive fines"? Not so, said the U.S. Supreme Court in a split decision in *Browning-Ferris Industries v Kelco* in 1989.[6] The court majority reasoned that the Eighth Amendment could be traced back to the English Bill of Rights of 1689 and through that back to the Magna Carta, and that the history consistently contemplated only those fines payable to the state. Justices O'Connor and Stevens dissented and felt that the Eighth Amendment should apply, just as it limits fines for criminal behavior. While ruling out (for the time being at least) Eighth Amendment challenges to unlimited punitive damages, Justices Brennan and Marshall expressed the view that the due process clause of the Fourteenth Amendment might apply to constrain punitive damages and expressed the opinion that due process was violated when "Punitive damages are imposed by juries guided by little more than an admonition to do what they think is best."

In two subsequent cases, *Pacific Mutual Life Insurance Company v Haslip*[28] and *TXO Production Corporation v Alliance Resources Corporation,*[38] the court majority declined to draw a clear line or multiple of actual damages as an upper limit. The court did affirm the authority of the trial judge to modify the damage award.

Punitive damages are not as frequently asserted in medical malpractice claims as in product liability suits, but they can be potent negotiating weapons for the plaintiff attorney. The reason for this powerful negotiating leverage is that punitive damages often are not covered by a physician's malpractice insurance carrier. In some states, this is because state law precludes insurance coverage for acts that public policy deems worthy of punishment. In other cases, insurance companies contractually exclude punitive damage coverage. In these instances, insurance companies are likely motivated by the impossibility of making rational actuarial projections about the size or frequency of punitive damages under current law and in the current legal climate. Whenever punitive damages are excluded from insurance coverage, a defendant physician finds himself or herself threatened with the potential of very large monetary damages which may be assessed at the whim of a jury and which will not be covered by his or her insurer. Not surprisingly, this is a powerful prod to force a settlement unfavorable to the defendant in return for dropping a punitive damage claim.

Several changes have been proposed to make civil punitive damages more consistent with the graded punitive function of criminal law and yet retain them in those special civil actions where compensatory damages alone seem inadequate. These include:

1. Requiring a higher burden of proof for punitive damages consistent with that required in criminal prosecutions. (The term "clear and convincing" evidence has been suggested.)

2. Restricting punitive damages to intentional torts or those cases evidencing near-criminal disregard for consequences to others.

3. Requiring all or most of punitive damages to be paid to a disciplinary board or some agency of government having a regulatory function over the subject of damages, rather than to the plaintiff and plaintiff's attorney personally. (This change might also bring punitive damages under the Eighth Amendment according to the reasoning of the *Browning-Ferris Industries v Kelco* case *{supra}*).

4. Applying a statutory ceiling to punitive damages (such as a fixed multiple of actual damages).

5. Allowing punitive damages to be assessed only once against a single tortfeasor. Currently, multiple plaintiffs can demand

punitive damages of the same defendant (e.g. Dalcon Shield, Silastic implants, asbestos cases.)

The Physician as Fiduciary

A fiduciary is a person holding the character of a trustee, or a character analogous to that of a trustee, in respect to the trust and confidence involved in it and the scrupulous good faith and candor which it requires.[5] The fiduciary relationship of physician to patient is recognized in case law both expressly and by clear implication:

> The relationship of patient and physician is a fiduciary one of the highest degree. It involves every element of trust and confidence and good faith.[24]

> The patient, being uninformed in medical sciences, has an abject dependence upon and trust in his physician for the information upon which he relies during the decisional process, thus raising an obligation in the physician that transcends arm's-length transactions.[8]

The fiduciary characteristic of the usual physician-patient relationship underlies most of the medical profession's ethical conflicts and legal exposure. Professional liability suits brought by patients almost invariably involve a claim of some failure to act consonant with the best interests of the patient, although they typically assert medical negligence or failure to inform rather than a breach of fiduciary duty. The label is more a matter of semantics and legal history than of substantive difference.

In addition to the familiar risk of malpractice litigation, newer areas of fiduciary conflict and potential legal entanglement include: 1) Managed-care insurers emphasis on reduction of medical costs rather than on providing the highest available quality of care (marketing brochures to the contrary notwithstanding); and 2) Referral of patients to medical support services in which the referring physician has an economic interest.

Wickline v California (1986)[40] was an important case in which cost containment efforts were pitted against medical judgment. Wickline, a Medi-Cal patient with severe arterial disease, underwent vascular repairs, a long hospital stay, and ultimately required a leg amputation. During the course of her initial hospitalization, her physician felt additional hospital observation was needed. This recommendation was denied by the California Welfare (Medi-Cal) office, and her surgeon acceded to a shortened stay without effective protest. At home, her condition worsened. Readmission, amputation, and lawsuit ensued. The California Supreme Court in its decision held that *a physician who complies with a third-party payer determination that is against his medical judgment cannot avoid his own liability*.

Less clear, but not reassuring to insurers, was the following dicta. (Dicta is gratuitous opinion included by the court but not necessary to the court's decision.)

> A patient who requires treatment and who is harmed when care which should have been provided is not provided should recover for the injuries suffered from all those responsible for the deprivation of such care, including, when appropriate, health care payers. Third party payers of health care services can be held legally accountable when medically inappropriate decisions result from defects in the design or implementation of cost containment mechanisms.

In this instance, the State of California managed to escape liability due to a particular statutory provision in California law.

The issue surfaced again in 1990 in *Wilson v Blue Cross of Southern California*.[42] Wilson was hospitalized by Dr. Taff for severe depression. Dr. Taff recommended 4 weeks of inpatient treatment, but the utilization review carried out by Blue Cross of Southern California concluded that the hospitalization was unnecessary and therefore not authorized. The final denial decision was made by a physician review agent for Blue Cross. Since neither the patient nor the patient's family could afford the hospitalization, Wilson left the hospital. Shortly thereafter, Wilson committed suicide. The estate brought suit against the insurer based on the utilization decision denying hospitalization. The trial court allowed summary judgment for the defendant based on the Wickline decision, and the plaintiff's family appealed based on the dicta *(supra)* from Wickline. The California Appellate

Court reversed the trial court and held that the insurer *could* be held liable for damages resulting from this medical utilization decision.

An important case that seemingly protects insurers under employer-provided insurance plans was decided in 1992 in *Corcoran v United Health Care, Inc*.[9] Corcoran, a South Central Bell Telephone Company employee, had a high-risk pregnancy. Her obstetrician, Dr. Jason Collins, recommended complete bed rest for the last few months of her pregnancy, and Mrs. Corcoran applied for temporary disability based on this medical recommendation. The company denied the temporary disability. Dr. Collins wrote the medical director for the Bell Telephone insurance carrier, and the medical director independently consulted another obstetrician who, it turned out, not only confirmed Dr. Collins' recommendations but specifically warned the company that it was at high risk of liability if it denied this request. Subsequently, near the end of her pregnancy, Mrs. Corcoran was hospitalized by Dr. Collins for the purpose of fetal monitoring. This hospitalization also was denied by the insurer, which instead authorized 10 hours per day of home health care. The patient, unable to afford the hospitalization on her own, went home on October 12. Fetal distress developed in the absence of monitoring and the fetus died on October 25 during the period when no nurse was present. The plaintiffs sued the utilization review company, which then had the case removed to the federal court on the theory that state law on the subject was pre-empted by the federal ERISA laws. The federal district trial court allowed summary judgment for the defendants based on the ERISA law, and this decision was upheld by the Fifth Circuit Court of Appeals. The plaintiffs then appealed to the U.S. Supreme Court, which declined review. The Fifth Circuit Appellate Court felt the wording of the ERISA law required this conclusion but noted that:

> Fundamental changes such as the widespread institution of utilization review would seem to warrant a re-evaluation of ERISA so that it can continue to serve its noble purpose of safeguarding the interests of employees.

This is a case in which the treating physician appears to have made the proper medical recommendations, and in which the insurer alone was responsible for the monitoring failure and likely for the death of the fetus. The court evidently sympathized with the plaintiffs but felt that the wording of the ERISA law required this result. This decision, while binding only within the Fifth Circuit, appears to confer immunity for utilization reviewers and insurers where the medical insurance is part of an ERISA-covered employer health insurance program.

Conflict with physician fiduciary duty seems almost "design inherent" in capitation plans in which a physician's income is maximized by providing the minimum of medical care. Only slightly less direct is the threat of preferred provider organizations (PPOs), health maintenance organizations (HMOs), and some hospitals applying economic credentialing retrospectively to the physician's clinical decisions. Such arrangements appear to be fertile ground for lawsuits that will pit physicians and managed-care entities against each other as defendants. Whether insurers will find safe or permanent haven in the Corcoran decision is not at all certain. Trial lawyers, and at least some appellate judges, have shown great inventiveness in expanding the range and theories of liability, and it is hard to believe that managed-care plans will really succeed in escaping liability where their cost-driven decisions have injured patients. A widely reported jury case decided in Riverside, California, in December of 1993 held an HMO insurer liable for $12 million in actual damages and an additional $77 million in punitive damages for denying the plaintiff insurance coverage for a bone marrow transplant. Although this case was brought under a breach of contract theory rather than for malfeasance in utilization review, the issues were very similar and all medical care insurers are viewing this case with increasing anxiety.[34] The conflict between cost containment and state-of-the-art medical care has attracted the attention of legal academia, and there are several law review articles addressing this subject.[20,25,27] Recognizing their potential exposure, insurers, employing hospitals, PPOs, and HMOs often attempt to disclaim their liability with contract terms such as:

> Nothing contained herein shall be construed as allowing the (hospital, PPO, HMO, insurance company, etc.) to engage in the practice of medicine, and it is agreed between the parties that any actions or medical decisions by the undersigned physician are solely those of the physician.

A currently organizing PPO contains (in separate sections of the agreement) the following terms in its participating physician's agreement:

> *Section 1.3*, PROVIDER shall be responsible for the provider relationship with each patient whom PROVIDER treats and shall be solely responsible to each patient for the health care provided. Participating PLANS are responsible for and shall maintain the PLAN-patient relationship. Neither COMPANY, PLANS, PROVIDER nor any of their respective employees shall be liable or responsible for any acts or omissions on the part of the other.

> *Section 3.3*, PROVIDER agrees to abide by the cost containment programs established by the COMPANY or PLANS for subscribers, including but not limited to, preadmission certification and length of stay review, outpatient surgery for designated procedures unless unusual circumstances are present, and second opinions for certain surgical procedures.

Some contracts also include hold-harmless clauses under which the insuring entity would be reimbursed by the physician for any legal expenses or judgments against it. Physicians are well advised to be very cautious about agreeing to such terms and should obtain their own independent legal counsel before agreeing to managed-care contracts containing provisions such as the above examples.

The Corcoran decision clearly will not protect physician "gatekeepers" whose decisions result in patient injury, and such primary care gatekeepers may find themselves at legal sword's point with specialists. Full and carefully written documentation of the specialist's recommendations will be the best defense for the specialist when these cases arise. Insurers no doubt see the advantage of using physician gatekeepers to shield themselves from adverse results of economically driven medical decisions. Physicians who willingly assume such gatekeeper roles will need to be particularly sensitive to their patient fiduciary obligations.

Moore v Regents of the University of California[26] is an interesting case in which a physician entrepreneur and his university employer were economic as well as medical fiduciaries. Moore was a patient at the University of California while undergoing treatment for hairy cell leukemia. In the course of his treatment, he had a splenectomy, and bone marrow and other tissues were removed on numerous occasions. Unknown to Moore during his active treatment and follow-up, his physician was using these body tissues for medical research and development. The physician developed, and the Regents of the university patented, an economically valuable cell line which was then used to produce lymphokines for the treatment of other patients. When Moore learned of this, he sued his oncologist and the University of California, claiming that he had an economic interest in the research products from his own body tissues and should share in the profits. The court, while denying damages for conversion, held that the treating physician and the University of California Regents did indeed have a fiduciary duty to the patient and that that duty had been breached.

Physicians have always functioned with the inherent conflict of making medical recommendations that can result in income to the recommending physician. This is recognized even in the ancient Hippocratic oath. If a neurosurgeon, for example, recommends a surgical procedure, the surgeon ordinarily stands to benefit more than if no surgery had been recommended. This everyday example goes to the very heart of a physician's fiduciary duty—the duty to recommend what is felt to be best for the patient regardless of any potential benefit to the surgeon. Although clinical recommendations may differ, motives should not. Probably, most physicians would say that this is simply inherent in the nature of a profession and is one of the factors differentiating a profession from a trade. But suspicion of clinical judgment (and of motives) has been the rationale for second opinion requirements and insurer managed-care decisions. Whether these have saved money or improved quality is unclear at this point, and some insurers now have discontinued mandatory second opinion requirements for most surgeries.

Much more attention has been focused lately on the issue of "self-referral," in which a physician has a financial interest in some diagnostic or treatment center to which he or she refers patients. This usually involves laboratories, imaging centers, physical therapy units, outpatient surgeries, or hospitals. In 1989, such self-referrals were restricted under the Medicare program. Several states also have enacted their own laws limiting such physician referrals, requiring disclosure of economic interest or making such referrals illegal altogether. The American Medical Association (AMA) jumped on this bandwagon in 1992. Why the self-referral issue is so "hot" as it applies to diagnostic and treatment centers and relatively "cold" as to medical and surgical recommendations by the physician is probably more a matter of practicality than reason and cannot easily be explained on a fiduciary theory. Most patients select their physicians for both consultation and treatment and probably have more confidence in their physician's professionalism than do the would-be regulators. Also, denying a patient the right to be treated by the same surgeon who carried out the consultation and made recommendations would interfere with the politically sensitive desire of many patients to choose their own physicians.

The Expert Witness

The general rule of evidence is that opinion testimony is not admissible. Fact witnesses are allowed to describe only their observations and any conclusions to be drawn from those observations are to be made by the jury. An exception is made for the opinions or conclusions of experts who have knowledge beyond the ken and experience of most jurors. Expert opinion offered in court goes through a two-step evaluation: The first is the question of admissibility, a judicial decision; the second is the weight to be given the evidence, a jury decision. (In a bench trial, the judge assumes both functions.) In a trial involving technical issues beyond the expertise of a jury, both the plaintiff and the defendant will need to present expert testimony. The admissibility of "expert" testimony of varying qualities has been a contentious issue for trial attorneys and other professionals for a very long time. Currently, there is little scientific guidance to assist a judge in the screening process, and there is a tendency to admit marginal evidence on the theory that the jury will "sort it out." Possibly, judges feel that they are less likely to be reversed for allowing evidence than for excluding it. *Frye v United States*[18] was not a very profound case, yet the so-called Frye test derived from that case became the measure of admissibility within the federal court until the First Amendment to the Federal Rules of Civil Procedure in 1975. Frye was a criminal case in which expert opinion testimony was proffered based on a blood pressure deception test (the forerunner of the modern polygraph lie detector test—itself not admissible in most jurisdictions today). The trial court excluded the evidence as not having been generally accepted by the scientific community, and the District of Columbia Circuit Court affirmed this decision in 1923. The federal courts and most state courts followed the Frye "general acceptance" rule until 1975 when Rule 702 of the amended Federal Rules of Civil Procedure permitted admission of any evidence that "might assist the trier of fact." Legal academicians argued for the next 18 years over whether Rule 702 overruled the Frye general acceptance test, but many judges throughout the country felt free to admit evidence that would not have been accepted under Frye. The latest word, at least within the federal courts, is found in the 1993 Supreme Court case of *Daubert v Merrill-Dow Pharmaceuticals, Inc.*[11]

Jason Daubert and Eric Schuller were born with congenital physical defects. Their mothers had taken Bendectin, an antinauseant medication, throughout their pregnancies. Merrill-Dow had been a defendant in many cases in which Bendectin was alleged to have caused birth defects and, despite convincing evidence that Bendectin was safe and effective, Merrill-Dow had finally withdrawn it from the market because profits from the drug were far less than the costs of the recurring litigation. Dr. Lamm, for the defendant Merrill-Dow, had reviewed all of the medical literature regarding Bendectin and birth defects. He discovered more than 30 published papers in peer-reviewed journals, involving more than 130,000 patients. No study had found a teratogenic effect from Bendectin. The plaintiff offered evidence based on a "re-analysis" of the same data

that had exonerated Bendectin and which reanalysis had not been peer-reviewed or otherwise accepted by the scientific community. The federal trial court refused to admit the testimony of the plaintiff's proposed experts based on the general acceptance test of the Frye rule and gave summary judgment to Merrill-Dow. The Ninth Circuit Court of Appeals affirmed and the plaintiff appealed to the U.S. Supreme Court, arguing that the Frye rule had been superseded by Rule 702 of the Federal Rules of Civil Procedure. In its decision, the U.S. Supreme Court concluded that the 1975 Federal Rules of Civil Procedure had overruled the Frye general acceptance test, but confirmed that the trial judge may screen evidence under Rule 702 and must ensure that the evidence is reliable. The court majority held that:

> General acceptance is not a necessary precondition to the admissibility of evidence under the Federal Rules of Evidence, but the rules of evidence—especially Rule 702—do assign to the trial judge the task of ensuring that an expert's testimony both rests on a reliable foundation and is relevant to the task at hand. Pertinent evidence based on scientifically valid principles will satisfy that demand.

In remanding the case for further proceedings consistent with the majority opinion, the court noted: "The inquiry of the district court and the court of appeals focused almost exclusively on 'general acceptance' as gauged by publication and the decisions of other courts." Two Supreme Court justices (Rehnquist and Stevens) concurred in part, but felt that the majority decision gave trial judges little or no guidance regarding their evidentiary gatekeeper role. One may indeed be left wondering if this is another legal "distinction without a difference" since the new requirement sounds much like the Frye test but without the words "general acceptance."

Most state court procedural rules are nearclones of the federal rules, and most personal injury claims are adjudicated under state rules and precedent. The Daubert case, for which the defense bar had had high hopes, probably is not going to result in any major changes. Judges retain broad discretion in the admission of expert witness testimony, and it is seldom that a judge is overruled for abuse of discretion.

The American Association of Neurological Surgeons and the American College of Surgeons maintain testimony files containing transcripts of testimony that can be used to impeach a witness who makes assertions inconsistent with some prior testimony. Plaintiff attorneys share with each other the names of witnesses who have been particularly effective in the past. Also available to attorneys, through the LEXIS and Westlaw computer system, is an expert witness file compiled by the National Forensic Center of Princeton, New Jersey. The technical advisory service for attorneys of Fort Washington, Pennsylvania, reports a list of more than 10,000 experts in 4,000 categories, and an annual growth rate of 15%. The legal battle of the experts appears likely to continue unless there is a significant change in the method of settling personal injury and commercial disputes.[14] In England and other countries, the judge routinely appoints expert witnesses—a suggestion that has not found favor with either plaintiff or defendant attorneys in the United States, and has been used rarely by U.S. judges. There is increasing interest in the use of alternative dispute resolution formats for medical liability disputes, including mediation, arbitration, and other administrative resolutions such as proposed by the AMA with The Specialty Society. These could be mechanisms for the increased use of independent expert witnesses not hired by either the plaintiff or defendant. Many trial attorneys feel that there is no such thing as an independent expert medical witness. The attorney's advocacy role leads him or her to think only in terms of the plaintiff's expert and the defendant's expert. Some even consider that a treating physician has a duty to assist his or her patient with supportive testimony at trial. I have tried in vain to convince some experienced plaintiff trial attorneys that the role of the expert medical witness is to evaluate the medical information and express an independent opinion, even in regard to his or her own patient, letting the "chips fall where they may." This difference in perception of the expert witness role, I believe, reflects a major conceptual difference between the practices of law and medicine.

Occasionally, an attorney will try to obtain an expert witness for the statutory witness fee. In most states, the issue probably would be determined by whether the questions put to the physician expert call for a medical opinion. Conceivably, an attorney could subpoena a physician and ask questions only about what transpired between a physician and patient. If no question requires a medical opinion answer, the physician might be considered only a fact witness and thus entitled only to a statutory witness fee. A 1990 Washington Appellate Court decision denied an expert witness fee for an accountant who had been employed to evaluate a dental practice for the purpose of sale.[4] The purchasing orthodontist defaulted on the sale agreement, and the accountant was deposed and appeared at trial. He was compensated only with a $20 statutory witness fee for preparation, deposition, and trial testimony. In a separate action, the trial court allowed the accountant his $575 billing fee, plus his attorney fees for bringing the action. The appellate court reversed, stating that:

> An expert person is not necessarily an expert witness as defined in CR 26 (b)(4). Professionals who have acquired or developed facts and opinions not in anticipation of litigation but from involvement as an actor in a transaction are not entitled to expert witness fees.

Physicians, in states where this has become a problem, may wish to demand prepayment by an attorney before scheduling a deposition or trial. This should at least smoke out the attorney's intentions and allow inquiry about whether opinion questions will be asked.

In the context of medical malpractice litigation, some neurosurgeons have proposed that medical testimony be provided as a service, without any fee. The proponents of this suggestion hope, thereby, to put professional witnesses out of business. That has not been generally adopted, but the suggestion is an interesting one.

Medical Malpractice Suits

The threat of a medical malpractice lawsuit is something physicians have come to accept with varying degrees of equanimity. The threat influences relationships with colleagues, hospitals, and the fraternity of personal injury lawyers. Sometimes, it spills over to relationships with the entire bar.

From time to time, there have been "crises" in which malpractice premiums have risen abruptly to alarming levels, or in which insurers have abandoned geographic markets or discontinued the medical liability line of business altogether. These crisis periods stimulated efforts both to change the laws and procedures governing medical tort claims and to find other sources of insurance coverage. Various tort reform efforts have been made (with varying results) in every state. Physicians in most states formed their own insurance companies, and physician-owned companies now write medical liability insurance for more than 60% of the private physicians in the United States. These companies operate independently but share data summaries through the Physician Insurers Association of America (PIAA). The commercial carriers, which at one time dominated the market, generally considered claims information proprietary and, even when sponsored by a state medical society, would not make the figures available to their insureds. The PIAA now has accumulated national claims data from its member companies dating back to 1985 and makes this available to its membership and interested physicians generally. The claims data in the following *Special Appendix* are from the May 1993 report of the PIAA and are reprinted through the courtesy of the PIAA (1130 Connecticut Avenue, NW, Washington, DC 20036).

Determination of claims frequency for specific procedures and for specific specialties obviously requires additional information, including the insured population breakdown of specialties and procedures. In the introductory notes to the published data, the PIAA warns that this statistical material does not by itself allow premium calculations and therefore cannot be used for rate setting. A study of the claims numbers compared with the population of various specialties does, however, provide an overview of frequency. Assuming that neurosurgeons constitute about 1% of practicing physicians, insurers seem to be on solid ground in rating neurosurgery among the highest risk specialties.

Special Appendix

<table>
<tr><td colspan="3" align="center">TABLE 1
Indemnity for Top Ten Specialties*</td></tr>
<tr><td>Specialty</td><td>Total</td><td>Average</td></tr>
<tr><td>Obstetrics/gynecology</td><td>$822,643,921</td><td>$180,841</td></tr>
<tr><td>General Surgery</td><td>429,263,775</td><td>119,042</td></tr>
<tr><td>Internal Medicine</td><td>399,216,989</td><td>131,973</td></tr>
<tr><td>General Practice/
   Family Practice</td><td>367,261,914</td><td>103,454</td></tr>
<tr><td>Orthopedic Surgery</td><td>315,582,296</td><td>111,513</td></tr>
<tr><td>Anesthesiology</td><td>212,750,984</td><td>149,614</td></tr>
<tr><td>Pediatrics</td><td>156,171,250</td><td>204,681</td></tr>
<tr><td>Radiology</td><td>131,736,584</td><td>101,336</td></tr>
<tr><td>Neurosurgery</td><td>118,727,171</td><td>199,207</td></tr>
<tr><td>Ophthalmologic Surgery</td><td>83,716,929</td><td>112,826</td></tr>
</table>

* Tables in Special Appendix reprinted courtesy of the Physician Insurers Association of America (PIAA).

<table>
<tr><td colspan="2" align="center">TABLE 2
Claim Counts for Top Ten Specialties</td></tr>
<tr><td>Specialty</td><td>Count</td></tr>
<tr><td>Obstetrics/Gynecology</td><td>14,388</td></tr>
<tr><td>Internal Medicine</td><td>12,868</td></tr>
<tr><td>General Surgery</td><td>11,446</td></tr>
<tr><td>Orthopedic Surgery</td><td>10,490</td></tr>
<tr><td>General Practice/
   Family Practice</td><td>10,176</td></tr>
<tr><td>Radiology</td><td>5,416</td></tr>
<tr><td>Anesthesiology</td><td>4,054</td></tr>
<tr><td>Plastic Surgery</td><td>3,515</td></tr>
<tr><td>Pediatrics</td><td>3,036</td></tr>
<tr><td>Ophthalmology</td><td>2,833</td></tr>
</table>

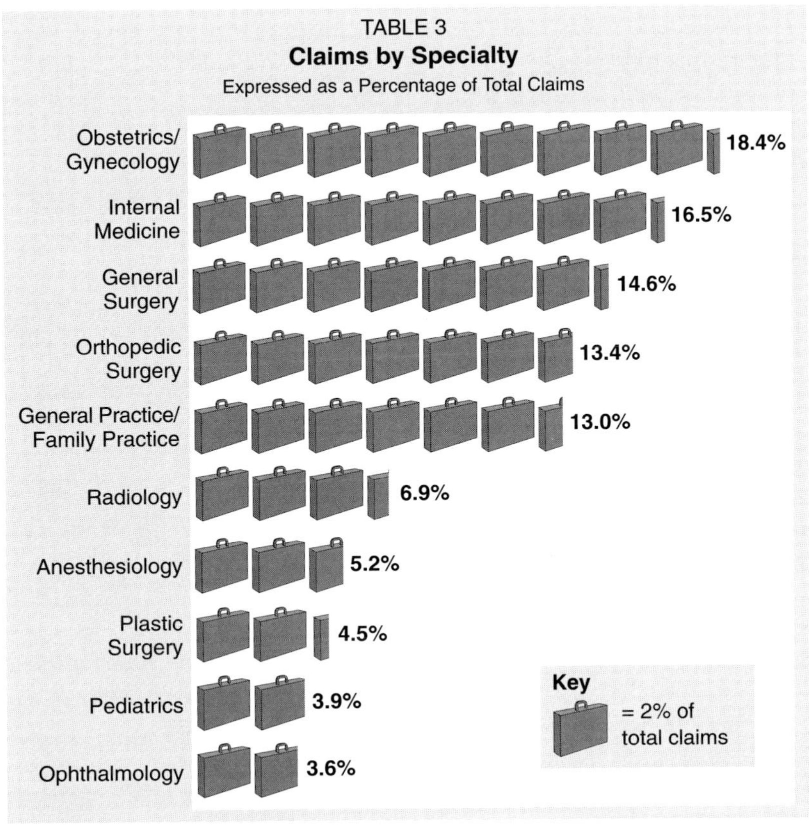
TABLE 3
Claims by Specialty
Expressed as a Percentage of Total Claims
Obstetrics/ Gynecology 18.4%
Internal Medicine 16.5%
General Surgery 14.6%
Orthopedic Surgery 13.4%
General Practice/ Family Practice 13.0%
Radiology 6.9%
Anesthesiology 5.2%
Plastic Surgery 4.5%
Pediatrics 3.9%
Ophthalmology 3.6%
Key
= 2% of total claims

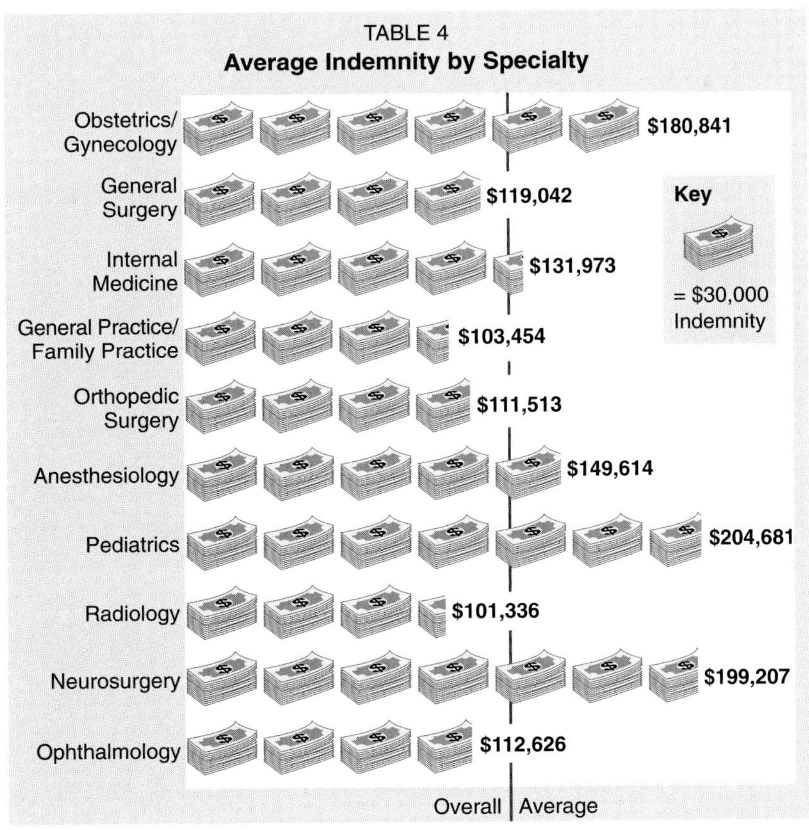
TABLE 4
Average Indemnity by Specialty
Obstetrics/ Gynecology $180,841
General Surgery $119,042
Internal Medicine $131,973
General Practice/ Family Practice $103,454
Orthopedic Surgery $111,513
Anesthesiology $149,614
Pediatrics $204,681
Radiology $101,336
Neurosurgery $199,207
Ophthalmology $112,626
Key
= $30,000 Indemnity
Overall Average

TABLE 5
PIAA Data Sharing System
Most Prevalent/Expensive Procedures and Conditions by Specialty*

SPECIALTY GROUP—Neurosurgery	No. of Files	No. of Closed Files	No. of Paid Files	% Paid of Closed Files	Indemnity Paid ($)	Average Indemnity Per Paid File ($)
PART I: Ten Most Prevalent Procedures						
1) EXCISION OF INTERVERTEBRAL DISC	528	462	150	32.47	22,471,654	149,811
Most prevalent misadventures this procedure and specialty						
Improper performance	280	244	87	35.66	14,117,499	162,270
No medical misadventure	106	96	3	3.13	216,784	72,261
Wrong patient or body part	34	27	18	66.67	1,884,265	104,681
Performed when not indicated or contraindicated	27	23	7	30.43	729,990	104,284
Errors in diagnosis	16	14	6	42.86	721,833	120,306
Most prevalent conditions this procedure and specialty						
Displacement of intervertebral disc	293	273	82	30.04	10,226,267	124,711
Disc disorder of unspecified region	44	30	6	20.00	521,500	86,917
Backache or back pain	23	18	7	38.89	540,000	77,143
Degeneration of intervertebral disc	15	14	8	57.14	932,274	116,534
Spondylosis	13	12	4	33.33	1,000,000	250,000
Most prevalent iatrogenic injuries this procedure and specialty						
Nerve root, injury to	11	10	4	40.00	882,500	220,625
Spinal cord, injury to	8	7	5	71.43	1,027,499	205,500
Abdomen or pelvis, blood vessel of, injury to	7	6	3	50.00	207,500	69,167
Ureter, accidental perforation or laceration of	2	2	2	100.00	624,004	312,002
Pelvis or lower limb, nerves of, injury to	2	2	2	100.00	59,998	29,999
2) EXPLORATION AND DECOMPRESSION OF SPINAL CANAL	353	305	112	36.72	24,330,469	217,236
Most prevalent misadventures this procedure and specialty						
Improper performance	176	153	62	40.52	12,952,771	208,916
No medical misadventure	76	64	3	4.69	280,000	93,333
Performed when not indicated or contraindicated	29	27	10	37.04	1,982,500	198,250
Errors in diagnosis	20	18	12	66.67	4,944,861	412,072
Failure to supervise or monitor case	12	11	8	72.73	2,025,750	253,219
Most prevalent conditions this procedure and specialty						
Displacement of intervertebral disc	78	72	26	36.11	4,228,629	162,640
Spondylosis	32	26	9	34.62	1,625,499	180,611
Disc disorder of unspecified region	23	22	5	22.73	138,499	27,700
Backache or back pain	19	17	7	41.18	874,222	124,889
Stenosis, spinal, other than cervical	19	17	6	35.29	839,431	139,905
Most prevalent iatrogenic injuries this procedure and specialty						
Nerve root, injury to	7	7	4	57.14	540,000	135,000
Spinal cord, injury to	5	5	3	60.00	493,831	164,610
Pelvis or lower limb, nerves of, injury to	2	2	2	100.00	700,000	350,000
Abdomen or pelvis, blood vessel of, injury to	1	1	1	100.00	636,629	636,629
Pain in limb	1	1	1	100.00	25,250	25,250
3) DIAGNOSTIC INTERVIEW AND EVALUATION	177	149	36	24.16	6,876,935	191,026
Most prevalent misadventures this procedure and specialty						
Errors in diagnosis	65	56	17	30.36	2,096,831	123,343
No medical misadventure	44	38	1	2.63	900,000	900,000
Improper performance	19	16	5	31.25	1,212,604	242,521
Delay in performance	14	9	4	44.44	1,462,500	365,625
Failure to supervise or monitor case	10	8	1	12.50	200,000	200,000
Most prevalent conditions this procedure and specialty						
Closed fracture of cervical vertebra	13	11	3	27.27	215,000	71,667
Subarachnoid hemorrhage, not following injury	8	7	3	42.86	123,333	41,111
Postoperative infection	7	3	2	66.67	187,500	93,750
Disc disorder of unspecified region	7	2	0	0.00	0	0
Intracranial hemorrhage following injury without mention	5	5	1	20.00	200,000	200,000

*From PIAA report #4, pp. 236-248, 5/8/93.

SPECIALTY GROUP—Neurosurgery	No. of Files	No. of Closed Files	No. of Paid Files	% Paid of Closed Files	Indemnity Paid ($)	Average Indemnity Per Paid File ($)
4) CONSULTATION	176	146	15	10.27	5,454,524	363,635
Most prevalent misadventures this procedure and specialty						
No medical misadventure	55	50	0	0.00	0	0
Errors in diagnosis	47	36	2	5.56	149,500	74,750
Improper performance	31	21	1	4.76	950,000	950,000
Delay in performance	10	10	4	40.00	1,670,824	417,706
Not performed	10	8	3	37.50	1,309,950	436,650
Most prevalent conditions this procedure and specialty						
Closed fracture of cervical vertebra	14	9	2	22.22	1,050,000	525,000
Displacement of intervertebral disc	9	8	0	0.00	0	0
Concussion	7	6	0	0.00	0	0
Intracranial hemorrhage following injury without mention	6	3	1	33.33	75,000	75,000
Subarachnoid hemorrhage, not following injury	6	5	1	20.00	50,000	50,000
5) CRANIOTOMY AND CRANIECTOMY	156	145	38	26.21	11,160,668	293,702
Most prevalent misadventures this procedure and specialty						
Improper performance	49	46	12	26.09	3,621,322	301,777
No medical misadventure	47	42	3	7.14	366,475	122,158
Errors in diagnosis	12	12	3	25.00	1,080,067	360,022
Delay in performance	11	10	7	70.00	3,225,958	460,851
Performed when not indicated or contraindicated	7	5	0	0.00	0	0
Most prevalent conditions this procedure and specialty						
Benign neoplasms of the brain	9	9	3	33.33	966,849	322,283
Subdural hemorrhage, following injury	9	9	1	11.11	5,000	5,000
Intracranial hemorrhage, following injury without mention	8	7	3	42.86	1,262,155	420,718
Subarachnoid hemorrhage, not following injury	8	8	1	12.50	480,000	480,000
Malignant neoplasms of the brain	8	7	1	14.29	22,500	22,500
Most prevalent iatrogenic injuries this procedure and specialty						
Mononeuritis	2	2	0	0.00	0	0
Paralysis	2	2	0	0.00	0	0
Cranial nerve, injury to	1	1	1	100.00	700,000	700,000
Head or neck, blood vessel of, injury to	1	1	0	0.00	0	0
Convulsions	1	1	0	0.00	0	0
6) SPINAL FUSION, NOT OTHERWISE SPECIFIED	126	96	31	32.29	8,529,499	275,145
Most prevalent misadventures this procedure and specialty						
Improper performance	68	48	16	33.33	3,720,068	232,504
No medical misadventure	17	13	0	0.00	0	0
Performed when not indicated or contraindicated	10	8	4	50.00	2,836,790	709,198
Wrong patient or body part	10	7	7	100.00	873,500	124,786
Failure to supervise or monitor case	6	6	0	0.00	0	0
Most prevalent conditions this procedure and specialty						
Displacement of intervertebral disc	25	20	8	40.00	1,875,422	234,428
Closed fracture of cervical vertebra	23	18	7	38.89	2,379,900	339,986
Spondylosis	12	8	3	37.50	180,000	60,000
Dislocation of vertebra, coccyx, or sacrum	10	8	2	25.00	1,385,000	692,500
Degeneration of intervertebral disc	6	4	4	100.00	274,415	68,604
Most prevalent latrogenic injuries this procedure and specialty						
Spinal cord, injury to	2	2	1	50.00	150,000	150,000
Accidental puncture or laceration during procedure	2	0	0	0.00	0	0
Cranial nerve, injury to	2	1	0	0.00	0	0
Injury to nerves	1	1	1	100.00	47,500	47,500
Intestine, accidental perforation or laceration of	1	1	0	0.00	0	0
7) NEUROLOGIC EXAMINATION	93	86	14	16.28	2,185,332	156,095
Most prevalent misadventures this procedure and specialty						
No medical misadventure	38	35	2	5.71	57,500	28,750
Errors in diagnosis	23	20	3	15.00	88,499	29,500
Failure to supervise or monitor case	15	14	8	57.14	1,239,333	154,917

SPECIALTY GROUP—Neurosurgery	No. of Files	No. of Closed Files	No. of Paid Files	% Paid of Closed Files	Indemnity Paid ($)	Average Indemnity Per Paid File ($)
Improper performance	5	5	0	0.00	0	0
Delay in performance	4	4	1	25.00	800,000	800,000
Most prevalent conditions this procedure and specialty						
Subdural hemorrhage, following injury	5	5	1	20.00	74,999	74,999
Closed fracture of cervical vertebra	5	4	0	0.00	0	0
Subarachnoid hemorrhage, not following injury	4	4	0	0.00	0	0
Epilepsy	3	3	1	33.33	683,333	683,333
Neoplasm of the spinal cord, unknown if malignant or benign	3	2	0	0.00	0	0
Most prevalent Iatrogenic injuries this procedure and specialty						
Lower extremity, blood vessel of, injury to	1	1	0	0.00	0	0
8) PRESCRIPTION OF MEDICATION	59	50	17	34.00	1,346,374	79,198
Most prevalent misadventures this procedure and specialty						
Medication errors	23	18	10	55.56	432,374	43,237
No medical misadventure	12	11	1	9.09	50,000	50,000
Errors in diagnosis	5	5	2	40.00	680,000	340,000
Performed when not indicated or contraindicated	4	4	2	50.00	160,000	80,000
Failure to supervise or monitor case	4	2	0	0.00	0	0
Most prevalent conditions this procedure and specialty						
Encephalopathy, not further defined	4	3	3	100.00	135,000	45,000
Lumbago	4	4	1	25.00	60,000	60,000
Headache	4	4	1	25.00	5,000	5,000
Convulsions	3	3	1	33.33	50,000	50,000
Subarachnoid hemorrhage, not following injury	3	3	1	33.33	29,999	29,999
9) NO CARE RENDERED	57	54	5	9.26	143,500	28,700
Most prevalent misadventures this procedure and specialty						
No medical misadventure	48	45	1	2.22	100,000	100,000
Errors in diagnosis	2	2	1	50.00	7,500	7,500
Improper supervision of residents/other staff	2	2	1	50.00	6,000	6,000
Improper performance	2	2	0	0.00	0	0
Surgical foreign body left in patient after procedure	1	1	1	100.00	20,000	20,000
Most prevalent conditions this procedure and specialty						
Displacement of intervertebral disc	9	9	0	0.00	0	0
Backache or back pain	3	3	1	33.33	6,000	6,000
Cerebral degeneration	3	3	0	0.00	0	0
Subarachnoid hemorrhage, not following injury	2	2	1	50.00	10,000	10,000
Postoperative infection	2	1	0	0.00	0	0
Most prevalent iatrogenic injuries this procedure and specialty						
Lung or bronchus, accidental perforation or laceration of	1	1	1	100.00	6,000	6,000
10) CONTRAST MYELOGRAM	53	44	12	27.27	3,319,773	276,648
Most prevalent misadventures this procedure and specialty						
No medical misadventure	18	16	2	12.50	281,338	140,669
Improper performance	15	12	4	33.33	1,156,500	289,125
Errors in diagnosis	7	5	1	20.00	36,666	36,666
Performed when not indicated or contraindicated	4	3	1	33.33	642,769	642,769
Failure to supervise or monitor case	4	4	1	25.00	7,500	7,500
Most prevalent conditions this procedure and specialty						
Displacement of intervertebral disc	12	9	1	11.11	6,338	6,338
Lumbago	5	4	2	50.00	152,500	76,250
Backache or back pain	3	2	0	0.00	0	0
Spondylosis	3	3	0	0.00	0	0
Disease of the spinal cord	2	2	2	100.00	1,900,000	950,000
Most prevalent iatrogenic injuries this procedure and specialty						
Nerve root, injury to	1	1	0	0.00	0	0
TOTALS	1778	1537	430	27.98	85,818,728	199,578

SPECIALTY GROUP—Neurosurgery	No. of Files	No. of Closed Files	No. of Paid Files	% Paid of Closed Files	Indemnity Paid ($)	Average Indemnity Per Paid File ($)
PART II: Ten Most Expensive Procedures						
1) EXPLORATION AND DECOMPRESSION OF SPINAL CANAL	353	305	112	36.72	24,330,469	217,236
Most expensive misadventures this procedure and specialty						
Improper performance	176	153	62	40.52	12,952,771	208,916
Errors in diagnosis	20	18	12	66.67	4,944,861	412,072
Failure to supervise or monitor case	12	11	8	72.73	2,025,750	253,219
Performed when not indicated or contraindicated	29	27	10	37.04	1,982,500	198,250
Delay in performance	8	6	2	33.33	628,932	314,466
Most expensive conditions this procedure and specialty						
Displacement of intervertebral disc	78	72	26	36.11	4,228,629	162,640
Paraplegia	12	10	7	70.00	2,746,912	392,416
Intraspinal abscess	3	3	3	100.00	2,230,000	743,333
Paralysis	7	7	3	42.86	2,140,000	713,333
Spondylosis	32	26	9	34.62	1,625,499	180,611
Most expensive iatrogenic injuries this procedure and specialty						
Pelvis or lower limb, nerves of, injury to	2	2	2	100.00	700,000	350,000
Abdomen or pelvis, blood vessel of, injury to	1	1	1	100.00	636,629	636,629
Nerve root, injury to	7	7	4	57.14	540,000	135,000
Spinal cord, injury to	5	5	3	60.00	493,831	164,610
Pain in limb	1	1	1	100.00	25,250	25,250
2) EXCISION OF INTERVERTEBRAL DISC	528	462	150	32.47	22,471,654	149,811
Most expensive misadventures this procedure and specialty						
Improper performance	280	244	87	35.66	14,117,499	162,270
Wrong patient or body part	34	27	18	66.67	1,884,265	104,681
Not performed	6	5	4	80.00	1,142,549	285,637
Delay in performance	7	6	5	83.33	1,060,000	212,000
Failure to instruct or communicate with patient	4	4	2	50.00	825,000	412,500
Most expensive conditions this procedure and specialty						
Displacement of intervertebral disc	293	273	82	30.04	10,226,267	124,711
Spondylosis	13	12	4	33.33	1,000,000	250,000
Nerve root, injury to	1	1	1	100.00	1,000,000	1,000,000
Degeneration of intervertebral disc	15	14	8	57.14	932,274	116,534
Lipoma	1	1	1	100.00	900,000	900,000
Most expensive iatrogenic injuries this procedure and specialty						
Spinal cord, injury to	8	7	5	71.43	1,027,499	205,500
Nerve root, injury to	11	10	4	40.00	882,500	220,625
Ureter, accidental perforation or laceration of	2	2	2	100.00	624,004	312,002
Intestine, accidental perforation or laceration of	1	1	1	100.00	524,004	524,004
Pancreas, accidental perforation or laceration of	1	1	1	100.00	500,000	500,000
3) CRANIOTOMY AND CRANIECTOMY	156	145	38	26.21	11,160,668	293,702
Most expensive misadventures this procedure and specialty						
Improper performance	49	46	12	26.09	3,621,322	301,777
Delay in performance	11	10	7	70.00	3,225,958	460,851
Errors in diagnosis	12	12	3	25.00	1,080,067	360,022
Failure to recognize a complication of treatment	4	4	1	25.00	900,000	900,000
Medication errors	1	1	1	100.00	831,849	831,849
Most expensive conditions this procedure and specialty						
Quadriplegia	2	2	2	100.00	1,899,250	949,625
Benign neoplasms of the cerebral meninges	4	4	4	100.00	1,742,566	435,642
Intracranial hemorrhage following injury without mention	8	7	3	42.86	1,262,155	420,718
Benign neoplasms of the brain	9	9	3	33.33	966,849	322,283
Extradural hemorrhage, following injury	4	4	1	25.00	788,303	788,303
Most expensive iatrogenic injuries this procedure and specialty						
Cranial nerve, injury to	1	1	1	100.00	700,000	700,000
Mononeuritis	2	2	0	0.00	0	0
Paralysis	2	2	0	0.00	0	0
Head or neck, blood vessel of, injury to	1	1	0	0.00	0	0
Convulsions	1	1	0	0.00	0	0

SPECIALTY GROUP—Neurosurgery	No. of Files	No. of Closed Files	No. of Paid Files	% Paid of Closed Files	Indemnity Paid ($)	Average Indemnity Per Paid File ($)
4) SPINAL FUSION, NOT OTHERWISE SPECIFIED	126	96	31	32.29	8,529,499	275,145
Most expensive misadventures this procedure and specialty						
Improper performance	68	48	16	33.33	3,720,068	232,504
Performed when not indicated or contraindicated	10	8	4	50.00	2,836,790	709,198
Patient positioning problem	1	1	1	100.00	974,141	974,141
Wrong patient or body part	10	7	7	100.00	873,500	124,786
Failure to recognize a complication of treatment	5	5	3	60.00	125,000	41,667
Most expensive conditions this procedure and specialty						
Closed fracture of cervical vertebra	23	18	7	38.89	2,379,900	339,986
Displacement of intervertebral disc	25	20	8	40.00	1,874,422	234,428
Quadriplegia	4	4	2	50.00	1,434,762	717,381
Dislocation of vertebra, coccyx, or sacrum	10	8	2	25.00	1,385,000	692,500
Spondylolisthesis, congenital	2	1	1	100.00	325,000	325,000
Most expensive iatrogenic injuries this procedure and specialty						
Spinal cord, injury to	2	2	1	50.00	150,000	150,000
Injury to nerves	1	1	1	100.00	47,500	47,500
Accidental puncture or laceration during a procedure	2	0	0	0.00	0	0
Cranial nerve, injury to	2	1	0	0.00	0	0
Intestine, accidental perforation or laceration of	1	1	0	0.00	0	0
5) DIAGNOSTIC INTERVIEW AND EVALUATION	177	149	36	24.16	6,876,935	191,026
Most expensive misadventures this procedure and specialty						
Errors in diagnosis	65	56	17	30.36	2,096,831	123,343
Delay in performance	14	9	4	44.44	1,462,500	365,625
Improper performance	19	16	5	31.25	1,212,604	242,521
No medical misadventure	44	38	1	2.63	900,000	900,000
Not performed	7	6	4	66.67	370,000	92,500
Most expensive conditions this procedure and specialty						
Extradural hemorrhage, following injury	1	1	1	100.00	1,100,000	1,100,000
Cerebrovascular accident	2	2	1	50.00	1,082,604	1,082,604
Intracerebral hemorrhage	1	1	1	100.00	1,000,000	1,000,000
Hemiplegia	1	1	1	100.00	900,000	900,000
Hydrocephalus, congenital	2	2	1	50.00	350,000	350,000
6) CONSULTATION	176	146	15	10.27	5,454,524	363,635
Most expensive misadventures this procedure and specialty						
Delay in performance	10	10	4	40.00	1,670,824	417,706
Not performed	10	8	3	37.50	1,309,950	436,650
Improper performance	31	21	1	4.76	950,000	950,000
Failure/delay in referral or consultation	2	1	1	100.00	480,000	480,000
Failure to supervise or monitor case	7	6	2	33.33	419,250	209,625
Most expensive conditions this procedure and specialty						
Herpes simplex	1	1	1	100.00	1,150,000	1,150,000
Intracranial abscess	4	4	2	50.00	1,094,250	547,125
Closed fracture of cervical vertebra	14	9	2	22.22	1,050,000	525,000
Spinal cord, injury to	2	2	1	50.00	480,000	480,000
Cerebral degeneration	1	1	1	100.00	375,000	375,000
7) CONTRAST MYELOGRAM	53	44	12	27.27	3,319,773	276,648
Most expensive misadventures this procedure and specialty						
Improper performance	15	12	4	33.33	1,156,500	289,125
Medication errors	2	2	2	100.00	1,020,000	510,000
Performed when not indicated or contraindicated	4	3	1	33.33	642,769	642,769
No medical misadventure	18	16	2	12.50	281,338	140,669
Delay in performance	1	1	1	100.00	175,000	175,000
Most expensive conditions this procedure and specialty						
Disease of the spinal cord	2	2	2	100.00	1,900,000	950,000
Neoplasm of the other endrocrine gland, unknown if malignant	1	1	1	100.00	642,769	642,769

SPECIALTY GROUP—Neurosurgery	No. of Files	No. of Closed Files	No. of Paid Files	% Paid of Closed Files	Indemnity Paid	Average Indemnity Per Paid File
Spinal cord, injury to	1	1	1	100.00	275,000	275,000
Acquired deformities of ankle and foot	2	2	1	50.00	175,000	175,000
Lumbago	5	4	2	50.00	152,500	76,250
Most expensive iatrogenic injuries this procedure and specialty						
Nerve root, injury to	1	1	0	0.00	0	0
8) REPLACEMENT OF VENTRICULAR SHUNT	13	13	5	38.46	2,599,274	519,855
Most expensive misadventures this procedure and specialty						
Delay in performance	3	3	2	66.67	1,544,336	772,168
Improper performance	5	5	2	40.00	754,938	377,469
Not performed	1	1	1	100.00	300,000	300,000
No medical misadventure	3	3	0	0.00	0	0
Failure to recognize a complication of treatment	1	1	0	0.00	0	0
Most expensive conditions this procedure and specialty						
Cerebral degeneration	3	3	1	33.33	1,000,000	1,000,000
Hydrocephalus, congenital	5	5	2	40.00	844,336	422,168
Epilepsy	2	2	2	100.00	754,938	377,469
Aphasia	1	1	0	0.00	0	0
Subdural or cerebral hemorrhage as a result of delivery	1	1	0	0.00	0	0
9) EXCISION OR DESTRUCTION OF LESION OR TISSUE OF BRAIN	37	30	9	30.00	2,325,551	258,395
Most expensive misadventures this procedure and specialty						
Errors in diagnosis	2	2	1	50.00	1,097,250	1,097,250
Failure to supervise or monitor case	4	4	2	50.00	720,801	360,401
Delay in performance	1	1	1	100.00	250,000	250,000
Wrong patient or body part	2	2	1	50.00	105,000	105,000
Improper performance	11	9	2	22.22	80,000	40,000
Most expensive conditions this procedure and specialty						
Demyelinating disease of central nervous system	2	2	1	50.00	1,097,250	1,097,250
Malignant neoplasms of the cerebral meninges	2	2	2	100.00	750,801	375,401
Malignant neoplasms of the brain	8	7	2	28.57	355,000	177,500
Benign neoplasms of the brain	8	8	3	37.50	117,500	39,167
Cerebellar or brain stem laceration	1	1	1	100.00	5,000	5,000
Most expensive iatrogenic injuries this procedure and specialty						
Optic nerve, injury to	2	1	1	100.00	105,000	105,000
Disorder of the pituitary gland and its hypothalamic connections	1	0	0	0.00	0	0
10) NEUROLOGIC EXAMINATION	93	86	14	16.28	2,185,332	156,095
Most expensive misadventures this procedure and specialty						
Failure to supervise or monitor case	15	14	8	57.14	1,239,333	154,917
Delay in performance	4	4	1	25.00	800,000	800,000
Errors in diagnosis	23	20	3	15.00	88,499	29,500
No medical misadventure	38	35	2	5.71	57,500	28,750
Improper performance	5	5	0	0.00	0	0
Most expensive conditions this procedure and specialty						
Benign neoplasms of the cerebral meninges	1	1	1	100.00	800,000	800,000
Epilepsy	3	3	1	33.33	683,333	683,333
Nonpsychotic mental disorder following organic brain damage	1	1	1	100.00	350,000	350,000
Paralysis	1	1	1	100.00	75,000	75,000
Subdural hemorrhage, following injury	5	5	1	20.00	74,999	74,999
Most expensive iatrogenic injuries this procedure and specialty						
Lower extremity, blood vessel of, injury to	1	1	0	0.00	0	0
TOTALS	1712	1476	422	28.59	89,253,679	211,502

There are clearly some factors, in addition to an excessively litigious society, that influence claims frequency. All medical liability insurers are aware that a few particular physicians are named in a disproportionate number of suits when compared to their colleagues. An analysis of these physicians' cases usually points to one or more factors contributing to the "outlier" status.

Rapport

Patients seldom sue physicians whom they like personally. Genuine human warmth in the physician-patient relationship is probably the most effective lawsuit deterrent. But a trust once breached, either in fact or in perception, is likely to cause much greater anger than in the case of a less trusting relationship. Failure to communicate and to be available for family discussions is a common source of conflict, especially after some real or perceived complication. An excessively busy practice is sometimes a factor, but a physician's personality and interpersonal communication skills are often the chief problem. There is the occasional physician whose personality renders him or her virtually uninsurable.

Negligence

The word "negligence" has acquired a more pejorative connotation than it deserves. Everyone is negligent in some manner and to some degree every day. Most negligent acts cause no injury and little attention is paid to them. When negligence does cause significant injury to others, the law usually assigns liability to the party causing that injury. The physician-patient relationship imposes a higher duty of care than between strangers, and the expectation of the patient is accordingly higher. Some physicians are more careful in their medical practices than others (perhaps they also drop things on their own feet less often), but those who are chronically less thoughtful or less attentive inevitably will cause more accidents. There is simply no way to defend operating on the wrong extremity, the wrong side of the spine or head, injecting the wrong substance (assuming proper labeling), and the like, and the significantly less careful physician invites more incidents and claims than his or her group-rated premiums can sustain.

Skills

Some physicians are marginal in certain skills (we all know of examples) and consequently experience more complications than the majority of their colleagues performing the same procedures. Unless these physicians have extraordinary rapport, they are also likely to incur more lawsuits.

Atypical Practices

When a practice contains an unusually high percentage of some procedure that is rarely performed by colleagues, this may be associated with an increased claims incidence (of course, it may also reflect a large referral pattern due to special expertise). A highly publicized lawsuit regarding such a disproportionately executed procedure may induce other dissatisfied patients to file their own suits.

These and other factors are not beyond individual control. Practice volumes and patterns can be altered. Personal communication skills can be improved and careful habits can be cultivated. Physicians who continually attract a disproportionate number of suits, even though they may be defensible, invite being dropped by their insurers, being required to self-insure to some level (perhaps the first $200,000 of claims per year), or perhaps being required to drop certain aspects of practice in return for continuing coverage.

There are a number of steps physicians can take to reduce the likelihood of a suit being filed and to increase the likelihood of a successful defense once a suit has been filed.

1. Informed consent usually connotes signing some form, but it really goes to the matter of communication. There is no foolproof consent form, whether it is a simple, all-inclusive statement or a multiple-page compendium of all conceivable complications. A written document usually does constitute evidence of consent that the plaintiff must then rebut. In addition, written evidence of the discussion of risks and benefits contained in office records or hospital progress notes is very important since a jury will credit such written evidence much higher than the physician's self-serving statement that he

or she remembers having said something long ago. Some states consider informed consent to be a question of the standard of practice. In those states, expert medical opinion is required to establish whether the information given met the medical standard of practice. A larger number of states take the view that informed consent is measured by what the hypothetically reasonable patient in the same circumstance would consider important in giving consent. In those states, the adequacy of consent is always a question for the jury to decide, regardless of the local practice standard. Full communication is the essence of real informed consent, but documentation (the more the better) will be necessary when the issue is in dispute.

2. Never alter medical records by erasure or re-entry. All corrections should be timely and legible and should be dated.

3. Notify your insurer early of potential claims. This allows interviews with witnesses who may be unavailable later and allows for preservation of evidence that might otherwise be lost or destroyed.

4. Do not communicate directly with the plaintiff attorney about a case in which you may be a defendant. All communications with the plaintiff attorney, under these circumstances, should be through your insurer or attorney. (An attorney defendant in a legal malpractice case should do the same thing.)

5. Attend all depositions of opposing experts. This generally causes deponents to be more circumspect. This also helps your attorney to challenge statements that are beyond his or her own expertise and knowledge, since most attorneys are not experts in the technical subject matter of a medical deposition.

6. Answer only what is asked. Do not volunteer additional information under cross examination in discovery depositions or at trial.

7. Do not become angry. Remain courteous and professional. A jury is evaluating your demeanor, at least as much as what you may say.

Many other do's and don'ts should be discussed early with your attorney and insurer. Independent defense counsel usually is not necessary but can be important when:

1. There are potential damages in excess of your insurance coverage.
2. Punitive damages are part of the case and not covered by insurance.
3. You have no confidence in the defense attorney assigned, and the insurer declines to assign an attorney acceptable to you.
4. Your insurer insists on a single attorney for you and a defendant with whom you have some conflict of interest.

A proposal contained in the American Law Institute (ALI) Reporters Study[2] called "Enterprise Liability" would transfer medical liability from individual physicians to prepaid insurers, hospitals, and other large institutions. This study, which contained many other proposals, was not adopted by the ALI, but the enterprise liability concept has shown up among recent suggestions for national health care reform. If generally adopted, it could provide relief from medical malpractice lawsuit threats against individual physicians but would likely be accompanied by a further loss of income and autonomy as the liable entity exerted greater control over physicians and their practices in its own attempt to minimize legal exposure. One might also wonder whether the Enterprise Liability model could transfer fiduciary duty from the physician-patient relationship to the enterprise-patient relationship. Fiduciary duty has been the chief reason many states have not permitted the corporate practice of medicine (professional service corporations of physicians excepted).

Antitrust

The antitrust laws forbid any two or more persons or other legal entities from combining in a manner that is anticompetitive. The Sherman Antitrust Act of 1890 was passed to counter the growing economic power of monopolies which, by their size, were able to fix prices, control markets, and destroy would-be competitors. This was followed in 1914 by the Clayton Act, which established the Federal Trade Commission (FTC), and in 1936 by the Robinson Patman Act. The Celler Kefauver Act of 1950 addressed the subject of acquisitions and mergers with greater specificity, and in 1974 the authority of the FTC was expanded by provisions of the Magnuson Moss Act.

Sections 1 and 2 of the Sherman Law (15 USC) forbid combinations that have an anticompetitive effect on trade in and among the states. Invoking the commerce clause of the U.S. Constitution permitted application of the federal antitrust laws to intrastate activities throughout the country. (It is not difficult to find some effect on interstate commerce, however tenuous, of almost any commercial activity within any state.) In addition, states have added their own layers of antitrust laws. Antitrust law has become a large legal specialty with its own subspecialists. Most major business decisions must now pass antitrust scrutiny lest they run afoul of expensive legal challenges and the threat of treble damages.

Federal enforcement of the antitrust laws may be under civil or criminal statutes and is assigned to the FTC or the antitrust division of the justice department. Private civil enforcement may be brought by companies or individuals who believe they have been or are likely to be injured by some act or contemplated act in violation of the laws. The provision for trebling of actual damages makes the threat of antitrust prosecution particularly intimidating. State antitrust laws further complicate the analysis of what may be acceptable or proscribed business activity.

Antitrust questions are analyzed by the courts as per se violations or as rule of reason violations. Per se violations, such as price fixing, are usually prosecuted under criminal statutes and are illegal without regard to any possible business reasons. The rule of reason test, which is applied to non per se violations, determines whether, on balance, the activity promotes or discourages competition. Retail competitors are considered to be in a horizontal relationship. Manufacturers, and retailers whom they supply, are considered to be in a vertical relationship for antitrust purposes.

Exceptions to the antitrust laws have been carved out for certain groups and businesses, including labor unions,[23] insurance companies,[22] agricultural cooperatives,[1] certain joint publishing ventures,[17] professional baseball teams,[35] and certain activities regulated by government agencies

such as the Interstate Commerce Commission, the Federal Communications Commission, and others. For the better part of a century, the practice of medicine and the other so-called "learned professions" were generally considered to be excluded from the reach of the antitrust laws, but this changed in 1975 with the decision in *Goldfarb v Virginia Bar.*[19] Within the State of Virginia, property title searches were required by law to be performed by or under the supervision of an attorney. The Virginia Bar (and the Fairfax County Bar) had established a minimum fee for this service and charging below this minimum was cause for disciplinary action against the offending attorney. The plaintiff, Goldfarb, had been unable to find a Virginia attorney willing to do this rather routine task for less than the statewide minimum fee. He brought suit alleging violation of Article 15 USC Section 7. Goldfarb lost at the trial court level and in the Fourth Circuit Court of Appeals, which held that the Virginia State Bar was exempt under the state action doctrine and that the county bar and the attorney were exempt under the learned professions exception. Appeal was taken to the U.S. Supreme Court, which reversed the Fourth Circuit decision and held that both the state and county bar associations were in violation of the antitrust laws. It held that the state action exception did not apply because no state law existed requiring attorneys to set a minimum fee. It further stated explicitly that *there is no antitrust exception for the learned professions.*

With the professions now clearly within the ambit of the antitrust laws and with minimum fee schedules illegal, what about *maximum* fee schedules? The answer came in 1982 in *Arizona v Maricopa County Medical Society.*[3] About 70% of Maricopa (Arizona) County physicians had agreed on a schedule of maximum fees for various medical procedures within the county. This arrangement was part of a foundation organized to negotiate with local insurance plans and to preserve and encourage the private fee-for-service practice of medicine. The foundation also established peer review procedures to assure medical necessity and the appropriateness of treatment plans. This was challenged by the State of Arizona on the theory that even maximum fee schedules were in violation of antitrust laws as they encouraged everyone to charge at the published maximum rate, and that periodic upward revisions assured increasing fees. The foundation physicians maintained that the fee schedule assisted insurers with actuarial calculations of premiums and that it effectively restrained inflation in medical fees. The U.S. Supreme Court held that the arrangement was a per se violation of the antitrust laws and was therefore illegal regardless of any possible benefits.

Attempts by physicians to bargain with large insuring organizations such as HMOs, PPOs, and other "managed-care" plans have run into numerous antitrust problems and have left physicians feeling powerless to protect their economic interests and their practice autonomy. In 1986–1987, a group of dentists in Tucson, Arizona, objected to a local prepaid insurance plan's remuneration for crowns and root canal procedures at about 30% of the usual and customary rate, a remuneration rate that had not been changed for 10 years. When the insurer refused an increased remuneration to cover increased costs, about 50 dentists met and sent identical letters to the insurer demanding increased reimbursement. The justice department's antitrust division brought a criminal indictment against the dentists for conspiring to fix prices and a jury subsequently convicted the dentists. The verdict was modified on appeal, but the appellate court confirmed that any concerted effort by professionals to set fees and any concerted threat by those professionals to withhold services from an insurer was a per se violation of the antitrust laws.[33]

At what point medical joint ventures can escape antitrust violation and yet offer some protection to physicians' interests is a close call. When physicians, who would otherwise be competitors and who, in the aggregate, do not exceed 20% of the market control, join in sharing the costs and the risks of adverse financial results, they *may* be able to avoid the charge of price fixing. These combinations can take the form of independent practice associations, PPOs, or even HMOs. All such physician plans should be advised by an experienced antitrust attorney if the regulatory minefield is to be successfully negotiated.

Physicians' antitrust problems also arise in the peer review process. The leading decision was the U.S. Supreme Court case of *Patrick v Burgett* (1988)[29] in which anticompetitive behavior was alleged in the context of peer review. Dr. Patrick

was employed as a surgeon by the Astoria Clinic of Astoria, Oregon. At the end of his employment year, he was offered a partnership in the clinic. He declined the offer and instead went into private practice in competition with the clinic in regard to general surgery patients. The clinic doctors then ceased to refer patients to him and eventually moved to restrict his hospital practice based on quality-of-care concerns. Dr. Patrick sued the reviewing physicians, alleging anticompetitive behavior. Patrick prevailed at the trial level, winning damages of $650,000 which were then trebled to $1,950,000. The Ninth Circuit Court of Appeals reversed the decision based on the state action doctrine, which holds that if the peer review is supervised and required by the state, there is no personal liability on the part of the reviewers. The U.S. Supreme Court accepted the case on certiorari. There were many amicus briefs, including those by the Oregon Medical Association and the AMA, asserting that effective peer review required protection from the threat of personal antitrust prosecution. The Supreme Court reversed the Ninth Circuit decision and reinstated the damages. It further defined the extent of the state action exception as requiring active state supervision of the peer review process, with the authority to make the final decision residing in the state.

More recently, Home Oxygen and Medical Equipment Company of San Leandro, California, and the Home Care Oxygen and Medical Equipment Company of Concord, California, entered into joint ventures with local pulmonologists to supply oxygen and oxygen delivery equipment to patients requiring outpatient oxygen therapy. The arrangement was challenged by the FTC, which claimed that the vendors controlled too much of the market for these services. A settlement agreement required the companies to include no more than 25% of the pulmonologists in the local area. Attorneys for the companies and physicians agreed to the settlement because "they were not in a financial position to fight the FTC."[12]

Antitrust issues are also present in the hospital accreditation process. Holders of certificates of special competence have tried to exclude nonholders from caring for patients in intensive care units. Radiologists may try to prevent neurosurgeons from performing endovascular procedures in the hospital x-ray facilities. Currently, lawsuits have been filed involving emergency medicine certification and exclusion from emergency room practice. Antitrust and accreditation concerns have become factors in the ongoing debate about recertification and subspecialty certification. Antitrust issues are often raised in disputes over surgical overlap areas, such as that between general vascular surgeons and neurosurgeons performing carotid artery procedures. Conflicts have been present for years between plastic and reconstructive surgeons and oral surgeons in regard to procedures involving the jaw, and with otolaryngologists in regard to facial cosmetic procedures.

The antitrust laws have been in continuous transition even as their reach has continually expanded. The best that a nonexpert can do is recognize where there may be problems and know enough to seek expert (and usually expensive) legal advice. Failure to anticipate potential antitrust problems can be even more expensive.

The Attorney's Perspective

Legal training emphasizes identifying legal issues and applying the appropriate law to the particular facts. Unlike a medical student's anatomy examination, which might require the student to describe the origins, course, and terminations of the vagus nerve, the law student's conclusions on the merits are not considered either right or wrong. The law student's application of the law to the facts must be reasonable, of course, but finding all or most of the legal issues embedded in a question is the essence of the test. For someone with a physical science background, the study of law is not just a new discipline but a completely different analytic approach. Fundamental differences between the practices of law and medicine probably contribute somewhat to the distrust that exists between the two professions; another minor factor may be a specialty language barrier. Perhaps the most significant difference, however, surrounds the concept of legal advocacy. An attorney is employed to represent his or her client's interests. This often entails giving advice on how to avoid legal problems; but at other times, when legal conflicts are unavoidable, it requires the attorney to represent his or her client as vigorously as possible. The

attorney must then take the facts as they are, or as they can best be interpreted, to support the client. (A physician expects no less of his own attorney.) He or she must play the hand that has been dealt and do so with every argument that favors the client. There is an unclear margin between zealous advocacy (as required by the canons of legal ethics and disciplinary rules) and misrepresentation either by emphasis or interpretation. Reasonable people may well differ as to whether that line has been crossed. The adversarial relationship is a consequence of, as well as an inherent part of, attorney advocacy. The tone of the entire dispute resolution process is set by the nature of the ultimate determinant: the adversarial trial process. Early proposals for settlement are measured by what would be the likely outcome if the dispute were to be taken all the way to trial. This means that even the earliest discussions and negotiations are imbued with an adversarial quality rather than a cooperative working together to identify and solve a possible problem. This adversarial relationship is further enhanced when the plaintiff attorney has taken a personal monetary interest in the size of the damages (the contingency fee rather than an hourly rate). Physicians, and particularly high-premium specialists such as neurosurgeons, often feel antagonistic toward medical malpractice lawyers and the manner in which they typically function. While this antagonism frequently becomes personalized, the conflict is driven by the requirements of the legal system to a considerable extent. If an attorney does not use the existing system effectively and to the best advantage, the attorney risks a legal malpractice claim against himself or herself. Astonishing as it may seem, many appellate courts hold that the plaintiff attorney does not owe any duty of reasonable care to the defendant party being sued.[7,16,31,36]

It may be useful to trace a medical malpractice suit from the plaintiff attorney's perspective. A typical claim will include, but is not limited to, the following activities and considerations.

Initial Interview

When a potential client is first interviewed, the attorney must listen to the recitation with some skepticism and obtain as much objective detail as possible regarding names, dates, personalities, and possible witnesses. Clients often are distraught and angry. It is necessary to make some estimate of the nature, extent, and monetary value of any damages. If damages are not substantial, there is no point in the attorney proceeding (at least on a contingency-fee basis) even though there may appear to be negligence. The busier and more successful the attorney, the higher this threshold of "substantial damages" is likely to be. The statute of limitations must be determined early because, if it is about to expire, the attorney must either decline the case, file suit immediately to preserve the patient's legal rights, or conceivably obtain a waiver of the statute by the defendant or defendants in return for not filing immediately. An attorney who misses a statute of limitations with an otherwise valid claim is vulnerable to a legal malpractice claim. While attorney malpractice premiums are a small fraction of what surgical specialists pay, they are increasing, and attorneys practice defensive law just as physicians practice defensive medicine. This same consideration extends to include all of the possible defendants in a suit since, if not all of the appropriate defendants are included, this may invite a successful "empty chair" defense by the defendant and a subsequent legal malpractice claim against the plaintiff attorney.

The potential client's veracity and credibility must be evaluated since the client will most likely be an important witness on his or her own behalf. A poor witness will reduce the value of the case along with the attorney's chance of winning a contingency fee. The jurisdiction and venue of the case must be considered and may influence the likelihood of success as well as legal and logistic difficulties of prosecuting the case. There may be a choice of venue which could influence the outcome of the case. If there are arbitration agreements that have been signed, a different approach will be required, although ultimately there may be recourse to the courts. If the attorney decides, on the basis of the initial interview, to take the case, he or she needs to discuss the fee agreement with the client (informed consent), and the client will be asked to sign a formal fee agreement. Almost all personal injury attorneys work only with a contingency-fee arrangement in which the at-

torney receives an agreed-upon portion of any settlement or judgment. This typically will range between 30% and 50%, with expenses subtracted from the client's portion of the award.

Collection of Documents

Hospital records often contain many of the pertinent records of a target physician. Client release for these records must be obtained, and sometimes the client will be asked to obtain these records directly so that the defendant will not be alerted early to the malpractice attorney's interest. Request for the target physician's records may be deferred for the same reason. Records must also be obtained from any other treating physicians. The client's prior tax records and other proof of earning potential are needed as they can be a measure of damages resulting from the client's inability to work. Eventually, the target physician's office records will need to be obtained, and all of the records (sometimes voluminous) must be organized in a logical sequence for analysis.

Analysis

Once all available records are assembled, the attorney must obtain expert medical evaluation. Most attorneys doing a substantial amount of medical malpractice litigation have relationships with physicians whose judgment they trust. Initial medical analysis may take the form of off-the-record consultations used only to determine the strengths and weaknesses of a claim and with no intent of using this expert as a witness. Some larger offices have physicians or registered nurses on retainer or even on salary for initial medical evaluations. At other times, a physician will be asked to review case material with the intent of testifying if in agreement with the attorney's theory of the case. There are "experts" for hire who will say whatever they are paid to say, but the better attorneys try to avoid these professional witnesses because they are often weak, inconsistent, and easily discredited by the defense. The preferred witness is a genuine expert with the stature and verbal skills to make a favorable impression on the jury. "Would I go to this doctor if I were ill?" is a good test, and one that will likely predict the impressions of jurors. Finding a good expert witness is often a frustrating and time-consuming job for the plaintiff attorney. The theory of the case may need to be revised to correspond to the opinion of the expert witness. An accounting of special damages must be made, and then a determination of general damages (pain and suffering) must be estimated. General (non-economic) damage estimates will vary with the nature of the injury and the historic tendency of juries in the particular venue of the trial. If the jurisdiction permits punitive damages, a decision must be made to determine whether the facts or inferences support a claim for punitive damages. If so, punitive damage demands can place significant additional pressure on a defendant physician to accept a settlement favorable to the plaintiff.

If, at this point, suit has not already been filed, a decision must be made whether to drop the case or to proceed. This is ultimately the client's decision but will probably be strongly influenced by the attorney's recommendations. The attorney may withdraw if the facts learned at this point do not support the initial claims of the client. Also at this point, the attorney probably has expended a substantial number of uncompensated hours and likely has advanced cash to collect data and expert evaluations. From here on, however, monetary advances are likely to become much larger due to the need for expert witnesses, travel expenses, etc., and the attorney's personal time involvement also will become much greater. If the decision is to continue, an affidavit of merit is advisable in many jurisdictions to protect the attorney and his client against a Rule 11 challenge by the defendant. In some areas, lawsuits must be preceded by a notice of intent to sue, and failure to make such timely notice can either delay the suit or leave the attorney exposed to damage claims against himself or herself.

Discovery

Interrogatories must be prepared and sent to the defendants, and return interrogatories from the defendant will be received and must be answered. At this point, the defendant can be expected to have conferred with his or her own attorney and experts, and will have his or her own evaluation and theory of the case. If the defendant wishes to settle, negotiation conferences with the defendant's representatives will be held to explore settlement possibilities. Most suits are either dropped or settled by negotiation by the time both sides have completed their evaluations and early discovery. If not, the process continues; at some point, both sides must inform each other of the identities of their respective expert witnesses. These experts will then be scheduled for oral deposition. The plaintiff attorney will need to schedule and take depositions of all of the defendant's fact and expert witnesses, and must prepare the plaintiff for deposition by the defense attorney(s). The extent of this preparation may vary considerably depending upon the plaintiff's sophistication, intelligence, and verbal skills. By the end of discovery, each side has gained a considerable knowledge about the strengths and weaknesses of each other's case. If there is a general agreement on liability and damages likely to be returned by a jury, the case will probably be settled. Included in settlement calculations by both sides must be the unpredictability of juries. Offers of settlement must be discussed with the plaintiff, and there may be several counter offers. If the parties are still far apart in their expectations, preparations for trial proceed. Most attorneys prefer settlement, but a plaintiff attorney does need at some time to prove that he or she is effective at trial before insurance companies develop sufficient respect for him or her. A defendant insurance company's evaluation of the plaintiff attorney's abilities and history of successes at trial is a factor in its evaluation of loss potential. The plaintiff attorney must also evaluate the jury appeal of the plaintiff and the defendant as witnesses. Some information about this will have been learned from the deponents' performances during discovery depositions.

Trial Planning

Trial preparation involves preparation of a trial notebook containing all pertinent information, supporting legal authority, motions, arguments against anticipated motions by the defendant, and supporting documents. Every aspect of the trial detail needs to be anticipated and organized for fast retrieval. Some attorneys do go to trial with less preparation and are pretty good at "winging it," but most agree that careful preparation, although time-consuming, does pay off. Subpoenas must be sent to all witnesses, and calendar scheduling and timing logistics must be worked out. Backup witnesses may be needed if critical primary witnesses become unavailable due to some emergency. The plaintiff and other plaintiff witnesses will need to be prepared for direct and cross-examination. This may mean hours of simulated trial questions with videotape recording and coaching to present the best possible impression for the jury. Some judges will require pretrial conferences to resolve procedural questions and simplify the issues.

Trial

A trial is a major effort for the attorney. Not everything will go as planned, and there are likely to be frequent decisions and modifications of plans that must be made in the course of trial developments. Trials are stressful and intensely competitive, yet many trial attorneys approach them with the same enthusiasm that most neurosurgeons bring to a difficult and challenging surgical operation. The trial begins with jury selection, which may be short or time-consuming depending on the local practice and the judge's preference.

Opening statements by the plaintiff and defense are designed to give the jury an overview of how each side views the dispute and what facts will be presented by each side in the course of the trial. The plaintiff then proceeds with direct examination of witnesses. The defendant then may cross-examine each of the plaintiff witnesses. Following this, the defense presents its witnesses, and the plaintiff attorney may cross-examine them. After both plaintiff and defendant have rested their cases, they present closing arguments to the jury. Jury instructions, drafted or selected by the plaintiff and defendant attorneys, will have been given to the judge, who then chooses the instructions that he or she will use. These instructions are given by the judge to the jury, and the jury retires to consider the case. A typical medical malpractice trial lasts a few days to a few weeks. The plaintiff attorney usually has invested many hours and often many thousands of dollars in cash advances. If unsuccessful at trial, a decision must be made about an appeal. If there were trial errors

and the right to appeal has been preserved through timely objections (judicial rulings, jury instruction choices, etc.), the likelihood of success on appeal must be evaluated with further legal research. The time required for this must be balanced against the additional costs, the likelihood of prevailing on appeal, and the importance of the issue to future cases. If there is a defense verdict (about 60% to 70% of medical malpractice trials result in defense verdicts) and no viable basis for appeal, the plaintiff attorney swallows his or her loss of cash and time and goes on to other cases. If the plaintiff wins at trial and the damages are large, the plaintiff attorney can celebrate another "big hit," as it is known in the vernacular of the plaintiff bar. Successful plaintiff attorneys are the highest earning lawyers in the country.[15]

While the current legal system does require plaintiff attorneys to do their jobs in ways physicians often find objectionable, it must also be said that most trial attorneys vehemently resist reforms that would substantially change their role or their income potential, or require them to change procedures with which they have become comfortable. They will not willingly be relegated to a less dominant position in the legal process. The legislative contests to change the method of resolving medical liability claims show no signs of abating. But, putting aside the confrontational relationship between plaintiff trial attorneys and the medical profession, it is worth noting that there is generally a good working relationship between physicians and the rest of the bar. There are now more than 20 neurosurgeons in the United States who have earned law degrees. There is an ever-expanding need for legal advice and representation in business relationships and in dealing with federal and local governments. We live in an increasingly complex age, and physicians and attorneys need each other's expertise on a fairly regular basis. Law school is an absorbing challenge and an excellent business education. I enthusiastically recommend it to any colleagues who have the opportunity and interest.

Conclusions

In this chapter, we reviewed some of the legal background affecting the interface of neurosurgeons with the legal system. These are as much a fundamental force in neurosurgical practice as scientific, technical, and clinical factors. Many neurosurgeons face legal confrontations as part of their routine practice within the clinical community. The philosophic trends shaping this legal milieu are an integral force in the philosophy of neurosurgery and deserve continuing analysis, study, and, at times, active involvement by the thinkers and leaders of the field, and by each and every neurosurgeon.

References

1. Agricultural Cooperatives, Clayton Act §6, 15 USC §17, 29 USC §101.
2. American Law Institute (ALI) Enterprise Liability for Personal Injury. *ALI Reporters Study*. Philadelphia, Pa: American Law Institute; 1991.
3. *Arizona v Maricopa County Medical Society*, 457 US 332 (1982).
4. *Baird v Larson*, 49 Wash App 715, 801 P2nd 247 (1990).
5. Black HC. *Black's Law Dictionary*. Rev 4th ed. St Paul, Minn: West Publishing; 1968.
6. *Browning-Ferris Industries v Kelco*, 109 SCt 2909, 292 US 257, 106 LEd2nd 219 (1989).
7. *Carroll v Kolor*, 112 Ariz 595, 545 P2nd 411 (1976).
8. *Cobbs v Grant*, 502 P2nd 1, 104 Cal Rptr 505 (1972).
9. *Corcoran v United Health Care, Inc.*, 965 F2nd 1321 (5th Cir), *cert denied*, 113 SCt 812 (1992).
10. *Dartmouth v Woodward*, US 4 Wheat 518, 4 LEd 629 (1819).
11. *Daubert v Merrill-Dow Pharmaceuticals, Inc.*, 113 SCt 2786, 125 LEd2nd 469 (1993).
12. Davidson J. Antitrust laws used by U.S. against doctors. *Wall Street Journal*. November 4, 1993:B6.
13. Ellis, 56 S Cal L Rev, Ed 2.
14. Expert witness: booming business for the specialists. *New York Times*. July 5, 1987:1, 13.
15. Fanning D. The best paid lawyers in America. *Forbes Magazine*. October 16, 1989:212-219.
16. *Feldhusen v Oudenhoven & Travelers Insurance Co*, Circuit Court Brown County Wisc No 64-233, July 20, 1977, 20 ATLA Law Rptr 387.
17. *Flood v Kuku*, 407 US 258, 92 SCt 2099, 32 LEd2nd 728 (1972).
18. *Frye v United States*, 292 F 1013 (DC Cir 1923).
19. *Goldfarb v Virginia Bar*, 431 US 773, 44 LEd2nd 572, 95 SCt 2004 (1975).
20. Grimes D. *Paying the Piper: Third Party Payer Liability for Medical Treatment Decisions*. 25 Ga L Rev 861 907-11 (1991).
21. *Hickle v Money*, 95 Eng Rep 768.
22. Insurance Organizations, 15 USC §1012.
23. Labor Unions, Clayton Act §6, 15 USC §17, 7 USC §291-292.
24. *Lockert v Goodill*, 430 P2nd, 589 71 NW2nd 654 (1967).
25. Macauley RC Jr. *Health Care Cost Containment and Medical Malpractice: On a Collision Course*. 21 Suffolk U L Rev 91 (1986).
26. *Moore v Regents of the University of California*, 793 P2nd 479 (Cal 1990).
27. Morreim EH. *Cost Containment and The Standard of Medical Care*. 75 Cal L Rev 1719,1749-50 (1987).
28. *Pacific Mutual Life Insurance Co. v Haslip*, 493 US 1014, 107 LEd2nd 731, 110 SCt 710 (1990).
29. *Patrick v Burgett*, 486 US 94, 100 LEd2nd 83, 108 SCt 1658 (1988).
30. *Pennoyer v Neff*, 95 US 714, 24 LEd 565 (1878).
31. *Pentone v Dema's*, Ill Cir Ct, Cook County Docket #76 L12425, December 3, 1976. Reported in Citation 128, March 15, 1977.
32. Peterson MA, Sarma S, Shanley MG. *Punitive Damages: Empirical Findings*. Santa Monica, Cal: Rand Corporation, Institute for Civil Justice; 1987:33-33-11-lCJ.
33. *PLT v United States*, 974 F2nd 1206 (9th Cir 1992).
34. Pollock EJ. HMO held liable for refusing coverage.*Wall Street Journal*. Western ed. December 28, 1993:B4.
35. *Professional Baseball Teams, Federal Baseball Club v National League of Professional Baseball Clubs*, 259 US 200, 42 SCt 465, 66 LEd 898 (1922).
36. *Spencer v Burglass*, 288 So2nd 68 (La App 1974).
37. *Texaco v Penzoil*, 729 SW2nd 768 (Tex App, Houston [lst Dist] 1987), *cert denied*, 108 SCt 1305, 485 US 994, 99 LEd2nd 686 (1988).
38. *TXO Production Corp. v Alliance Resources Corp.*, 113 SCt 2711 (1993).
39. U.S. Constitution, Article 111, §2.
40. *Wickline v California*, 183 Cal App 1175, 228 Cal Rptr, 661 (1986).
41. *Wiles v Wood*, 98 Eng Rep 489 498-499 (1793).
42. *Wilson v Blue Cross of Southern California*, 271 Cal Rptr 876 (Cal App 2nd 1990), 222 CalApp3rd 663.
43. York KH, Broman JA. *Remedies, Cases, and Materials*. 2nd ed. St. Paul, Minn: West Publishing; 1973:43.

CHAPTER 16

The Neurosurgeon and Health Care Policy

Clark Watts, MD, JD, and Charles Plante, PhD

To discuss any relationship between neurosurgeons and *health care policy*, it is necessary to focus on what is health care policy, in this form a most amorphous phrase. To begin to understand the subject, it is important to point out that the subject is one of policy related to health care. *Webster's Ninth New Collegiate Dictionary* (1990) defines "policy" in a number of ways. Considering the tenor of the present debate on health care reform and the general concerns of people regarding the increased involvement of the government in an industry comprising approximately one-seventh of the gross domestic product of the United States, one definition of the word "policy" has a fatalistically humorous appeal: "A daily lottery in which participants bet that certain numbers will be drawn from a lottery wheel." However, this is not a useful definition from which can be developed a serious discussion of the involvement of neurosurgeons in the formulation and implementation of health care policy in the United States. Another definition can be had by combining two seemingly separate definitions provided by this dictionary into one: 1) "A definite course or method of action selected from among alternatives and in light of given conditions to guide and determine present and future decisions"; and 2) "a high level overall plan embracing the general goals and acceptable procedures, especially of a governmental body." In this chapter, affecting health care policy will involve both influencing the creation of policy by governmental bodies, to include the actions and activities flowing therefrom, and the execution of activities that have significant health care impact on the population.

Governmental bodies include judicial, legislative, and executive branches of government as well as agencies of these branches.

To describe and explain how neurosurgeons have interacted with other societal groups over health care policy, it is not necessary to be historically all-inclusive or nondiscriminative regarding issues. Major examples of health care policy issues in which neurosurgeons have invested significant time, energy, and capital include provider manpower, medical liability tort reform, reimbursement, research legislation, injury prevention, brain death and organ donation, medical and postgraduate medical education, indigent care, drug legislation, and military medicine. In affecting health care policy, neurosurgeons have testified before congressional committees regarding pending legislation, filed friend-of-the-court briefs in important litigation, worked with executive agencies such as the Food and Drug Administration (FDA) developing and implementing rules and regulations, and provided leadership in medical organizations from local to national levels. It is not possible, in the space available, to chronicle each specific effort. Rather, this chapter will describe in a generic sense, with examples, how neurosurgeons have in the past influenced health care policy, and why in the present and future they should continue to attempt to do so.

When delving into the past to understand its history, we find that neurosurgery consistently begins with the efforts of its founder in this country, Harvey Cushing. Indeed, Harvey Cushing was very active in attempting to influence, as well as to implement, health care policy. Early in this century, most practical health care policy was articulated and implemented, not by the various levels of government, but by nongovernmental entities, including the American Medical Association (AMA) and the American College of Surgeons (ACS), who often were at odds. Parenthetically, from this vantage point, it is difficult to determine from the nature of the debates conducted in the early part of this century whether policies regarding the development of standards of health care delivery were articulated out of altruism or from some other more political reason.

In 1913, the ACS was established with the aim, among others, of improving the standard of practice by surgeons and providing the public a means for discriminatingly selecting a qualified surgeon. Harvey Cushing was "... staunchly in favor ..." of the establishment of the ACS, and spoke against the attempts by the AMA to suppress the developing college.[15] However, Cushing did continue to support certain policies of the AMA. Early in President Franklin Roosevelt's tenure, the AMA openly and vehemently opposed compulsory health insurance. Cushing, as a member of the President's Committee on Economic Security, upheld the view of the AMA and thus could "claim to have had a large part in the exclusion of health from the Social Security Act of 1935."[4]

Of course, the participation of Cushing in the formulation and implementation of health care policy by both the private and public sectors does not stop here. However, it is not necessary in this chapter to annotate his many contributions to neurosurgery and medicine. These range from the laboratory and his clinical practice to the realm of education and the development of residency education programs. The latter have had a great impact on the development of the health care system today, and include the rise of academic centers and their roles in the provision of health care to the indigent.[6,10]

Often it has been left to others to address, in the literature, efforts by neurosurgeons to affect health care policy. An exception is the work by Morley, *Current Controversies in Neurosurgery*.[8] Included in this timely book are discussions of issues that have significant importance today: the role of government in the production of neurosurgeons (i.e. manpower), animal experimentation, psychosurgery, tort reform.

A major event in the story of how neurosurgeons have been involved in affecting health care policy was the creation of the Washington Committee. The next section of this chapter will describe that event and its impact on the way the neurosurgical leadership has responded to health care policy issues. The final section will highlight present and emerging thought regarding the process of neurosurgical involvement in health care policy activity.

The Washington Committee

In 1975, the American Association of Neurological Surgeons (AANS) and the Congress of Neurological Surgeons (CNS) jointly made a decision to explore the suggestion of certain members and some state societies to open a socioeconomic office in Washington, D.C. There was a general feeling that a number of issues specific to the practice of neurological surgery were not being addressed by primary umbrella organizations, namely, the AMA and the ACS. In particular, there was widespread concern among neurosurgeons that issues of professional liability and antitrust were not receiving the needed attention by the national organizations. In addition, the leadership of the AANS and CNS felt a Washington presence would enhance their position with the AMA and the ACS.

A small committee was formed, with Drs. Louis Finney, Donald Steward, Russel Patterson, and Charles Fager as members, charged with the responsibility of exploring options available to the two organizations. The committee contacted a number of individuals and organizations concerning the specifics of opening a Washington office. One of the individuals contacted was Jay Constantine, a professional staff person on the Senate Finance Committee. He recommended that they interview a former member of Congress, Slick Rutherford, and Charles Plante, a former Senate administrative assistant.

An agreement was reached with Plante to provide a part-time presence in Washington for organized neurosurgery, with an emphasis on monitoring legislative, executive, and regulatory matters relevant to neurological surgery. Plante set out basic criteria for a working relationship with the two organizations. First, a small socio-economic committee was formed with no more than eight members who would serve for at least 4 years. The members would be senior members of the Societies and would be expected to have a strong interest in federal affairs. Plante insisted that there be a long-term commitment to a Washington presence, because a small society needs to stay the course if there is to be any hope of success. Finally, he suggested that the committee needed wide authority to act for the two organizations since the federal process timetable was not predictable.

The office was opened in 1976 with a six-member committee, Dr. Finney serving as its first chairman. The Washington Committee decided to meet four times a year to set priorities and address issues. The first years, 1976–1980, were spent determining the extent to which organized neurosurgery would become involved in issues, and when and if it would assume a leadership role on specific issues. The opening of the Washington office coincided with two events that influenced the direction of the Committee and the perception of its effectiveness by the leadership of the two organizations. One of these was the professional liability premium crisis and the other was the government's review of the medical manpower needs of the nation.

The malpractice crisis obviously was focused on the states in general, and a few in particular such as California, New York, and Florida. The Committee attempted to be a resource to the various states while at the same time providing a modicum of leadership in defining the critical problem and possible state-by-state solution. This led to several attempts to form coalitions, for example, in Pennsylvania and New York. The broad-based coalitions were able to identify reforms, but when asked to present specific legislative agendas in both states, lacked the cohesiveness to speak with a single voice. The result of this was disarray and failure. The Committee did discuss exploring the possibility of national tort reform and met with Congressman Tom Floria of New Jersey, then the strongest advocate of product liability reform, but the effort came to no end. In fairness to the Committee on this issue, it did much to focus the debate within organized neurosurgery, in fact providing the vehicle to eventu-

ally persuade organized neurosurgery to switch its emphasis from state to national reform.

In reference to manpower, the Committee took a leadership position in addressing neurosurgical manpower issues by developing specific recommendations to the AANS and CNS leadership which, unfortunately, were largely ignored (see below).

During the period between 1980 and 1985, the Committee greatly expanded its agenda of neurosurgical-specific concerns. Included in the new initiatives was proactive support for increased neuroscience research at the National Institutes of Health (NIH), reimbursement for specific procedures, expanding the numbers of neurosurgeons appointed to various federal advisory positions, and the more global issues of national health insurance. This in turn led to more tangible results related to more specific concerns of organized neurosurgery. It was also during the period from 1980 to 1985 that the Committee struggled to gain credibility inside the two organizations. It was widely held that the Committee was the preserve of a few leaders and ex-presidents of the AANS. This led to the first meaningful reform of the Committee and its function for the membership.

The period between 1986 and 1993 saw an explosion of involvement of the Washington Committee in a broad range of issues and activities. The critical issues of liability, reimbursement, manpower, and science continued to have the highest priority. However, the Committee began to consider trauma, peer review, practice guidelines, FDA regulatory problems, Veteran's Administration affairs (e.g. dumping, regionalization), Department of Defense issues (Feres doctrine), highway safety (seat belts and helmets), animals in research, quality of care, fetal tissue research, and organ transplantation. It was also during this period that a formalized structure was developed between the Committee and the boards of the AANS and CNS. The Committee chairman and Plante reported to the boards semiannually and the president and president-elect of the two parent organizations became ad hoc members of the Committee, thus increasing the membership from 6 to 10.

This reorganization also implied that the Washington Committee would become an initiator of programs for the two organizations. One example worth noting was the development of the head and spinal cord injury prevention program, subsequently to be renamed "THINK FIRST." The idea of a national program was introduced at the Washington Committee and nurtured there for a few years before it was embraced and given a life of its own by the national organizations (see below). Such was the case for the "Decade of the Brain" and several state-related issues. Still another result of the reorganization was a substantial outreach to other joint committees and sections. The idea was to provide resources and information on their specific charges as the federal government impacted on their work.

The Committee is beginning still another period in 1994 as critical issues of reimbursement, manpower (including graduate medical education) and national health care reform are being considered by the federal government. The joint officers have established special socioeconomic working groups to assess the future involvement of organized neurosurgery in these issues and what additional resources are needed to adequately address them.

Present and Future

Neurosurgery, as it looks to its responsibilities in the present and the future to affect and implement health care policy in the United States, is at a crossroads. As evident from the discussion in the previous section, neurosurgery has its plate full and overflowing. Its leaders must ask serious questions about the extent to which it should devote its time, energy, finances, and reputation to the various socioeconomic and political matters that affect medicine in general and neurosurgery specifically. Neurosurgery must realize, as Don Quixote did not, that it does not have the capital to tilt all windmills created by health care reform. Neurosurgery must be discriminating. It must address those issues that immediately and decidedly impact upon neurosurgeons and their patients. Its leaders must develop the wisdom—and the intestinal fortitude—to define and exclude those issues that may be better left primarily to other political segments of the health care industry and other elements of our society.

For example, should neurosurgery through its representatives focus on the budget of the NIH, or should it use its expertise to focus the attention of elected and appointed government officials on the needs within the National Institute of Neurological Disorders and Stroke (NINDS)? One might argue that these two issues are inseparable. However, by focusing on the portion of the budget for NINDS alone, the elected and appointed officials might become more educated regarding neurologic disease specifically, and in so doing, the needs of scientific research generally. As a building is constructed one brick at a time, a policy may be created by focusing on one issue at a time. Another issue involves whether neurosurgery should spend its time on gun control policies or take those resources and focus on altering policies that drive trauma care in this country.

A final question: Should neurosurgery provide resources in one forum after another, attempting to develop ways to alter the tort system in this country in general because of its specific impact on medicine, or should it instead be more actively involved in providing educational input in specific legal engagements that more directly impact the practice of neurosurgery? A recent example was when the AANS joined with the AMA in an amicus curiae brief in *Cruzan v Director, Missouri Department of Health*, a right-to-die case, heard by the U.S. Supreme Court.[1]

The AMA has elevated the issue of tort reform to a level of debate occupied by that surrounding the health care policy considerations of health care reform. In intelligently participating in the debate on tort reform, neurosurgery must, as must the rest of medicine, understand that the tort system is primarily a common law system that has grown out of the courts, as opposed to the legislatures, and any attempt to alter that system dramatically is immediately engulfed in the political tension between legislative and judicial branches of government. The process of reform is less messy when the issue of reform is confined solely within the scope of responsibility of the individual branches than when the issue is one in which one branch purports to define for the other branch its responsibility. For example, within reasonable limits, the judicial branch has little concern when the legislative branch develops statutes of limitations on the filing of causes of action in a court. Nor does the legislative branch feel threatened when the judicial branch provides a new interpretation of some common law principle, such as the definition of "reasonableness." The leaders of neurosurgery must understand this separation and also must understand that it often is easier to influence the opinion of one judge (or a group of judges), who can in turn influence the law through the rendering of decisions that establish precedents, than to influence dozens of individual legislators who have agendas, often disparate, based more on political than on social needs.

Illustrative of this point is a recent change in the law that will have a significant impact on the ability of medical experts to establish their credentials in the courtroom. The U.S. Supreme Court in *Daubert v Merrill-Dow Pharmaceuticals, Inc.* held that scientific (to include medical) testimony must not only be generally accepted by the scientific community, as had been the previous law, but it must, among other accomplishments, have established itself through the peer-review scientific process.[2] This means that experts for both the plaintiff and the defendant must be able to justify their medical conclusions on the basis of peer-review data instead of just experience. A number of scientific organizations, including the AMA, provided briefs in this case and the conclusion of the court can be traced directly to the language in some of those briefs.

It is tempting for neurosurgery to focus on socioeconomic issues that directly impact practicing neurosurgeons. After all, neurosurgery is represented by professional organizations made up of members who pay dues and elect the leadership. However, there is a reality to be considered. The total number of neurosurgeons in this country is less than one–one-hundredth of the total number of physicians in this country.[11] Extrapolating from economic data and limiting the extrapolation to the diseases that neurosurgeons directly affect (for example, the craniotomy for epidural hematoma as opposed to the long-term consequences of the brain injury resulting from the hematoma), neurosurgery accounts for approximately 3.5% of the surgical component of the health care dollar,[14] which is somewhat less than 50% of the health care costs.[13] It is, therefore, not difficult to challenge the assertion that neurosurgery itself should address each socioeconomic issue it faces. Rather, it is reasonable to hold that neurosurgery primarily should address only those issues facing the public in which neurosurgery has particular expertise and experience, thus enhancing its reputation with the public for social responsibility. That enhanced reputation will permit the voice of neurosurgery to be heard at a lower decibel level than would otherwise be the case. This premise is substantiated by two endeavors, both in the past and one extending through the present to the future. These endeavors relate to physician manpower and injury prevention.

In the mid-1970s, before the uproar over the rising physician manpower "glut" in this country, neurosurgery was one of the few specialties that began to study itself. The AANS obtained an NIH grant allowing it to conduct the first extensive neurosurgical manpower survey in its history.[9] As a result, the neurosurgery leadership decided that it was appropriate to slow down the rate of increase in the production of neurosurgeons by reducing the size of some existing programs and curtailing the development of others. Although this fact escaped public notice at the time, it was recognized in the late 1970s and early 1980s. Neurosurgery's experience and expertise was sought during the studies of the Graduate Medical Education Advisory Committee, as well as by the Mendenhall studies that defined the manpower levels in all specialties in this country.[7,16] To this day, that experience by neurosurgery is pointed to as a model for the study of physician manpower in this country. Unfortunately, neurosurgery missed an excellent opportunity to go further at that time, and consequently finds itself today in a difficult situation.

In 1980, the Board of Directors of the AANS received a recommendation from the neurosurgical manpower committee of the AANS that it, as the organization speaking for neurosurgery, consider and support changes in the neurosurgical residency training program that would formalize the development of subspecialization within neurosurgery.[12] Under this concept, every neurosurgery resident in a program, reduced to a minimum of 4 years from a minimum of 5, would be taught the neurologic basis for neurosurgery and the surgical skills to deal with approximately 75% to 80% of neurosurgical problems presented by the public. Additional training in the management of high-risk/low-volume problems would be provided to a selected, much smaller group of neurosurgeons in fewer selected institutions. These institutions would include the major academic centers and associated health care institutions of excellence. Through this process the management of neurosurgical problems in the United States would be altered so that the high-risk/low-volume cases would be diverted to these centers of excellence and out of the general community hospitals.

The concept was rejected as creating two classes of neurosurgeons and limiting the practice opportunities of all neurosurgeons. Coupled with a loosening of the reins on the growth of neurosurgery training positions, this rejection has resulted in a density of neurosurgeons in the United States which is difficult to equate with the goals of health care reform. Today, there is approximately one neurosurgeon for every 65,000 potential patients in this country. Health care planners who are looking at the future of "managed care" and "managed competition" estimate that one neurosurgeon will be necessary for each 150,000 to 200,000 potential patients.[5] It appears neurosurgery, both leadership and individuals, has a health care policy challenge presented by this dichotomy. The leadership of neurosurgery, especially the academic leadership responsible for the training of neurosurgeons, acting on its reputation for social responsibility, should energetically and objectively look at its manpower policies and define necessary modifications. Individual neurosurgeons must be very proactive in finding ways to protect themselves economically, as health care reform alters the density and distribution of physicians in general.

Neurosurgery has a voice in injury prevention that far exceeds its size and resources. In 1986, with the help of then-Surgeon General C. Everett Koop, the AANS and the CNS introduced to the nation an injury-prevention program that focused on the adolescent and young adult. The National Head and Spinal Cord Injury Prevention Program of the AANS and the CNS, later to be renamed "THINK FIRST," was launched. The nucleus of the program was educational, based on the simple premise that the targeted audience could be taught rational decision-making in risk-taking

behavior.[3] In the ensuing 8 years, this country has seen a dramatic fall in the number of unintentional injuries, attributable not only to safer design and legislation (e.g. seat belts, motorcycle helmets), but also education. Neurosurgery's prevention program has received positive recognition and acceptance, as evidenced by several public-service awards and the more than 200 chapters of the injury-prevention program sponsored by neurosurgeons in every state of the United States. Included in the program was the production of a film entitled "Harm's Way," which received a number of national and international awards. Recent preliminary studies indicate that this approach has resulted not only in the alteration of knowledge, attitude, and behavior about risk-taking in the targeted group, but also in a reduced number of injuries in the targeted group.[17] In keeping with its social responsibility, the program is currently developing additional means of studying its efficacy.

Final Thoughts

Neurosurgery clearly has both a present and future role in the establishment and implementation of health care policy in this country. Because it is a relatively small specialty with limited resources, it must, however, make major decisions about where and when it will enter the debate on health care policy. While it is important for the leadership of neurosurgery to attend to the socioeconomic concerns of its members, by and large these concerns are little different from those of physicians in general who may collectively address them with a greater voice and more political power through such organizations as the AMA, the American College of Physicians, and the ACS. Neurosurgery should ensure that it is well represented within these organizations and that it speaks with a clear and concise voice that can be judged as representing the interest of the patient versus the self-interest of the neurosurgeon. It should learn, however, from its past record and reputation for social responsibility, and address those health care and other issues of interest to the public that neurosurgeons, because of their expertise based on training, education, and experience, can speak to with a unique voice. Based on its experience with the National Head and Spinal Cord Injury Prevention Program, it could work to alter the health education system in general in this country. Because of its experience and reputation with physician manpower concerns, it should address not only the current institutional residency education process but also how that process relates to the provision of health care in this country, as Cushing did at the beginning of the 20th century.

References

1. *Cruzan v Director, Missouri Department of Health*, 110 SCt 2841 (1990).
2. *Daubert v Merrill-Dow Pharmaceticals, Inc.*, 113 SCt 2786 (1993).
3. Eyster EF, Watts C. An update of the National Head and Spinal Cord Injury Prevention Program of the American Association of Neurological Surgeons and the Congress of Neurological Surgeons: THINK FIRST. *Clin Neurosurg*. 1992;38:252-260.
4. Fulton JF. *Harvey Cushing: A Biography*. Springfield, Ill: Charles C Thomas; 1946;649-657.
5. Grant PN, Tremaine DW. Integrated delivery systems: a national perspective. Presented at Texas Health Law Conference; October 8, 1993; Austin, Tex.
6. Lyons AS, Pertrucelli RJ II. *Medicine. An Illustrated History*. New York, NY: HN Abrams; 1978;600.
7. Mendenhall RC, Watts C, Radecki SE, et al. Neurosurgery in the United States: a log-diary study. *Neurosurgery*. 1981;8:267-276.
8. Morley TP. *Current Controversies in Neurosurgery*. Philadelphia, Pa: WB Saunders; 1976.
9. National Institute of Neurological Disorders and Stroke. Publication #72-2308. Park Ridge, Ill: Archives of the American Association of Neurological Surgeons; 1976.
10. Nuland SB. *Doctors: the Biography of Medicine*. New York, NY: Alfred A Knopf; 1988;419.
11. *Report of the Graduate Medical Education National Advisory Committee to the Secretary, Department of Health and Human Services: Vol 1*. Washington, DC: GMENAC Summary Report; 1981. US Government Printing Office publication 1980-0-721-748/266.
12. *Report of the National Neurosurgical Manpower Commission to the Board of Directors of the American Association of Neurological Surgeons*. Presented on April 18–20, 1980; action item #14, Park Ridge, Ill.
13. Rich S. Don't blame health care costs for what ails U.S. industry. *The Washington Post National Weekly*. January 22–28, 1990;34.
14. Rutkow LM. *Socioeconomics of Surgery*. St. Louis, Mo: CV Mosby; 1989;3-29.
15. Stevens R. *American Medicine and the Public Interest*. New Haven, Conn: Yale University Press; 1971;88.
16. Watts C. Neurosurgical manpower requirements for 1990: an estimate of the Graduate Medical Education National Advisory Committee. *Neurosurgery*. 1981;8:277-279.
17. Watts C, Eyster EF. National Head and Spinal Cord Injury Prevention Program of the American Association of Neurological Surgeons and the Congress of Neurological Surgeons. *J Neurotrauma*. 1992;9(suppl 1):S307-S312.

CHAPTER 17

The Neurosurgeon and Modern Technology

M. Peter Heilbrun, MD

> *. . . whenever new technology is introduced into society, there must be a counterbalancing human response—the "high touch"—or the technology is rejected. . . . The response to more technology is not to stop it, but to accommodate it, to respond to it, to shape it.*
>
> —John Naisbitt

Technology in Neurosurgical Practice

In our daily lives as neurosurgeons, we increasingly depend on sophisticated tools and technologies to maximize the intuitive creativity of the human mind and the dexterity of the human hand in order to improve the outcome of surgery. At the same time, the inventiveness that creates new means to alleviate suffering and to cure disease can curiously also result in new suffering and disease. Technologies can destroy as well as enrich, sometimes simultaneously; witness the many surgeons who have honed their skills on the crude battlefield.

More and more, I believe in the Ghia proposition that the world is a single organism. Any act—whether of the scientist manipulating a gene to express a protein, of a leader seeking to conquer an enemy tribe, of nature's force, or of isolated individuals seemingly alone—effects the whole organism. All of our lives, as well as the lives of future generations, are touched.

What does this mean to the neurosurgeon practicing his or her skills through long years of training and experience? Obviously, it is neither new nor original to base the physician's responsibility on the Hippocratic oath. Among Hippocrates' many teachings, two tenets are particularly important to my own philosophy. The first is to do no harm. The second is that in order to treat and to alter the course of a disease, one must have a profound understanding of the natural course of that disease.

Thus, I must use technology not simply for intervention, but also to gather information that will increase my understanding of the natural course of a disease and therefore make it possible to attempt to alter that disease. I must use technology to improve my specific understanding of a disease without increasing the patient's pain or fear. I must balance the application of a surgical therapy with the understanding that to apply a surgical therapy without the ability to alleviate suffering and pain or to cure a disease is an act of assault. Finally, I must fully inform the individual suffering from a disease so that the patient and family can participate in the decision to alter the disease's natural history. That is, I must explain which treatment interventions may be pursued to cure a disease and which may only temporarily abate pain and suffering. Only with full communication can the expectations of the physician and the patient be in harmony.

Keeping these premises in mind, I will discuss in this chapter the role of technology in my own career as a physician and surgeon, analyzing my approaches to the neurosurgical treatment of four diseases: occlusive cerebrovascular disease, malignant central nervous system (CNS) tumors, epilepsy, and Parkinson's disease.

Cerebrovascular Disease

In 1967, I went to the laboratory to study the effect of middle cerebral artery occlusion in a dog stroke model, with the specific goal of analyzing the electrophysiologic pattern of spreading cortical depression. An unused Zeiss operating microscope was sitting in the laboratory. Having just read a *Journal of Neurosurgery* article by Lawrence Pool[3] on using the microscope to better visualize aneurysms, I started dissecting dog middle cerebral arteries under magnification and quickly noticed the improvement in hand-eye coordination. This observation, duplicated around the country, was immediate and irrefutable. No prospective randomized evaluation was necessary, and there was no returning to the world of dissection without magnification.

The magnified view of the vascular supply of the brain and its relationship to brain function as manifest by changes in electrical potentials induced me to explore other methods of quantification of cerebral function. So, after my residency, I traveled to Copenhagen to learn methods of xenon measurement of cerebral blood flow. There, I studied possible roles for cerebral blood flow measurements in the management of patients with subarachnoid hemorrhage and severe trauma. At that time, Yasargil was describing his initial results with anastomosis of a branch of the superficial temporal artery to a cortical arterial branch (extracranial-intracranial [EC-IC] bypass) for inaccessible occlusive disease. Chater and Reichman were initiating studies of this elegant operation in San Francisco and Salt Lake City, respectively. It seemed a natural extension of the technologies I was exploring. The operation required magnification, specialized surgical instruments, and a most important engineering advance, namely, the technique of attaching a 10-0 monofilament nylon suture to a

needle. In addition, if the operation worked, good clinical results could be correlated with improvements in cerebral blood flow.

The word was out. Neurosurgeons now had a new operation which was an exquisite technical feat. I was soon on the faculty of the University of Utah, exploring the vagaries of the EC-IC bypass operation, with Reichman, Roberts, and Anderson.

Optimists in the field of neurosurgery equated this new operation to the new operations of the cardiovascular surgeons. Now we could create new routes of blood flow to the brain wherever an artery is narrowed or occluded. Added to carotid endarterectomy and aneurysm surgery, the EC-IC bypass significantly advanced neurosurgery's expansion into the subspecialty of neurovascular surgery. The cynics said otherwise: "Too bad there isn't a disease that needs to be treated with this exquisite operation."

The controversy had started. Our own skepticism grew as our first cerebral blood flow measurements showed no significant improvement in regional postoperative cerebral blood flow, even though the patients' clinical status remained stable. We were also very aware that a credible understanding did not yet exist of the natural history of patients with carotid artery occlusions, carotid siphon stenoses, and middle cerebral artery occlusions and stenoses.

This controversy was resolved in the best spirit of science. Five to 6 years after the operation was introduced, a group of neurosurgeons, neurologists, and neuroradiologists initiated a prospective randomized study of the EC-IC bypass procedure.[2] The formula for the study was a more sophisticated version of the study completed during the 1960s evaluating carotid endarterectomy. Patients who were candidates for EC-IC bypass were prospectively randomly assigned to one of two groups: one group received the best medical treatment available, including treatment of risk factors, while the other group underwent both the best medical treatment available and EC-IC bypass. Outcome endpoints were well defined: new ischemic events and death. The study was initiated quickly through funding from the National Institutes of Health. The first patients were enrolled in 1978, a full cohort was enrolled by 1981, and the results of 5-year follow-up announced in 1985.[1]

The study provided the neurologic community with a relatively clear understanding of the outcome of treated inaccessible occlusive disease of the brain. There was a significant stroke and death rate, but it was not significantly altered in any of the subgroups studied by adding an EC-IC bypass operation. This conclusion was statistically acceptable. Nonetheless, many neurosurgeons felt that the study was flawed, because some study centers failed to randomly assign certain patients who were determined to have a life-threatening need for the EC-IC bypass operation. However, this criticism was not really a proper condemnation of the study results. The art and science of medicine still allow for the individual patient in whom all other therapies have been ineffective and for whom a last resort EC-IC bypass operation is worth trying. Today, the EC-IC bypass is still used for narrowly selected indications; however, the operation is rarely used for the largest group of patients who were once primary candidates, namely, patients with transient ischemic attacks (TIAs) or mild completed strokes with internal artery occlusion.

The operation was conceived in the late 1960s; it was subjected to a sophisticated scientific analysis by 1978 and, based on that analysis, by 1986 it was limited to a few specific indications. Nonetheless, the operation was responsible for introducing neurosurgeons to a critical technology that is now standard in all operating rooms—the operating microscope.

The results of the EC-IC bypass study provided the impetus for a re-analysis of indications for carotid endarterectomy starting in the mid-1980s. Even though the initial study carried out in the 1960s suggested that carotid endarterectomy reduced the stroke and death rate only in patients with TIAs ipsilateral to a significantly stenotic internal carotid artery, it took a repeat of this study under more rigorous conditions in the late 1980s and early 1990s to come to the same conclusion—hopefully reducing the explosion of carotid endarterectomies being performed in this country. The story of the EC-IC bypass procedure taught us to analyze a new technology to gain an understanding of how poorly understood disease processes can be impacted by treatment.

Malignant CNS Tumors

Malignant brain tumors also provide us with a lesson in the impact of technology. Understanding the natural outcome of the disease is not an issue. Without treatment, death comes rapidly. Generally, with treatment, life is prolonged. The quality of that prolonged life is variable. Survival is rarely altered. Yet, as neurosurgeons surrounded by modern technologies of imaging, precision tissue ablation, and modern molecular biology and immunology, we are challenged to discover methods of curing the devastating glioblastoma.

During my days as a neurosurgical resident, treatment of a malignant astrocytoma consisted of aspirating it, stopping the bleeding, and administering postoperative irradiation. Some might say we have not come very far since then. However, the treatment has been beneficially impacted by computed tomography (CT) which improved our appreciation of the three-dimensional relationship of the tumor mass to other brain structures. This, in turn, suggested techniques of stereotactic localization, previously limited to functional procedures, to accomplish precision biopsy.

Kelly demonstrated that integration of computerized reformatting of CT scans, coupled with cross-registration of image coordinates with stereotactic frame coordinates, permitted precision volumetric resection of tumor masses through smaller openings in the cranial vault. This less invasive procedure reduced operative morbidity, and lowered patient costs for the acute phase of the treatment by decreasing the length of hospital stays.

Magnetic resonance imaging (MRI) gave us an even better appreciation of the distribution of a focal malignancy through the brain. Precision resection and biopsy brought a new understanding of the histopathologic differences between the solid tumor that displaces or replaces normal brain, the infiltrating tumor that is mixed with normal functioning brain tissue, and the diffuse distribution of isolated tumor cells situated long distances from the tumor nidus. This better-defined differentiation explained why local treatment therapies provide predominantly palliation and rarely long-term cure. Moreover, the ability to sample tissue with precision, based on imaging, has provided us with new insights. We can now extend classic histopathologic analysis based on morphologic changes, differentiating tumor cells and tissue from normal brain through the technologies of molecular biology. We are beginning to define the differences in DNA, RNA, and protein expression of tumor tissue compared to normal brain tissue, and to look at cytokines, growth factors, and excitatory and inhibitory mechanisms. We are starting to understand mechanisms of normal and abnormal growth and to differentiate factors that allow some growing tumors to displace and push aside normal tissues while others invade and infiltrate. We can start to look at biologic therapies with the goal of replacing factors at the level of gene and protein expression to suppress tumor growth.

Yes, our technology can provide us with the tools to understand the dynamic etiology of abnormal uncontrolled growth. We will need to perform the human experiments to define the effectiveness of new therapies. And we must always remember the Hippocratic mandate of doing no harm. It may be easy to make the statement. We do not have a good treatment for glioblastoma, so it is reasonable to try a new experiment. However, it is essential that any investigator who proposes a new experiment understand the implications of that experiment, and that the patient and the family also understand that the treatment is an experiment and that it could, in fact, be harmful and not fulfill its desired effect.

We must be thoughtful when we participate in surgical trials that involve a placebo operation. Are such trials fair to a patient? Are there no other means to satisfy the statisticians and yet gain useful information? We do have historical controls. Yet I shudder when I read a report of a tumor study protocol concluding that the treatment being tested is statistically significant when compared to controls, while the actual details disclose that the average survival of the malignant glioma cohort was increased by 3 months. This may be good science, but it does not justify the treatment or reflect the art of medicine unless it becomes clear that the increased survival was also associated with a significantly improved quality of life.

My premise to do no harm means that most experiments, particularly our continued trials of new combinations of drugs, must be used only if there is an excellent rationale based on prior ex-

perimentation that a significantly improved survival time and a good quality of life can be attained. Thus, although we know the devastating endpoint of the glioblastoma, our use of technology must clearly be based on a reasonable expectation of success, even if the goal is palliation rather than cure.

Epilepsy

My residency exposed me to Goldring's expertise in the surgical management of epilepsy. However, because invasive diagnostics required long hospitalizations, only a limited number of adults with medically intractable epilepsy were offered surgery, and then only at a few medical centers. Today's refinement of established techniques such as electroencephalography (EEG) and detailed clinical history-taking, along with the careful application of new imaging modalities such as MRI, now provide cost-effective diagnosis and surgery to increasing numbers of adult patients with intractable seizures of temporal lobe onset.

Modern imaging and digital methods of EEG recording show that the majority of adults who are good surgical candidates, whose epilepsy is not associated with an MRI- or CT-defined mass lesion, have foci in the mesiotemporal lobe structures. These patients present with a relatively stereotypical clinical history. An aura almost always precedes the seizure. During the seizure (which generally lasts seconds to minutes and often occurs in clusters), there is a complete loss of awareness but no loss of consciousness. Witnesses describe a wide range of motor automatisms, easily distinguished from the tonic-clonic motor activity of generalized seizures.

The paradigm for cost-effective diagnosis confirms the clinical impression of seizures of mesiotemporal origin with a battery of outpatient studies. Several hours of digital EEG recordings capture seizures and interictal events to demonstrate the correct side of origin. A computer program analyzes the interictal spiking to identify three-dimensionally the source of electrical signals. Volumetric analysis of the uncus, hippocampus, and parahippocampal gyrus generally confirms atrophy consistent with the histopathologic diagnosis of mesiotemporal sclerosis. What we once deduced from pneumoencephalography we can now see with special MRI sequences that provide exquisite anatomic detail of mesiotemporal structures—namely, that hippocampal atrophy is generally ipsilateral to the side of seizure origin as determined from EEG studies. In addition, a number of cognitive components of temporal lobe function are evaluated with a neuropsychometric battery. The most useful predictors have been intelligence and visual-spatial and verbal memory. An angiogram and Wada test confirm speech dominance and the capability of the side opposite the planned resection to support verbal memory.

In surgery, electrocorticography permits a limited, customized temporal lobe resection for removing the uncus, the anterior two centimeters of the hippocampus, and the parahippocampal gyrus. Selective mesiotemporal resection on the appropriate side will eliminate seizures in over 80% of patients who are generally hospitalized 3 to 4 days following the surgery and tapered off their medication over a 2-year period. The results suggest that even in the middle-aged adult, surgical control of seizures is an important outcome that significantly improves the quality of life in patients who have endured seizures throughout their lives.

In the near future, stereotactically guided, minimally invasive mesiotemporal resections, radiofrequency, and radiosurgical lesions have the potential of further reducing morbidity and hospital stays. In addition, physiologic mapping of brain dysfunction using modern supercomputers for visualization of magneto- and electroencephalographic source dipoles, functional MRI, and MRI spectroscopic signals will make surgical cure a possibility for an even larger number of patients. As our methods of noninvasive evaluation become more sophisticated and our methods of surgical ablation become less invasive, we can attain a higher cure rate for a greater number of patients, and we can eliminate diagnostic and surgical techniques that occasionally cause harm without cure.

Parkinson's Disease

Today, the majority of the computerized databases, such as MEDLINE, perform a literature search going back only a few years. Certainly, this is convenient and helpful, as the information we seek is often found in the latest article. However, to do a full search, it is also important to go back to the old books—to analyze old procedures and ideas that have been discarded, before exploring what might be new.

An important contemporary example of this premise is Laitinen's recent relook at ventroposterolateral pallidotomy (VPL) for Parkinson's disease. Three years ago, I listened to him report his results with VPL pallidotomy and then visited him in Sweden. In the mid-1980s, Laitinen became intrigued with a 1960 report[4] on Leksell's experience with lesions in the VPL portion of the globus pallidus to relieve the rigidity and bradykinesia of Parkinson's disease. This is a significantly different effect on the disease than tremor relief which can be accomplished with thalamic lesions. Why Leksell's favorable experience with VPL pallidotomy was discarded or not taken up by other neurosurgeons is not clear.

The differences in the indications for the application of pallidotomy over thalamotomy are quite striking. Since the introduction of dopamine-replacement medications, thalamotomy is now performed predominantly on younger patients with unilateral tremor. Although thalamotomy has some beneficial effect on rigidity and bradykinesia, the effect is not dramatic. On the other hand, pallidotomy can reverse many of the late disabling symptoms of Parkinson's disease. Specifically, patients with late-stage Parkinson's disease may have an annoying tremor, but generally the tremor is not incapacitating. Instead, it is the rigidity and bradykinesia that often make the patients wheelchair-bound, because they have difficulty initiating programmed movements such as moving from lying down to sitting, from sitting to standing, and then from standing in place to walking. Often the L-dopamine-type drugs reduce the rigidity and bradykinesia so that the patients can move and walk for brief periods of time. During this "on" phase, many patients do relatively well and feel quite good. However, in many patients, the beneficial effect of the medications lasts for shorter and shorter periods and includes uncomfortable involuntary choreoathetoid-like dyskinesias. Some patients get to the point where the only way they can move with any kind of efficiency is if their mobile periods are accompanied by severe dyskinesias. Often these patients with end-stage Parkinson's disease alternate between two states; either they are rigid, stiff, and unable to move or they have hyperactive movements associated with disfiguring uncomfortable dyskinesias. Laitinen has demonstrated that VPL pallidotomy not only relieves much of the rigidity and bradykinesia but also allows patients to reduce their medication dosage so that relatively fluid movements are not associated with off-cycle dyskinesias. In addition, most tremor is relieved. The preliminary experience of other surgeons confirms Laitinen's results. It is my early conclusion that this rediscovered and reapplied known operative procedure will have a significant positive impact on a large number of Parkinson's patients with incapacitating end-stage disease. This increased application is in contrast to the experience with thalamotomy, which has been reserved for unmanageable unilateral tremor.

Thus, as we learn new technology, we should also re-examine old technologies and approaches that have been discarded. This is particularly important in Parkinson's disease as we explore neural restoration accomplished with fetal or genetically engineered cells grafted into the nervous system.

Conclusion

I have attempted to relate some thoughts regarding the role of technology in the context of several specific disease entities that I deal with on a daily basis as a practicing neurosurgeon with the additional responsibility of defining the direction of a neurosurgical training program. This discussion has not been inclusive. I have not addressed spine disease, trauma, and perioperative care in the intensive care environment, areas of neurosurgery in which technologic advances often bring up philosophic and ethical questions related to life and death. The challenges facing us as physicians and neurosurgeons today in applying technologies to improve the human condition demonstrate at the same time more possibilities and options, yet more potential for doing harm if they are not used with reason and thought. If we undertake the use of any new technology, we must do so with an understanding of how the disease we are proposing to treat impacts the individual harboring that disease, and we must be aware of how our decisions impact the patient, his or her family, our society, our specialty of neurosurgery, and our own egos as physicians. Thus can we fulfill our responsibility to alleviate suffering yet do no harm.

References

1. The EC/IC Bypass Study Group. Failure of extracranial-intracranial arterial bypass to reduce the risk of ischemic stroke. Results of an international trial. *N Engl J Med.* 1985;313:1191-1200.
2. The EC/IC Bypass Study Group. The International Cooperative Study of Extracranial/Intracranial Arterial Anastomosis (EC/IC Bypass Study): methodology and entry characteristics. *Stroke.* 1985:16: 397-406.
3. Pool JL, Colton RP. The dissecting microscope for intracranial vascular surgery. *J Neurosurg.* 1966:25: 315-318.
4. Svennilson E, Torvak A, Lower R, et al. Treatment of parkinsonism by stereotactic thermolesions in the pallidal region. A clinical evaluation of 81 cases. *Acta Psychiatr Scand.* 1960;35:358-377.

CHAPTER 18

The Paradox of Success and the Neurosurgeon—Competing Currents and Allegiances

Joseph C. Maroon, MD

Neurosurgeons occupy a unique and elite position in the United States. Approximately 3500 are available to meet the surgical needs of over 250 million people. Admission to this distinguished "club" requires such extraordinary personal characteristics as insatiable curiosity, steadfast perseverance, self-denial, perfectionism, and an ardent desire to achieve a place among what one believes to be the brightest and best in the field of medicine.

But these same laudable qualities, reflected so well in Greek tragedies, often turn out to be the hero's Achilles' heel. Perseverance against seemingly insurmountable obstacles, for example, may require time away from family, friends, and others of importance. Discipline and self-denial, so necessary for survival in the forge of a neurosurgery residency, may result in disdain for those who seem to lack such qualities, projecting an air of arrogance. Finally, the quest for perfection and "success" often leads to a unidimensional individual, successful in neurosurgery, but unbalanced and often a failure in many of life's other pursuits.

While a balanced life is highly desirable, it is ironic that society most richly rewards those who are unbalanced, because we are much more useful to society when a small part of ourselves is overdeveloped. The amulets of worldly success—prestige and power, possessions and pecuniary acquisitions—are strung about the neck as compensation for the unique qualities of the neurosurgeon, emblems of membership in such an elite club.

What neurosurgeon has not asked: "Why do I work so hard?" "Why am I so consumed by the internecine warfare of hospital politics?" "Will the Clinton Administration's health plan destroy me financially?" "Why do I have no time to enjoy the arts, take up a sport, or just spend with my family?"

In this chapter, I explore and attempt to define the driving force—the "engine"—that propels neurosurgeons to such extraordinary accomplishments, as well as to overwork, self-sacrifice, and perfectionism. I also attempt to define what is perceived to be "success" for the neurosurgeon and to illustrate the great paradox therein. Finally, I suggest the framework for a mindset through which one may attain a degree of balance or equanimity among the opposing currents and competing allegiances we face today.

Motivation: The Engine

To determine the motivating factors for any human endeavor, in this case a career choice, the most direct approach is to question the individual as to his or her own driving force for choosing a specific discipline. A second technique would be to look at behavioral traits shared by individuals pursuing a particular career and to attempt to deduce a common denominator.

In speaking to many neurosurgical colleagues, frequent responses to the question

"Why did you choose neurosurgery?" included: "I was fascinated by the nervous system"; "I was overwhelmed by the challenge of operating on the human brain"; "Neurosurgery represented the most challenging field of medicine"; "It was clearly the most prestigious and demanding field I could choose"; "I was motivated by Doctor X, a neurosurgeon, who selflessly devoted his entire life to helping others"; "It was my favorite rotation as a medical student." With persistent further questioning, it became apparent that relatively little introspection of a detailed nature was given by most for choosing neurosurgery. Also, when I spoke to cardiovascular surgeons, thoracic surgeons, general surgeons, and others, the reasons for choosing their fields were often similarly vague.

I wondered next whether there might be common character traits among those who are considered successful by society's standards and who have been rewarded for outstanding accomplishment in a specific area. This group included chief executive officers of major corporations, "top" lawyers, engineers, and other professionals, as well as "successful" physicians. Overall, the most successful individuals in all careers shared qualities of perfectionism, self-denial, and overwork. All were highly competitive, achievement-oriented, easily frustrated, impatient, time-pressed, and constantly under deadlines.

The search for "the engine" of motivation then narrowed to a quest for the origin of the incredible drive that leads to a continual striving for perfection, in which one is never satisfied with any accomplishment before moving on to another. What inner need leads to the self-denial of other pleasures of life for 10 to 15 years until "I finish my residency" only to find new goals demanding further self-denial? What is the force that leads to 16-hour workdays, as well as to the neglect of family and friends, and physical and spiritual needs?

Psychiatrist Glenn Gabbard, Director of the Menninger Memorial Hospital, offers an answer.[12] Dr. Gabbard has treated hundreds of physicians for clinical depression, substance abuse, and sexual boundary violations—physicians whose marriages and lives imploded upon experiencing the "emptiness of success." He concluded that, in any field, the most successful individuals (as determined by society's acceptance and approval) are those who have experienced the most significant childhood deprivation. Deprivation of what? In most cases, it is the deprivation of approval or acceptance irrespective of performance. In the formative years, the message heard—either real or perceived—was not "I love you because you are you," but that self-worth, love, acceptance, and approval were earned only if one lived up to the expectations of others (parents, teachers, and subsequently society at large). In other words, they were *not* good and *not* worth very much, no matter how mightily they would strive to meet these expectations, often with only variable success.

This deprivation does not necessarily mean that they were unloved or uncared for. Perhaps in many cases, there were unrealistic needs for approval due to birth order, family economic factors, sibling status, or parental pressure. Regardless, rather than learning to trust and depend on themselves for their own self-esteem and value, they came to depend on others to validate their intrinsic goodness and worth. Consequently, they may spend their entire lives seeking the imprimatur of others, never satisfied, never content with any accomplishment, always looking toward the next challenge or goal.

This engine of real or perceived childhood deprivation and the subconscious inner craving for society's approbation results in a highly competitive, achievement-oriented individual with ultra-high standards and a perfectionistic mindset. In their book *The Perfectionist Predicament: How to Stop Driving Yourself and Others Crazy*, Elliott and Meltsner[7] describe the results of such behavior.

> Hooked on the praise, applause, recognition, or other tangible rewards, "playing the game" is no more than an inconvenience on the way to victory. Yet, each time you emerge victorious your thoughts immediately turn to sustaining your success, surpassing it, or finding fault with the way you played the game. You have become your own carrot dangler, both the donkey pursuing the carrot and the driver holding that reward just beyond your own grasp. Disappointment and dissatisfaction are virtually guaranteed.

If one can only perform perfectly, one feels that he will get the reward he deserves. But that reward always remains just beyond reach. . . .

The pain of deprivation of love and approval, whether real or imagined, results in a profound fear of emotional dependence on and commitment to others. In reaction to this fear, physicians often demonstrate selfless giving—the opposite of dependency and a reaction formed as a defense. This interaction results in dependency by patients on their physician, indirectly fulfilling the physician's unmet needs and allowing him to remain "in control."

Such physicians become hard-working, high-achieving, self-denying, and devoted to the welfare of others. At times, they may neglect their family, friends, health, and anything else not directly related to their "magnificent obsession." In short, they become perfect candidates for neurosurgical practice.

At some point, usually in our late 30s or early 40s, we may face a great void: something is missing. Where is the next challenge? We have spent selfless, perfectionistic professional lives taking care of everyone else, pleasing teachers, parents, patients, family members—but who will offer the same in return? We have done everything that we were supposed to do: suffered an arduous residency and struggled to support a family and to build a practice. But the hollow feeling persists. We ask, as the song says, "Is that all there is?"

At this stage, the anxiety and longing may lead to unhealthy, destructive coping mechanisms. Infidelity, substance abuse, clinical depression, poorly inhibited anger, or hyper-religiosity become manifest as modes of escape. Each of these has its own disastrous consequence: divorce, addiction, injuring patients and possibly family members, feelings of futility with life, and even self-destruction.

The late Jesuit priest Anthony DeMello,[6] who was schooled in Aristotelian and Christian thought as well as Eastern religions, wrote extensively about the genesis of this emptiness and suggested a more appropriate reaction.

As children, we were given a set of programs and a taste for the drugs called approval, appreciation, attention, making it to the top, prestige [getting our names in journals], power, being the boss, being the captain of the team, leading the band. Having a taste for these drugs, we became addicted and began to dread losing them. Recall the lack of control and terror at the prospect of failure or making mistakes [an operative complication], at the prospect of criticism of others [the anguish of a malpractice suit]. We became cravenly dependent on others and lost our freedom. We gave others the power to make us happy or to make us miserable.

Although we may not consciously articulate it as such, this is the genesis of the emptiness. No matter how great our successes, acquisitions, titles, or publications, we are never satisfied and remain "deprived" because very early on we abrogated our self-esteem to the whims of others, although not necessarily through any fault of our own.

This is clearly seen at national neurosurgical meetings. We experience intense anxiety during the weeks and months of preparation to give a 10-minute presentation, upon the completion of which we either soar with the elation of acclaim or become depressed—possibly infuriated—with any negative review. Even with a startlingly creative piece of work, little time is spent truly savoring the accomplishment before we are busy preparing for next year's meeting, pursuing yet another "fix" that will depend again on the assessments and reactions of others rather than of ourselves.

To break this dependency we must become "deprogrammed," releasing ourselves from the programming that we experienced as children. Change will occur only through awareness and understanding. We need to break out of the prison of programming and conditioning and into the freedom of reality. With awareness, we may still perform the same activities, present the same papers, engage in the same research, and work just as hard. But as Freud once said, "What I once did out of compulsion or neuroses before therapy (or awakening or enlightenment) I now do by volition." The outward behavior may appear the same, but there is an amazing difference when we do it by conscious choice and not out of neurotic compulsion. We then may laugh at our activities and not rise and fall like a yo-yo, dependent on the "Great job, Joe" or "That was terrible, Joe," of others. Or as St. Paul preached, we need to be in the world, but not of it.

We must ask ourselves if it is possible to work hard, to compete, to take risks, to have influence, authority, or wealth, and still experience the joy of fulfillment. The answer is unequivocally "yes"—as long as these are not the *primary* source of our happiness. To seek excellence in all we do, to derive satisfaction and self-esteem from our efforts is healthy and desirable. To be perfectionistic, with all of its attendant downsides, is neurotic.

Seeking Excellence vs. Pursuing Perfection

People who pursue excellence can be as careful, meticulous, and thorough as any perfectionist. Although they may have their share of fears and insecurities, they are willing to venture into unfamiliar territory and to take certain risks. In comparing perfectionists with seekers of excellence, certain character and personality traits become evident (Table 1).[7]

The pursuit of flawless accomplishments, technical or intellectual, is still the highest goal. But a balanced approach to our profession and to

TABLE 1

Traits of Excellence Seekers vs. Perfectionists

Excellence Seekers	Perfectionists
• Self-accepting, aware of their strengths and limitations and know that both contribute to their unique personalities; believe that they are basically worthwhile and valuable human beings.	• Self-absorbed, acutely aware of their flaws and deficiencies; minimize their virtues and work hard to conceal their inadequacies; because everything is a potential threat to their façade, they are constantly on the defensive.
• They can lose and still have a positive self-image.	• They must always win and be infallible in order to believe they have any worth or value at all.
• They set goals and standards that take into account their limitations and strengths, increasing the likelihood of success.	• They demand a higher level of performance than is humanly possible; this reduces their chance of success and meeting goals.
• When facing a challenge, they focus on their strengths and on how to do well.	• When facing a challenge (which they usually see as a problem), they focus on their deficiencies and concentrate on how not to do poorly or make any mistakes.
• They try new ventures, take risks, and learn from their experiences and mistakes.	• They avoid new experiences and fear risk-taking for fear of looking foolish or incompetent, focusing on how not to make the same mistakes again.
• They are relaxed and careful when undertaking new tasks. They feel excited and clear about what needs to be done and emotionally charged when entering unfamiliar territory.	• They are tense and deliberate in new, unfamiliar, unpredictable situations, and may devote so much energy to worrying about new tasks ahead of time that they feel anxious, confused, or exhausted before they even begin.
• They are open to direction and constructive criticism.	• They take criticism as a personal attack and tend to think that people would not make suggestions unless they doubted their competence in the first place.
• They derive a sense of satisfaction and enhanced self-esteem from their efforts. They appreciate a job well done and feel free to be less painstaking or results-oriented.	• They rarely, if ever, see their efforts—including their best ones—as good enough. They do not appreciate a job well done, believing that they could and should always do better. They derive little satisfaction from their accomplishments—even truly remarkable ones.
• <u>Balanced</u>. They are able to relax, have satisfying personal relationships, participating in and enjoying activities that are not even remotely related to their goals.	• <u>Unbalanced</u>. They are single-mindedly devoted to certain areas of their lives to the exclusion of all else, distinctly lacking in close personal relationships, relaxation, or purely pleasurable pursuits.

our lives becomes the talisman and the *sine qua non* for personal satisfaction and happiness.

Attaining Balance

Twenty-three hundred years ago, Aristotle reasoned that the primary end of all human activity is a good life or happiness.[1] Happiness, however, is an enigma. "Ask yourself whether you are happy," said J. S. Mill, "and you cease to be so."[4] "Happiness cannot be pursued; it must ensue . . . as the unintended side-effect of one's personal dedication to a course greater than oneself," said Viktor Frankl in his book, *Man's Search For Meaning*.[8] So how do we reach this elusive goal of a good life if it cannot be attained by a direct conscious route? I believe that it ensues from accepting our human nature and imperfections (even laughing at them), leading a balanced life, and living in the "now."

Several years ago, distressed from being in a state of chronic imbalance, I chose as the subject of a presidential address the topic of balance or *aequanimitas* in a physician's life: the importance of it, the consequences of not possessing it (although unaware that I was an expert in the field!), and the methods of attaining it.[10] *Aequanimitas* derives from the Latin words *aequus* or "even" and *animus,* meaning "mind" or "spirit." Thus it defines evenness in mind, temperament, and composure or, combined in modern parlance with imperturbability, means "balance" or "equanimity."

Philosophic literature is replete with the importance of a balanced life. Aristotle urged in his writings to "always seek the mean between extremes." The Roman prescription was *mens sana en corporare sano* (a healthy mind and a healthy body). The Native Americans of the Southwest sought "hozho," which referred to the natural balance between the earth, the sky, the waters, and the soul of the American Indian. In the late 1800s, Claude Bernard[2] wrote: "It is the fixity of the *milieu interieur* which is the primary condition for a free and independent life. All the vital mechanisms of the body, varied as they are, have only one object: that of preserving balance and equilibrium." Walter Cannon,[3] several years later, maintained that an organism's *milieu interieur* should be called "homeostasis" or "physiological equanimity."

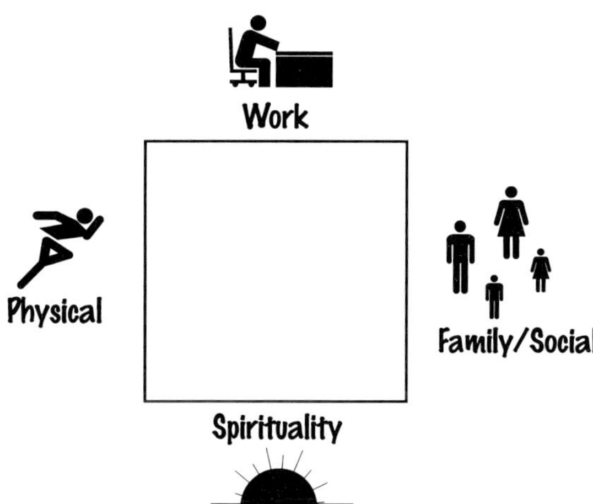

Figure 1. *The balanced square depicting symmetry in the commitment to each of four areas in a person's daily life: the professional, the family/social, the spiritual, and the physical.*

What then are the areas to be "balanced" in our daily lives to attain this inner homeostasis or *aequanimitas*? There are essentially four: the professional, the family/social, the spiritual, and the physical. In 1954, in a most simplistic way, William Danforth,[5] President of the Purina Company in St. Louis, Missouri, challenged his employees and subsequently students throughout the county to be the best they could be by "balancing" their lives. He proposed that each individual consider these four major areas of personal commitment and determine the extent to which they were devoted to each. A figure could then be constructed with the length of each arm proportionate to the degree of commitment to that area of life (Figure 1). Such a drawing would clearly reflect the symmetry or "balance" of their existence.

Ideally, the sides of the figure should be equal in length, forming a perfect square. At different points of my own life, my square has looked more like a trapezoid—or anything but a square (Figure 2). In terms of commitment, the professional arm is usually at least two times longer than any of the other three. I have experienced the cataclysmic personal consequences of such imbalance. This has prompted the introspective search for the engine or motivating force giving rise to the perfectionism, self-denial, and overwork that has characterized the professional arm of my own square.

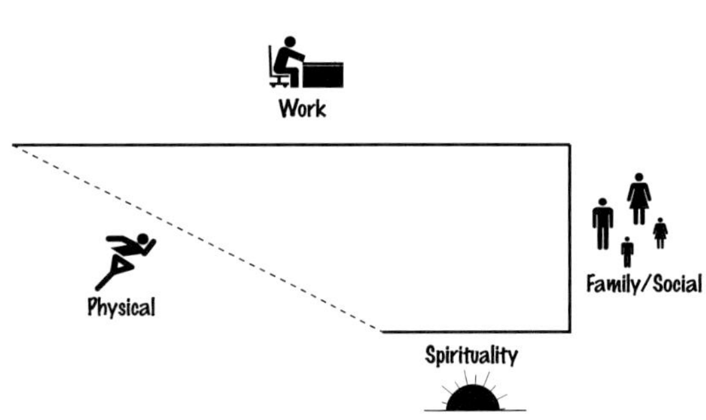

Figure 2. The unbalanced "square" of a typical neurosurgeon illustrating the overcommitment to work (the professional area) to the diminution of the other aspects of life.

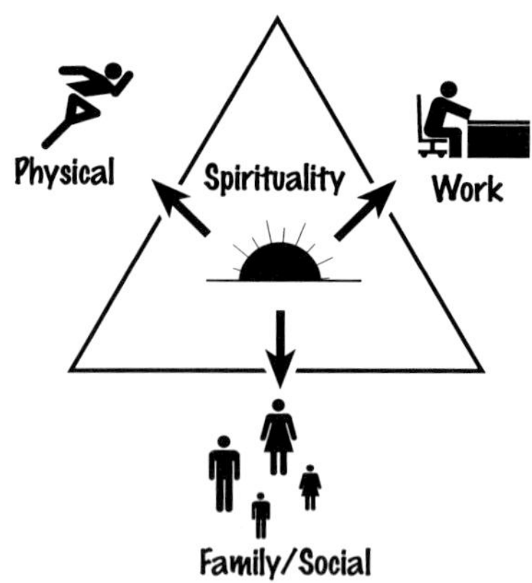

Figure 3. A triangle with spirituality permeating all aspects of one's life.

The discovery of unrecognized childhood deprivation and the subsequent years of unconscious dependence on (addiction to?) external affirmation had a profound effect on my own decision-making. At last I could look at the four sides of my square and consciously, on a daily basis, choose specific areas to which to commit my time. The family/social, physical, and spiritual sides became, for the first time—consciously—of primary concern.

In discussing these concepts with different colleagues, I discovered in myself and in others the ability to function satisfactorily, but not optimally, with a deficiency in one of the areas of commitment. It is axiomatic, however, that if two sides of the square are neglected (e.g. the spiritual and the family or the physical and the spiritual), major emotional problems from the "imbalance" are imminent, if not already present. Depression, anxiety, and overall poor concentration result. Relief may be sought in unhealthy ways such as substance abuse, destructive relationships, and excessive physical or religious addictions.

Eventually, however, the road to recovery—and balance—demands a re-assessment of the role of spirituality or religion in our lives to help answer the incessant philosophic question "What's it all about?" At this point, we may discover the distinction between "religion" (as we were taught as children) and "spirituality," which is much more encompassing.[13]

Religion, in the most generic sense, includes acknowledgement of a divine or supernatural power, usually expressed in specific beliefs, codes of conduct, and ritual practices. This contrasts with generic spirituality, which penetrates beyond creeds and practices. Spirituality is not immediately concerned with the specifics of a single religion, but with the transcendent aspects of all creeds. Spiritual existence sees beyond appearances and is in touch with a higher dimension, one that is not readily available to most people. Spirituality focuses on a vision, whereas religion concentrates on beliefs and actions.

Contemplatives and mystics of the major religions are in touch with a plane of being, a vital core of faith, that lies behind and beyond external existence. They share a sense of awe experienced when they are in contact with the divine at the center of the soul and in the wonders of nature. Spirituality is therefore independent of the constraints of the world's creeds, such as Buddhism, Christianity, Hinduism, Islam, or Judaism. Neither does it depend on the words and deeds of Buddha, Jesus, Krishna, Mohammed, or Moses. It exists entirely in how we "see beyond appearances."

With these thoughts in mind, I submit that the best depiction of the neurosurgeon's approach toward equilibrium is a triangle—with spirituality permeating all aspects of our professional, familial, and physical lives (Figure 3). Indeed, our days are infused with spiritual experiences that enhance our being: a walk through a cool forest, a swim in a placid lake, a bicycle ride along back-country roads, the first words of a child, the intimacy shared with a loved one, or the total trust in the eyes of an elderly widow crippled by pain that may be eased by our gift of healing.

Living in the "Now"

With an understanding of some of the motivating factors propelling us through life, and a simple (yet not really so simple) formula for helping us attain balance, there remains what I have found to be perhaps the most difficult task of all—that is, living in the "now" or today. Far too often, as someone said, "Life is something that happens to us while we are busily engaged in something else."

But life is really a series of moments; to live each one fully is to truly succeed. Success in living is found not in the accomplishment of a few great deeds but in the performance of thousands of little ones moment by moment.

How difficult it is to stay focused on the present! Consider a typical scenario at the symphony. The orchestra is playing and you settle in your seat. As you prepare to enjoy the music, you suddenly remember that you forgot to lock your car. What do you do now? You cannot leave since it would be too disturbing, and you cannot enjoy the music because you are obsessed with your car. You are caught in the middle. That is the image of life for most people—constant anxiety. How do I deal with this? How do I get out of it?

Robert Hastings' "The Station" even more succinctly defines the problem and suggests a solution:

> Tucked away in our subconsciousness is an idyllic vision, we see ourselves on a long trip that spans the continent, we are travelling by train. Out of the wonders we drink in the passing scenes of cars on nearby highways, of children waving at a crossing, of cattle grazing on a distant hillside, of smoke pouring from a power plant or row upon row of corn and wheat, of flatlands or valleys, of mountains and rolling hillsides, or city skylines and village halls, but uppermost in our minds is the final destination.

> On a certain day at a certain hour we will pull into the station, bands will be playing and flags waving.

> Once we get there so many wonderful dreams will come true, and the pieces of our lives will fit together like a completed jigsaw puzzle. How restlessly we pace the aisles, damning them, minutes of loitering, minutes of waiting, waiting, and waiting for the station. Sooner or later we must realize there is no station, no one place to arrive at once and for all. The true joy in life is in the trip, the station is only a dream, it constantly outdistances us. This is the day which the Lord hath made, we rejoice and be glad in it.

> It isn't the burdens of today that drive men mad, it is the regrets over yesterday and the fear of tomorrow. Regret and fear are twin thieves that rob us of today. So stop pacing the aisles and counting the miles, instead, climb more mountains, eat more ice cream, go barefoot more often, swim more rivers, watch more sunsets, laugh more, cry less. Life must be lived as we go along, the Station will come soon enough.[9]

Life must be seized at the moment—*carpe diem*. The time to live is now! By living in the present, we are in full contact with ourselves and our environment. Our energy is not dissipated. It is always available. In the present, there are no regrets for the past, no dilution by the future. As long as we are doing at the moment exactly what we are at that moment, we are one in being and action—that is the essence of Zen. WE are accomplishing to the fullest. Our focus of being is *NOW*. How difficult that is to carry out: to escape the regrets of the past and the problems of tomorrow.

The paradox of attaining success and also of living in the present is perhaps best summarized in the Zen riddle, "When you seek it, you cannot find it." The happiest people seem to be those who work at being kind, helpful, and reliable. Hans Selye[11] described this state as "altruistic egotism." Happiness sneaks into their lives while they are busy doing something else—the paradox. Happiness is a by-product of something else that is good and worthwhile. It cannot be pursued. It is like the proverbial butterfly: the more you chase it, the more it flies away from you. Stop chasing and it sneaks up and perches on your shoulder. "True happiness cannot be defined. It must ensue . . . as the unintended side effect of one's personal dedication to a course greater than oneself"[8]—again, the paradox. We know not what sight is until the eye is unobstructed. We know not what happiness is until we live in the present, drop the attachments of the past, and the longings for the future. Happiness, then, ensues.

As Tennyson said in his great work *Ulysses*, "I am a part of all I have met." I have attempted to put into words the feelings and thoughts that I have experienced during periods of tears and laughter in my life. Many of these words have come from those much wiser than I. However, I have found that, of all of them, the Socratic admonition "know thyself" is indeed the hardest task we face. As the Buddhist master states, "Knowing others is wisdom, knowing yourself is enlightenment."

I have come to recognize many of the paradoxes of life. During those intermittent times when I am in balance with the spiritual, physical, social, and professional aspects of my life, the quality of existence is dramatically enhanced. Relationships with others are enriched. I am in awe of nature and in closer touch with myself. I have come to understand that enlightenment—and success—simply mean recognizing the inherent balance and harmony of ordinary life and living in the "now."

And one might therefore say of me, that in this book I have only made up a bunch of other people's flowers, and that of my own, I have only provided the string that ties them together.

—Montaigne[11]

References

1. Adler MJ. *Aristotle for Everybody*. New York, NY: Macmillan; 1978: 80.
2. Bernard C. *An Introduction to the Study of Experimental Medicine*. New York, NY: Macmillan; 1927.
3. Cannon WD. *The Wisdom of the Body*. New York, NY: WW Norton & Co; 1932.
4. Csikszentmihalyi M. *Flow: The Psychology of Optimal Experience*. New York, NY: Harper & Row; 1990:2.
5. Danforth W. *I Dare You*. St. Louis, Mo: Privately printed; 1954.
6. DeMello A. *Awareness: The Perils and Opportunities of Reality*. New York, NY: Doubleday; 1990.
7. Elliott M, Meltsner S. *The Perfectionist Predicament: How to Stop Driving Yourself and Others Crazy*. New York, NY: Berkeley Books; 1991:50-51.
8. Frankl VE. *Man's Search for Meaning*, New York, NY: Washington Square; 1960:12,18.
9. Kelly DL Jr. AANS Presidential Address, 1991: Now is our time. *J Neurosurg*. 1991;75:677-684.
10. Maroon JC. Presidential Address: from Icarus to Aequanimitas. *Neurosurgery*. 1987;21:1-6.
11. Selye H. *Stress Without Distress*. Philadelphia, Pa: JB Lippincott; 1974: 115,136.
12. Skelly FJ. Mapping medicine's mind field: Dr. Gabbard explores physicians' psychological vulnerabilities. *AMA News*. October 11, 1993;11-15.
13. Somerville JM. *The Mystical Sense of the Gospels XII: Religions and Generic Spirituality in the Rolle*. Pfafftown, NC: Schola; 1993;3:96-107.

CHAPTER 19

International Neurosurgery: Philosophic Issues in the Global Context

Jeffrey V. Rosenfeld, MBBS, MS, FRACS, FRCS(Ed), and
Issam A. Awad, MD, MSc, FACS

The woods are lovely, dark and deep,
But I have promises to keep
And miles to go before I sleep,
And miles to go before I sleep.

—Robert Frost
(An inspiration to Indian sciences[20])

We few Nigerian neurosurgeons accept our assignment with humor and humility and
with hope that tomorrow will be better than today.
—A. Adeloye, Nigerian neurosurgeon

Astonishing advances in neurosurgery and neuroscience have occurred in the last 20 years. Interactive image-guided neurosurgery utilizing frameless stereotaxy and robotics, neural replacement therapy, and molecular neurosurgery are evolving and may become standard practice in the developed world in the third millennium.[3] However, at the other end of the spectrum, millions of the world's population are lacking in any specialized neurosurgical services, or even basic neurosurgery performed by general surgeons. The afflicted and their families suffer great hardship and tragedy as a result of this inequity, which remains a blemish on the developed world. Neurosurgery and cardiothoracic surgery are perceived to be the most sophisticated tertiary care specialties and are widely believed to be unaffordable in much of the developing world.

Over the last two decades, the focus of neurosurgery has been inward-looking and technology-driven, with increased precision and lower morbidity being the driving forces. Considera-tion of the development and provision of neurosurgical services in the developing world has been severely neglected by neurosurgeons in the developed world. Surprisingly, this subject is not discussed in any of the major neurosurgery text books. Neurosurgeons of the developed world bear a strong responsibility to try and redress this dreadful situation.

The developing world has a burgeoning population in poor general health, with meager resources for health care. Despite improvements in life expectancy and health, enormous health problems remain. Infectious diseases such as malaria, tuberculosis (TB), human immunodeficiency disease, schistosomiasis, and gastroenteritis are still rife, and increasing drug resistance is producing greater problems of control. The prevalence of Western diseases, particularly cancer and heart disease, is increasing in the Third World as life expectancy increases and Western diets and habits, such as smoking, are preferred. Smoking is already commonplace in the Third

World. Inequity, inefficiency, and exploding health costs are also ongoing problems. Political instability and government corruption result in the funneling of enormous funds away from health care. The developing world spends $170 billion (4% of the gross national product) on health services or an average of $41.00 per person, which is less than one–thirtieth the amount spent by rich countries.[33]

In general, people of underdeveloped countries have low expectations of advanced health care because of a lack of knowledge and previous experience with treatments available in the developed world. It is likely that the demand for these procedures will increase dramatically as the people become more informed.

The Problem

Economic Considerations

The developing world varies markedly in its political stability, and this often results in grossly deficient health service delivery (Table 1). Not even primary care is available where famine and war are endemic. However, many developing countries have a relatively stable government that is able to provide some element of health care, albeit with meager internal resources and foreign aid. However, the inequitable distribution of financial resources within many developing countries renders the development of a satisfactory health service an impossibility.

TABLE 1

Economic Considerations Affecting Health Care in Underdeveloped Countries

- Budgetary allocation—inadequate, inequitable, wide fluctuations
- Exclusive focus on primary care
- Neglect of hospital infrastructure
- Poor staff remuneration
- Maldistribution of health resources to the wealthy
- Centralized decision-making
- Harmful effect of war, famine, political repression, corruption

The World Bank report "Investing in Health,"[33] written in conjunction with World Health Organization (WHO) data, offers at least a partial solution to this tragic situation, by emphasizing primary health care to the exclusion of specialist care. This is a potentially insensitive policy, seemingly based on broad macroeconomic considerations. If more humane solutions to the health problems of developing countries are to be found, particularly when considering the worth of neurosurgery, the individual and the family unit deserve much greater consideration, rather than the entire focus for health care policy being directed to society as a whole.

The focus of the primary health care advocate is largely population-based, whereas the specialist surgeon deals with the individual patient and his or her family. When it comes to the allocation of health care resources and the development of health care policy, there is a fundamental philosophic dichotomy between the hospital-based medical and surgical specialists, and the health department and foreign-aid bureaucrats. The World Bank report argues that spending on cancer and heart disease would be a misallocation of funding and would tend to withdraw funds from health intervention of low cost and high efficacy.[33] This is a short-sighted view that fails to take into account the increasing prevalence of these diseases, or their humanitarian aspects .

The World Bank report also argues that government hospitals and clinics in low-income countries are often inefficient, suffering from highly centralized decision-making, wide fluctuations in budgetary allocations, and poor motivation of facility managers and health workers.[33] This, however, is not an argument for decreasing the budgetary allocation to government hospitals and clinics. Drugs and equipment for surgery and for the wards in these hospitals are in short supply, usually with a poorly functioning ordering system. This creates a vicious cycle of declining staff morale and poor quality of care. These are arguments for breaking the vicious cycle and improving the administrative structure of these hospitals, improving their budgetary allocation, and improving the standard of specialized care by training specialists who are citizens of that country, will take pride in their work, and want to maintain the health care system and develop it further.

The shift of funds and more advanced health care toward the upper income groups of the Third World, which also often involves fraud and bribes, does make it more difficult for the poor to have access to the health system. This also is not an argument for reduction in services to the poor.

The World Bank report recommends that developing countries should spend on average about 50% less than they do currently on less cost-effective interventions and correspondingly increase spending on public health programs such as immunization, AIDS prevention, and "essential clinical services."[33] This economic advice is sound, but should not be advocated to the total detriment of hospital-based specialties, such as neurosurgery. The public health programs, such as pediatric care, TB treatment, and obstetric care, all rely on specialist input in so-called tertiary hospitals to handle the problem patients in these groups. For instance, women in obstructed labor or patients with the complications of TB, such as meningitis, cerebral abscess, and spinal TB with Pott's paraplegia, and many pediatric patients with neurosurgical conditions are readily treatable. Treatment can result in a normal life span and earning capacity, or prevent a life of invalidism and great economic burden to the community. These humanitarian concerns and economic benefits of specialist care to the individual have been neglected in the World Bank report.

The World Bank report argues that if tertiary services benefit only the wealthy, then they should be phased out,[33] but this is illogical. It is the political and administrative systems that require changing, so that the poor will also benefit from the tertiary services. There is a great difference in complexity and expense of various procedures in specialist hospitals, ranging from organ transplantation to the insertion of a ventriculoperitoneal shunt or closure of a low myelomeningocele, both simple and cost-effective procedures. It would be impossible to downgrade some specialist services further than their present state, e.g. neurosurgery in Papua New Guinea or Bangladesh. Therefore, recommendations for further reductions in these and other countries are ludicrous.

Equipment Availability

Even basic equipment and instruments are often lacking in many parts of the developing world, and those that are available are often inappropriate, outdated, or in a state of disrepair (Table 2). Operating room facilities are often primitive, and ancillary supports underdeveloped in the extreme.

Many of the procedures of modern neurosurgery can, however, be performed using minimal levels of technology and instrumentation.[7,11,12,23,35] A basic craniotomy set including perforators, burrs, and Gigli saw, and a laminectomy set including rongeurs and punches are all that is required for many neurosurgical procedures, and these are relatively inexpensive. However, microinstruments, computed tomography (CT) scanners, and electrical—or compressed air-driven craniotomy would be essential equipment for a consultant neurosurgeon.

The practice of multinational companies selling poor-quality, out-of-date, or inappropriate equipment must be eliminated through competition and more efficient ordering. These multinational companies should be selling good-quality equipment at discounted prices to the Third World, particularly because of the bulk orders that could result.

Radiology

Almost two-thirds of the world population lacks access to diagnostic imaging services.[10] There is a gross maldistribution of services, with approximately 80% to 90% of the imaging specialists and equipment located in a few large cities.[10] In underdeveloped countries, inadequate performance of procedures is a problem; 30% to

TABLE 2
Equipment Availability in Underdeveloped Health Care Systems

- Shortages of equipment, drugs, disposables
- Disorganized ordering system
- Expensive, poor-quality imported products
- Inadequate provision for new equipment and replacement of faulty equipment

60% of the equipment is nonfunctional because there is no budget for maintenance, spare parts, and consumables; and radiation protection services are insufficient.[2,9,10] The WHO has developed a Basic Radiological System, which includes training manuals and a simple x-ray unit.[10]

High-technology radiology such as angiography and CT should be available in tertiary centers and is necessary for the development of a neurosurgical service. The acquisition of this technology correlates closely with national political and economic status.[32] Although CT is established in some underdeveloped countries, the ratio of machines to population is significantly lower compared with the developed nations,[32] and CT is still non-existent in many developing countries. When CT is introduced, it requires at least one local technician to maintain the equipment, and an adequate ongoing budget allocation. Magnetic resonance imaging (MRI) is even less available than CT,[32] and is currently an unattainable luxury in many areas. There is one MRI machine for every 15 million people in Central America.[4]

Neurosurgical Practice

Surgery in the developing world is largely performed by generalists and encompasses a broad range of pathology. Patients often present late in the course of their disease, and there is a lack of equipment and aids regarded as essential in affluent countries.[5] The vast problems of developing surgical services in the Third World have been previously outlined.[17,28,29] The scope of neurosurgery in the developing world (Table 3) and the difficulties with training and setting up a neurosurgical service have also been described.[1,5–7,12,16,22] The ratios of neurosurgeons to the general population in the developing world are in stark contrast to the ratios in the developed countries, where one or more neurosurgeons per 200,000 of the population is commonplace (Table 4).

In the developing world, general surgery is better developed than the specialist branches of surgery, such as otorhinolaryngology, ophthamology, and neurosurgery, that require more specialized training. Plastics and orthopedic surgery can often be performed by general surgeons with some additional training, whereas otorhinolaryn-

TABLE 3
Neurosurgical Practice in Underdeveloped Health Care Systems

- Late presentation of disease
- Shortage or unavailability of neurosurgeons
- Lack of trained nursing or ancillary staff
- Poor morale
- Lack of training opportunity
- Inadequate neurology, oncology, radiology, and laboratory investigative services

gology, ophthalmology, and neurosurgery require, for the most part, total devotion to those specialties. However, some basic neurosurgery, particularly neurotrauma, is usually performed by general surgeons.[30] Even the critically ill patient can be catered to adequately in the Third World with meager resources.[27,31]

There is a misconception among primary care advocates that neurosurgical conditions are by-and-large untreatable with poor prognoses. However, much in neurosurgery is eminently treatable with excellent results and often long-term cure, e.g. hydrocephalus, neurotrauma, central nervous system infection, benign cerebral tumors, and congenital and degenerative spinal disorders. The nontreatment of neurosurgical conditions is tragic and results in long-lasting misery or early death for the patient and much distress and disruption to the family, and remains all too common a phenomenon in the developing world. Just a few examples of this are congenital hydrocephalus, frontal encephalocele, spinal cord compression, pituitary tumor, and craniosynostosis. Untreated neurosurgical conditions may produce cosmetic deformity that causes mental anguish and rejection by society. In addition, mental subnormality and behavioral and personality deficits are a cost to the community in terms of institutional care and social service support for the family. Physical deformity and chronic illness destroy the patient's ability to work and support the family. A ruptured disc causing disabling sciatica, TB of the spine causing gibbus deformity and neurologic problems, and chronic lesional epilepsy are examples. Early death from trauma, tumor, or cerebral infection are often preventable by the use

TABLE 4
Neurosurgery Survey in a Number of Diverse Countries with Underdeveloped Health Care

Country*	Total No. of Neurosurgeons	Ratio of Neurosurgeons: Population (millions)	Total Population (millions)†	Reference
Tanzania	0	0:25	25	M Choux, personal communication, 1994
Mozambique	0	0:16	16	M Choux, personal communication, 1994
Angola	0	0:10	10	M Choux, personal communication, 1994
Papua New Guinea	0	0:4	4	JV Rosenfeld
Bangladesh	3	1:35.7	107	G Fabinyi, personal communication, 1994
Nepal	1	1:19	19	RG Lee[16]
Ghana	1	1:18	18	ER Laws[14]
Nigeria	8	1:12	96	A Adeloye[1]
Kenya	4	1:6	24	J Dar[6]
Indonesia	36	1:4.9	178	G Fabinyi, personal communication, 1994
Vietnam	15	1:4.4	66	A Kaye, personal communication, 1994
India	210	1:3.6	850	O Sato[24] and AP Karapurkar[12]
Malaysia	6	1:3	18	M Nachiappan, personal communication, 1994
China	443	1:2.4	1060	O Sato[24]
Philippines	60	1:1	61	A Cedillo, personal communication, 1994
Egypt	74	1:0.7	52	O Sorour[26]

* The selection of these countries was made on the information available to the authors. Inclusion does not imply any distinction from those countries not selected.

† According to the World Bank report.[33]

of timely and straightforward neurosurgery. Treatment of malignant tumors may allow the breadwinner to continue working for a considerable period and enjoy the time remaining with the family. The inability of the breadwinner to work is a reason for producing more children and increasing the population burden. It is thus imperative that simple corrective neurosurgery is available so that pain and suffering are relieved and permanent disability avoided, particularly in a child or a young adult.[7,11,23]

It is not generally appreciated that cancer is a common cause of death in the developing world. In 1985, 56% of the world's 5 million cancer deaths occurred in developing countries.[21] Radiotherapy and chemotherapy programs are also required for any comprehensive oncology service, which would also provide access to palliative radiotherapy of brain and spine malignancies.

The number of neurotrauma cases in the developing world is likely to increase significantly as the number of motor vehicles and thus the number of motor vehicle accidents increase.[18,25,34] The number of fatal road accidents in Papua New Guinea rose more than 400% between 1968 and 1978,[25] and 65.5% of road fatalities involved head injuries.[34]

The prevalence of cerebrovascular disease is likely to increase as life expectancy increases in the developing world. As the prevalence of neurotrauma, cancer, and cerebrovascular disease increases in the developing world, there will be a proportionate increase in the need for neurosurgical services.

A Paradigm for Progress

The Schism of Primary and Specialty Care

The World Bank report[33] advocates a threefold approach to improving the health of the developing world: 1) to foster an economic environment that enables households to improve their own health, with growth policies within the Third World ensuring income growth of the poor; 2) to develop more cost-effective government spending programs that do more to help the poor; and 3) to promote greater diversity and competition in the financing and delivery of health services. Developing world governments are to encourage private sector involvement.

It is proposed that these reforms will translate into longer, healthier, and more productive lives for poor people. It is also claimed that too much of the health care budget currently goes to specialist care in tertiary facilities that provide little gain for the money spent, and that too little money is spent on low-cost, highly effective programs, such as control and treatment of infectious disease and malnutrition.[33]

On the contrary, the primary care movement has maintained pre-eminent influence with granting bodies.[33] The proportion of the grants going to secondary and tertiary care have traditionally been overwhelmed by grants distributed to primary health care and preventive strategies. It is important that this imbalance is redressed. Some grants should be targeted for hospital-based care, so that hospital infrastructure is strengthened and the necessary equipment purchased. However, the disadvantage of targeting grants is

that the developing nation may perceive that "colonial powers" are dictating terms and being too meddlesome in their internal affairs.

In developing strategies for delivery of neurosurgical services to the developing countries, the neurosurgeons in the developed country should first ask the question "Does the country want help?" Imperious and paternalistic thrusting of health care services on developing countries who guard their independence vigorously is an all too frequent mistake. Respect for local customs and culture, language, and medical practice is an essential prerequisite for any health care aid. Delicate and step-wise diplomacy is needed.[8] Policy that promotes managerial, medical, and nursing self-reliance in the developing world is the essence of the solution to developing neurosurgery in underserved areas. Enhancement of pride in the work and development of a sense of achievement among the local care-givers is vital for success. Sending sophisticated teams to the Third World on whirlwind tours to display surgical virtuosity may be of little worth in developing such specialist services. However, great gains will be made from the visits of individual neurosurgeons who can show the local medical and nursing staff and health administration what good can come of neurosurgery. Mutual respect will evolve, which will help to stimulate future neurosurgical and related endeavors.

The excessive bias toward primary health care and preventive strategies at the expense of specialist interventions, such as neurosurgery, requires intense lobbying from neurosurgical organizations to influence the main funding bodies, such as the World Bank and the WHO.

Most countries view access to basic health care as a human right. Perhaps the word "basic" should be removed from this phrase, so that *health care becomes a human right.*

"Health care for all by the year 2000" was a goal of the Alma-Ata conference of the WHO and United Nations Children's Fund in 1978.[33] This goal should include access to specialized hospital facilities in countries where there is political stability and the administrative structure to develop such a plan. The World Bank report describes advances in income and education creating advances in health; economic policies that lead to sustained growth improve health standards in the Third

World. Education of children, especially girls, leads to improved health standards. It is stated that prevention is the mainstay of a health care program.[33] This may be so, but diseases that have already occurred also require adequate treatment.

The World Bank has proposed five "essential clinical services" of high cost-effectiveness: obstetric and antenatal care, family planning, TB control, control of sexually transmitted diseases, and treatment of common pediatric illness.[33] The treatment of infection and trauma is included in this group. General surgeons perform much of this treatment in the developing world. However, input from neurosurgeons, orthopedic surgeons, and other surgical specialists, and the provision of adequate resources and facilities are required to optimize this treatment. The practice of the medical and surgical specialties is intimately enmeshed with these essential clinical services and adequate coverage of the population with the full range of these essential clinical services cannot be achieved unless specialty care is also available. The World Bank predicts saving 9 million infants with the introduction of their policies, but these infants may still require more advanced care from neurosurgeons and other specialists later in life.

Creating an Infrastructure for Future Development

Adoption of the package for essential clinical services would require a quadrupling of expenditures on public health.[33] The method of paying for the package invokes a shifting of resources down the pyramid to the community facilities and health centers, but this would create a disaster for the care of patients with problems requiring a specialist. These patients are already struggling or unable to be treated in the hospitals of the Third World. Watters and Bayley[28] have outlined the training required for doctors and surgeons to meet the surgical needs of Africa. These surgeons should be trained to perform a wide variety of procedures, including some neurosurgery.

Clearly, the training of subspecialist surgeons must continue and be fostered by specialized surgical organizations. Specialist physicians and surgeons should be carefully selected from the most able of local medical graduates and be trained with financial and intellectual aid from the developed nations. These surgical trainees should train in their own countries and receive a strong grounding in general surgery. Having completed some basic specialized surgical training in their own country, if it is available, they should then be encouraged to do additional training in sponsoring countries. Fellowships are already available through WHO and other surgical and medical organizations. Hands-on experience should be a prominent feature of the fellowship experience. Observational and supernumerary status are not sufficient to make the experience worthwhile. Particular experience in neuroradiology, including the performance and interpretation of angiograms, is essential.[22] A strong grounding in neurology, neuropathology, and neuroanesthesiology are also highly desirable.[7] Neurosurgery training programs are already established in several developing countries,[1,13] but until a surgical specialty such as neurosurgery is established in the developing country, the trainee chosen to become a neurosurgeon will have to do all the higher training abroad. As the service is developed, the trainees will spend more of their training time in their own country. In this way, the countries of the developing world retain ultimate control of their destiny and develop more self-sufficiency in health care. Viable employment contracts should be forthcoming on the return of the trainees, otherwise many will wish to remain abroad (as has happened in the past) or return to an exclusively private practice. However, even if these graduates choose to practice privately in their home country, they will invariably contribute to the local medical infrastructure, which eventually serves all patients to some degree.

According to the World Bank report:[33] "Scaling back public spending for tertiary care facilities, specialist training and clinical care with lower cost effectiveness would help to increase the effectiveness of health spending." This may free up some money for the essential clinical services, but that would be at the expense of specialized care, which is still a necessary part of the health system. "Health care for all by 2000" cannot be achieved by scaling down advanced care or eliminating it altogether.

Selective development of a specialized infrastructure, including neurosurgery, at regional centers in underdeveloped countries will help keep private patients (notably the local wealthy) at home, and help invest their money in the local health care economy. This can benefit all patients. For example, the partial subsidy of a CT scanner (purchase and operation) by local governments and academic centers will allow local paying patients to undergo such scanning locally, and perhaps further care as well. This will help stem the common practice of such paying patients obtaining their care abroad, thereby draining the local health care economy of much needed hard currency. It is a common observance in many regions overseas for the local wealthy and middle class (as rare and relatively poor as they may be) to spend precious and limited hard currency overseas on the care of a single patient—at times selling cattle or land to care for a son or daughter with a brain tumor in London, Paris, Cairo, or Santiago, for example. This money, invested locally, will contribute to the success and viability of local centers, transforming health care in poorer countries from *underdeveloped* ("sous-developpé") to *developing* ("en voie de developpement"). Selective strategic investment in nuclei of specialized health care will insure against a permanent institutionalization of inferiority and will give real hope to the poor for a true framework of health care development.

The Role of Neurosurgical Organizations

The neurosurgical organizations of an advanced nation already closely associated with a particular developing country should enter into direct negotiation with the government of a developing country to lobby for improved neurosurgical facilities and to offer assistance with neurosurgical training and neurosurgical care by promoting visits from neurosurgeons for short periods and allowing trainees from the developing countries to visit their neurosurgical centers. The Federation for International Education in Neurosurgery is helping to develop indigenous neurosurgical training programs in underdeveloped countries.[14,15] There are also other programs under the auspices of the World Federation of Neurosurgical Societies, The International Committee of the Congress of Neurological Surgeons, and British and French-Speaking Neurosurgical Societies.

Visiting surgeons need to spend enough time in the developing world to teach the local surgeons, surgical trainees, medical students, and nurses the art and science of neurosurgery, and its value and place in the overall health care of their people. A minimum of 2 weeks and preferably longer is recommended. An extended period of employment as an expatriate may be the stimulus required to establish a neurosurgical service. The visiting neurosurgeon should work under the same conditions as the local surgeons to prove that neurosurgery can be performed successfully with basic equipment and resources. Good standards in neurosurgery can be achieved with limited equipment.[11,23,35] The visiting neurosurgeon could then better advise his or her hosts on what additional equipment is required.

Experience and personal relationships will be developed, enabling the visiting neurosurgeon to better appreciate what is required to train a neurosurgeon in that environment, and enabling the local staff to develop respect and trust for the visitor and his or her own institution and country of origin. The expansion of personal horizons, intellectual maturity, and respect for humanity that comes from such a visit cannot be over-emphasized, and favorably adds to the persona of whoever experiences it.

Neurosurgical care should remain within a regionalized (government or academic) hospital system of the developing world. Patients with the ability to pay for their care should be required to recompense the health system so that this money can be used to support and develop the health system.

Donation of equipment and books is appreciated and is an important component of developing neurosurgical services, but should not be regarded as an excuse for local health authorities to neglect their responsibilities. Lists of essential equipment for neurosurgical operating rooms and wards in the Third World should be developed, with appropriate consultative advice, by the neurosurgical bodies of the advanced nations. The multinational drug and medical equipment companies, particularly those involved in neurosurgical supplies, should be lobbied to improve the quality of products being sold to the Third World. Bulk purchases should be encouraged to enable reduced prices. The local manufacture of disposables and prostheses, such as shunts,[19] is economically very attractive, and should be encouraged by the targeting of seeding grants.

Universities and large specialized medical centers in the United States and other developed countries have initiated focused nuclei of international development activities through foreign trainees and graduates, or the care of selected wealthy patients from otherwise massively poor or underserved regions. These have resulted in sustained contacts, focused assistance programs, the training of successive generations from the same country, and frequent visits among an expanding network of colleagues. Such experiences by centers such as the Henry Ford Hospital in Detroit, The Cleveland Clinic Foundation, and Yale University have advanced in a small and sustained fashion the neurosurgical care in many regions of the world. These and other efforts by individuals and organizations should not be discouraged by well-intended but ill-fated broad macroeconomic policies that result in the crushing of these promising seeds of specialist development.

Nongovernment foreign aid is often misdirected and carries high administrative costs. Increased development aid needs to be directed to health care, but the distribution needs to be worked out very carefully so that specialist services and training receive some of this help, with the aim of nurturing local access and expertise.

Greater reliance on the private sector to deliver services would improve efficiency, but potential overservicing is a danger. Government regulation of the private sector and the health insurance system is an important goal. Charging wealthy local patients for treatment in government hospitals would significantly increase the income in these institutions, allow for upgrading of their standards, and aid those who cannot afford to pay. The World Bank recommendation that competition be introduced to improve efficiency and that there be performance incentives, decentralization, competition between suppliers, and government regulation of private services would all work to improve health care delivery to the poor. This cannot be accomplished without a focused investment in a specialized infrastructure, including neurosurgery.

Allocation of limited grants or even a minor reduction in the massive primary health care budget would have a significant effect in redressing the current imbalance in resources to specialized surgical services versus those directed to primary and preventive care.

A Global Neurosurgical Perspective

Primary health care is of overriding importance in the development and maintenance of health care services, but this should not be developed and supported to the exclusion of specialized hospital-based services. Patients with neurosurgical problems can often be cured or helped significantly by having the opportunity to undergo neurosurgery, even if at a basic level. Pain, suffering, disability, employment prospects, and longevity can often be significantly improved by the neurosurgeon. There is a desperate shortage of trained neurosurgeons in the developing world.

Neurosurgeons of the advanced and prosperous nations have a great responsibility to assist in the development of neurosurgical services in the developing world. This will produce lasting benefits to all mankind. Neurosurgical organizations need to lobby the governments of the developing world, the humanitarian aid organizations, and the World Bank to implement change.

Philosophically, neurosurgeons of the prosperous world cannot accept the premise that their professional contribution is a luxury that cannot be afforded by mankind. Nor can we condemn to a perpetual double standard the vast populations with limited access to any modern health care resources. The macroeconomic "equation" that has determined that neurosurgery is an unnecessary and unaffordable service ignores a fundamental variable—namely, the right of underdeveloped peoples to a chance to develop. Without this variable, international health care initiatives will be as shortsighted and destructive as "well-meaning and rationalized" colonial determinations of yesteryear. The world is becoming closer through effective communications and more affordable technology. We should aim toward similar standards of health care throughout the globe, far-reaching as this goal may be, rather than arbitrary sentencing of vast masses to perpetual underdevelopment.

A paradigm for progress toward this goal should not ignore the vast and urgent primary care needs of utmost epidemiologic impact. However, a true battle against poverty and neglect cannot be waged without a modest and focused investment in the infrastructure for future development. Such an investment should not be obstructed by other health care strategies, and can be viewed as a small part of a multifaceted strategy for improved health care. Neurosurgeons, in individual and coordinated efforts, and professional and academic organizations can and should share their perspective, vision, knowledge, and resources toward this end. Let us dream that a resected benign neoplasm, a clipped aneurysm, or a spinal cord injury carefully nursed to full recovery are not cures that belong only to the wealthy.

References

1. Adeloye A. Perspectives in international neurosurgery: neurosurgery in Nigeria. *Neurosurgery.* 1983;13:333–336.
2. Aggarwal SK. Problems of radiology in the Indian subcontinent. *Invest Radiol.* 1993;28(suppl 3): S32–S33.
3. Apuzzo ML, ed. *Neurosurgery for the Third Millennium.* Park Ridge, Ill: American Association of Neurological Surgeons; 1992.
4. Arredondo F. Technology and practice of radiology in central America. *Invest Radiol.* 1993;28(suppl 3):S30.
5. Clezy JKA. Surgery in the tropics. *Med J Aust.* 1993;159:552–555.
6. Dar J. Perspectives in international neurosurgery: neurosurgery in Kenya. *Neurosurgery.* 1985;16: 267–269.
7. Djhnga S. Perspectives in international neurosurgery: neurosurgery in Zaire. *Neurosurgery.* 1983; 13:95–97.
8. Durham Smith E. The responsibility of established colleges to the developing world. *Aust NZ J Surg.* 1994;64:1-3. Editorial.
9. Fuchs WA. Radiology in developing countries. *Invest Radiol.* 1993;28(suppl 3):S27
10. Hanson GP, Volodin V. Developing world. World Health Organization programs in third world countries. *Invest Radiol.* 1993;28(suppl 3):S24-S25.
11. Jacob OJ, Rosenfeld JV, Watters DAK. The repair of frontal encephaloceles in Papua New Guinea. *Aust NZ J Surg.* 1994. In press.
12. Karapurkar AP, Pandya SK. Neurosurgery in India. *Neurosurg Rev.* 1983;6:85-92.
13. Kiryabwire JWM. Neurosurgery in Uganda. *Neurosurgery.* 1987;20:664–665.
14. Laws ER Jr. Report of the activities of the Foundation for International Education in Neurological Surgery. *Neurosurgery.* 1993;33:775.
15. Laws ER. Foundation for International Education in Neurosurgery. *J Neurosurg.* 1994:80;352. Letter.
16. Lee RG, Gongal DN. Neurology and neurosurgery in Nepal. *Can J Neurol Sci.* 1983;10:117-118.
17. Loefler IJP. Surgery in the third world. *Clin Trop Med Comm Dis.* 1988;3:173-189.
18. Lourie JA. Use of seat-belts in Port Moresby. *Papua New Guinea Med J.* 1982;25:214-218.
19. Oliver MJ, Museta F. Treatment of hydrocephalus using the Harare valve. *Proc Assoc Surg E Africa.* 1989; 12:80-82.
20. Pandya SK, ed. *Neurosciences in India: Retrospect and Prospect.* Trivandrum, India: The Neurology Society of India; New Dehli, India: Council of Scientific and Industrial Research; 1989.
21. Pisani P, Parkin DM, Ferlay J. Estimates of the worldwide mortality from eighteen major cancers in 1985. Implications for prevention and projections of future burden. *Int J Cancer.* 1993;55:891–903.
22. Puplampu B. Perspectives in international neurosurgery: neurosurgery in Ghana. *Neurosurgery.* 1983; 12:241.
23. Rosenfeld JV, Kevau I, Jacob O, et al. Dumbbell schwannoma causing acute spinal cord compression: case report. *Papau New Guinea Med J.* 1994; 37:47–50.
24. Sato O. Pediatric neurosurgery around the world—Asia and Australia. *Childs Nerv Syst.* 1988;4: 317–320.
25. Sinha SN, Sengupta SK, Purohit RC. A five year review of deaths following trauma. *Papua New Guinea Med J.* 1981;24:222-228.
26. Sorour O. Neurosurgery in Egypt. *Neurosurgery.* 1986;19:142-143.
27. Watters DAK. Organisation and management. In: Watters DAK, Wilson IH, Leaver RJ, et al, eds. *Care of the Critically Ill Patient in the Tropics and Subtropics.* London, England: Macmillan; 1991;2 94–306.
28. Watters DAK, Bayley AC. Training doctors and surgeons to meet the surgical needs of Africa. *Br Med J.* 1987;295:761-763.
29. Watters DAK, Bem C, Echun DA, et al. Audit of 'surgery in general' in an African teaching hospital. *J R Coll Surg Edinb.* 1991;36:402–404.
30. Watters DAK, Sinclair JR. Outcome of severe head injuries in central Africa. *J R Coll Surg Edinb.* 1988;33:35–38.
31. Watters DAK, Sinclair JR, Warren I. Care for the critically ill in Africa. *Proc Assoc Surgeons E Africa.* 1987;10:57-62.
32. Wittenberg J. Radiology in South America. Contrasting political/economic imperatives and opportunities. *Invest Radiol.* 1993;(suppl 3):S28-S29.
33. World Bank: World Bank Development Report 1993. Investing in Health. Executive Summary. Washington, DC: The World Bank; 1993.
34. Wyatt GB. The epidemiology of road accidents in Papua New Guinea. *Papau New Guinea Med J.* 1980;23:60–65.
35. Zeng-fu J. A brief history of the development of neurosurgery in China. *Chinese Med J.* 1987; 100: 503–508.

Conceptual Synthesis: Elements of a Philosophy of Neurological Surgery

Issam A. Awad, MD, MSc, FACS

The preceding chapters of this book have outlined the basic elements of a philosophy of neurological surgery. These are summarized in this conceptual synthesis, including the defining questions, the dimensions of the neurosurgical identity, the scope of the neurosurgical mission and challenges, and a universal concept of the neurosurgical school. These elements are presented briefly and conceptually in this chapter; the reader is referred for more detailed consideration to the individual chapters of the book. It is also clear that our examination in this book of many of these elements has been limited in scope, depth, and perspective, and that additional study and detailed analysis of each element is required. This synthesis represents a glimpse of where we are in the consideration of defining questions of our field, and plants the seeds for future scholarship and thoughtful discussion on our identity, our method, and our purpose.

Defining Questions and the Neurosurgical Identity

Most philosophic questions can be articulated within the scope of metaphysics, epistemology, and ethics. In the first realm, we must discuss the notions of the neurosurgical system, including a clear statement of our identity and our purpose. We are the product of a proud heritage, taking on the task of manipulating the nervous system so as to alleviate suffering or to cure disease involving this system. This heritage includes notions of medicine, of surgery, and features unique to surgeons who study and tackle the human nervous system. It is a heritage of science, of technical precision and determination, of art, of supreme responsibility and accountability, and of empathy. There is little room for error in our work, recognizing a sense of elitist selection of those few who will dedicate more than half of their lives to attaining the knowledge and skills required from our profession, and the rest of their lives in the continuing thrust to learn, to apply new techniques, and to re-examine strategies and approaches. Our system is based on intense knowledge, attention to detail, and careful technical performance. It is also a system of urgent and decisive action within narrow therapeutic time windows. The outcome of our work is measured by the impact on the human mind, intelligence, cognition, independence, physical ability, and life's worth in the highest and most demanding sense. We are the products of this heritage, and of these requirements inherently imposed upon us and also embraced and adopted by us.

These notions of the neurosurgical system impose a theory of neurosurgical knowledge, and a method of articulating questions and relating them to our experience. In an epistemologic sense, we possess a method, a science. This is intimately related in heritage, theory, and application to biologic and also clinical science. The neurosurgeon uses the concepts, knowledge, and techniques of the biologist and the clinical scientist. The neurosurgeon also contributes to the broad scope of biologic and clinical science through unique experiential observations, skills, and perspective.

The neurosurgeon is also an artist, contributing to beauty, perfection, and harmony in technical work, and in the very implication of his work on order and harmony in the nervous system and in the patient's life. The neurosurgeon is a part of a complex interaction of vectors known as the clinical community—patients, other physicians, administrators, and political, legal, and economic forces. The neurosurgeon works for a purpose that is foremost and inherently patient-centered, and therefore considers and evaluates each experience, concept, and method in reference to the patient, the patient's well-being, and the possible effects on society as a conglomerate of patients or potential patients harboring or risking neurosurgical disease.

Neurosurgical disease is defined in the existential tradition as a set of clinical entities where the opinion or action of a neurosurgeon contributes to advanced knowledge, better prognosis, or more effective treatment than in the absence of such an opinion or action. Hence, neurosurgical disease and the role of the neurosurgeon are not defined by the narrow scope of one or another neurosurgical intervention, but rather by the broader potential for good through such intervention, and also through refining, avoiding, or limiting—or precisely timing or imposing—such intervention. The neurosurgeon aims to understand the disease, the technology, and the potential as well as the limitations of surgical intervention. The scientific dimensions of neurosurgical disease include the formulation of hypotheses through experiential observations, and the methodologic testing of these hypotheses to confirm or exclude them, and hence to advance scientific knowledge and the practice of neurosurgery. Hypotheses include epidemiologic perspectives and mechanistic questions based on system, cell, and molecular biologic concepts, aiming to explain and also to predict clinical behavior. They also include conceptual queries and question-driven technology assessment aimed at modifying the disease, including detection, diagnosis, prognostication, and treatment. These encompass most certainly, but are not limited to, the assessment of neurosurgical intervention itself and the objective evaluation of the strengths, weaknesses, and limitations of our concepts, our methods, and our tools. The neurosurgical system, as in Karl Popper's view of any scientific system, is a set of hypotheses rather than a body of knowledge.

Lastly, our philosophy is shaped by an ethical perspective. Our patient-centered mission imposes a moral dimension on our work, including our methods, tools, and objectives. Yet, our altruism cannot be accepted a priori. We are challenged to reflect on our moral excellence as we do on our technical and scientific excellence. We must justify to ourselves, to individual patients, to the clinical community, and to society as a whole the worth of our contribution. This worth is measured not only in terms of individual human wellness, but also in the common good and purpose, and increasingly also on a socioeconomic scale. Competing currents and allegiances must be balanced, including a foremost role as the individual patient's advocate, but also the role as an advocate for society, the clinical community, and the purposes of truth and knowledge. To do so, the neurosurgeon must master the mature wisdom of philosophers and remain content and generous in his view of himself and in his relationship to his family and to the medical and human community. Ethics, etiquette, and personal harmony must converge in the life and work of neurosurgeons, as highlighted in the Discourses of the stoic philosopher Epictetus: "To achieve the good life, a man must master his desires, perform his duties, and think correctly concerning himself and the world. Every man has a duty to others because each man is a citizen of the world, and one of its principal parts. Duties are universally measured by relations, and relations by understanding one's role and acting well the part that is given to you." The understanding of a neurosurgeon's role and harmonizing it with the roles of others must be an integral part of our reflection on our self-worth, our contribution, and our moral excellence.

In summary, the neurosurgical identity includes a historical heritage and role models, and a method of science and biology, cognizant of the universality of truth and also of doubt. It embodies an art, with dimensions of esthetics and expression, and the responsible application of technology. It also includes a noble purpose committed to the well-being of man and of society, a mission of service, and a quest toward harmony with our fellow man. The universality of Perfection is recognized in scientific pursuits and in the decisiveness of healing. The same ideal of Beauty is sought in art, in love, in human relations, and in the truths of science. Being a neurosurgeon is the ultimate embodiment of this vision.

Diversity and the Global Challenge

The universality of our identity, the defined neurosurgical method integrating and balancing science and the surgical art, and the common ideals and harmony of our mission conceal an equally remarkable diversity in neurological surgery. Modern neurological surgery evolved in several countries almost simultaneously, driven undoubtedly by a revolution in communications and cross-fertilization of ideas. This represented a splendid triumph of human ideals and common purpose during a century when those same countries were torn by two great wars and a prolonged ideologic chill. The temporal leadership and technical superiority of one group of neurosurgeons did not translate into supreme intellectual dominance of the field. Instead, tremendous cross-cultural fertilization created a dynamic and highly eclectic medium with local cultural and traditional colors.

The Industrialized World

Continental and British neurosurgeons and scientists influenced the fathers of modern neurological surgery in America. These men in turn trained many leaders of neurosurgical departments throughout the world. European neurosurgery reasserted its leadership through technical and intellectual giants including Yasargil, who in turn influenced the next generation of neurosurgeons through microsurgical technique. Also, European functional neurosurgeons, including Leksell and Taillerach, had a tremendous impact on the renaissance of stereotactic and functional neurosurgery in North America. American and Canadian neurosurgical centers maintained at the same time a leadership role in the science and technology of modern neurosurgery, subspecialization, multidisciplinary interface, and defining standards of neurosurgical outcome assessment and education. Yet the same academic centers of excellence that cradled modern neurological surgery in North America were themselves influenced by the German model of the university as a center for both teaching *and* research.

Japanese neurosurgery evolved from native roots, but also with strong European and American influence. In less than one generation, the tremendous influence of this school was noted worldwide, notably in technique and in neurovascular surgery.

It is accurate to note that modern neurosurgery developed almost simultaneously and with a balance and diversity of influence among the industrialized countries in the 20th century, despite the conflicts tearing these countries apart and the varied traditions of medicine and science and strong ethnic and cultural colors. This remarkable diversity reflected what Harvey Cushing described as "the kind of sympathetic and encouraging interest in one another's activities . . . (which) held the respect of the Profession as a whole." This evolved because of common purpose—unique and formidable challenges requiring collaboration—and also because of the universality of neurosurgical ideals.

Major ongoing challenges facing neurological surgery in these developed nations relate to the responsible use of technology, the integration and application of explosive scientific information, and the self-examination of the neurosurgical mission in relation to the expectations of society. Opportunities abound in these same areas, aiming to further enhance safety and effectiveness and to decrease risks and costs of neurosurgical intervention through advanced technology, including computer modeling and robotics, and to develop innovative neurosurgical strategies through cellular and molecular neurosurgery while better predicting—and explaining—disease behavior.

A sober reassessment of our worth to society is being imposed on us on purely socioeconomic terms. It must be answered by self-assessment on these same terms through better awareness and active participation in these aspects important to society, and also on equally important moral and ethical grounds. There are unique opportunities in public health and medical education about neurosurgical disease in our own societies, and also more magnificent opportunities in international neurosurgical education and development.

The Developing Nations

Simultaneously, students of the founding schools of neurosurgery established neurosurgical departments in many countries and regions of the world, reflecting the training, traditions, and aspirations of their respective mentors. The same neurosurgical seed prevalent in industrialized nations was now planted in diverse soils and climates. Within a generation, the practice of neurosurgery in these less-developed countries had evolved and adapted to local constraints of education, culture, and economic pressures. It also evolved to meet special public health needs of local populations in harmony with local traditions and medical, socioeconomic, and religious forces. The neurosurgical schools of India, The Middle East, and South America represent examples of such traditions.

These schools have adapted the most advanced neurosurgical concepts and techniques despite formidable economic and cultural barriers. Ingenious uses of private capital have allowed the development of a sophisticated local medical infrastructure—initially private, then resulting in local investment of hard currency in health care (hard currency that would have been spent by the local wealthy abroad to seek the same services). This infrastructure has surprisingly become accessible to an increasing fraction of the middle class, and often at a cost quite affordable through local means.

However, local problems have permeated this promising developing neurosurgical infrastructure: rampant inflation and an increasing gap between the haves and the have-nots, local corruption, and the absence of investment in the endowment of academic institutions, even by some local neurosurgical leaders who amassed substantial personal wealth through the private sector as described above. In some countries, many among the cast of senior neurosurgeons have not invested in the development of a local academic neurosurgical hierarchy, nor have they been willing to entrust more junior colleagues with subspecialization, program development, or education. They have not embraced later in their careers the same progressive philosophy that allowed them to establish and lead the local schools. Problems of access of the poor to even trivial neurosurgical services are often compounded by the lack of well-trained neurosurgeons in public service or the lack of technology availability to these patients. These problems are worsening with poorer per capita income, cruel inflation, and an absent public health care infrastructure.

Yet these nations harbor the seeds of a neurosurgical renaissance in view of the number of native neurosurgeons superbly trained abroad who may consider returning to work locally as the incentives of neurosurgical practice in Western countries are rapidly declining. This native talent is further attracted by improving economic and political conditions in much of the Middle East, Eastern Europe, and South America, and by the decline of the power and expertise of many existing medical forces in these countries, hence the appeal of opportunities not possible in yesteryears. These younger neurosurgeons understand the potential effectiveness and limitations of technology and of subspecialization. Many are computer literate, and can potentially develop innovative and inexpensive access to the world information revolution. They potentially can develop real-time audiovisual satellite consultative links with major Western centers at the cost of telephone communication.

This future generation of local neurosurgical leaders may also hope to play a strong role in academic institutions of excellence that have existed in many of the countries, and may hopefully strive toward the same neurosurgical universal ideals articulated previously. They can adapt these same ideals to local needs and aspirations, and mobilize local resources and cultural assets toward these ideals.

The Underdeveloped World

The economic and cultural gaps that can realistically be closed in many developing countries are grossly unsurmountable in much of the underdeveloped world. An increasing *majority* of our planet harbors stark poverty, hunger, poor basic health and hygiene, a sobering illiteracy and lack of technical infrastructure, and a rapidly growing population in increasing misery. Resources available for health care are in fact shrinking on a per capita basis in much of the underdeveloped world, with many people able to watch real-time international news service on local television while being denied access to basic immunizations and minimal nutrition. This sobering economic and sociopolitical milieu prevents all but the most rudimentary neurosurgical services in many regions, without the faint hope of a favorable change in the near future.

Yet there is a surplus of neurosurgical knowledge in more developed countries, and even in some regions of the same continents. There is also a surplus of usable equipment and materials rejected by Western standards. There have been procedural, legal, and local cultural barriers that have prevented distribution of these human and material resources, barriers that must be eliminated, along with local fraud, so as to allow a bare minimum standard of neurosurgical access to these masses.

World health organizations have operated on macroeconomic assumptions that any neurosurgical infrastructure is too expensive and would shunt scarce resources away from more pressing nutritional and public health needs. Yet, organized neurosurgery must rise to this challenge of purpose, asserting that a minimal and modest specialized technical infrastructure can achieve tremendous individual and public welfare, and can represent the seed of future modern medical development. We cannot afford to further widen the technical and knowledge gap lest we condemn vast masses to perpetual underdevelopment. This challenge belongs to neurosurgeons, and we must meet it with our own human and material resources, so vastly maldistributed among the human pool that these resources must serve.

Toward the Future: A Framework of Neurosurgical Development

On the eve of the third millennium, the future of neurological surgery must depend on a sense of identity from within, a keen awareness of our purpose, and a commitment to re-examine and continually improve our system in response to the needs of society and the dynamic challenges and opportunities presented to us. Our heritage is solid and proud, and our accomplishments in the past decades have been exemplary. We cannot and should not consider any compromise of these values; such compromise is incompatible with and would betray our greatness. Our patient-centered philosophy, the stringent self-imposed standards of moral excellence, competence, and conduct, our intellectual honesty through objectivity and science, and our commitment to universal ideals are formidable assets that society and mankind hold in highest esteem. They are our most splendid weapon in the societal battle of self-worth.

Yet we do not have access to limitless resources commensurate with this identity and with our dreams. We must justify to society the worth of what we take in return for our "contribution," and this must be expressed in individual human terms as well as in relation to mankind. We must carefully define local needs and the local and global resources—in a world where the sharing of knowledge is easier and less expensive than ever. We must articulate specific goals and achievable objectives consistent with our clear mission and purpose, but also with those needs and resources.

Such is the framework of a strategy of neurosurgical development, motivated by a common identity and ideals and driven by local needs and available resources. Our heritage, the demanding mastery of the art and of extraordinary performance and service, and the tremendous surplus—and also maldistribution of information and knowledge—should fuel this development. Its elements are to a certain degree technical and material, but to a greater extent moral and intellectual. Investment in meaningful local schools of neurosurgery will perpetuate this commitment to our universal ideals and will allow it to sprout local roots in response to local cultural wealth, needs, and aspirations.

Questions for *Philosophy of Neurological Surgery*

The following questions have been provided to give physicians the option of testing their comprehension of the material provided in *Philosophy of Neurological Surgery*. The test is to be self-scored. Answers may be found in the back of this book. A Continuing Medical Education (CME) certificate will be mailed upon the return of the enclosed test evaluation/feedback card along with a $25 administrative fee. Telephone 708-692-9500 to order additional evaluation/ feedback cards or information about other CME products from the American Association of Neurological Surgeons.

After reading this book, a physician should be able to:
- identify a historical and philosophic framework for the discipline of neurological surgery
- formulate relevant historical references that have shaped the field
- conceptualize the scientific and clinical methods of neurological surgery
- integrate historical, clinical, scientific, artistic, ethical, and legal perspectives into the current and future directions of the field.

Philosophy of Neurological Surgery

1. The research university is:
   (A) an ancient format in use in medical education since the Greeks.
   (B) a product of funds available from the National Institutes of Health.
   (C) a revolutionary concept that began in Germany about 100 years ago.
   (D) the product of a committee of deans organized in 1890.
   (Chapter 1)

2. The revolutionary changes in medical education introduced by William Welch included:
   (A) an undergraduate degree, competitive examinations before acceptance, formal examination during the educational process, and entrance of women into medicine.
   (B) a men-only medical school, preference for children of physicians, a 4-year curriculum, and practical medical training at the bedside.
   (C) a required research experience during medical school, competitive entrance for all races, no examinations, and a pass/fail system.
   (D) emphasis upon bedside teaching rather than science, teaching to be done by full professors, specific positions set aside for women, and a formal lecture program.
   (Chapter 1)

3. William Halsted created the following as the primary new fields of specialization in surgery:
   (A) neurosurgery, ophthalmology, and neurology
   (B) orthopedics, urology, and otolaryngology
   (C) orthopedics, urology, otolaryngology, and ophthalmology
   (D) orthopedics, urology, neurosurgery, and ophthalmology
   (Chapter 1)

4. Harvey Cushing's career in neurosurgery was likely because of:
   (A) the influence of William Osler and Theodore Kocher during his training.
   (B) a long-standing interest in the nervous system present even as a medical student.
   (C) an assignment by Halsted against his will.
   (D) an assignment given by William Welch.
   (Chapter 1)

5. Walter Dandy became Chief of Neurosurgery at Johns Hopkins after Harvey Cushing because:
   (A) he was personally chosen by Dr. Cushing and installed in his place.
   (B) he was personally chosen by William Welch and trained to follow Cushing.
   (C) of his own inclination to fill a void after Cushing left.
   (D) he was personally chosen by William Halsted and trained specifically for the position.
   (Chapter 1)

For each of the phrases concerning theories of ethical behavior, choose from the list below the person or persons whose concepts most closely fit the phrase.

6. categorical imperative

7. utilitarian for society

8. theologically based

9. a theory acceptable to all
   (A) David Hume
   (B) Immanuel Kant
   (C) Jean-Jacques Rousseau
   (D) none of the above
   (Chapter 5)

Match the phrase with the most appropriate response below.

10. rules delineating behavior and conduct

11. passive life-ending decisions for justified cause

12. best for both medicine and society

13. consideration of how to proceed toward a decision
    (A) medical ethics
    (B) medical etiquette
    (C) both A and B
    (D) neither A nor B

(Chapter 5)

Determine if the following statements are *true* or *false.*

14. There is no significant difference between morals and ethics.

15. Medical ethics have evolved in part because there is no universally acceptable concept of ethics.
    (A) The statement is *true.*
    (B) The statement is *false.*

(Chapter 5)

16. The following are *true* regarding Aristotle's understanding of brain function *except:*
    (A) it closely resembled, in general, modern neurologic/physiologic views.
    (B) it identified the brain as an organ to cool the blood.
    (C) it considered the heart as the seat of the emotions and sensations.
    (D) it included the observation that the brain was cold and bloodless.

(Chapter 6)

17. The Greek physician Galen:
    (A) lived in the same century as Hippocrates.
    (B) considered the ventricles as the seat of mental activity and memory.
    (C) described reflex action for the first time.
    (D) thought epilepsy originated in the heart.

(Chapter 6)

18. The following is true about Leonardo da Vinci *except:*
    (A) he accepted the medieval "cellular doctrine" of brain function.
    (B) he was the first to demonstrate the anatomy of the ventricles.
    (C) he considered the cerebral cortex important for higher brain function.
    (D) he depicted reasonably well the anatomy of the skull and the foramina for the cranial nerves.

(Chapter 6)

19. René Descartes:
    (A) was a contemporary of Shakespeare.
    (B) discovered the pituitary as a hormonal gland.
    (C) described the elements of reflex action.
    (D) viewed the thalamus as a relay center for pain sensation.

(Chapter 6)

20. The 17th century physician Thomas Willis:
    (A) accepted the views of Aristotle on brain function.
    (B) was a general practitioner who had little interest in medical science.
    (C) considered the cerebral cortex to be important for intellectual activity.
    (D) agreed fully with Descartes on the role of the pineal gland as the central seat of sensation.

(Chapter 6)

21. The field of phrenology:
    (A) flourished in the latter part of the 19th century.
    (B) had little influence on the development of cerebral localization.
    (C) postulated correctly the localization of sensory, motor, and speech areas of the cortex as we know them today.
    (D) promoted as a spin-off the increase of anatomic knowledge of the brain.
    (E) provided a sound basis for modern functional neurosurgery.

(Chapter 6)

22. Sir Charles Sherrington:

    (A) considered that the knowledge of physiology of the brain can ultimately explain mind.

    (B) took the position of a "dualist" and considered that there are two separable components, brain and mind.

    (C) was a purely laboratory neuroexperimentalist with no interest outside his research area.

    (D) died in his early 60s, too soon to summarize his philosophic views on brain and mind.

    (E) carried out the major part of his research at Cambridge University.

    (Chapter 6)

23. The term "mind":

    (A) was introduced in the late 19th century by William James.

    (B) has a precise and clear meaning as provided in the *Oxford English Dictionary,* being distinguished from the terms "memory" and "consciousness."

    (C) can be traced back etymologically to Sanskrit.

    (D) has been used interchangeably in meaning with "memory."

    (E) answers C and D.

    (Chapter 6)

24. The following are *true* about Wilder Penfield *except:*

    (A) he showed, with Hebb, that large surgical ablations of frontal cortex for focal epilepsy or tumor produced severe deficit in intellectual function.

    (B) he introduced the concept of the centrencephalic system as an integrating system between the brain stem and the two cerebral hemispheres.

    (C) he viewed the diencephalon rather than the cerebral cortex as the seat of "the highest level" of brain activity.

    (D) he considered that epileptic automatism inactivated the "highest brain mechanism" to produce an automaton without capacity to make new decisions.

    (Chapter 6)

25. Contemporary views of mind include the following observations *except:*

    (A) the amygdala plays an important role in epileptic automatism and amnesia.

    (B) radical unilateral removal of the amygdala for temporal lobe epilepsy produces a devastating loss of memory input.

    (C) the amygdala and its widespread cortical-subcortical connections can act as a substrate for the functional expression of mind and memory.

    (D) some modern investigators hypothesize that problems of brain and mind can ultimately be resolved by detailed understanding of the physiology and anatomy of the brain.

    (Chapter 6)

26. Aspects of a patient's life that can be affected by neurosurgical complications include:

    (A) mortality.

    (B) personality and emotions.

    (C) pain and comfort.

    (D) convenience in daily living.

    (E) all of the above.

    (Chapter 7)

27. Neurosurgeons may tend to overlook complications affecting cognition because:

    (A) cognitive complications are unimportant to patients.

    (B) patients can perform activities of daily living with cognitive deficits.

    (C) neuropsychologic understanding of and probes for cognitive deficits are relatively new and sometimes unfamiliar to neurosurgeons.

    (D) cognitive deficits are seldom as severe as motor or sensory deficits.

    (E) patients exaggerate and misinterpret the significance of slight alterations in their cognition.

    (Chapter 7)

28. Acceptance by the neurosurgeon of responsibility for a surgical complication:
    (A) undermines the authority role necessary between the neurosurgeon and the patient.
    (B) enhances the neurosurgeon's appreciation of how errors have been made and can be avoided in the future.
    (C) weakens the neurosurgeon's ability to face difficult clinical situations in the future.
    (D) increases the likelihood of litigation.
    (E) decreases the esteem of neurosurgical peers.

    (Chapter 7)

29. A neurosurgeon's religious attitudes:
    (A) should not be suppressed when a neurosurgeon faces a complication.
    (B) should be shared with atheist patients having difficulty coming to terms with a neurosurgical complication.
    (C) influence the importance attached by a neurosurgeon to a given complication.
    (D) require revision when the neurosurgeon is unable to empathize with a patient's reaction to a complication.

    (Chapter 7)

30. An informed philosophy of complications is more important for current than early neurosurgeons because:
    (A) society has become more litigious.
    (B) technical advances enable interventions that result in a broader spectrum of deficits.
    (C) patients have become more sophisticated about neurosurgical procedures.
    (D) societal expectations for outcome are more demanding.
    (E) all of the above.

    (Chapter 7)

31. A major dehumanizing factor in neurosurgery is:
    (A) government intervention.
    (B) time constraints.
    (C) lack of tort reform.
    (D) focus of attention and energy on technical advances.
    (E) lack of compassion witnessed during residency.

    (Chapter 7)

32. Neurosurgeons born and raised in Third World countries:
    (A) are more likely to be racist toward white patients.
    (B) are less likely to be racist toward white patients.
    (C) have less compassion for patient suffering than their American-born counterparts.
    (D) are more likely to perform invasive procedures that result in complications and less likely to accept responsibility for these complications.
    (E) must come to terms with American attitudes toward many aspects of human existence affecting attitudes toward complications.

    (Chapter 7)

33. The patient's attitudes toward a complication:
    (A) are less valid because the patient is too closely affected by the complication.
    (B) must be respected even if incompletely understood.
    (C) should guide the neurosurgeon in all choices of subsequent therapy.
    (D) are usually biased by family members and friends.
    (E) should be probed by a psychologist or psychiatrist and dealt with according to that professional's recommendation.

    (Chapter 7)

34. The neurosurgeon who, despite all due care, causes a serious complication yet continues to operate:
    (A) should be rigorously and severely reprimanded through the peer review process.
    (B) has done nothing wrong and should give the matter no further thought.
    (C) must remediate by available mechanisms to bring his or her skill level up to par.
    (D) is dangerous in failing to appreciate that he or she is a danger to society.
    (E) should reconcile the event internally and with the patient involved.
    (Chapter 7)

35. There is no single philosophy of neurosurgical complications because:
    (A) all neurosurgeons are different.
    (B) neurosurgery is a rapidly changing discipline.
    (C) organized medicine has traditionally avoided philosophic issues.
    (D) philosophers disagree on the definition of "complication."
    (Chapter 7)

36. Dying involves:
    (A) the ultimate crisis.
    (B) extinction.
    (C) physical anguish.
    (D) mental anguish.
    (E) all of the above.
    (Chapter 8)

37. Bioethics is:
    (A) a term coined by Van Renussean Potter.
    (B) a combination of "bio" representing biological knowledge, and "ethics" representing knowledge of human value systems.
    (C) a form of moral philosophy.
    (D) all of the above.
    (Chapter 8)

38. The theories of bioethics:
    (A) are utilitarian and deontologic.
    (B) can be proven by facts.
    (C) can be proven by human reason.
    (D) are exactly the same for all cultures.
    (E) must be universally accepted.
    (Chapter 8)

39. In the United States, medical decision-making:
    (A) is left to the decision of the patient.
    (B) is left to the judgment of the physician.
    (C) is discussed rationally.
    (D) must conform to decisions of the Supreme Court.
    (E) is systematically reviewed by legislatures.
    (Chapter 8)

40. The population of the United States is:
    (A) of uniform ethnic background.
    (B) of uniform religious background.
    (C) of uniform level of schooling.
    (D) of uniform financial status.
    (E) heterogeneous.
    (Chapter 8)

41. There is agreement about when life must be preserved:
    (A) in the fetus.
    (B) in the severely impaired infant.
    (C) in the vegetative adult.
    (D) in the severely demented.
    (E) in most circumstances.
    (Chapter 8)

42. In the United States, the patient has a right to:
    (A) commit suicide.
    (B) request aid in committing suicide.
    (C) ask for help in dying.
    (D) refuse care.
    (E) always refuse blood.
    (Chapter 8)

43. In the United States, scarce resources:
    (A) are not an issue.
    (B) are an issue that has been addressed.
    (C) are regulated by states.
    (D) need to be addressed rationally.
    (E) are becoming less of a problem.

    (Chapter 8)

44. Dementia:
    (A) is becoming less common.
    (B) is becoming more common.
    (C) is not age-related.
    (D) is simple to deal with.
    (E) is an issue that is being addressed
        satisfactorily.

    (Chapter 8)

45. Patients may be dangerous:
    (A) because of their behavior.
    (B) because of their disease.
    (C) but are still the moral responsibility of
        physicians.
    (D) but must be treated by law.
    (E) all of the above.

    (Chapter 8)

46. Which of the following is *true* about the
    status of medical science in the United States
    in the 19th century?
    (A) There was no scientific observation
        regarding human disease.
    (B) There were no clinical research
        laboratories.
    (C) There was excellent training of physicians
        in the scientific method.
    (D) The German model of academic medicine
        was firmly established in U.S. medical
        schools.

    (Chapter 9)

47. Which of the following areas accounts for the
    greatest contributions of neurological surgery
    to biologic science during the second half of
    the 20th century?
    (A) molecular biology
    (B) methodology of clinical trials
    (C) the case report
    (D) medical application of technology

    (Chapter 9)

48. Which of the following is/are examples of
    German academic influence in U.S.
    institutions?
    (A) Heidelberg influence in the Sheffield
        Laboratory at Yale
    (B) Leipzig influence in Bowditch's
        experimental physiology laboratory at
        Harvard
    (C) both of the above
    (D) neither of the above

    (Chapter 9)

49. The concept of "paradigm shift" in the
    evolution of science was championed by:
    (A) Osler.
    (B) Kühne.
    (C) Ludwig.
    (D) Popper.

    (Chapter 9)

50. Future contributions of neurosurgeons to
    biologic science are most likely to occur in
    which of the following settings?
    (A) neurosurgeons rotating in basic science
        laboratories
    (B) "separate but equal" laboratories of
        neurosurgery and basic science
    (C) integrated research teams including
        neurosurgeons
    (D) basic science research in the operating
        room

    (Chapter 9)

Match each of the contributions to the philosophy of science with the individual most responsible for it.

51. experimental medicine

52. the operating room as the surgeon's special laboratory

53. the role of hypothesis

54. space-time interchangeability

   (A) Albert Einstein

   (B) Claude Bernard

   (C) Henri Poincaré

   (D) Wilder Penfield

(Chapter 10)

Match the clinical research methodology with the description or phenomenon most related to it.

55. stratification

56. randomization

57. statistical power

58. blinding

   (A) sample size

   (B) observer bias

   (C) selection bias

   (D) cohort characteristics

(Chapter 10)

59. The precise clinical behavior of a neurosurgical lesion is best predicted as follows.

   (A) natural history profile

   (B) host factors affecting lesion behavior

   (C) lesion factors affecting clinical behavior

   (D) all of the above

(Chapter 10)

60. The dimensions of neurosurgical science include:

   (A) predicting lesion behavior.

   (B) explaining lesion behavior.

   (C) both A and B.

   (D) neither A nor B.

(Chapter 10)

61. In a pterional craniotomy, the first retractor position is:

   (A) perpendicular to the temporal lobe.

   (B) in the long axis of the carotid artery.

   (C) perpendicular to the carotid artery.

   (D) in the long axis of the optic nerve.

   (E) none of the above.

(Chapter 11)

62. In stereotactic surgery, target position is relative to:

   (A) external anatomic landmarks.

   (B) internal anatomic landmarks.

   (C) the boundaries of stereotactic space (the frame).

   (D) the boundaries of the scanner gantry.

   (E) none of the above.

(Chapter 11)

63. In a pterional craniotomy for an aneurysm, temporal lobe retraction is:

   (A) safe when the dome sits above the tentorial edge.

   (B) used to expose the A_1 segment.

   (C) used to expose the optic nerve.

   (D) used to expose the olfactory nerve.

   (E) sometimes not needed.

(Chapter 11)

64. Aneurysm mangement today resembles the approach of 25 years ago in:

   (A) the use of early surgery.

   (B) the introduction of new steroid agents.

   (C) the use of temporary clips.

   (D) attention to blood rheology.

   (E) all of the above.

(Chapter 11)

65. In the history of painting, which of the following is *true?*
    (A) Change has occurred more slowly with each century.
    (B) Art sometimes anticipates technology.
    (C) Conceptual art preceded abstract expressionism.
    (D) Cubism preceded French impressionism.
    (E) Art ignored Einsteinian relativity.
                                (Chapter 11)

66. Which of these pairs goes together?
    (A) one-point perspective/cubism
    (B) virtual reality/operating microscope
    (C) shallow space or flatness/abstract expressionism
    (D) Renaissance painting/multiple points of view
    (E) linear or direct vision/stereotactic surgery
                                (Chapter 11)

67. Neurosurgery can be considered an art because:
    (A) it creates artifacts.
    (B) it resembles the subjects of the trivium.
    (C) it is the practical application of science.
    (D) it is difficult.
    (E) it is life-saving and creates value.
                                (Chapter 11)

68. Which statement is *not true* about Art and Science?
    (A) They use the same criteria to judge the value of work.
    (B) They usually develop in a common zeitgeist (cultural moment).
    (C) Either Art or Science may anticipate developments in the other field.
    (D) Their practitioners share many personality traits.
    (E) all of the above.
                                (Chapter 11)

69. Which of the following statements about contemporary painting is *true?*
    (A) The painters are often critical of modern technology.
    (B) The painters use technology to create their works.
    (C) Paintings are often photography-based.
    (D) The paintings are more expressionistic and less abstract.
    (E) all of the above.
                                (Chapter 11)

70. Neurosurgeons can be considered artists because:
    (A) they creatively solve unique problems.
    (B) they use skill and judgment to mend the world.
    (C) they share traits with both artists and scientists.
    (D) their practice depends on developing new ways of seeing.
    (E) all of the above.
                                (Chapter 11)

71. Resident training in surgery, as it is currently designed, was started by:
    (A) Osler.
    (B) Virchow.
    (C) Cushing.
    (D) Halsted.
    (E) Billroth.
                                (Chapter 12)

72. Harvey Cushing established the first training program for neurosurgeons in:
    (A) Cleveland.
    (B) Baltimore.
    (C) Boston.
    (D) New York.
    (E) Philadelphia.
                                (Chapter 12)

73. The first neurological surgery association was established in 1920 as the:
    (A) Society of Neurological Surgeons.
    (B) American Association of Neurological Surgeons.
    (C) American Academy of Neurological Surgeons.
    (D) Congress of Neurological Surgeons.
    (E) Harvey Cushing Society.

    (Chapter 12)

74. The American Board of Neurological Surgery was created in 1940 to:
    (A) adjudicate professional disputes.
    (B) certify fully-trained neurosurgeons.
    (C) accredit training programs in neurosurgery.
    (D) advise medical schools about neurosurgery.
    (E) control the neurosurgery manpower problem.

    (Chapter 12)

75. The Residency Review Committee for Neurosurgery concerns itself with:
    (A) accreditation of training programs in neurosurgery.
    (B) certification of neurosurgeons.
    (C) medical school curriculum design.
    (D) resident salary programs.
    (E) manpower control.

    (Chapter 12)

76. Neurosurgical residency programs are *required* to offer experience in:
    (A) neurology.
    (B) neurochemistry.
    (C) neuropharmacology.
    (D) electrophysiology.
    (E) neurogenetics.

    (Chapter 12)

77. Periodic evaluation of performance in training programs is required of:
    (A) residents.
    (B) faculty.
    (C) neither A nor B.
    (D) both A and B.

    (Chapter 12)

78. Pediatric neurosurgery began as a subspecialty because of the focused practice of its founder:
    (A) John Shillito.
    (B) Frank Ingraham.
    (C) Robert McLaurin.
    (D) Anthony Raimondi.
    (E) Kenneth Till.

    (Chapter 12)

79. Features of an "ideal" training program include all of the following *except:*
    (A) progressive responsibility.
    (B) protected time for study.
    (C) fundamental clinical skills.
    (D) solo responsibility as Chief Resident.
    (E) supervised responsibility as Chief Resident.

    (Chapter 12)

80. Accredited continuing education of neurosurgeons may include all of the following except:
    (A) home-study courses.
    (B) journal reading.
    (C) annual scientific meetings.
    (D) industry-sponsored hands-on courses.
    (E) grand rounds.

    (Chapter 12)

81. The patient must be at the center of the health care process because:
   - (A) it is the patient who "owns" the disease or illness.
   - (B) it is the patient's body that has the potential to heal.
   - (C) it enhances the patient-doctor relationship.
   - (D) all of the above.

   (Chapter 13)

82. The neurosurgeon's role with respect to the patient is:
   - (A) to augment healing and recovery from an illness/disease or traumatic incident.
   - (B) to tell the patient as little as possible about the diagnosis and treatment.
   - (C) to treat the patient.
   - (D) to assume responsibility for the patient's healing.

   (Chapter 13)

83. The technologic revolution in neurosurgery has:
   - (A) enhanced the doctor-patient relationship.
   - (B) caused a paradigm shift from patient-centered to doctor-centered care.
   - **(C) made neurosurgical procedures more cost-effective.**
   - (D) supports doctor-centered care.

   (Chapter 13)

84. Philosophically, biology teaches us that:
   - (A) there is a correlation between healing and the mind.
   - (B) it is the patient who has the inherent capabilities for healing and recovery.
   - (C) our immune system will become weak and vulnerable without challenge.
   - (D) all of the above.

   (Chapter 13)

85. Neurosurgery can be viewed as:
   - (A) a three-legged stool.
   - (B) a pedestal stool.
   - (C) a source of revenue for trial attorneys.
   - (D) having reached its highest potential in the Decade of the Brain.

   (Chapter 13)

86. Patient education must be an integral part of the treatment process because:
   - (A) patients must be able to weigh the risks of the disease versus the risks of surgery.
   - (B) it enables patients to make informed, empowered decisions.
   - (C) it helps patients to understand the medical process and that all management of disease is based on statistical outcomes.
   - (D) all of the above.

   (Chapter 13)

87. Economic issues are important to neurosurgery because:
   - (A) it is imperative to support neurosurgical research and teaching programs.
   - (B) it supports clinical neurosurgery.
   - (C) it may impact on physician performance.
   - (D) all of the above.

   (Chapter 13)

88. Patient-centered care enhances the role of the neurosurgeon by:
   - (A) allowing patients to see him or her as omnipotent.
   - (B) continuing a paternal approach to treatment.
   - (C) allowing the neurosurgeon to focus his or her energies and skills to augment healing and recovery.
   - (D) all of the above.

   (Chapter 13)

89. There is a unique link between spirituality and healing because:
    (A) patients who have a spiritual base will invariably heal and recover more quickly and are more trusting and appreciative patients to care for.
    (B) Hippocrates commanded "do no harm."
    (C) spirituality is synonymous with religious beliefs.
    (D) the holistic approach is superior to the technical approach.

    (Chapter 13)

90. We can help patients to become our *partners in healing* rather than victims of disease by:
    (A) sharing the common goal of healing and recovery through patient education.
    (B) collaborating with all involved to promote physical, emotional, and spiritual healing.
    (C) helping patients understand that disease and healing are inherent parts of life and may actually strengthen them as human beings.
    (D) all of the above.

    (Chapter 13)

91. Equitable remedies operate:
    (A) in rem.
    (B) in personum.
    (C) neither in rem nor in personum.
    (D) both in rem and in personum.

    (Chapter 15)

92. Due process includes requirements of:
    (A) notice.
    (B) jurisdiction.
    (C) the right to appear in person.
    (D) equal protection before the law.
    (E) all of the above.

    (Chapter 15)

93. Punitive damages are:
    (A) subject to the VIII amendment.
    (B) consistently applied.
    (C) a fixed multiple of economic damages.
    (D) usually covered by professional liability insurance.
    (E) none of the above.
    (F) answers A and B only.

    (Chapter 15)

94. Physician fiduciary duty:
    (A) is entirely financial.
    (B) may conflict with managed care.
    (C) is relieved by ERISA.
    (D) is usually shared with the patient's insurer.

    (Chapter 15)

95. Expert witness evidence:
    (A) must be generally accepted by the scientific community.
    (B) must be admitted by the judge.
    (C) must be consistent with other expert testimony in the same case.
    (D) usually is from experts selected by the judge.

    (Chapter 15)

96. When you are a defendant in a medical malpractice lawsuit:
    (A) avoid direct contact with the plaintiff's attorney.
    (B) attend depositions of opposing experts.
    (C) answer only what is asked by opposing counsel.
    (D) all of the above.

    (Chapter 15)

97. Antitrust laws:
    (A) are enforced by the justice department.
    (B) are enforced by the Federal Trade Commission.
    (C) are enforced privately.
    (D) all of the above.
    (Chapter 15)

98. There is antitrust immunity for:
    (A) insurance companies.
    (B) professional baseball teams.
    (C) learned professions.
    (D) agricultural cooperatives.
    (E) all of the above.
    (F) some of the above.
    (Chapter 15)

99. The attorney advocacy role:
    (A) is essential to conflict resolution.
    (B) is probably influenced by the contingency fee.
    (C) is a legal requirement.
    (D) all of the above.
    (E) some of the above.
    (Chapter 15)

100. Lawyers:
    (A) have their own malpractice exposure to consider.
    (B) usually do plaintiff personal injury representation on a contingent fee basis.
    (C) often must advance money in the evaluation of personal injury cases.
    (D) need to establish their trial skill credibility to achieve maximum negotiating leverage.
    (E) all of the above.
    (Chapter 15)

101. An American neurosurgeon who was active in formulating and implementing health care policy was:
    (A) William Macewen.
    (B) Otfrid Foerster.
    (C) Harvey Cushing.
    (D) Edward Busch.
    (Chapter 16)

102. Early at odds over health care policy in this country were:
    (A) the American Medical Association (AMA) and the American College of Surgeons.
    (B) the AMA and the American College of Physicians.
    (C) the AMA and the American Association of Neurological Surgeons (AANS).
    (D) the AANS and the Congress of Neurological Surgeons (CNS).
    (Chapter 16)

103. The Washington Committee is:
    (A) a not-for-profit arm of the AMA to which the AANS provides funding.
    (B) a joint committee of the AANS and the CNS.
    (C) a cell of the national office of the AANS.
    (D) a committee of the Joint Council of State Neurosurgical Societies.
    (Chapter 16)

104. As a result of the debate, within neurosurgery, on malpractice reform:
    (A) Congress passed the Physician Protection Act.
    (B) emphasis within neurosurgery shifted from state to national reform.
    (C) organized neurosurgery incorporated a physician-owned liability company.
    (D) federal legislation passed that pre-empted state statutes.
    (Chapter 16)

105. The primary focus by neurosurgery on health care policy should be:
    (A) to support efforts of organized medicine.
    (B) to ensure an adequate supply of well-trained neurosurgeons in the future.
    (C) the costs of health care.
    (D) on those issues that immediately and decidedly impact upon neurosurgeons and their patients.

    (Chapter 16)

106. A major purpose of the Washington Committee is to monitor:
    (A) pending Congressional legislation.
    (B) executive-branch health care policy.
    (C) regulations of health agencies.
    (D) all of the above.

    (Chapter 16)

107. *Cruzan v Director, Missouri Department of Health* was about:
    (A) bad-faith insurance coverage.
    (B) third-trimester abortion.
    (C) gun control.
    (D) right-to-die.

    (Chapter 16)

108. The study by neurosurgery of its manpower in the mid-1970s:
    (A) was funded by the PEW Foundation.
    (B) was eventually recognized as a model of physician manpower studies.
    (C) led to a mandatory 25% reduction in residency positions in U.S. programs.
    (D) led to the creation of the ACGME.

    (Chapter 16)

109. Two issues addressed early by the Washington Committee were:
    (A) welfare reform and handgun legislation.
    (B) the Feres doctrine and Medicare legislation.
    (C) medical liability and physician manpower.
    (D) the need for orphan drug and medical device legislation.

    (Chapter 16)

110. An example of where organized neurosurgery should place its resources in a cost-effective attempt to influence emerging health care policy in this country is:
    (A) Vice President Gore's Waste in Government initiative.
    (B) funding for AIDS vaccine research.
    (C) residency education.
    (D) restructuring of the health care delivery system in the military.

    (Chapter 16)

Match the elements of local infrastructure with the most appropriate statement in relation to neurosurgical development.

111. advanced technology
112. immediate public health need
113. local talent
114. international communications
    (A) necessary for neurosurgical development
    (B) sufficient for neurosurgical development
    (C) both A and B
    (D) neither A nor B

    (Chapter 19)

From a perspective of the developed world, analyze the following observations as either *true* or *false*.

115. Much of the world population is underserved by neurosurgeons.

116. Maldistribution of neurosurgical resources is unique to poor countries.

117. Limiting specialized medical services can inhibit future development.

118. Local spending on neurosurgical services invariably shunts resources from public health needs.

    (A) The statement is *true*.

    (B) The statement is *false*.

(Chapter 19)

Which of the following statements apply to global neurosurgical challenges?

119. technical and material resources

120. educational and information resources from public health needs

    (A) in surplus in the developed world

    (B) in need in underdeveloped countries

    (C) both A and B

    (D) neither A nor B

(Chapter 19)

Match each of the philosophic contributions with the philosopher who originated it.

121. intuitional philosophy

122. empirical philosophy

123. positivism

124. the primacy of hypothesis

    (A) Henri Poincaré

    (B) Aristotle

    (C) Plato

    (D) Auguste Comte

(Chapter 20)

Match each of the elements of philosophy with the most appropriate description.

125. metaphysics

126. epistemology

127. ethics

128. scientific method

    (A) formulation of general notions

    (B) moral judgment

    (C) theory of knowledge

    (D) hypothesis and doubt

(Chapter 20)

129. Which of the following elements are a part of the neurosurgical identity?

    (A) the art and methods of science

    (B) unlimited altruism

    (C) resistance to change as a danger to heritage

    (D) all of the above

(Chapter 20)

130. Which of the following are essential to future neurosurgical development?

    (A) question-driven technology assessment

    (B) correcting maldistribution of resources

    (C) cultivating local leadership

    (D) all of the above

(Chapter 20)

Index

Previously Published Books in the *Neurosurgical Topics* Series

For order information call (708) 692-9500.

Philosophy of Neurological Surgery

Answers to Questions

Chapter 1

1. C   2. A   3. B   4. A   5. C

Chapter 5

6. B   7. A   8. C   9. D   10. B   11. D   12. A
13. A   14. B   15. A

Chapter 6

16. A   17. B   18. C   19. C   20. C   21. D
22. B   23. E   24. A   25. B

Chapter 7

26. E   27. C   28. B   29. C   30. E   31. D
32. E   33. B   34. E   35. A

Chapter 8

36. E   37. D   38. A   39. D   40. E   41. E
42. D   43. D   44. B   45. E

Chapter 9

46. B   47. D   48. C   49. B   50. C

Chapter 10

51. B   52. D   53. C   54. A   55. D   56. C
57. A   58. B   59. D   60. C

Chapter 11

61. E   62. C   63. E   64. E   65. B   66. C
67. C   68. A   69. E   70. E

Chapter 12

71. D   72. C   73. A   74. B   75. A   76. A
77. D   78. B   79. D   80. D

Chapter 13

81. D   82. A   83. B   84. D   85. B   86. D
87. D   88. C   89. A   90. D

Chapter 15

91. B   92. E   93. E   94. B   95. B   96. D
97. D   98. F   99. E   100. E

Chapter 16

101. C   102. A   103. B   104. B   105. D
106. D   107. D   108. B   109. C   110. C

Chapter 19

111. A   112. A   113. A   114. A   115. A
116. B   117. A   118. B   119. C   120. C

Chapter 20

121. C   122. B   123. D   124. A   125. A
126. C   127. B   128. D   129. A   130. D

Contents

List of Contributors

Zh.I. Alferov
Ioffe Physico-Technical Institute
26 Polytechnicheskaya str.
St. Petersburg 194021
Russia
Zhores.Alferov@mail.ioffe.ru

V.M. Andreev
Ioffe Physico-Technical Institute
26 Polytechnicheskaya str.
St. Petersburg 194021
Russia
vmandreev@mail.ioffe.ru

C.J. Brabec
CTO Konarka Technologies Inc.
Altenbergerstr. 69
A-4040 Linz
Austria
cbrabec@conarka.com

G. Dennler
Konarka Austria GmbH
Altenbergerstr. 69
A-4040 Linz
Austria

A. Goetzberger
Fraunhofer Institute
    for Solar Energy Systems
Heidenhofstr. 2
D-79110 Freiburg
Germany
adolf.goetzberger@
ise.fraunhofer.de

K. Hesse
Wacker Chemie AG
WACKER POLYSILICON
Johannes-Hess-Straße 24
D-84489 Burghausen
Germany
karl.hesse@wacker.com

G. Hey
DLR – Deutsches Zentrum
    für Luft- und Raumfahrt e.V.
Direktion Raumfahrt
Postfach 30 03 64
D-53183 Bonn
Germany

R. Hezel
University of Hannover
Josef-Heppner-Straße 26
D-82049 Pullach
Germany
rudolf.hezel@t-online.de

W. Hoffmann
Vice President and CTO EES
Applied Materials GmbH & Co.KG
Siemensstraße 100
D-63755 Alzenau
Germany
winfried_hoffmann@amat.com

M. Koppe
Konarka Austria GmbH
Altenbergerstr. 69
A-4040 Linz
Austria

G. LaRoche
AZUR SPACE Solar Power GmbH
Theresienstr. 2
D-74072 Heilbronn
Germany

O. Mayer
GE Global Research
Freisinger Landstrasse 50
D-85748 Garching
Germany
oliver.mayer@research.ge.com

E.W. Merkle
Bayerische Solar AG
Dachauerstr. 37
D-80335 München
Germany
merkle@bayerische-solar.de

M. Morana
Konarka Austria GmbH
Altenbergerstr. 69
A-4040 Linz
Austria

D. Mühlbacher
Konarka Austria GmbH
Altenbergerstr. 69
A-4040 Linz
Austria

V. Petrova-Koch
Gate East
Schleissheimerst 17
D-85748 Garching/Munich
Germany
vpkoch@yahoo.de

K.-D. Rasch
AZUR SPACE Solar Power GmbH
Theresienstr. 2
D-74072 Heilbronn
Germany

V.D. Rumyantsev
Ioffe Physico-Technical Institute
26 Polytechnicheskaya str.
St. Petersburg 194021
Russia
rumyan@scell.ioffe.rssi.ru

M.C. Scharber
Konarka Austria GmbH
Altenbergerstr. 69
A-4040 Linz
Austria

I.A. Schwirtlich
SCHOTT Solar GmbH,
D-63755 Alzenau
Germany

G.F.X. Strobl
AZUR SPACE Solar Power GmbH
Theresienstr. 2
D-74072 Heilbronn
Germany

M. Sturm
Solar*Tec AG
Uhlandstr. 13
D-85609 Aschheim b. München
Germany
sturm@solartecag.de

R. Tölle
Solar*Tec AG
Uhlamstr. 13
D-85609 Aschheim b. München
Germany
toelle@solartecag.de

L. Waldmann
Public Relations
SCHOTT Solar GmbH
Carl-Zeiss-Straße 4
D-63755 Alzenau
Germany

D. Waller
Konarka Technologies Inc.
100 Foot of John Street
Boott Mill South, 3rd Floor
Lowell, MA 01852
USA

Z. Zhu
Konarka Technologies Inc.
100 Foot of John Street
Boott Mill South, 3rd Floor
Lowell, MA 01852
USA

1 Milestones of Solar Conversion and Photovoltaics

V. Petrova-Koch

1.1 Prehistory

Seventh century BC: In ancient *Egypt* the houses were built so that the solar radiation could be collected during the day and used during the night.

Fifth century BC: The *Greeks* oriented their houses so that they could receive solar energy in the winter time *to heat the buildings*.

Third century BC: *Archimedes* used *mirrors* to reflect *direct sun radiation* and to defend Syracuse from invasion by the Romans.

Second century BC: the first *windows* made out of *transparent mica* were inserted in houses in northern Italy, with the aim to increase the use of solar radiation in winter time.

First century AD: the so called *heliocaminos* started to be used. These solar baths with big mica windows oriented to the south found their maximum application in Italy around the fifth century.

Fourteenth century: the first *solar law* was introduced in Italy.

1767 in Russia: *M.V. Lomonossov* suggested the use of lenses to concentrate the solar radiation.

1767 in Switzerland: *Horace de Saussure* discovers the amplification and increased heat efficiency in Matjoshka-type five-folded glass boxes.

1830 in South Africa: *J. Hershel* uses the first *solar cooker*.

Around 1830: *H. Repton* constructs the first (*glass*) *greenhouses* in Europe.

1.2 Milestones of Photovoltaics

1839: *Alexandre-Edmund Becquerel*, a young experimental physicist in France, discovered the photovoltaic effect at age of 19, while assisting his father, experimenting with electrolytic cells made up of two metal electrodes.

1873: *W. Smith, working in the UK*, discovered the photoconductivity of selenium, which led to the invention of the photoconductive cell.

1876: *W.G. Adams and R.E. Day, USA*, observed the photovoltaic effect in solid selenium.

1883: *Ch. Frits*, an American inventor, described the first solar cell made from Se wafers.

1887: *H. Hertz* discovered in Germany that ultraviolet light altered the lowest voltage capable of causing a spark between two metal electrodes.

1888: *Ed. Weston* receives the first patent for solar cells (U.S. 389124 and US3891-25).

1904: *W. Hallwachs* discovered the photosensitivity in a copper/cuprous oxide pair.

1904: *A. Einstein* publishes his pioneering theoretical work on the photoelectric effect (he received the Nobel Prize in 1921 for this work).

1916: *R.A. Millikan* provides experimental proof of the photoelectric effect.

1916: *Y. Czochralski* (Polish scientist) develops a new method to grow single-crystal silicon.

1930: *W. Schottky* discovers a new cuprous oxide photoelectric cell.

1931: *A.F. Ioffe* guides a project at the Physico-Technical Institute in St. Petersburg on thallium sulphide photocells, which reach a record efficiency at that time of more than 1%. He submitted a proposal to the Soviet government concerning the use of solar PV roofs for providing electricity.

1932: *Audobert and Stora* discover the photovoltaic effect in CdS.

1948: *W. Schottky* presents the first theoretical concept for semiconductor PV.

1951: at *Bell Labs* the first p–n junction was grown in germanium.

1953: *D. Trivich* publishes the first theoretical calculations on the conversion efficiency of the solar spectrum with materials of different band gaps.

1953: *G. Pearson at Bell Labs* begins research of Li-doped Si solar cells.

1953: *D. Chapin; C. Fuller and G. Pearson* realized a two cm^2 Si solar cell with an efficiency of 4% (published on *NY Times* cover page).

1954: *D. Chapin, C. Fuller and G. Pearson* improve the efficiency of a Si Cell to 6%; first AT&T solar cell demonstration in Murray Hill, NJ.

1954: At *Siemens in Germany, G. Spenke* and his team develop an efficient *method for poly-Si growth*: Scientists and experts from *Wacker* and TU Munich participate in this work as part of a joint team with Siemens. The so-called *Siemens Method* is the main technology for the production of solar and semiconductor grade Si.

1954: *J.J. Loferski and Jenny* at RCA reported a pronounced PV effect in CdS.

1954: *The International Solar Energy Society (ISES) was founded in Phoenix, AZ, 1970. Its headquarters was later moved to Melbourne, Australia, and in 1995 it was moved again to Freiburg, Germany.*

1957–1959: *Hoffmann Electronics* achieves 8, 9 and 10% efficiency and develops the grid contact, significantly reducing the series resistance of the device.

1960: *Hoffmann Electronics* makes a jump to 14% efficient PV cells, mainly used for satellite technology and space applications.

1960/1961: *H. Mori* in Japan and *A.K. Zaitseva & O.P. Fedoseeva* in Russia independently proposed bifacial PV modules.

1961: *W. Shockley and H. Queisser* developed a thermodynamic theory on the principle of *detailed balance* for one-junction solar cell.

1961: *First IEEE PV Specialists Conf.* is initiated in *Philadelphia, USA.*

1963: *Sharp in Japan* installs the world largest array for *terrestrial applications*, with a power of 242 W!

1966: *The first 1 kW PV Array* was installed on the Orbiting Astronomic Observatory.

1966: *Zh.I. Alferov, V.B. Khalfin and R.F. Kazarinov* discovered "the superinjection-effect" in a *double heterostructure (DHS)*.

1970: *Zh.I. Alferov, V.M. Andreev and a team* at Ioffe Institute St. Petersburg demonstrated the first efficient *GaAs heterostructure solar cell.*

1973: *Solarex was founded in the USA. This produced the first commercial polycrystalline solar cell and the first commercial amorphous solar cell. Solarex was later acquired by Amoco/Emron and then by BP Solar.*

1974: *Japan* formulates *Project Sunshine* at the beginning of the *first oil crisis.*

1976/1977: The first *fluorescent collector for solar applications* is suggested independently by *A. Goetzberger* and *W. Greubel*, and by *W.H. Weber* and *J. Lambe.*

1976: *D. Carlson and Ch. Wronsky at RCI, USA* demonstrate the first a-Si:H thin-film solar cell with an efficiency of around 1%.

1977: The *Solar Energy Research Institute (SERI)*, later to become the *National Renewable Energy Laboratory (NREL),* opens in Golden, CO, USA.

1977: *EC PV Solar Energy Conference* starts *in Luxembourg.*

1978: The first lab *for Solar Energy and Renewable Energy Sources (SENES)* starts operations in Europe at the *Bulgarian Academy of Sciences in Sofia.*

1980: *M. Riel* starts the famous *1,000 solar roof program in Zurich*, Switzerland.

1980: *BP enters solar business.*

1981: *The Fraunhofer Institute for Solar Energy ISE* in Freiburg Germany founded by A. Goetzberger.

1981: *R. Hezel introduced Plasma Silicon Nitride (PECVD)* as *antireflection and passivation layer*, which is presently applied for almost all commercial silicon solar cells.

1981: *Reflective solar concentrators* used for the first time with solar cells at Ioffe Institute St. Petersburg.

1982: *The PV Production* worldwide reaches the value *of 10 MW!*

1982: *A 1-MW PV plant* – built by *ARCO Solar* with 100 Dual-Axis trackers with c-Si modules – goes online in *California.*

1983: The PV production worldwide exceeds *20 MW, and sales exceed* $250 million U.S.!

1983: *International Science and Engineering Conference* (the Asian ISE-Conference) is started.

1984: *M.A. Green and S. Wenham* introduced the *laser-grooved buried-contact* solar cell (*LGBC*).

1985: *M. Green* at the University of New South Wales Australia, *breaks the 20% efficiency barrier for c-Si solar cell under one sun* in the research lab.

1985: *R. Swanson* founded *Sun Power in CA* with the goal to commercialize the high-efficiency c-Si solar cell.

1986: *ARCO Solar* releases the first *commercial thin-film power module.*

1987: The Solar Challenge is inaugurated, and *PV-powered cars* race across Australia.

1989: *V.D. Rumyantsev at Ioffe Institute St. Petersburg* introduces a *solar concentrator lens-cell system with radically reduced size.*

1990: *ARCO Solar* is sold to *Siemens* and renamed *to Siemens Solar.*

1991: *Nukem GmbH* (*now Schott Solar*) built *1 MW pilot PV plant* out of *mono- and bifacial MIS-inversion-layer solar cells*, developed by the team of *R. Hezel at the University of Erlangen.*

1991: *M. Graetzel* invents the *dye-sensitized electrochemical solar cell.* An efficiency more than 10% was obtained within five years after the discovery.

1992: *BP* commercializes the *Laser Grooved c-Si Solar Cell* (*patented by M.A. Green and S. Wenham*).

1994: *NREL* develops and demonstrates *a two-terminal, high-efficiency GaInAsP/ GaAs solar cell*, which under 180 suns shows more than 30% efficiency. The third generation CPV was born.

1997: *The biggest PV roof* with more than 3 MW is installed in Munich, Germany.

1997: *Sanyo* starts mass production of its *high-efficiency HIT c-Si/a-Si:H PV cells.*

1998: *SolarWorld A.G.* is founded in Germany, the *first vertically integrated PV company.*

1999: *M.A. Green and J. Zhao* achieved a *record efficiency of 24.7% for laboratory c-Si solar cells.*

1999: *Total PV power* installed worldwide exceeds *1 GW*!

2000: *April: Germany* introduces the *new EEG* (*feed-in law*), the law which, in 2008, was translated into more than 40 languages. Germany becomes the largest PV market worldwide.

2002: *First Solar Silicon Conference* dealing with the crisis of Si feedstock *was* organized by Photon in Munich, Germany.

2002: *Cypress Corp. and Sun Power* in the USA start pilot production of the high-efficiency c-Si Sun Power PV cell. Mass production set up in the Philippines.

2002: *Siemens Solar* sold its solar activities to *Shell Solar*, *in 2004 Shell Solar* c-Si solar cell activities were divested to *SolarWorld.*

2004: *General Electric* enters PV, after becoming owner of *AstroPower.*

2005: *Sharp* remains *the biggest producer* of PV cells worldwide.

2005: *Q-Cells*, which was founded in 2002, is the *fastest growing PV cell producer* worldwide.

2006: *A PV Roadmap for Europe* is proposed by WCRE.

2006: More than *25% of the PV Modules* produced worldwide are installed in Germany.

2006: *SolFocus in USA, Concentrix-Solar in Freiburg, Germany, and SolarTec AG in Munich, Germany,* start *pilot-production of concentrator III–V PV (CPV).* CPV Modules consisting of GaAs triple cells on Ge substrates with efficiency more than 35%, and Fresnel concentrator lenses made out of UV-resistive silicone, capable of providing up to 800 suns; system will be available in 2008.

2006: *Wacker* expands the production of solar-grade poly-Si in *Burghausen*, Germany, up to 16,000 tonnes per year to become the second biggest company in this field worldwide. The new investment is about 500 million €.

2006: *First Int. Solar Glass Conference* is organized by Photon in Munich.

2007: *Hemlock* announces its mega-expansion of poly-Si production up to 3,600 metric tonnes per year in *MI, USA*, and will start producing in 2010. The investment is about $1 billion U.S. Hemlock remains the biggest poly-Si producer worldwide.

2006: *InterSolar*, the *biggest International Solar Fair* takes place for a 10th and last time in Freiburg, Germany. In 2008 it will continue to operate in Munich.

2007: *SunPower* and *Sanyo* both announce the *highest efficiency* for mass produced Solar Cell under one sun solar radiation of *22%.*

2007: *Al Gore and IPCC* receive the *Nobel Peace Price.*

2007: *UN-Conference* devoted to climate change takes place *in Bali.*

2008: *Q-Cells* bypasses *Sharp* to becomes the world biggest PV cell producer.

2 From Extraterrestrial to Terrestrial Applications

G.F.X. Strobl, G. LaRoche, K.-D. Rasch, and G. Hey

2.1 Introduction

In the early 1950s, Bell Laboratories in the USA investigated possible applications of silicon semiconductors in electronics. While improving transistors, Bell scientists Gerald Pearson and Calvin Fuller invented the first silicon solar cell. That first effort was further improved for applications in remote humid locations by Darryl Chapin [1]. The first experiment with silicon yielded an efficiency of 2.3%. Improvements with regard to the dopants, the metallic contacts to the p- and n-side and the application of an antireflection coating led to efficiencies of 4%. In 1954, cells with 6% efficiency could be reliably manufactured.

The first solar battery was presented to the public by Bell Laboratories on April 25, 1954. The battery powered a 21-inch Ferris wheel one day and a solar-powered radio transmitter the next. Technical progress continued and the cell efficiency doubled within two years. Even then, Bell representatives dreamt of a limitless power supply. But this progress could be achieved only with high-purity, single-crystal silicon which was expensive. Thus, a commercial breakthrough was prevented with the exception of some applications by Western Electric to run telephone lines in rural areas. The price at that time was more than $300/W.

Commercialization efforts were undertaken by the National Fabrication Products Company with their chief Scientist Dr. Martin Wolf. But the company did not succeed in bringing the price down and was bought in 1956 by Hoffmann Electronics of El Monte, CA. They developed a 25 W sun-power-to-electricity converter module which no one bought. Its only application was in toys.

At the same time, the U.S. Army Signal Corps investigated possible applications for solar energy converters and found one preferred application: satellites in space! The U.S. Army signal corps was responsible for the design of a solar cell power system for the satellite project Vanguard to be built by the U.S. Navy. They contacted Hoffmann Electronics, and its chief engineer, Eugene Ralph, assembled some of their cells. On St Patrick's Day 1958, Vanguard 1, the first satellite with solar cells aboard, went into orbit. Two months later, SPUTNIK III, also equipped with silicon solar cells, was launched. After six years in orbit, Vanguard 1 was still sending radio messages back to Earth [2].

Despite some early applications on oil platforms, the astronomical price of silicon solar cells limited their use to space. So the onset of the Space Age was the salvation of the solar cell industry (M. Wolf). From 1958 to 1969 the U.S. government spent more than $50 million on solar cell research and development.

2.2 Solar Cells for Space

Space cells had to be extremely overengineered to withstand the harsh space environment – charged particles, micrometeoroids, hard UV radiation, and temperature extremes due to change of daylight and eclipses all posed challenges. Those challenges required a special design for each satellite, due to individual layout, limited area, storage volume and mass. The solar cell power supplies grew steadily and reached 500 W with the Nimbus Spacecraft in 1964; 1,000 W on the Orbiting Astronomical Observatory in 1966; and 20 kW for the Orbiting Laboratory Skylab in 1972. The upper limit to the size of photovoltaic solar converter arrays in space was given by the capacity of the available launch vehicles. It was found that a high power-to-mass ratio of the solar array was the most important factor which could be increased by improving the solar cell efficiency and/or lowering the solar array mass.

In Germany on August 23, 1962, the "Gesellschaft für Weltraumforschung GfW" was founded to manage and coordinate space activities with the goal of building the first German satellite "AZUR". The satellite's mission was to study cosmic rays and their interference with the Earth's magnetosphere, the northern lights and the time variation of the solar wind due to solar flares. German industry was invited to develop and manufacture the required subsystems and to make the satellite ready for launch. It was launched on November 8, 1969, with a Scout rocket from Cape Canaveral. For this application the solar cell development also took place in Germany at Siemens and Telefunken. These activities benefited from progress made in the U.S. and published in dedicated technical journals and conference proceedings. Importantly, the cells delivered by Telefunken were 2 cm by 2 cm and delivered efficiencies of more than 10%. Moreover, with the introduction of titanium-silver contacts, a technology was developed that became the baseline for all future silicon solar cells for space applications.

Improved understanding of the theory of device operation led to increased efficiency and cost reduction of silicon solar cells (Fig. 2.1 from [2]). But the efficiencies achieved were still far below the theoretical ones. Moreover, theory stated that materials other than Si – like GaAs or CdTe – would give better efficiencies in the Sun spectrum, especially at increased temperatures (Fig. 2.2). Given that Si was the most developed and best understood material, most efforts were directed toward further improvements of Si solar cells. In parallel, other materials like cadmium sulfide, cadmium telluride, and gallium arsenide were investigated but did not achieve better results than silicon. Other thin-film technologies – one based on amorphous silicon and the other on the ternary compound $CuInSe_2$ (CIS) – found applications in electronics and to some extent in power plants.

One advantage of GaAs-based solar cells over Si was their better temperature stability and higher radiation resistance, giving them preference for special

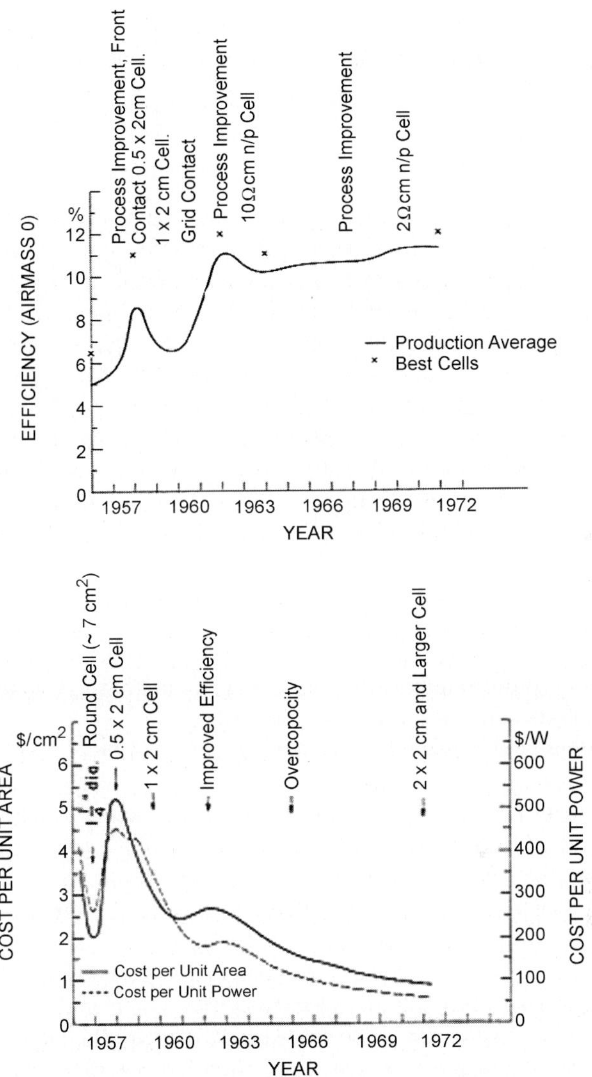

Fig. 2.1. Early historical development of silicon solar cell efficiency (*top*) and cell prices (*bottom*)

applications despite their higher costs. One of the first space applications of the temperature-stable GaAs solar cells took place on the Russian spacecrafts Venera-2 and Venera-3, launched in November 1965 to the "hot" planet Venus. The area of each GaAs solar array fabricated by the Russian Enterprise KVANT for these spacecrafts was $2\,\text{m}^2$. Then, the Russian moon cars were launched in 1970 (Lunokhod-1) and in 1972 (Lunokhod-2) with GaAs $4\,\text{m}^2$ solar arrays in each. The operating temperature of these arrays on the illuminated surface of the Moon was about $130\,°\text{C}$.

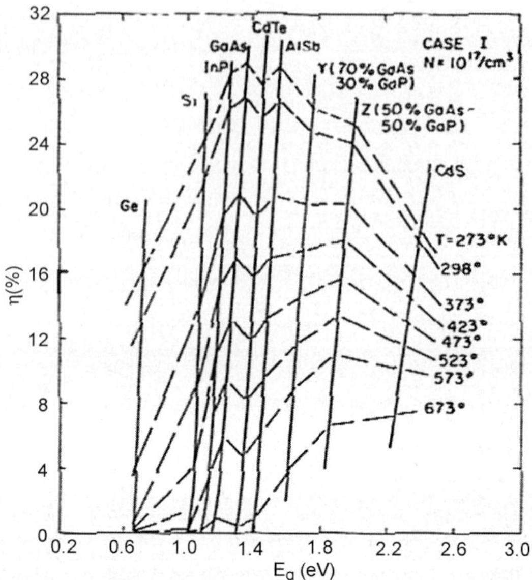

Fig. 2.2. Theoretical efficiencies of different materials at various temperatures (from [3])

The solar arrays demonstrated an efficiency of 11% and have provided the energy supply during the life-time of these moon cars [4].

Further progress was achieved by the development of AlGaAs/GaAs heterostructures, the combination of materials with different energy gaps. Their AM0 efficiency was increased up to 18–19% [5]. A solar array with a total area of 70 m^2 was installed in the Russian space station MIR launched in 1986 (Fig. 2.3). During 15 years in orbit, the array degradation appeared to be lower than 30% under hard operating conditions with appreciable shadowing, the effects of numerous dockings, and a challenging ambient environment of the station.

But GaAs solar cells were more expensive than Si solar cells by a factor 5 to 10, and therefore were used only for special applications. Compared to silicon, the use of GaAs solar cells was considered profitable only if their efficiency would exceed 20%. This was not realistic in the near-term. Therefore, main emphasis was given to further improving the Si technology.

2.3 Closer to the Limit

An analysis of the main loss mechanisms of Si solar cells by M. Wolf [6] yielded the following power-limiting factors:

1. Optical reflection of incident light on the cell surface.
2. Crystal quality limiting quantum efficiency of electron – hole pair production.
3. Loss of excess energy of the majority of absorbed photons necessary to generate electron – hole pairs.

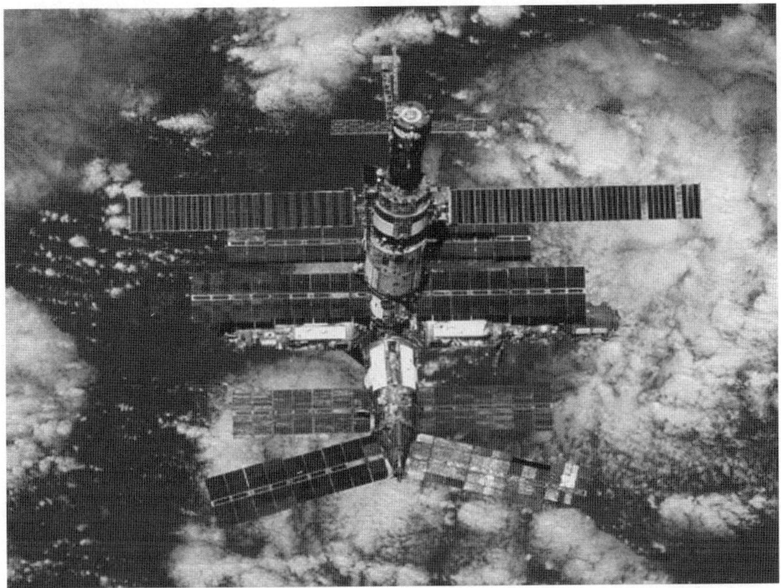

Fig. 2.3. AlGaAs/GaAs solar array on the MIR Space Station (from [4])

4. Low optical absorption coefficient.
5. Recombination of minority carriers on the surfaces, by impurities, dislocations and on the back contact.
6. Reduced barrier height of the junction by the distance of the Fermi levels from the band edges.
7. Loss and leakage currents across the junction and recombination within the depletion layer.
8. Series resistances in the base region and the cell contacts.

The improvement of each factor should bring the real solar cell efficiency closer to the theoretical one. For space applications, the impact of charged particle irradiation had to also be considered. The following main developments were milestones in the improvement of Si solar cells to their present status.

2.3.1 Material Quality

Impurities in the solar cell material generally introduce traps into the crystal. These traps act as recombination centers. An increased density of such centers decreases the minority carrier lifetime and the cell efficiency. On the other hand, silicon must not only be very pure, but it must also be in a single-crystal form with essentially zero defects in the crystal structure. To achieve the required purity the metallurgical grade silicon extracted from silicon dioxide (quartzite) by reduction in large arc furnaces must be further purified by fractional distillation of the condensed volatile compound SiHCl$_3$ and reduced by hydrogen. This semiconductor grade material is then melted in a crucible with trace levels of the dopant required (normally boron for p-type silicon) and, by means of a seed crystal, large cylindrical single crystals are pulled from the melt (Czochralski process). These so-called boules are sliced up into wafers forming the ingot for the manufacture of solar cells.

Refinements of the above processes improved the wafer quality continuously, allowing higher doping levels which resulted in remarkable efficiency improvements ($10\,\Omega$ cm versus $2\,\Omega$ cm base resistivity). The increase of the crystal diameters from 5.0 cm to more than 12.5 cm allowed the manufacture of large-area solar cells. Though small cells are using the wafer area better (minimum material loss), large area cells were preferred for the subsequent processing steps of cover glassing, cell interconnection and substrate bonding due to cost savings.

2.3.2 Back Surface Reflector (BSR)

The absorption of photons from the incident sunlight depends on the absorption coefficient, which is high for short wavelengths and low for longer wavelengths. Accordingly red and infrared light penetrate deeper into the silicon material and a big portion is scattered or absorbed at the rear side contact. Polishing and coating the rear side with a thin aluminum reflector makes the back contact reflective giving the longer wavelengths a second chance at being absorbed and the energy which is not absorbed is re-emitted through the front surface leading to a reduction in cell absorbance. This is a critical parameter controlling the device's operating temperature.

Such back surface reflectors (BSR) gave a boost to the performance of thin cells and lowered the cell temperature considerably. Thin cells are making solar cells more resistant to charged particle radiation, since minority charge carriers have a higher chance of reaching the pn-junction even in the presence of recombination centers.

2.3.3 Back Surface Field (BSF)

The primary mechanism for the movement of minority carriers toward the pn-junction is the diffusion process. An additional moving mechanism was found to be the drift of minority carriers caused by a built-in electrostatic field arising from gradients of the impurity density. While a positive effect in the diffused region of the cell is found only with a deep junction, which stands against the enhancement of blue response (see violet cell), a drift field is advantageous in the bulk area in order to reduce minority carrier recombination at the rear side. It was found by Wolf [7] that the inclusion of a narrow layer with a drift field in the base region has a marked effect on the performance of the cell and the degradation rates due to nuclear particle radiation. The efficiency of silicon solar cells could be improved by the introduction of a back surface field by up to 17% (e.g., Spectrolab K4700- type compared to Spectrolab K6700-type [8]).

Technologies developed at Telefunken in Germany to form back surface fields consisted of boron diffusion, boron ion implantation and evaporated aluminum paste processes [9]. While the diffusion and implantation processes yielded equal efficiencies at beginning of life, implanted BSF cells showed lower degradation after particle irradiation (end of life EOL condition).

2.3.4 The Violet Cell [10]

Former cells were very limited in the short wavelength region and their diode characteristics were far from ideal. By the existing diffusion process the front regime of a cell consisted of three regions: a shallow region, called the dead layer, with an extremely short lifetime of the minority carriers. This was due to high dopant concentration above the solid solubility limit, a high field region maintained by the impurity profile, and the space charge region. An improvement of the short wavelength response had to eliminate the dead layer, and the recombination states in the space charge region caused by stresses and defects originating in the silicon front surface. Because the dislocation density decreases sharply toward the diffusion front, the dead layer could be eliminated by shallow diffusion. This minimized the total density of dislocations in the diffusion region. This reduction of the emitter thickness caused an increase in the lateral resistance which could be compensated for by increasing the grid lines, thus keeping the solar cell active area constant to avoid shading losses. These improvements in solar cell efficiency increase efficiency by 30% compared with typical commercial cells without changing the degradation behavior under particle irradiation.

2.3.5 Textured Surfaces

Aside from optical coating optimization, another approach to reduce reflection losses is to use textured surfaces. Texturization is achieved by creating a topology of small, densely packed tetrahedral grooves, V-grooves or random pyramids [11] that act as light traps on the solar cell's surface. When light impinges on this textured surface, reflection occurs at such an angle that it is deflected into a new point on the surface. Multiple interactions occur with the silicon, thus reducing the amount of light normally lost through reflection. Together with an antireflection coating the reflection of sunlight can be kept well under 3%, making the cell appear black ("black cell"). The textured surface also provides a reduction in path length to the junction which is most pronounced for longer wavelength light, thereby increasing longer wavelength collection efficiency (an important factor for thin devices) and radiation tolerance. As bulk region diffusion length is reduced by the effects of radiation, the reduced effective path length enables a contoured surface device to maintain more of the lower wavelength response than a comparable smooth cell.

Texturization increases solar absorbance also in the wavelength region not contributing to the carrier generation. To compensate for the resulting higher temperature special infrared (IR) or blue-red-reflecting (BRR) coverglass coatings have been developed.

2.3.6 Contacts

Titanium-silver and nickel-gold with solder on the interconnector pads were used for the solar cell contacts in the early stages [12]. Later, when the welding technique replaced the soldering technique, the solder layer was eliminated and the titanium was protected against electro-corrosion by an intermediate palladium layer. Today the standard contacts consist of Ti/Pd/Ag applied by vacuum evaporation with a subsequent sintering process and photolithographic process for grid forming. A similar process is applied for the rear side with an additional Al-layer serving as BSR.

2.3.7 Bypass Function [13]

Cell breakage or shadowing of solar cells could cause the solar cell to operate in reverse, forming a so-called "hot spot" with temperatures up to 400 °C. This unwanted effect can be avoided by applying a bypass diode in parallel to the cell but in opposite polarity. By special n^+/p^+-doping through the diffusion layer, this bypass diode could be integrated into the cell structure thus saving the additional expense for separate diode application. The application of a bypass function is an indispensable requirement for modern sophisticated GaAs-based multijunction solar cells.

2.3.8 Surface Passivation

Exposed surfaces – such as between gridlines at the top of the cell or the interface between ohmic metal contacts and semiconductor – are generally regions of high carrier recombination velocity. Drift fields prevent the minority carriers from reaching the wrong surface by forming an electric field between highly doped and lightly doped material like for the BSF; these are already effective at reducing recombination velocity.

Another effective method of surface passivation is the growth of a high purity siliconoxide coating in micro-electronic quality. The purer the oxide the higher the passivation effect. This requires special cleaning provisions prior to the growth of the oxide.

A combination of both methods is the local back surface field [14] minimizing recombination at the metallic rear side point contacts while the majority of the cell rear side is passivated by silicon oxide (Fig. 2.9).

2.3.9 Low-Intensity, Low-Temperature Operation

For the ESA deep space mission ROSETTA ASE, the former Telefunken developed a silicon solar cell which did not show power reduction effects under extreme low-intensity, low-temperature (LILT) conditions. The cell possessed all the characteristics for high efficiency, such as a shallow emitter, passivation oxides on front and rear side, textured front side with inverted pyramids, local back surface field and optimum gridline design realized by means of photolithography. The introduction of a p^+-channel stopper in contact with the emitter provided very good diode characteristics and reverse protection because the n^+/p^+ diode operated like a Zener diode with reverse breakthrough voltages between -6 V and -8 V [15].

2.3.10 Solar Cell Assembly

For space applications, the solar cells use a coverglass for protection against charged particle irradiation and micrometeorites. The cells also require an interconnector to allow solar cell interconnection. The interconnector has to match the solar cell contacts and survive the thermal stresses which can cause multiple gap variations between adjacent cells. Therefore the preferred interconnector material is pure silver, silver coated Kovar or Molybdenum, the latter matching the thermal expansion coefficient of silicon very close. The interconnectors incorporate stress relief measures in order to withstand the mechanical and thermal stresses. In general, resistance welding is applied for the interconnector integration allowing, in connection with a thin interconnector thickness, a 100% coverage of the solar cell by the coverglass.

The coverglass is adhesively bonded to the solar cell front side. It is coated with an anti-reflection coating on the upper side and a UV-reflective coating on the inner side to protect the coverglass adhesive from darkening. Coverglasses with cerium oxide doping absorb the UV and don't need a UV-coating.

Bonding on the substrate, which is in general a carbon-fiber/Al-honeycomb structure with a polyimide foil insulation, is performed with an elastic cement leaving the gaps between the cells free in order to allow the cells undisturbed linear change. The costs for the silicon solar cell assembly and array integration and test are typically three to four times the solar cell costs.

2.3.11 High Efficiency Solar Cells

Figure 2.4a shows the advances in silicon solar cell performance that led to improved current and the voltage. Figure 2.4b shows improvements in electrical power, and Fig. 2.8 shows gains in efficiency. In Fig. 2.4b, 10 mW/cm^2 corresponds to an efficiency of 7.32% at standard air mass zero (AM0) illumination, averaging the sun spectrum and intensity in the air-free space close to the Earth. It should be pointed out that the reference sun spectrum and intensity for terrestrial applications (AM1.5) is different from the AM0 due to absorption and scattering in the atmosphere. This enhances the relative red portion in the spectrum leading to higher silicon solar cell efficiencies.

The production efficiency of a series product with optimized design (Fig. 2.5) achieved 17.5% in the 1980s (Sharp, Telefunken). At that point the development of space solar cells concentrated more and more on Gallium-Arsenide solar cells on Germanium substrate, which were offered by U.S. manufacturers Spectrolab and Tecstar with efficiencies over 19%. These cells were available for a reasonable price and had the potential to realize higher efficiencies. This potential was based on the possibility of using a special epitaxial process to grow several cells monolithically on top of each other, forming a so-called multijunction solar cell [16]. Such cells

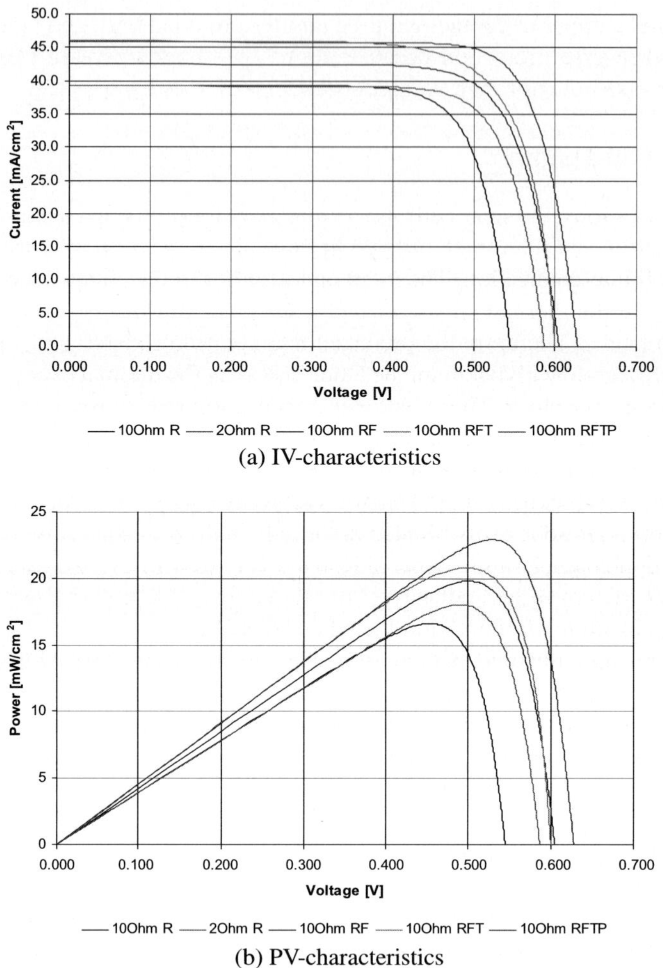

(a) IV-characteristics

(b) PV-characteristics

Fig. 2.4. Advances in silicon solar cell performance valued at the IV and PV characteristics. Legend: R: back surface reflector; F: back surface field; T: texture; P: passivation

use the sun spectrum much better and operate at much higher voltages. As a consequence, in space applications, silicon solar cells were more and more replaced by GaAs-based solar cells. Nevertheless, the potential of silicon solar cells was not exhausted, and developers found a similar challenging field in terrestrial applications.

Manufacture of multijunction solar cells on the basis of materials from the III/V-groups of the periodic system is possible because the materials can be composed with different band gaps but identical lattice constant. This is necessary for monolithically growing materials on top of each other. Figure 2.6 shows that, for silicon, no suitable crystalline partner can be found limiting the efficiency of silicon solar cells to the monojunction maximum.

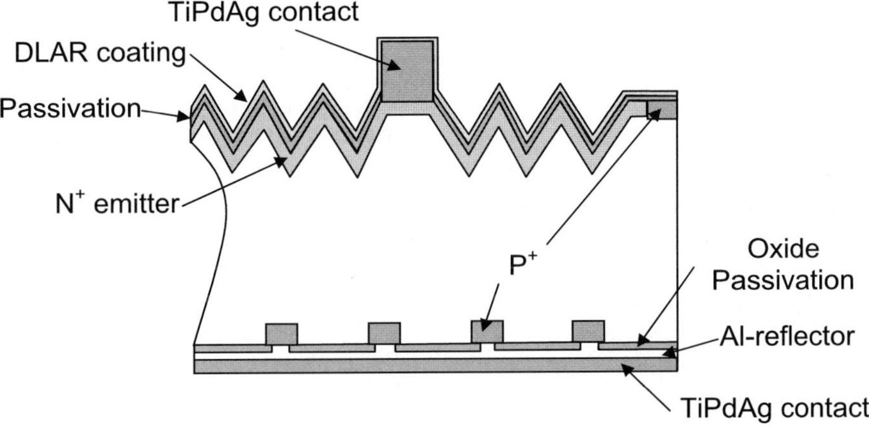

Fig. 2.5. Telefunken 17.5% high-efficiency space solar cell 2wiTHI-ETA®3-ID/ 130

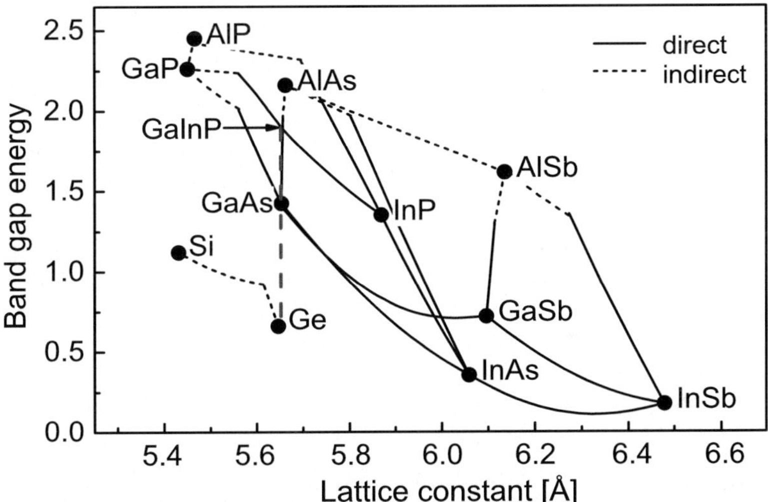

Fig. 2.6. Band gap of some semiconducting materials over their lattice constant. Only materials with same lattice constant like, e.g., Ge – GaAs – GaInP are intermateable

A multijunction solar cell is formed by stacking solar cells of different bandgap on top of one another. With the highest bandgap cell uppermost, light is automatically filtered as it passes through the stack. Each cell absorbs the light it can most efficiently convert, with the rest passing through to underlying cells (Fig. 2.7).

The first monolithic multijunction solar cells came onto the market in middle of the 1990s. These cells featured a dual junction solar cell consisting of a GaInP-top cell and a GaInAs-bottom cell epitaxially grown on a passive Ge-substrate by means of a chemical vapor deposition process using metalorganic precursors (MOCVD).

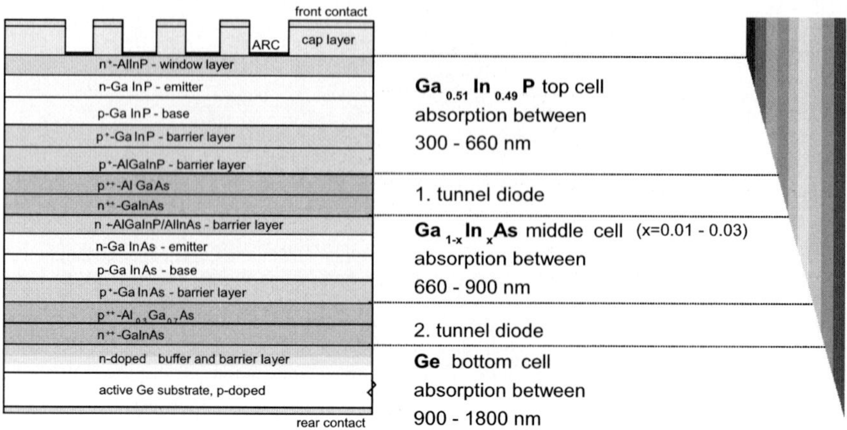

Fig. 2.7. Typical structure of a triple junction solar cell

The improvement compared to a single junction GaAs solar cell was more than 30% and yielded AM0-efficiencies of up to 24%. The first triple junction solar cells were developed at the end of the 1990s and consisted of a GaInP top cell, a GaInAs middle cell and a Ge bottom cell. By continuous improvements in the material, the growth conditions and especially the tunnel diodes separating the subcells from each other, the AM0-efficiency of triple junction cells has been improved from 25% in 2002 to 28.5% in 2006 (see Fig. 2.8). By optimizing the subcell design, the sensitivity to particle irradiation is only half that of silicon solar cells [17, 18]. Both high efficiency and high radiation hardness make the GaAs-based multijunction solar cells ideal for powering spacecrafts. But the price, which is more than five times that of a high-efficiency silicon solar cell (due to the sophisticated cell structure reflected in Fig. 2.7) limits terrestrial applications to concentrating systems.

Terrestrial applications started by adapting the technology developed for space as far as feasible. The developers of terrestrial photovoltaics did not have to consider the harsh space environment impacts and the mass requirements imposed on the design of space grade solar generators. Instead, the modules required encapsulation to protect the metallic cell contacts and interconnectors from corrosion and from mechanical damage caused by handling, hail, birds, and objects dropped or thrown on them. Additional requirements were UV stability, tolerance against terrestrial temperature extremes, abrasion hardness and self-cleaning ability. These requirements were met by a substrate consisting of aluminum, steel, epoxy board or window glass, a glass window, and as an encapsulant silicone adhesive or, alternatively, polyvinyl butyral (PVB) or ethylene/vinyl acetate (EVA).

But these solutions could not be realized in very large quantities at costs that allow solar-generated electricity to compete with wholesale electricity prices. To do so required not only low-cost approaches and low energy consumption during cell fabrication, but also high energy conversion efficiency to offset unavoidable area-related material and installation costs.

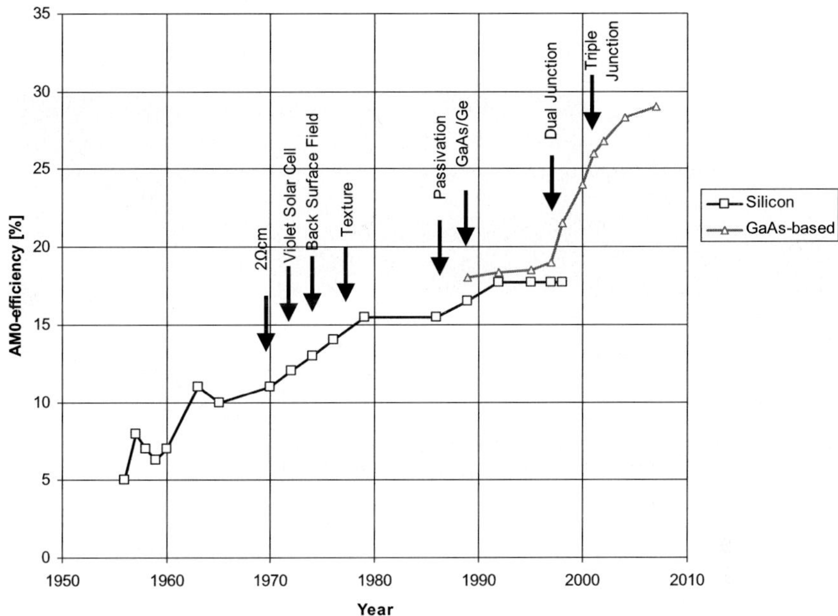

Fig. 2.8. Development of AM0-efficiency for space solar cells

To further improve the silicon solar cell efficiency, the following features have been introduced step-by-step:

- Highly doped bulk material (1 Ω cm base resistivity compared to 2–10 Ω cm for space solar cells).
- Use of float zone (FZ) silicon crystals instead of crucible grown (CZ). Due to the absence of oxygen in the molten silicon during the FZ process, there are no effects of thermal donors or oxygen precipitates. This produces a silicon wafer that has extremely stable resistivity performance and high carrier lifetimes. For space applications FZ material degrades more under combined particle/UV-radiation than CZ.
- Optimized emitter. In order to gain the full benefit of improved emitter surface passivation on cell performance, it is necessary to tailor the emitter doping profile so that the emitter is lightly doped between the gridlines, yet heavily doped under them.
- Shorter and narrower grid lines allow higher fill factors. Another approach for an improved fill factor is a shingled array design. Cells overlap in the module and the cell busbar area is shaded by the following row of cells. This allows a wide busbar design.
- Laser-grooved grid contacts followed by a second enhanced phosphorous diffusion producing selective doping in the contact areas.

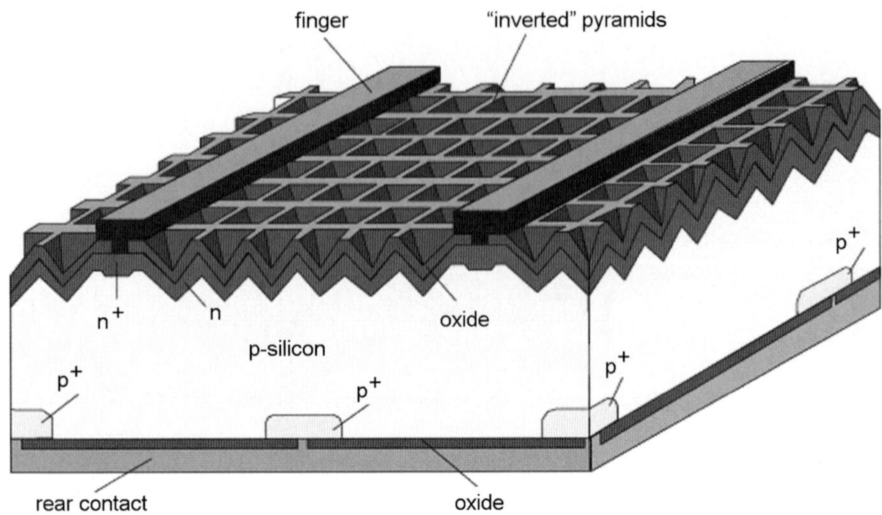

Fig. 2.9. Schematic of a PERL silicon solar cell (www.udel.edu/igert/pvcdrom)

A cell incorporating all of these improvements – in addition to the achievements of the space industry – is the passivated emitter with rear locally diffused (PERL) cell. This cell was developed by the University of New South Wales (Australia) (Fig. 2.9 and [19, 20]). It uses micro-electronic techniques to produce cells with efficiencies approaching 25% under the standard terrestrial AM1.5 spectrum. The passivated emitter refers to the high-quality oxide at the front surface that significantly lowers the number of carriers recombining at the surface. The rear is locally diffused only at the metal contacts to minimize recombination while maintaining good electrical contact.

Such extremely high-efficiency solar cells are very suitable for special applications, such as solar car racing, research and other applications where efficiency is the prime consideration. They are not a cost-competitive solution to most domestic and commercial solar cell applications. Achieving 23–25% efficiency, their price at ca. $400 U.S./W is about 100 times the cost of a standard commercial solar cell. They are cost prohibitive even for space applications.

The 1990 World Solar Challenge (WSC_solar-powered car race was won by "The Spirit of Biel" from the Engineering University of Biel, in Switzerland. Biel's winning time was 46 hours and eight minutes (65.3 ave. kmph). Biel's array was composed of laser-grooved aerospace cells that were connected by overlapping them in shingle style. The combination of high-efficiency cells with a high packing density (97.5%) resulted in an impressive 170 watts per square meter. The sleek, colorful, 182 kg solar racing car was clocked at 101 km/h during qualification trials and cruised at 72.4 km/h under mid-day sun [21].

2.4 Cost Reduction Measures

The efforts toward cost reduction had to consider design, materials and processes while keeping cell performance as high as possible. The most important parameter became the power-to-cost ratio replacing the power-to-weight ratio applicable for space solar generators. Compared with the highly sophisticated space technology, the following simplifications have been achieved step-by-step.

The major portion of the material costs is the expensive purification of the raw silicon and the single-crystal growing processes. Therefore numerous efforts have been undertaken to create basic material using less-pure silicon and a lower degree of crystalline perfection than the semiconductor-grade silicon.

2.4.1 Silicon Production

Alternative processes have been developed that, at a fraction of the cost of conventional semiconductor-grade silicon, create cells capable of adequate performance. The most common process applies the so-called fluid bed principle, using Trichlorosilane Cl_3HSi as the charge material which is then transferred into Monosilane SiH_4. From this the solar-grade silicon is extracted by cracking. This process is capable of reducing the costs required for semiconductor-grade material by 70%.

2.4.2 Bulk Material

A lot of material is lost by cutting the wafers into rectangular shapes. This waste of material can be avoided by using circular cells for the module assembly at the cost of low packing density. Waste can also be reduced by growing the ingots in square cross-sections to begin with. This can be achieved by casting silicon into boules or bricks. This process saves money compared to the CZ single-crystal growth technology but produces polycrystalline material instead of monocrystalline [22]. It has been demonstrated that a cell made of cast silicon can produce 12% to 14% efficiency and cost about 60% of a typical CZ cell. However, the slicing process is still necessary by which 50% of the material is lost.

A process that avoids material loss by slicing is the edge-defined, film-fed growth (EFG) of silicon [23]. This process consists of a slotted die of carbon or quartz which is partly dipped into molten silicon. The liquid silicon wets the die and is attracted into the slot by capillary action, forming a ribbon with the cross-section of the slot. Ten-cm wide ribbons at speeds up to 4 cm/min. were successfully grown in 1980 [24]. The process has been optimized by SCHOTT Solar (formerly RWE Solar), growing polycrystalline ribbons with a width of 15 cm at a growth speed of more than 10 cm/min. applying octagonally shaped dies.

2.4.3 Cell Contacts

Alternative developments replacing the expensive evaporation process were nickel plating followed by solder dipping and screen printing of metal pastes. Using the latter method, thin layers of a paste with fine-grained metal powder are printed on the cell surface by silkscreen technique and fired afterwards in a continuous sintering furnace under inert atmosphere. Fine glass particles dispersed in the paste act as binders for the metal powder after firing. This process reduced costs by replacing the expensive, high-purity titanium – silver with an aluminum – silver mix and the discontinuous evaporation procedure by a continuous process. On the rear side, the addition of aluminum increases the doping level in the surface region with the alloy forming a back surface field. There are several disadvantages to this technology, including a restricted width of the gridlines, a high contact resistance between paste and silicon, and low conductivity of the sintered material.

These disadvantages were extensively reduced by employing a buried contact design. Grooves, cut into the top surface emitter by laser scribing, mechanical or chemical approaches, provide for increased contact area and grid finger cross-section. The metal application is either by screen printing or is electroless by immersing the wafers in a plating solution. Grooved contacts give a 30% performance advantage over screen printed cells without grooves.

2.4.4 Encapsulation

The encapsulation of the modules has to guarantee long life operation under extreme weather conditions. For the transparent front side, safety glass is commonly used; its thickness results from a trade-off between material cost savings and additional costs due to increased breakage rate. The rear side is made either of glass, like the front side, or of a weather- and waterproof foil back. The cells are embedded in silicone or in ethylene vinyl acetate (EVA). For edge protection and mounting the assembly is firmly bordered with a sturdy, fully closed aluminum frame. An automated production line with high throughput ensures consistent product quality and low costs.

2.5 Concentrating Systems – A New Opportunity for High Efficiency Space Solar Cells

The power-to-weight ratio of a terrestrial module is typically more than 10 W/kg compared to 100 W/kg for a typical space solar array. Launch costs in the range of 20,000 €/kg justify the application of highly sophisticated technology for space.

Nevertheless, high-efficiency space grade solar cells have a good chance of entering the terrestrial market. The primary impediment to direct application is the high price. But this can be drastically reduced by operating the solar cells in a concentrated system. This has two advantages: On the one hand, the cell size is reduced approximately proportional to the concentration factor; on the other hand, the efficiency is increased by a factor proportional to the logarithm of the concentration. These facts have prompted a resurgence of research in multijunction cells and commercial interest in concentrator III–V photovoltaics. Of particular interest are high

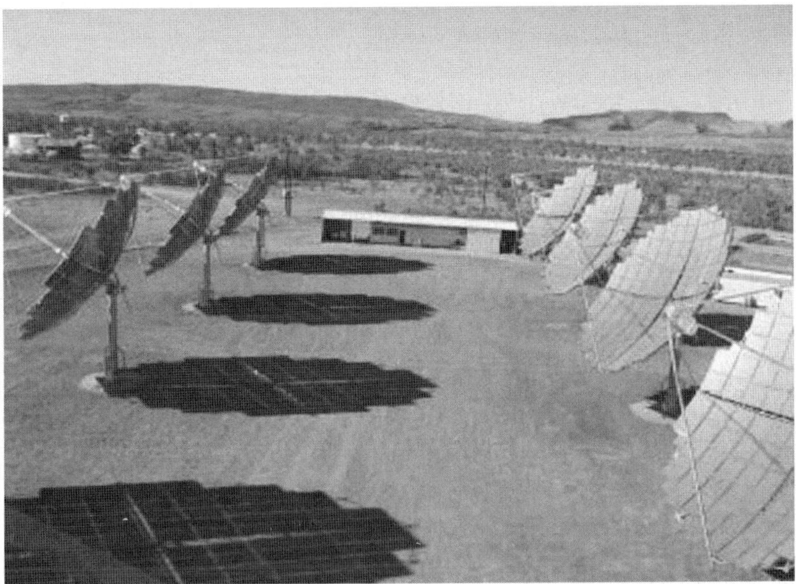

Fig. 2.10. 190 kWp power station by Solar Systems [27]

concentration systems. A record 40.7% efficiency at 240 suns was reported at the Madrid Conference in 2007 [25].

Over more than 30 years many research groups were engaged in developing concentrator photovoltaic systems (CPV). In the first concentrator modules and installations, large-area mirrors (0.5–1 m in diameter) focused the sunlight on cells of several square centimeters in area. Cooling by water or by means of thermal pipes was necessary [26]. Several reliable and efficient CPV power stations have been demonstrated, e.g., by Solar Systems in Australia (Fig. 2.10 and [27]). For this system, a new triple junction receiver was developed to replace the current silicon point-contact solar cells. The new receiver technology is based on high-efficiency (>35%) concentrator triple junction solar cells from Spectrolab, resulting in system power and energy performance improvement of more than 50% compared to the silicon cells. This is also due to the fact that multijunction cells exhibit lower ohmic losses because they operate at lower currents.

Appearance of the technology accessible for Fresnel lens fabrication has determined revision of the photovoltaic module design. Solar cells could be placed behind the concentrators in this case. The module housing could serve as a protector from the environment and provided for cooling by thermal conductivity. Since the Fresnel lenses had smaller dimensions (25×25 cm^2), the photocell dimensions were also decreased down to less than 1 cm^2.

In the late 1980s, the Ioffe Physico-Technical Institute, St. Petersburg [28] proposed the concept of a radical decrease in the concentrator dimensions while retaining a high sunlight concentration ratio. The first experimental modules of such a

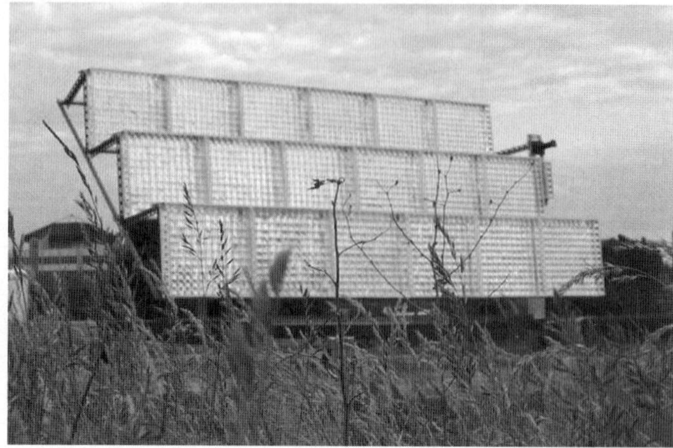

Fig. 2.11. Array of the Ioffe full-size concentrator modules with small aperture area Fresnel lenses

type consisted of a panel of lenses, each of 1×1 or 2×2 cm^2, focusing radiation on AlGaAs/GaAs cells of submillimeter size. At that time, the main advantages of a module with small-aperture area concentrators were: the requirements imposed on the capability of heat-sinking material to conduct heat, on its thermal expansion coefficient and on its thickness are essentially relieved. The focal distance of such lenses appeared to be comparable with the structural thickness of the conventional modules without concentrators.

The team at the Ioffe Institute has developed concentrator modules [29] in which Fresnel lenses are arranged on a common superstrate to form a panel of 12×12 lenses. Cells as small as 2×2 mm^2 and 1.7 mm, in a designated area diameter and operating at a mean concentration ratio of about $700\times$, are used (Fig. 2.11). The lens profile was optimized, taking into account the refraction index of the lens material and its dependence on wavelength, focal distance, receiver diameter, sun illumination spectrum, and the sensitivity spectra of the subcells in a multijunction cell. The lens structure consists of a sheet of silicate glass and refracting microprisms formed of transparent silicone on the inner side of the glass. The microprisms themselves are formed by polymerization of the silicone compound directly on the glass sheet with the use of a negatively profiled mold. The advantages of this concentrator technology are based on the high UV stability of silicone, its excellent resistance to thermal shocks and high/low temperatures, good adhesive properties in a stack with silicate glass, simplicity and very high accuracy of the formation method. The accuracy of cell position is of great importance because each cell must be placed in the center of the focal spot of a corresponding lens. This accuracy has to be about 100 μm, which is realized by using automatic processes and standard electronic industry machines.

The overall module outdoor conversion efficiency as high as 24.6% was measured on a 2×4 lenses module. But the outdoor efficiency could exceed 28% at

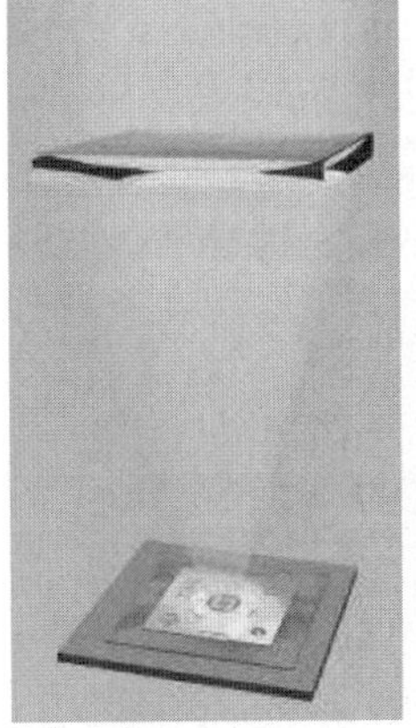
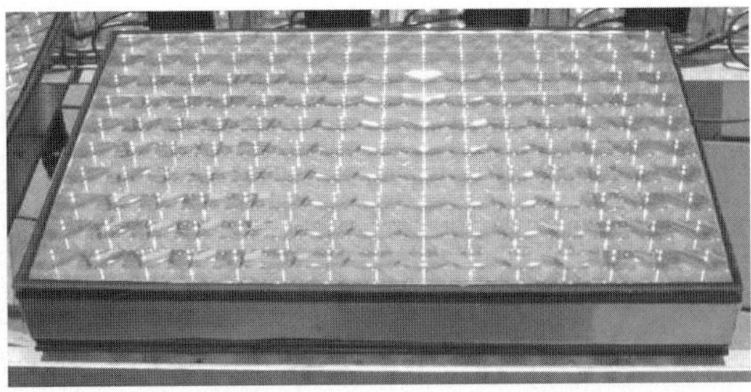

Principle   Module with 10x15 assemblies

Fig. 2.12. FLATCON®-module Technology [31]

lower ambient temperature, or at the use of the cells with indoor efficiencies in the range of 39–40% instead of used ones with 32.34%.

Concentrix Solar, Germany, also uses high-efficiency triple junction solar cells in their FLATCON®-modules [30, 31]. Figure 2.12 shows the principle of the FLAT-CON technology and a photo of a module consisting of 150 Fresnel lenses made of embossed silicone on a $4 \times 4\,cm^2$ glass plate equipped with circular triple junction cells with an active area diameter of 2.3 mm and a grid design optimized for the inhomogeneous illumination under the Fresnel lens. Under standard test conditions the efficiency is 33.0% at 300–500 suns. Typical operating module efficiency is 25.5%.

Most of the progress in solar cell development has been made for space use to the benefit of terrestrial applications. However, some of the technological improvements are starting to flow the other way, with discussion of solar cells made from copper-indiumdiselenide (CIS) material. This thin-film technology is very resistant to charged particle degradation and could be considered for space missions exposed to extremely difficult charged particle environment, e.g. those near the Jupiter moon Europa.

References

1. J. Perlin, *From Space to Earth: the Story of Solar Electricity, AATEC Publications* (Ann Arbor, Michigan, 1999). ISBN 0-937948-14-4
2. M. Wolf, Historical development of solar cells, in *Proc. 25th Power Sources Symposium*, 23–25 May 1972
3. J.J. Wysocki, P. Rappaport, Effect of temperature on photovoltaic solar energy conversion. J. Appl. Phys. **31** (1960)

4. Z.I. Alferov, V.M. Andreev, V.D. Rumyantsev, *III–V solar cells and concentrator arrays*, Ioffe Physico-Technical Institute, 26 Polytechnicheskaya str., St. Petersburg 194021, Russia
5. V.M. Andreev, V.R. Larionov, V.D. Rumyantsev, O.M. Fedorova, Sh.Sh. Shamukhamedov, P AlGaAs – pGaAs – nGaAs solar cells with efficiencies of 19% at AM0 and 24% at AM1.5. Sov. Tech. Phys. Lett. **9**(10), 537–538 (1983)
6. M. Wolf, A new look at silicon solar cell performance. Energy Convers. **11** (1971)
7. M. Wolf, Drift fields in photovoltaic solar energy converter cells, in *Proc. IEEE*, vol. 51, May 1963
8. Spectrolab Inc. Spectrolab production solar cell design data, 10 August 1981
9. G. Strobl et al., Experiences with implanted BSF solar cells, in *Proc. 4th European Symposium "Solar Generators in Space" Cannes*, 18–20 Sept. 1984 (ESA SP-210)
10. J. Lindmayer, J.F. Allison, The violet cell: an improved silicon solar cell, in *Ninth IEEE Photovoltaic Specialists Conference*, Silver Spring, Md., 2–4 May 1972
11. C.R. Baraona, H.W. Brandhorst, V grooved silicon solar cells, in *Proceedings of 11th Photovoltaic Specialists Conference*, 1975
12. P. Iles, Present state of solar cell production, in *Proc. 5th PVSC, NASA-GSFC*, Greenbelt, MD, 1965
13. T. Hisamatsu, H. Washio et al., Reverse bias characteristics of modules made of solar cells with and without integrated bypass function (IBF), in *Proc. 25th PVSC*, Washington, D.C., 13–17 May 1996
14. AZUR Patent DE 3815512C2
15. G. Strobl, H. Fiebrich, Production experience with LILT silicon solar cells for ROSETTA qualification, in *Proc. of 2nd WCPSEC*, Vienna, July 6–10 1998
16. B. Beaumont, J.P. Contour, P. Gibart, J.C. Guillaume, C. Vèrié, Conversion photovoltaique à haut rendement: le projet quadrispectral, in *Proc. 4th Europ. Symp. "Photovoltaic Generators in Space"*, Cannes, 18–20 Sept. 1984 (ESA – SP-210 Nov. 1984)
17. M. Meusel et al., Development status of European multi-junction space solar cells with high radiation hardness, in *Proc. 20th EPSEC*, Barcelona, 2005
18. G. Strobl et al., European roadmap of multijunction solar cells and qualification status, in *IEEE 4th World Conference on Photovoltaic Energy Conversion*, Waikoloa, Hawaii, 7–12 May 2006
19. J. Zhao, A. Wang, E. Abbaspour-Sani, F. Yun, M.A. Green, 22.3% efficient silicon solar cell module, in *25th PVSC*, Washington, DC, 13–17 May 1996
20. M.A. Green, *Silicon Solar Cells – Advanced Principles & Practice* (Sydney, 1996)
21. R.J. King, Recent car technology developments including Australian world solar challenge results, in *Proc. of 22nd IEEE PVSC*, 1991
22. K. Roy, K.-D. Rasch, H. Fischer, Growth structure of cast silicon and related photovoltaic properties of solar cells, in *Proc. 14th PVSC*, San Diego, CA, 1980
23. H.E. Bates, D.N. Jewett, V.E. White, Growth of silicon ribbon by edge defined, film-fed growth, in *Proc. 10th IEEE PVSC*, 13–15 Nov. 1973
24. J.P. Kalejs, B.H. Mackintosh, E.M. Sachs, F.V. Wald, Progress in the growth of wide silicon ribbons by the EFG technique at high speed using multiple growth stations, in *Proc. 14th IEEE PVSC*, San Diego, CA, 1980
25. R.R. King et al., Metamorphic concentrator solar cells with over 40% conversion efficiency, ECSC-4, in *4th International Conference on Solar Concentrators*, Madrid, 12–16 March 2007
26. Z.I. Alferov, V.M. Andreev, Kh.K. Aripov, V.R. Larionov, V.D. Rumyantsev, Pattern of autonomal solar installation with heterostructure solar cells and concentrators. Geliotechnica **2**, 3–6 (1981). Appl. Solar Energy **2** (1981)

27. P.J. Verlinden et al., Performance and reliability of multijunction III–V modules for concentrating dish and central receiver applications, in *IEEE 4th World Conference on Photovoltaic Energy Conversion*, Waikoloa, Hawaii, 7–12 May 2006
28. V.M. Andreev, V.R. Larionov, V.D. Rumyantsev, M.Z. Shvarts, High-efficiency solar concentrating GaAs-AlGaAs modules with small-size lens units, in *11th European Photovoltaic Solar Energy Conference and Exhibition – Book of Abstracts; abstract No. 1A. 15*, Montreux, Switzerland, 12–16 October 1992
29. V.M. Andreev, E.A. Ionova, V.D. Rumyantsev, N.A. Sadchikov, M.Z. Shvarts, Concentrator PV modules of "all-glass" design with modified structure, in *Proceedings of 3rd World Conference on Photovoltaic Energy Conversion 3P-C3-72*, 2003
30. A.W. Bett et al., High-concentration PV using III–V solar cells, in *2006 IEEE 4th World Conference on Photovoltaic Energy Conversion*, Waikoloa, Hawaii, on 7–12 May 2006
31. H. Lerchenmüller et al., From FLATCON® pilot systems to the first power plant, ECSC-4, in *4th International Conference on Solar Concentrators*, Madrid, 12–16 March 2007

3 PV Solar Electricity:
From a Niche Market to One
of the Most Important Mainstream Markets
for Electricity

W. Hoffmann and L. Waldmann

3.1 General Overview

PV solar electricity is seen as one of the few booming markets, today and in the coming decades. This market has grown globally at a rate of about 40% per year over the past 10 years. Related industries have realized a two-digit, billion-dollar (U.S.) turnover worldwide. PV solar electricity is a high-tech industry with high performance potential in the coming decades, leaving even the electronics industries behind and approaching the automotive industry.

The PV history and future can be differentiated into the following four phases, each phase lasting roughly two decades.

1960 to 1980: PV solar technology was developed as an energy supply for satellites in the early 1960s. Companies like Tecstar in the United States, AEG (one of the roots of today's SCHOTT Solar) in Germany and Sharp in Japan were the leading manufacturers in this technology. This first phase ended in the 1980s, as PV technology for satellites was well established and feasible. In this period, the price per watt of PV power came down to earth.

1980 to 2000: This second phase can be characterized by tremendous progress in research, development and demonstration, driven by investment aimed at employing PV technology for terrestrial use. Pilot projects to manufacture solar cells and modules were tested. Sales mainly were in small kW applications with even some MW projects; for example, the 6 MW Carrissa Plains plant in the U.S. in the early 1980s. In remote areas, PV was already cost effective for many applications. Market activities increased markedly, first in the U.S. in the 1980s and followed by Germany in the 1990s. Japan also adopted a specific industry policy in the 1990s. With the market support programs in Japan and following in Germany (starting in 1990 and extended with the feed-in tariff by 2000) these three countries developed an emerging industry.

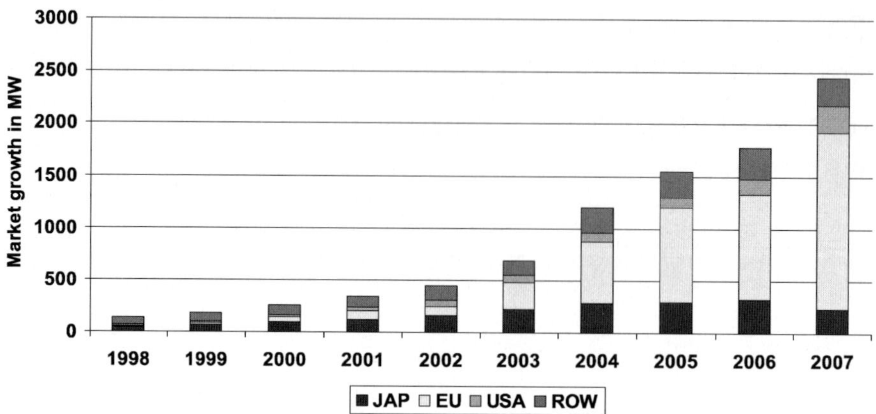

Fig. 3.1. Historical market development of PV solar electricity installation according to regions

2000 to 2020: This third phase could be named as a transition phase. In this period the benefits of the former political framework, as well as public awareness for the necessity of renewable energies go together with PV solar technology, which comes toward cost effectiveness in all market segments. Market support programs in more and more countries enable the local production industry for PV Solar technology to grow accordingly. With leading markets in Germany, the US and Japan, Spain, several new markets will emerge in Asia, Europe and the Americas.

2020 to 2040: In the fourth phase, finally PV solar electricity will be established on the world market. Due to the growing worldwide industrial production and thus falling costs, PV is competitive in all market segments and cost effective compared to most conventional energy sources.

PV solar electricity is a major technology and will play a significant role in the future development of economies worldwide. PV can help provide both industrial growth and the chance for at least 2 billion people to get access at all to energy by using clean electricity. In turn, this will open doors for education and development in poor and rural areas. Solar electricity technology might emerge as a key technology to represent the new industrial drive. Provided a growth rate of around 25% in the coming years, a total turnover of PV Systems worldwide can be estimated at around 100 billion Euros in 2020 and well above in the following years.

The PV vision of the European Commission for 2030 is to realize all the socio-economic benefits provided by (1) in the short-term, employment in large-scale, high-tech production; (2) in the mid-term, raising a viable industry that creates revenues and pays taxes; and last but not least (3) in the long-term supplying a significant contribution to global energy need with clean PV solar electricity. Thereby, in addition, PV contributes to reducing dependence on oil and gas imports and to help secure local energy supplies. Given recent political instability in the Middle

East, and after the crisis of gas supply between Russia and Ukraine, the premises of energy supply have changed crucially. Costs for risks and dependency have to be calculated on top of rising prices. The further growth will also cut significantly carbon dioxide emission by replacing power from fossil fuels.

The common goal of the PV industry and the European Commission is to create a self-sustaining market for solar electricity products by 2020. To attain this ambitious goal all instruments for market stimulation, technological development and system changes have to intertwine internationally.

3.2 PV Solar Electricity Market History

The annual market, which crossed the impressive number of one gigawatt, in average had an overall growth since 1998 by about 40%. The PV market for terrestrial applications may be divided into four major segments serving different customer needs:

- *Consumer*: Application in consumer goods such as calculators, wristwatches, garden lights, automotive applications etc.
- *Off-grid* Industrial: Remote industrial applications e.g. telecommunication repeater stations.
  Off-grid Residential: Rural electrification in developing countries providing for light, refrigeration and communication.
- *On-grid*: All applications connected to a national electricity grid.
- *High efficiency application*.

Consumer products powered by small solar applications will stay a niche market in terms of megawatt output. Nevertheless, intelligent housing and mobile communication provide growing demands for these applications in the future.

Also important are markets that are small in terms of number of applications, but that have high potential in terms of power output; this is the market for highest efficiency PV. Satellite powering and concentrator plants are typical applications for the highest efficiency segment.

While three market segments – off-grid industrial, residential and consumer – are already competitive today (these grew at a modest 18% p.a.), the fourth market segment of grid-connected systems increased by astonishing 63% p.a. The latter growth started in the USA in the 1980s, followed by Japan in the mid 1990s with Europe, in particular Germany, in the year 2000. The different growth rates catapulted the contribution of grid-connected systems in relation to the total market from about one quarter eight years ago towards more than three quarters today. The shares of these applications in the total market turned bottom up. The reason for this development is basically due to industry-politically induced market-support programs in the aforementioned countries. Today we find the feed-in tariff system in Germany, Spain, Italy, Greece, South Korea and India and some more to come in Europe as well as investment subsidies in Japan, U.S. and some other countries.

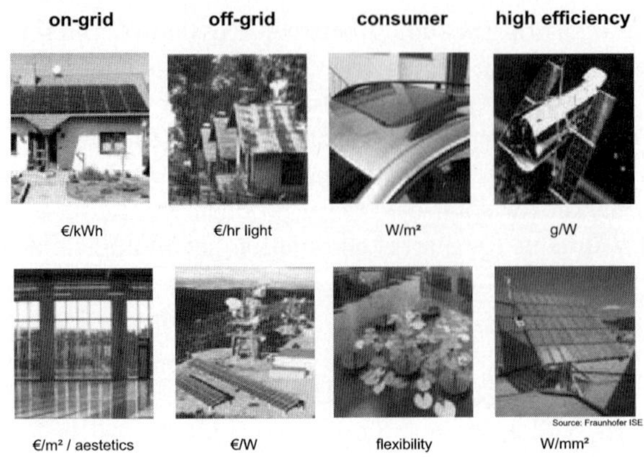

Fig. 3.2. Customer needs for different PV technologies

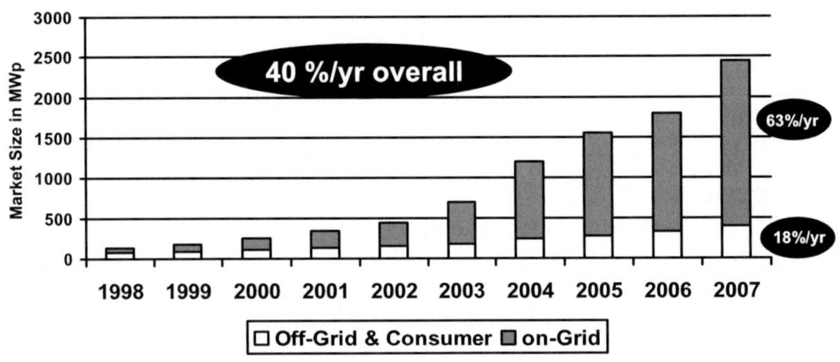

Fig. 3.3. Historic growth according to application

In 2004 Germany became the world leader in newly installed systems, with a total of more than 600 MW, leaving Japan far behind with 280 MW. But this development was not always foreseeable. The lessons learned from all the ups and downs in the German PV market can be summarized as follows: First, to create a fruitful environment and good conditions for a strong PV market, reliable long-term conditions must be requested. Second, financial incentives and an attractive feed-in tariff can actually compete with each other, especially when the financial incentive is restricted, capped or has to be applied for. In the latter case the customer follows the principle of maximizing benefits and waits for the additional incentive even when the feed-in tariff alone is sufficient for a return on investment rate of 6–8%. This effect is to be avoided. And third, the bureaucratic obstacles must be removed. In Spain, for example, it still takes more than 12 months to get all the permissions needed to install a PV plant.

These support schemes are necessary to have the market growth as described in the next section.

Table 3.1. Subsidy schemes of important European PV markets

	Feed in Tariff [€ct/kWh] Subsidy programm	Market size 2007	Targets
Germany	35.49–51.75	1,100 MWp	28% RES-E in 2020
Spain	23–44	623 MWp	400 MWp in 2010
Italy	36–49	50 MWp	3,000 MWp
France	31.19–57.19 50% tax reduction max 8000/16000 € grants in some regions	45 MWp	490 MWp in 2015
Greece	40–50 20%–60% grants for commercial plants	2 MWp (25% grid connected)	700 MWp in 2020

After all it has to be kept in mind that the estimated market growth in Europe can only be realized when the Spanish market opens up and other European countries follow. It is quite important to outline under which boundary conditions grid-connected systems will be competitive without support programs. The interaction of market growth, module price and competitiveness of PV solar electricity is discussed in Sect. 3.4.

3.3 Price and Competitiveness of PV Solar Electricity

In a more and more liberalized utility market, electricity produced by PV solar electricity systems worldwide will be able to compete with their generating cost first against peak power prices from utilities. This situation is most likely to happen within the next decade in more southern areas with higher solar irradiation (1,500–1,800 kWh/kW) while it may take about one decade more in places like Germany with lower insolation (800–1,000 kWh/kW). The point of time for this competitiveness is determined mainly by three major facts:

- Price decrease for PV solar electric systems leading to an equivalent decrease in the actual cost for PV generated electricity.
- Development of a truly liberalized electricity market.
- Correlation of higher priced peak power delivery from utilities and output of a PV solar electricity system.

Looking at electricity spot markets, clear price spikes can be seen that directly correspond with the energy yield of an installed PV solar array. The correspondence

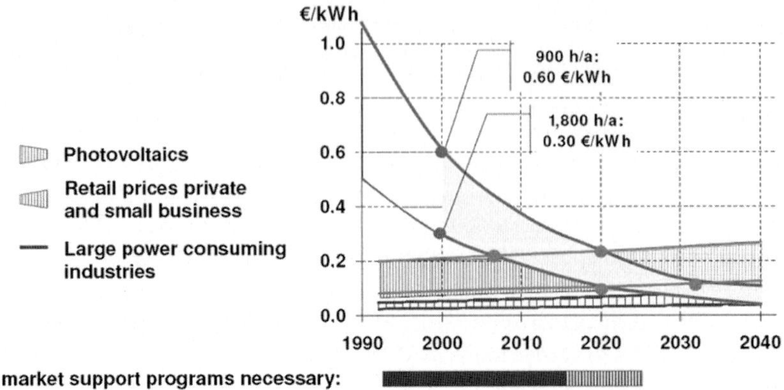

Fig. 3.4. Competitiveness of PV solar electricity

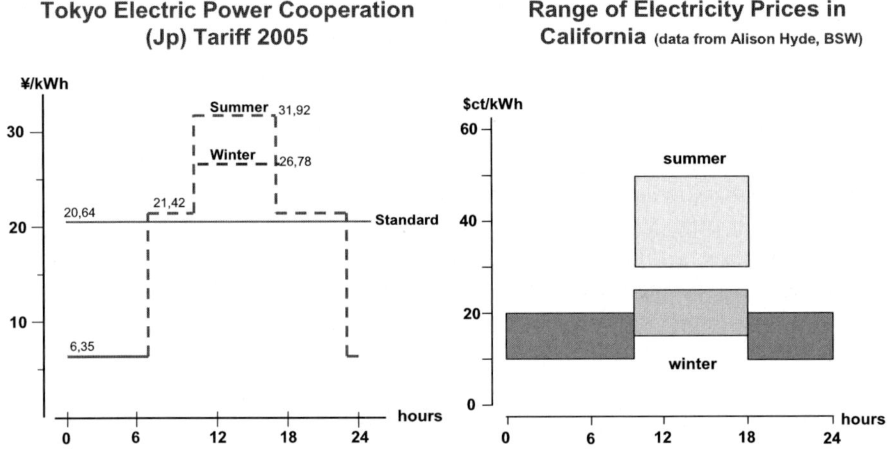

Fig. 3.5. Electricity retail prices for various countries

is remarkable with respect to time when one considers that the electricity is generated directly on the rooftop of the building where the energy is required. So the generation costs of PV solar electricity and the price of conventional electricity has to be compared at the point of sale, which is the power outlet. The electricity tariff of Tokyo Electric Power Corporation (TEPCO) provides a differentiated tariff that changes during the daytime and over the seasons. Thus, during the summer and at daytime, PV solar electricity in Tokyo is already cost effective for the customer. For this reason the Japanese market is still not collapsing, even though the incentives for PV in Japan went down to zero. A very similar situation can be observed in the liberalized electricity market of California. Differentiated tariffs show the highest price at summer during daytime. In these market situations, PV solar electricity is already cost competitive compared with the price at the private power socket.

Conventional energy costs are more likely to increase due to higher prices for gas, oil and coal and for the internalization of external costs as for the sequestration and storage of carbon dioxide. At the same time, prices for the technology-driven PV solar electricity will decrease. That gives us a clear picture for the future market.

For PV solar modules, there exists a good model for future price expectations derived from price experience curves. In analogy to production cost learning curves, a price experience curve in a double logarithmic plot shows the dependence of the component price versus the cumulative sold volume of said product. Typically one obtains a straight line whose slope determines the so-called experience factor, that being the price decrease in % by doubling the accumulated sold volume. This experience factor has been determined for a number of industries. The general finding is that for products where the smaller part of production cost is material-driven and the remaining, greater cost is "intelligence", one obtains experience factors at and above 30%. Examples are electronic devices with experience factors of 30 to 40% and, as a specific example, light-guided fiber cables with experience factors of 45%. Such experience factors in most cases typically stay constant for a given product and for quite a long time. In contrast, products with dominant material costs – e.g. float glass, steel, etc. – show almost no decrease in price; in fact, sometimes these products increase in price with more volume sold.

The price experience curve for PV solar modules currently shows a 20% decrease of price by doubling the cumulative volume. The material contribution for the product, the PV solar module, within the value-added steps is roughly two thirds for materials like glass, frame or plastic. The other one third is more "intelligence" driven, like cell efficiency or productivity by economy of scale. No surprise, in total there is then a 20% experience factor obtained.

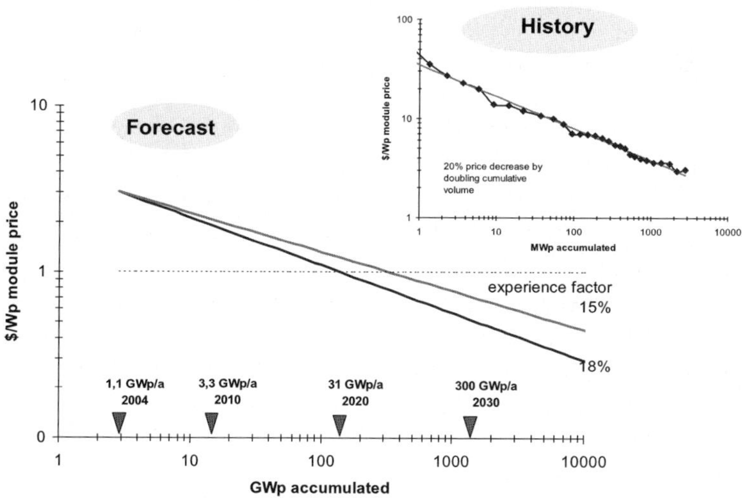

Fig. 3.6. Price experience curve for PV solar modules

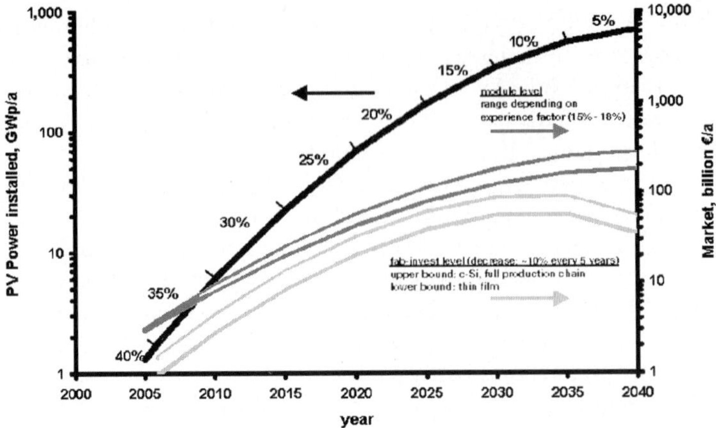

Fig. 3.7. Future growth of global PV solar electricity market in GWp and Bn€ turnover

As the proportion of material cost contribution increases with further production volumes, the experience factor may decrease from 20 to 18% or even 15%, just so we do not overestimate future cost decreases. On the shortfall of solar-grade poly silicon, a slight deviation of the ideal line is observed as the price for poly silicon more than tripled. After the massive investments and the boost in production capacity for poly silicon in 2008 the actual price points will most likely go back forwards the projected line. Whether Thin Film technologies will demonstrate a higher experience factor remains to be seen in the coming years.

It is important to realize that a price experience curve does not give us any answer as to the time when certain price levels will be reached. This can be obtained by assuming an annual growth rate from which an accumulated volume of sold products can be calculated and inserted as points in time when respective volumes will be reached. Taken together, the 25% annual growth and the experience factor of 15 to 18% would lead one to estimate an expected price decrease of about 5–7% per year, which is equivalent to half the price every 10 to 13 years.

The future generating cost for electricity was examined by the European Association of Utilities, Eurelectric, together with VGB Power Tech. As a result a study on electricity generation cost was released. The study compares different energy transforming processes:

- Fossil (coal, gas, lignite)
- Advanced fossil
- Nuclear
- Hydro
- Wind (off shore)

These processes were investigated at three different points in time: 2005, 2030 and 2050.

Price decrease by technological progress is taken into account, in addition to the development of prices for fuels and resources during that time period.

Table 3.2. Cost of electricity production with various technologies

	Cost of Electricity – Overlook			
	2005	2030	2030 CC	2050 CC
Hard Coal	4.11	6.18	6.72	6.46
Natural	4.44	6.95	7.06	8.76
Gas Lignite	3.72	6.47	6.21	6.19
IGCC	4.79	6.54	5.72	5.43
OxyFuel			6.09	5.95
Nuclear	4.30	4.70		4.90
Hydro run river	4.10		4.10+	
Wind off shore	7.62		7.57	
Cost of Electricity figures are in €-ct/kWh in prices of 2005				
Source: Eurelectric 2007				

Electricity generating cost [ct€/kWh]	Today 2005	Tomorrow 2030	Day after tomorrow 2050
Wind, off- on-shore	9/7.5[*]	6/5[*]	3/4
Solar thermal power	17[*]	6[*]	3
PV solar south/north	20/40	5/10	3/6

Source: Own estimates
[*] Eurelectric 2007

A clear increase is assumed in all fossil technologies. Today one kWh power output from coal or gas can be generated at a price level of 4 to 4.5 cent Euros. At 2030 this price will go up to 6–7 ct€ and leads to 6.5–9 ct€ in 2050.

The range for nuclear power starts at 4.3 ct€ and will likely stay stable until 2050 at 4.9 ct€. Hydro stays stable at 4.1 ct€ for the whole period.

Not surprisingly, wind power is represented by off-shore applications. But there is no significant price decrease through technological development indicated. Off-shore wind starts at 7.62 ct€, coming down to 7.57 ct€/kWh in 2030 and 2050.

Solar thermal power plants and PV solar electricity are not seen to have a significant contribution.

Other renewables were not subject to this study.

In fact there must be made some adjustments in this study from the point of view of the renewable energy sector.

As shown above the price experience curve will have its impact on the electricity generating cost. Of course, the rate is different with different technologies. PV solar electricity has a proven rate of around 20% price decrease by doubling the production output. Translated to a time scheme that assumes a growth rate of 25% for the PV sector, the 20% price experience curve leads us to estimate at least a 5% price decrease per year. That is to halve the generation cost every 12 years and, as a side effect, produce clean electricity without fuel cost. Solar thermal power plants today are calculated to have electricity generating costs at 17 ct€/kWh falling to 3 ct€ according to existing production and research-and-development roadmaps in this industry. At this point we want to appeal to the energy sector not to underestimate the PV solar mainstream market power and the potential of concentrated solar thermal power.

3.4 Future Market Development

PV solar electricity in total has a huge potential to ease the upcoming energy problems. Looking closer into the PV solar electricity business we see several customer needs to be served by different technologies and products. These needs depend on the kind of application and the functions which are intended by using PV solar power. Each of these customer needs are covered by specific products and PV technologies. First and fastest growing today is the grid-connected segment. Here we see mainly rooftop applications, but also a growing awareness for building-integrated PV systems (BIPV). With BIPV, cost savings can be realized by replacing functional parts of a building with PV components and thus diminishing installation and material costs. Provided an existing feed-in tariff, the price per kWh tells the profitability of the investment in the PV system. The on-grid market definitely left the niche category in 2000 and entered the mainstream in 2004.

But in fact there are several other criteria the customer may have in mind depending on the purpose of the PV system. Off-grid applications are the second market. For an energy supply to a remote facility – for example, for a telecommunication repeater set in a desert area – long-term reliability will be taken into account. For rural electrification, the decentralized and modular structure of PV offers the best solutions, especially for light and small solar home systems. Having in mind the growing number of people without fair access to clean energy, we can assume that this segment will follow the on-grid segment, moving from niche status to mainstream. Rural electrification will become a real mainstream market in two decades. So the picture today will change from a few regional markets and low share for rural into many widespread markets and a 50% share for rural applications.

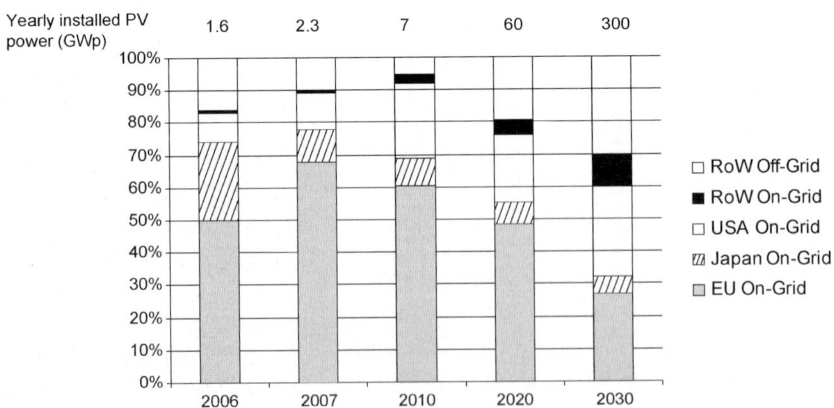

Fig. 3.8. Split of PV market according to region for on-grid and off-grid applications

Currently there are about 2–3 billion people in the world who are still without electric light and other amenities of the industrial world; this figure is not likely to change until 2030, due to the continuing population growth in these remote rural areas. Off-grid PV electricity supplies, such as PV-driven water-pumping systems, small solar home systems (SHS), and small village grids are aimed at greatly alleviating this situation.

For solar home systems in developing countries, both cost and service are important. The average monthly cost has been estimated by the Deutsche Gesellschaft für Technische Zusammenarbeit (GTZ), a federal Association for technical cooperation. For nonequipped homes the expenses for batteries, candles and kerosene amount to $6 to 8 (U.S.) per month. A 50 W PV solar electricity system with battery and charge controller represents an investment of about $500 (U.S.). That results in about $7 (U.S.) per month over six to eight years under the assumption of a low-interest loan (World Bank, national institutions, or banks supporting developing countries such as KfW). Microfinance is the core issue for this market segment. In the case of solar home systems, the performance, the operational lifetime and the price per service are more important than any considerations of PV module efficiency.

The need for solar villages in rural areas is eminently important due to the increase in global electricity consumption according to IEA, from 16,000 TWh in 2001 towards 36,000 TWh in 2040; the growth of the population in third-world regions will result in a need for more than 20,000 TWh within 35 years. More than half of the people will live in rural areas have not been connected to a main grid for decades due to prohibitive cost.

Decentralized power by renewable energies is the only choice. The PV solar technology employed for solar villages in rural areas is technology similar to grid-connected systems, e.g., in Germany. All cost and price decreases will be able to contribute to a faster and more widespread installation of decentralized power in these most needed applications.

3.5 Technology Evolution

All the existing technologies can be compared in terms of relative prices and module efficiencies. The crystalline wafer silicon technology with monocrystalline Czochralski wafers have a market share of around 30%; multicrystalline wafers make up around 60% of the market; and ribbon silicon wafers come close to 3% market share. These crystalline technologies (c-Si) show module efficiencies between 12 and 18% and have a total market share of 95%. The thin-film technologies like amorphous silicon with 4% market share and other thin-film technologies – e.g., CIS and CdTe – add up to the remaining 1% market share.

Setting a point of reference for module cost of 100% for modules containing ribbon silicon wafers with efficiency of 14.3%, the cost of the different technologies can be compared on relative terms. Modules with mainstream multicrystalline technology come to 111%, monocrystalline in conventional processing end up at 116%.

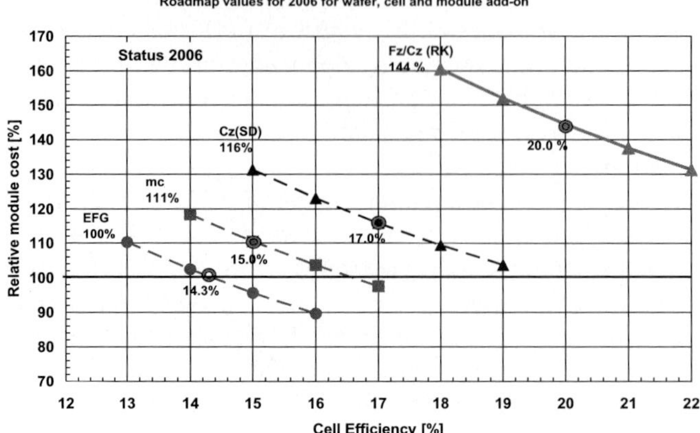

Fig. 3.9. Relative module cost by technology

In 2008 the curves will all be shifted by about 1.5% absolute to higher efficiencies, hence the same relative cost comparison applies.

Higher efficiencies lead to higher total cost by adding higher wafer and cell-processing cost and higher module add-on cost. Looking at the module cost relative to the efficiency of different technologies in 2006, the picture shows clear favorites. The very high efficiencies in monocrystalline cell technology – with 20% cell efficiency gained through rear contacting – have relative module costs that are up to 44% above the reference point of ribbon silicon technology, which has 14.3% cell efficiency. (Estimates by SCHOTT Solar on the basis of the technology roadmap.) This example shows that the technological pathway is also a function of market and economy. Highest efficiencies do not necessarily lead to lowest module prices per power output.

As time progresses, the module efficiencies will shift towards higher values and new technologies, like dye and organic cells may evolve.

To compare prices we set arbitrarily the highest price module with monocrystalline wafers and highest efficiencies to 100, then the price range shifts in relative terms from 70–100 in the year 2000 down to 35–60 in 2010 and 15–35 in 2020, corresponding well to the forecast in the price experience curve which we mentioned earlier. Looking to the split for the three major technologies we see 95% for c-Si and 5% for thin film in 2000. Toward 2020 we might find some two thirds c-Si technology and one third of thin film and new technologies, respectively. Even in 2030 we predict at least a share of one third for c-Si wafer technology. Altogether, there is good evidence that the price decrease for PV solar electricity produced kWh will decrease as assumed before.

Several side and synergy effects out of the TFT flat-panel display technology can be used for thin-film technology. Some of the processes handle similar material so basically the same machinery can be used.

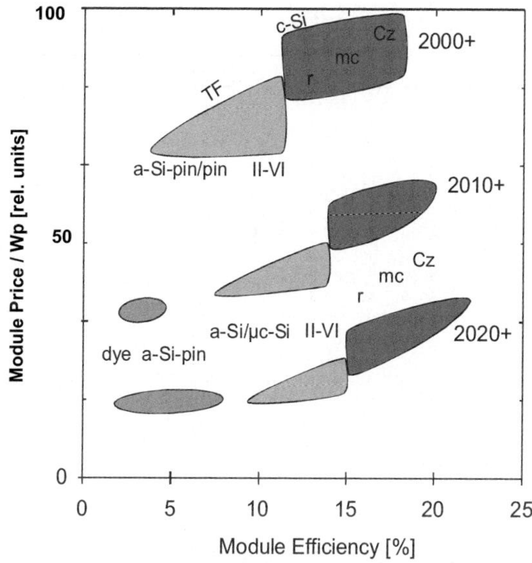

Fig. 3.10. Development for relative cost and module efficiency for various PV technologies

As a consequence of employing different technologies, different customer needs in separate markets can be served. The crystalline technology with high power per area and efficiencies between 25 and 40% will be a very niche product for space and concentrator applications.

The higher middle range, with efficiencies from 16 to 25% and premium price level covers the high power needs also in niche markets. The largest market share by far will have the mainstream multicrystalline and ribbon technology. With efficiencies from 14 to 16% these modules will be the PV workhorse in cost-effective applications. Both the high-efficiency and the medium-efficiency crystalline segment together will most likely take 95% of the market share within the next decade till 2015. Thin film and new concepts are going to catch up in the following decade until 2025, covering the largest market share starting in 2030.

With new concepts, in the future new materials and applications might be possible. Whereas the solar revolution in remote rural areas of our globe will literally mean "power to the people", the same solar revolution in industrialized areas must be a revolution of design in the building sector, urban planning and architectural solutions. This pathway has begun today.

This is in concert with a thorough study done by the German Advisory Council on Global Change (Towards Sustainable Energy Systems). In this study a share of more than one third of the global primary energy consumption in 2040 is predicted to be covered by renewable energies, in total with an approximate 10% share for combined PV solar electricity and solar thermal power stations. In 2100 the same study assumes an 85% coverage of primary energy consumption by renewables, with two thirds of that delivered by solar thermal power plants and PV solar elec-

Table 3.3. Various PV technologies in comparison

(a) Crystalline silicon		(b) Thin film	
Cz, Fz	High power/area @ premium price eta 16–25% space, niche markets	II–VI compound (CIS CTS) a-Si/µc-Si and thin Si films	Additional solutions for cost effective power applications eta 8–18%
mc & ribbon (EFG)	Cost effective power application eta 14–16% "The PV workhorse"	pin-ASI and ASI-THRU®	Low price/area @ low eta eta 4–6% "Solar electricity glass"
(c) III–V compounds (GaAs)		(d) New concepts	
Highest power/area @ very high price		Dye cells	"Color to PV" (eta 3–10%)
Multi bandgap	eta 25–40%	Organic cells	"Low material cost option"
	Space, concentrating systems	Scientific high eta approaches aiming for eta 30–60%	Utilization of hot electrons, intermediate band cells, up/down conversion, quantum wells, nanostructures etc.

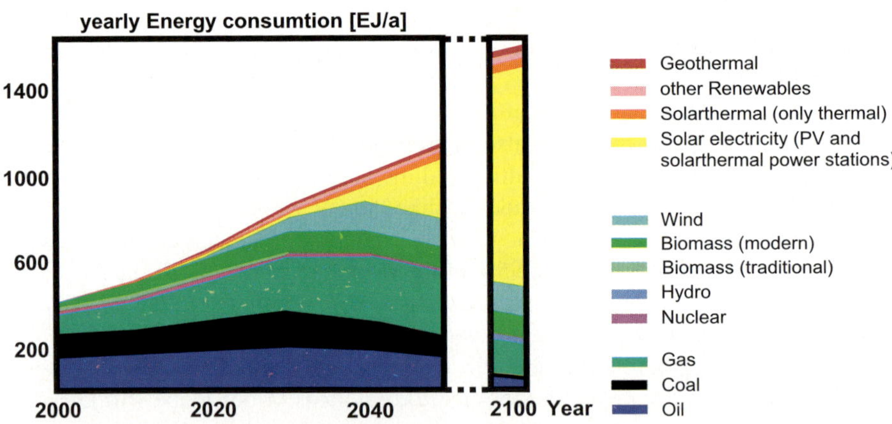

Fig. 3.11. Contribution of various technologies for global prime energy consumption

tricity systems. Although such long-term extrapolations always contain uncertainty, it is quite useful to examine highly probable boundary conditions – i.e. world population growth, prime energy split into applications and energy usage by region and application, environmental constraints etc. All these predictions tell us the tremendous need to act toward a major energy supply with PV solar electricity.

References

1. EPIA Roadmap, June 2004, http://www.epia.org/index.php?id=18
2. EREC "Renewable Energy Scenario to 2040", May 2004, http://www.erec.org/documents/publications/2040-scenario.html
3. German Advisory Council on Global Change, World in Transitions: Towards sustainable energy systems, Earthscan, London and Sterling, 2004
4. Sarasin Study "Solarenergie – ungetrübter Sonnenschein?", November 2004, Study "Solarenergie 2005", December 2005, Study "Solarenergie 2006", December 2006
5. SolarBuzz, MarketBuzz^{TM} 2005 "Annual World PV Solar Market Report 2005", March 2005 and MarketBuzz^{TM} 2006, "Annual World PV Solar Market Report 2006", March 2006
6. Strategies Unlimited, "Photovoltaics manufacturer shipments 2004, 2005 and 2006" published each April of following years

4 Advanced Solar-Grade Si Material

K. Hesse

4.1 Introduction

For three decades scientists around the world have been searching for the right technology to produce silicon feedstock for the photovoltaic industry, feedstock that fulfills the need for "low cost" as well as the need for sufficient quality. The urgency of this task has intensified since 1998, when it became clear that the PV demand could no longer be met with by-products from the electronics industry. The established producers of polysilicon developed specific products for the solar industry, but for the time being cannot catch up with the exploding demand. The actual Si shortage resulted in very high spot prices for solar-grade silicon and led to discussions on whether existing producers with their production methods will be able to cover the future demand of the solar industry. There are, again, opinions being expressed that alternative production methods are more suitable to fill the gap at lower costs. Here, requirements and possibilities have to be checked very carefully. In addition, old knowledge and experience about the different possibilities to produce silicon should not be forgotten. The future supply of silicon to the PV industry has to be seen in the tense environment of quality, costs and time of implementation.

4.2 Production Pathways for Solar Silicon Feedstock

4.2.1 Metallurgical Grade Silicon: Carbothermic Reduction of Silica as a Starting Point for Most Pathways

Most pathways for the production of solar silicon feedstock start with metallurgical silicon ("silicon metal", purity $> 98\%$) and end with hyperpure silicon (purity in the parts per billion range), so the challenge is to do this purification as efficiently as possible. The silicon metal is produced in submerged electric arc furnaces (electrical consumption between 10 to 30 MW) according to the formula

$$SiO_2 + 2C = Si + 2CO.$$

The feedstock includes woodchips, high-purity quartz lumps and high-purity coal, respectively charcoal and coke.

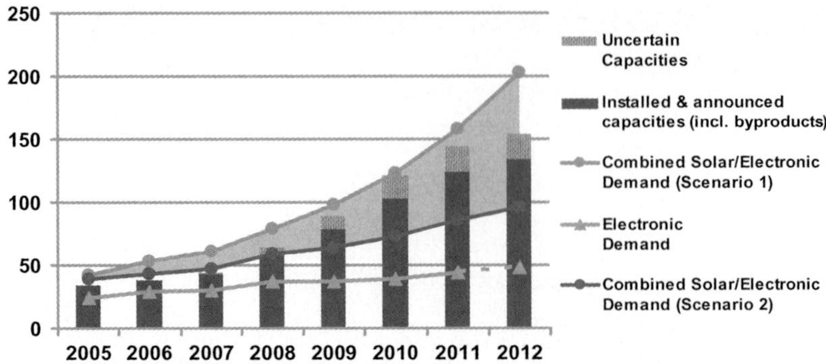

Fig. 4.1. Global polysilicon supply and demand (in ktons; mg-Si included) Status: June 2006

The silicon melt has to refined, is solidified in the casting process to get a multicrystalline structure and then crushed.

An important byproduct are silica fumes, formed in an side reaction according to the formulas

$$2Si + O_2 = 2SiO,$$
$$2SiO + O_2 = 2SiO_2.$$

Due to economy of scale and process improvements, the electric consumption of 10–11 KWh per kg has been achieved, compared to more than 14 KWh/kg in the past [1].

As the worldwide production capacity for metallurgical silicon is far more than 1 mio mto/a (most of it for the metal/aluminum industry) there is no foreseen supply bottleneck.

Regarding the quartz as feedstock, it is certainly true that SiO_2 is one of the most abundant materials available on Earth (as sand). But if you are looking for high-purity quartz – as is necessary for high-purity metallurgical silicon – the availability is much more limited to special mines, e.g. in Spain or Brazil. This is not so much an issue of availability, but of costs (for mining and transport). So the often-used saying "from sand to electric energy" is misleading, because fine sand cannot be used easily in the furnaces and, in addition, usually has too many contaminants.

The purity of a typical metallurgical-grade silicon with respect to metallic impurities is approximately six orders of magnitude worse than that of a typical solar-grade silicon. So purification for solar needs is an inevitability.

4.2.2 Established Production Methods: Purification of Metallurgical Silicon via the "Silane Route" is Dominating

The extreme purity required for silicon in photovoltaic or electronics applications is achieved by converting metallurgical grade silicon into silanes (large scale industrial

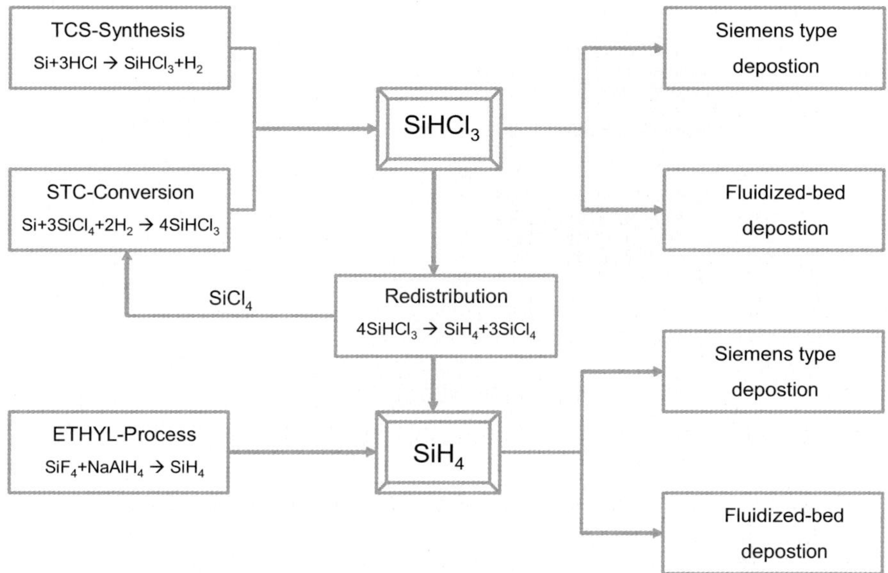

Fig. 4.2. Pathways for polysilicon production

processes are based on trichlorosilane or monosilane), which are then distilled and decomposed to yield hyperpure silicon. The conventional method is the so-called Siemens process, in which TCS is decomposed in bell jar-type reactors in the presence of hydrogen with the deposition of polysilicon on thin silicon rods [2]. The silicon tetrachloride (STC) produced as a byproduct is hydrogenated back to TCS or is used as a feedstock for pyrogenic silica. The fluidized-bed CVD process used to deposit polysilicon appears to be a very attractive alternative to the Siemens deposition process. WACKER has developed a successful fluidized-bed deposition process for granular solar-grade polysilicon based on TCS [3]. In contrast, two completely different processes use monosilane (SiH_4) as the feedstock for deposition of polysilicon. As shown in Fig. 4.2, one of these processes uses TCS as a feedstock to afford SiH_4, whereas the other process is based on SiF_4, a byproduct from the production of superphosphate fertilizers. Semiconductor-grade monosilane can be used in a modified low-temperature Siemens process or in a fluidized-bed deposition reactor to produce polysilicon.

According to a study by Pichel [4] in 2005, approximately 73% of the global capacity of polysilicon was produced using the Siemens process and TCS as a feedstock (Fig. 4.3).

4.2.3 Differences in Using TCS or Silane as Feedstock

Lobreyer [5] demonstrated that comparable qualities of semiconductor-grade polysilicon could be obtained from Siemens deposition of polysilicon, regardless of the type of silane feedstock (TCS or monosilane).

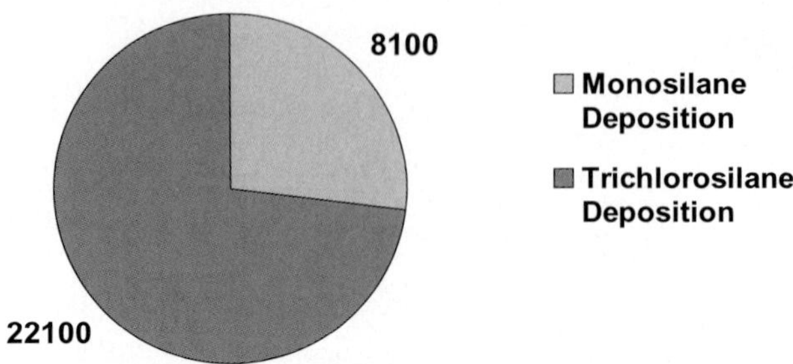

Fig. 4.3. Global capacity of polycrystalline silicon in 2005 [4]

There are pros and cons associated with the use of both monosilane and TCS to deposit polysilicon. Breneman [6] published a detailed review discussing the key advantages and disadvantages.

The deposition of polysilicon from monosilane can be carried out at a temperature as low as 650 °C, whereas temperatures >900 °C are necessary for TCS. If monosilane is used, the main problem appears to be the production of silicon dust by homogeneous vapor deposition, which decreases yields and limits deposition rates; it also negatively affects product morphology (pores, density, microroughness). If TCS is used, approximately 1/4 reacts to form silicon, 3/4 is converted into STC, and the remainder leaves the reactor as off-gas. On the other hand, if monosilane is used, conversion rates of nearly 100% are obtained and hydrogen is practically the only byproduct. The main pathway to produce monosilane is redistribution of TCS to monosilane and STC; here 1/4 of the TCS reacts to Monosilane and 3/4 is converted to STC; so the system with monosilane deposition has to deal with the same amounts of chlorosilanes as the TCS-based deposition system. There are also major differences in handling of the individual silanes. The self-ignition and the very low boiling point of monosilane necessitate extremely strict safety engineering requirements and a complex cryodistillation system.

Regarding the process complexity, the WACKER TCS-process achieves a closed loop production system based on only three chemical reactions:

$$mgSi + 3HCl \rightarrow SiHCl_3 + H_2 \qquad \text{metallurgical Si to TCS,} \qquad (4.1)$$
$$4SiHCl_3 \rightarrow Si + 3SiCl_4 + 2H_2 \qquad \text{deposition of Si,} \qquad (4.2)$$
$$3SiCl_4 + 3H_2 \rightarrow 3SiHCl_3 + 3HCl \qquad \text{hydrogenation of STC,} \qquad (4.3)$$

$mgSi \rightarrow Si$ sum: purification of metallurgical silicon to hyper-pure silicon, closed loops of hydrogen and chlorine

So the decisive point appears to be how the polysilicon deposition process is integrated into the manufacturer's particular product flow. The objective here is to either recycle all byproducts and waste products or to use them to synthesize other products to minimize losses of silicon, chlorine and hydrogen. It is also important

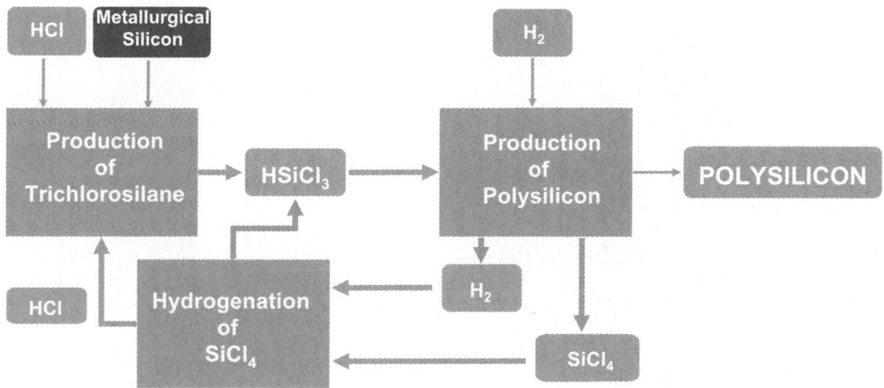

Fig. 4.4. WACKER polysilicon: Closed loops for hydrogen and chlorine yield significant cost advantages

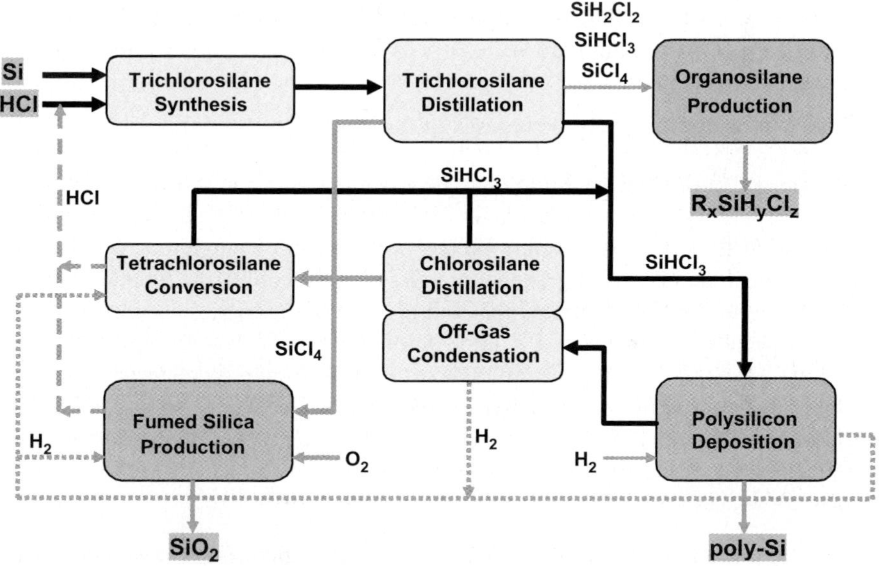

Fig. 4.5. Integrated product flow at Wacker Chemie AG, besides polysilicon, production of other value-added products is possible

to use any waste heat arising from the various processes within the integrated system.

The integrated product system used at the WACKER production site in Burghausen takes additional advantage of value-added products by linking the production of polysilicon to that of pyrogenic silica, organofunctional silanes, silicates and silicones (Fig. 4.5).

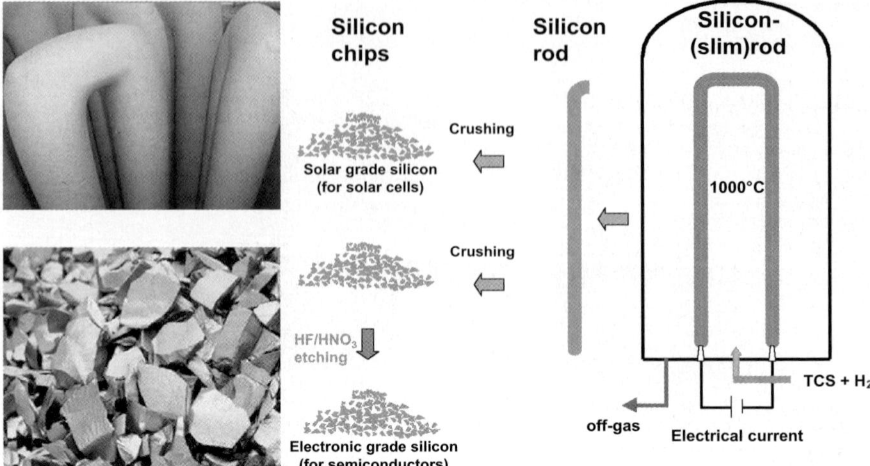

Fig. 4.6. Rod deposition: Optimized process of deposition handling and crushing for the solar industry

4.2.4 Accommodation of the Processes to the PV Requirements

An alternative to the "silane route" has been sought for many years, particularly for the production of solar-grade silicon. The purity of solar-grade silicon with respect to metallic impurities is approximately six orders of magnitude higher than that of a typical metallurgical-grade silicon. It is questionable as to whether there is an alternative to the "silane route" that can achieve this purity at acceptable costs. A very important parameter in PV applications is photovoltaic-system efficiency (generally 14–16%). The highest efficiencies with low specific material usage are possible only via high-quality feedstocks. For the production of solar grade feedstock, Wacker Chemie AG has optimized its production process taking into account the requirements of the solar industry for lower cost at somewhat lower quality requirements:

- The deposition process was modified for maximum deposition rate. The resulting rougher morphology does not impact the solar application.
- The purification of the surface by chemical cleaning or etching after crushing of the rods could be avoided by a new crushing process. This process leads to fewer contaminants, especially for metals, so that the solar requirements (metals contaminations in the low parts per billion per atom (ppba-) range can be fulfilled; the metal contamination of cleaned prime electronic-grade polysilicon are two orders of magnitude lower).

These modifications are allowing for economic production of solar feedstock, an important prerequisite for the actual capacity expansions at WACKER.

Deposition of granular polysilicon with trichlorosilane

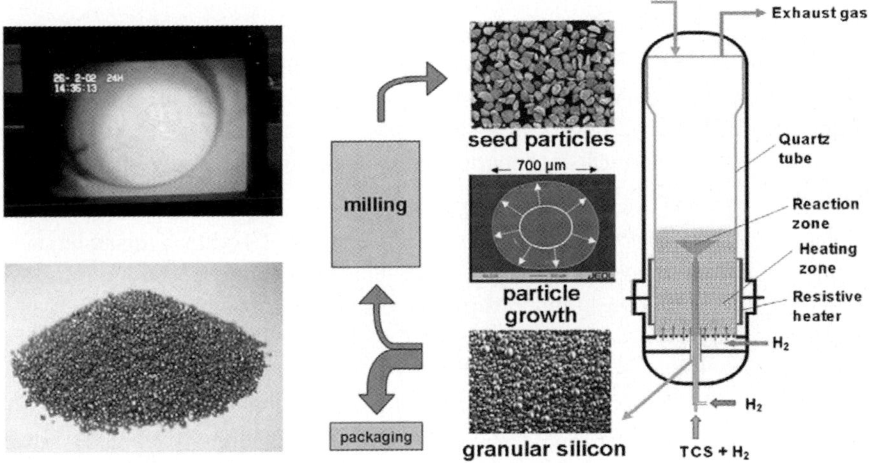

Fig. 4.7. Granular deposition

The fundamentals for cost-effective production of solar-grade silicon at WACKER POLYSILICON are:

- Highly integrated, but flexible production system: value-added use of byproducts.
- Economy of scale: investments, costs, productivity.
- Advanced reactor technology: high output, yield, quality.
- Flexible reactor technology: solar or electronic polysilicon according to demand.
- Fast realization time for new capacities with qualified personnel.

A fluidized bed deposition process might be a reasonable supplement to the "main route" rod deposition technology. In this process a fluidized bed of silicon particles is heated to the necessary decomposition temperature of the silicon containing gas which is passed through the bed. Ideally, elemental silicon is deposited on the silicon particles which hence are growing. It is possible to operate this process continuously by regularly withdrawing particles from the fluidized bed and adding smaller seed particles to the bed. The withdrawn particles are a ready-to-use product. Seed particles can be obtained, for example, by milling product granules. Besides the advantage of continuous operation, the process has the potential of lower specific energy consumption. For customers, granular polysilicon has a lot of advantages regarding handling, for high crucible filling grade (in combination with chunk material) and for applications that need a finely tunable continuous recharging. WACKER POLYSILICON is establishing this granular product to supplement its product portfolio.

4.2.5 The Myths of the "High-Energy/High-Cost" Rating of Established Silane-Based Polysilicon Deposition Technologies

There is a common perception that the production of solar- grade feedstock via gas-phase deposition is "too costly" because of the "high" energy consumption of the deposition process. And purification of silicon via metallurgical processes – i.e. different melting and crystallization steps, slag refining, treatment with different gases etc. – consumes much less energy and is therefore less expensive. But is this really true?

Myth 1: *High Temperature = high energy consumption*? The first misunderstanding is that high temperature in a process equals high energy consumption. But if there is no energy consuming reaction involved, the consumed energy is mainly influenced by the *energy losses* – a thermos bottle with hot fluid inside is also hot inside without being *"energy intensive"*. It is a similar situation with the gas-phase deposition. Energy consumption can be influenced a lot by scale, reactor design and process design. So the energy consumption figures given by Hunt et al. [2] are now much lower. Also the general belief that monosilane deposition is less energy consuming than trichlorosilane deposition, because of the lower deposition temperature, is not correct if you consider the maximum possible deposition rate: the trichlorosilane deposition rate can be much higher because the heterogeneous monosilane deposition rate is limited by the homogeneous gas-phase deposition (i.e. dust formation). The faster the deposition rate, the lower the energy losses. Also the high energy consumption for monosilane cryodistillation and storage has to be taken into account.

Myth 2: *The sum of chemical reactions, condensation and distillation steps of the silicon purification via silanes is more energy intensive than "direct" metallurgical purification.* Let us compare the trichlorosilane-based purification with a typical metallurgical purification involving at least two melting/crystallization steps (e.g. JFE-Process, Apollon Solar process [14, 15]) to reach the minimum required purity regarding metals by segregation. At WACKER the total energy consumption of the total TCS process is much lower than 100 kWh/kg with a total silicon yield of much more than 90%. In metallurgical refining, one melting /directed solidification step of silicon needs about 40 kWh/kg (relating to the usable end product). To reach a similar metal purity as the TCS-process you need at least three melting/solidification steps and still some elements cannot be efficiently removed due to their unfavorable segregation coefficient. In addition you have energy losses by treating the melt, e.g., with slag refining, gases, electron beam guns (for elimination of phosphorus), plasma torches (removal of boron) etc. to bring the dopant concentrations to an acceptable level. The remaining purity regarding carbon and dopants will still be worse compared to the TCS process. And you have high yield losses by slag and metal-contaminated parts after segregation. So there is no reason to condemn the "chemical" silicon purification methods in favor of "metallurgical" methods with respect to the needed energy or yield.

4.2.6 Alternative Technologies for the Production of Solar-Grade Feedstock: Purification of Metallurgical Silicon via Melt Treatment/Crystallization is Dominating

If you look at metallurgical methods you'll find that they need energy-intensive melting and crystallization processes and special treatments to remove dopants which are connected with yield losses. The achievable quality is still far lower as compared to gas-phase deposition processes. The situation is similar for the carbothermic direct reduction of pure quartz with pure carbon as well for the melt electrolysis of quartz. Other, previously evaluated and practiced methods – like the reduction of silicon compounds with metals, e.g. $SiCl_4$ with zinc in vapor phase or aluminothermic reduction – proved to be not competitive with regard to the achievable quality and costs. Important, limiting factors are the purities of the feed materials, contamination during the process steps, low yields of reaction steps and complex reprocessing of byproducts [9].

4.2.7 Alternative Vapor-Phase Deposition Technologies?

In a closed loop chlorosilane system the above-mentioned problems are already solved in large-scale production; the dominant technology is the heterogeneous vapor-phase deposition on rods. Thereby maximum purity is achieved. For solar-grade silicon, fluid bed deposition of granules is also a possibility. WACKER is testing this technology in a pilot project. Others are testing the deposition of silicon on hot surfaces with temperatures above melting point – "vapor-to-liquid" deposition [14]. The extremely corrosive nature of fluid silicon is limiting the achievable quality. The lowest energy consumption in deposition is reached in so-called "free space" reactors; here silanes are decomposed in a homogeneous gas phase reaction. But the resulting silicon is in the form of very fine particles ("dust"), which was not usable in the past because of the highly reactive oxidized surface and the low density which led to melting problems. There were also problems with contamination during handling of the material.

4.2.8 Time to Market

Very important is the period of time needed to develop new technologies to the point where they can be put into large-scale production. To come from a working concept in the lab to the pilot project and finally to production scale takes at least 10 years. This is a very long time frame compared to actual, extremely dynamic growth of the solar industry. That growth sets demanding targets regarding quality and especially costs. Based on its proven technology, WACKER actually almost tripled its capacity within four years, showing that it can keep up with the growth of the solar industry.

4.3 Summary

TCS will remain one of the semiconductor and photovoltaic industries' most important feedstocks in the future, regardless of whether it is used as a direct feedstock

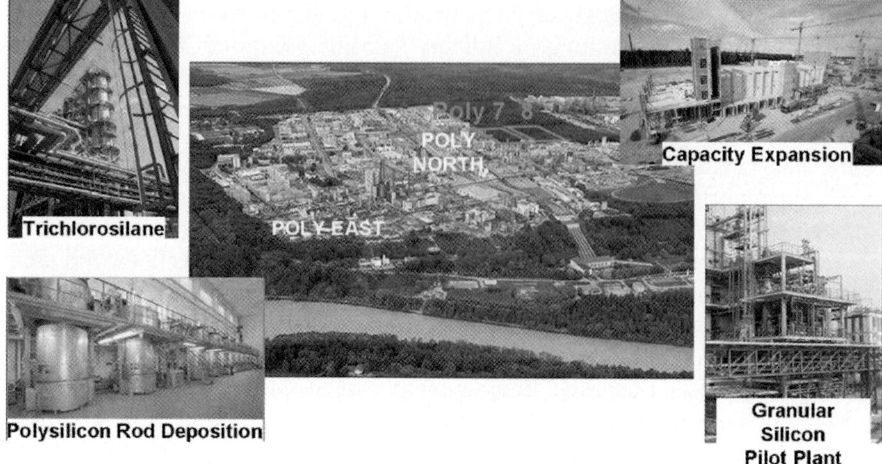

Fig. 4.8. Integrated polysilicon production of WACKER chemie AG in Burghausen, Germany

to produce polysilicon in the Siemens and granulated processes or as a raw material for monosilane production. For more than 50 years the WACKER group has used and improved polysilicon production based on vapor phase deposition of TCS in a closed loop process. Hydrogen and chlorine are processed in a cycle, and process heat is used efficiently in the chemical plant system. This process is safe and environmentally friendly and has further improvement potential. So it is suitable to meeting the future demand of the solar industry up to several hundred thousand tons. The capacity expansions to balance the actual shortage of polysilicon are under construction. In parallel, the downstream users are continuously improving the specific consumption of the precious polysilicon. Through higher cell efficiencies (based on high-quality feedstock), improved crystallization techniques, smaller wafer thicknesses, lower kerf loss during sawing and overall higher process yields, there is still the potential to lower the specific silicon consumption of about 10 g/Wp by almost half in the next several years [12].

References

1. A. Schei, J. Tuset, H. Tveit, *Production of High Silicon Alloys* (1998)
2. W.C. O'Mara, R.B. Herring, L.P. Hunt (eds.), *Handbook of Semiconductor Silicon Technology* (1990)
3. D. Weidhaus, E. Schindlbeck, K. Hesse, *Silicon for the Chemical Industry VII* (2004), p. 165, ISBN 82-90265-25-5
4. J. Pichel, M. Yang, *Renewable Energy Access*, Piper Jaffray, 11 January 2006
5. T. Lobreyer, K. Hesse, *Silicon for the Chemical Industry IV* (1998), p. 93, ISBN 82-90265-20-4
6. W. C Breneman, H.J. Dawson, *Silicon for the Chemical Industry IV* (1998), p. 101, ISBN 82-90265-20-4

7. I. Araki, T. Yamamoto, Y. Tokuda, H. Momose, *Silicon for the Chemical Industry VI* (2002), p. 197, ISBN 82-90265-24-7
8. H. Kohno, T. Kuroko, H. Itoh, *Silicon for the Chemical Industry II* (1994), p. 165, ISBN 82-519-1444-2
9. Flat-Plate Solar Array Project Final Report, vol. II: Silicon Material, JPL Publication 86-31, October 1986
10. Prometheus Institute, Polysilicon: Supply, Demand & Implications for the PV Industry, 2006
11. Ryan's Notes, Ferrous and Nonferrous News and Prices
12. EPIA, Capacity and market potential, Dez. 2006
13. Sun Screen II, CLSA, Juli 2005
14. 3rd Solar Silicon Conference, 2, München, April 2006
15. 21st European Photovoltaic Solar Energy Conference, Dresden, 4–8 Sept. 2006
16. Hesse, K.: Feedstock for the PV Industry. Photon 2nd Solar Silicon Conference, 11 April 2005
17. PHOTON International, May 2005

5 EFG Ribbon Technology

I.A. Schwirtlich

5.1 Introduction

Since the beginning of solar cell development based on crystalline silicon, there have been efforts to produce wafers directly from the melt instead of through crystallization of ingots. Ingots require slicing into the blocs and wafers which form the basis of solar cells. In the last 30 years, several dozen processes have been published that describe a variety of concepts. Only few of these processes could be developed to an acceptable degree of technical maturity. Among those successful technologies are the Dendritic Web process, the Edge Supported Pulling (ESP) process and the Edge-Defined-Film-Fed-Growth (EFG) process. The EFG Process was originally developed by Mobil Solar and, since the mid-1990s, belongs to SCHOTT Solar GmbH and its predecessors, respectively. The Ribbon Growth on Substrate (RGS) process was originally developed by Bayer AG and is now in a pilot project at the ECN, Petten. Considering the past 20 to 30 years, the EFG process has reached the most advanced state in terms of industrialization.

5.2 EFG process

The publicly known silicon ribbon growth processes can be categorized into two basic concepts despite their totally different designs:

(a) Pulling direction *vertical* to the melt surface
(b) Pulling direction *parallel* to the melt surface

Ribbon technologies belonging to category (a) are the ESP, Dendritic Web and the EFG processes. The RGS process should be placed in category (b) (see Fig. 5.1).

The processes due to concept (a) benefit from the good heat radiation by the two large surfaces of the ribbon. As the crystallization direction is directed into the melt, the segregation leads to enrichment of the remaining impurities in the residual melt. The feedstock material should therefore be relatively pure. The pulling speed and the crystallization speed are identical in absolute value but the direction is opposite. Processes following concept (b) have the advantage that the crystallization speed is

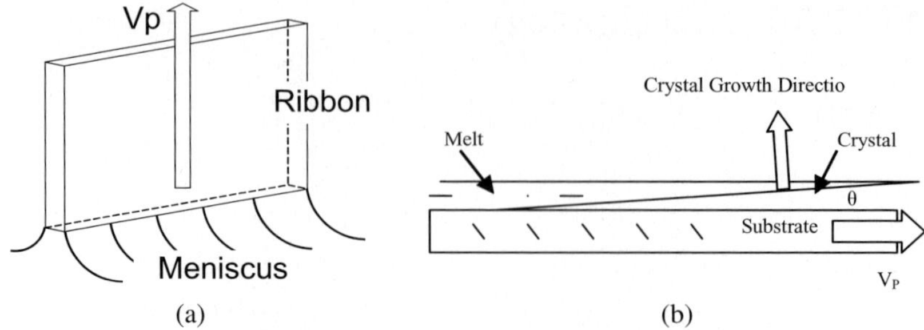

Fig. 5.1. Ribbon pulling direction vertical (**a**) and parallel (**b**) to the melt surface

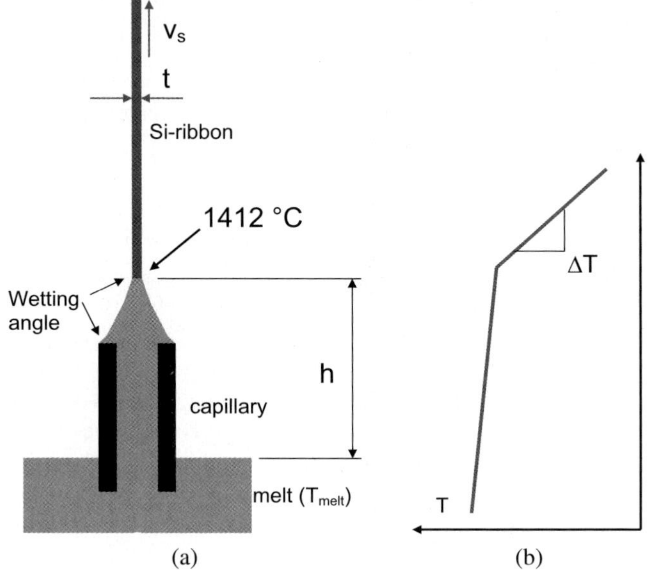

Fig. 5.2. Schematic drawing of the EFG process

directed nearly perpendicular to the pulling direction. As a consequence the segregation of impurities leads to a collection of impurities on the upper side of the ribbon that can be removed later by etching. Because of a potentially much higher pulling speed than crystallization speed, productivity can be much higher than in concept (a) processes. In addition to these basic differences, the quality of the produced wafers is decisive. Highest efficiencies – i.e., a conversion rate of sunlight into electricity of more than 15% – has been obtained with processes following concept (a).

To stabilize the melt meniscus, the EFG process uses a capillary die made of a material that is very well wetted by the melt. Due to the capillary effect of the wetting material the feeding of the meniscus with melt from the volume of the die is realized. Figure 5.2 shows this principle schematically.

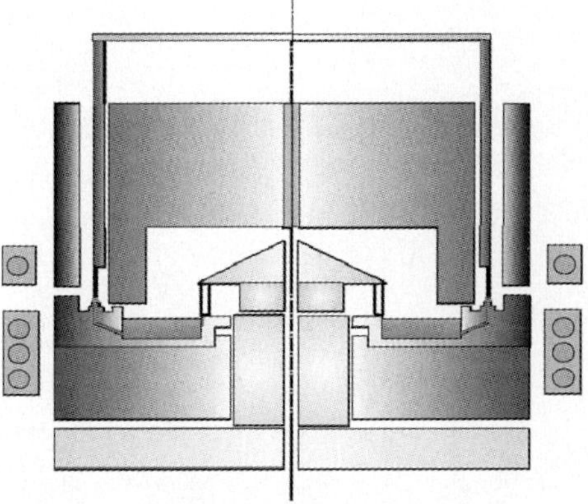

Fig. 5.3. Schematic drawing of the melt crucible with melt reservoir and capillary

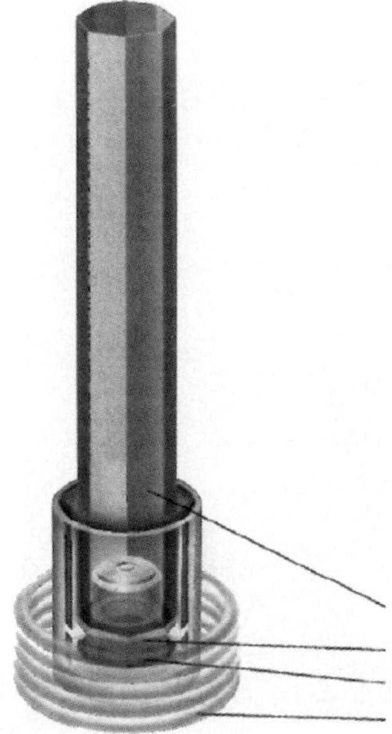

Fig. 5.4. Simplified presentation of an EFG pulling device

The thickness of the ribbon depends on the wetting angle of the capillary material and the melt, the height h between meniscus and surface of the melt, the temperature difference ΔT between meniscus and crystal temperature as well as the pulling speed v_s.

A more detailed schematic drawing of the EFG crucible with capillary and melt reservoir is shown in Fig. 5.3. The crucible rests on a construction that carries the total set up including susceptor and cooling distance. Figure 5.4 shows a simplified presentation of the equipment as it is used in the production.

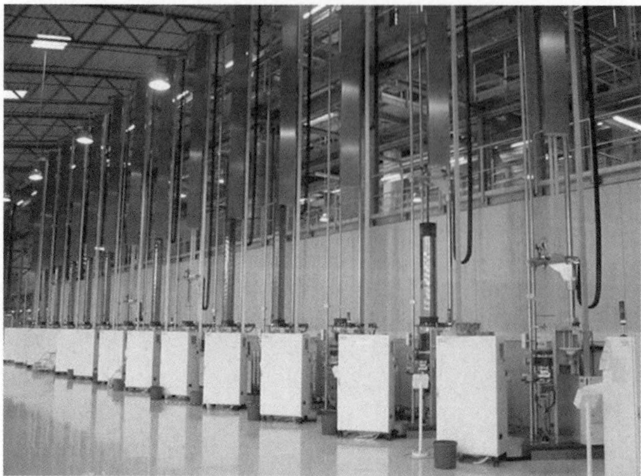

Fig. 5.5. View of the EFG production hall at SCHOTT Solar in Alzenau

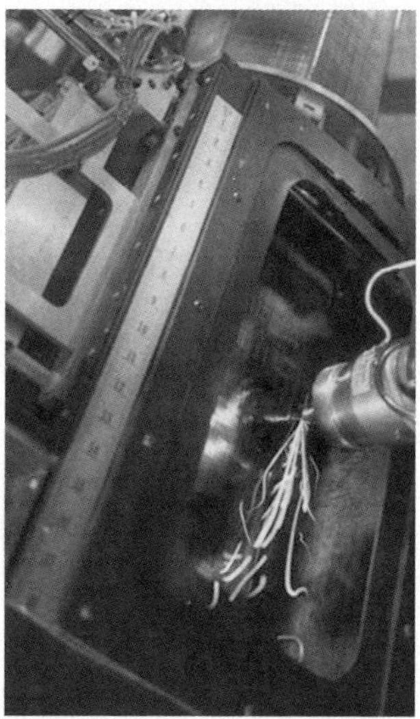

Fig. 5.6. Wafer production by separating

Figure 5.5 shows a view of the production hall at SCHOTT Solar in Alzenau, where octagon tubes with a length up to 6.5 m are produced. The control of the pulling process is mainly automatic.

The faces of the EFG-tubes are cut by laser beams into single wafers, shown in Fig. 5.6 along with details of the laser cutting equipment. Figure 5.7 shows an EFG wafer cut from one of the tube faces by laser.

To improve the productivity of the EFG process, developments have been made to extend the side facets of the tubes from 100 mm to 125 mm. 125-mm octagon

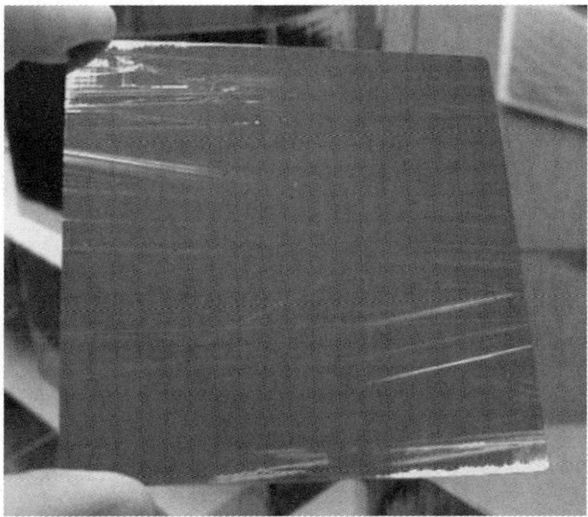

Fig. 5.7. EFG wafer produced by using a laser to cut the octagon tubes with a laser

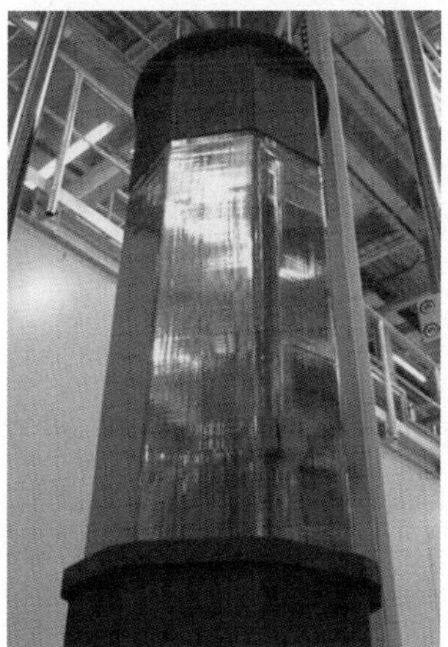

Fig. 5.8. Octagonal tube with 8 × 125-mm wide facets

tubes are now the main production. The dimension of the wafers cut from these tubes is 125 mm × 125 mm.

Figure 5.8 shows an octagonal tube with 8 × 125-mm wide facets. The progress in productivity is shown by the increase in diameter from octagons with 8 × 10 cm faces to 8 × 125 mm up to the latest development to dodecagons with 12 × 125 mm faces (Fig. 5.9(a), (b)).

The wafers' electrical properties are important for the production of solar cells. The minority carrier lifetime is especially key for high efficiencies. Figure 5.10 shows a topography of the minority lifetime of an EFG wafer. Clearly visible are

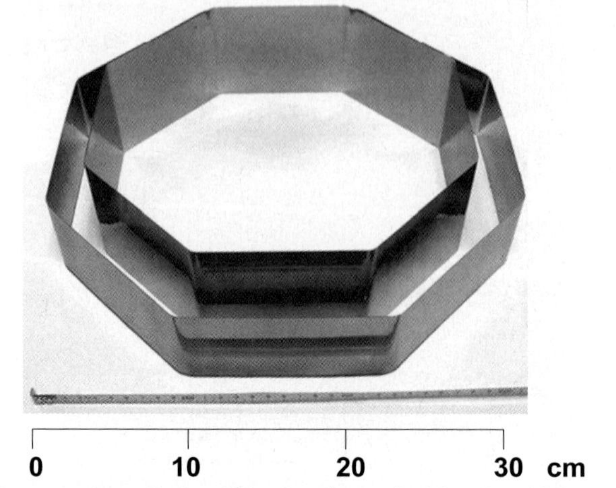

(a) Cross-section of a 8 × 100 mm tube put inside a 8 × 125 mm tube

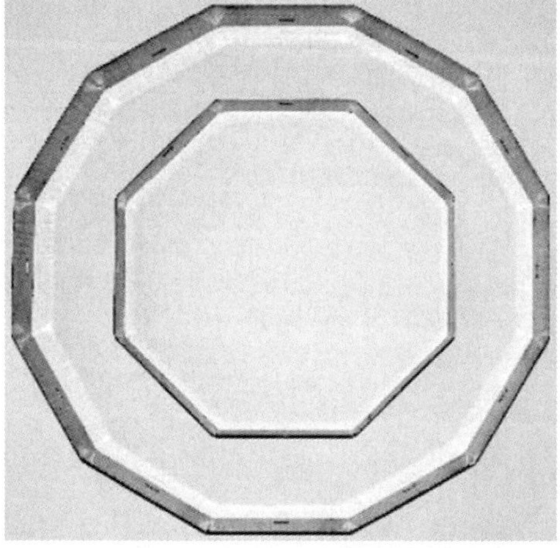

(b) Two cross-sections of tubes put together: A 8 × 125 mm tube inside a 12 × 125 mm tube

Fig. 5.9. (**a**) shows the difference in circumference of 8 × 100 mm tubes compared to 8 × 25 mm tubes. Because the tubes have the same growth rate, productivity is higher accordingly. The latest efforts to improve productivity resulted in the first experimental runs of dodecagon tubes with 12 × 125 mm facets grown at the same growth rate (**b**)

the different zones in the direction of crystal growing. The blue areas show good values at about 10 µs, the red in the range of 5 µs.

Solar cells produced from EFG wafers show efficiencies of up to 15% in production and offer an economical alternative to state-of-the-art multicrystalline wafers.

Research and development has obtained efficiencies of up to 18.2%, which shows the material's potential. Figure 5.11 shows the results obtained at NREL.

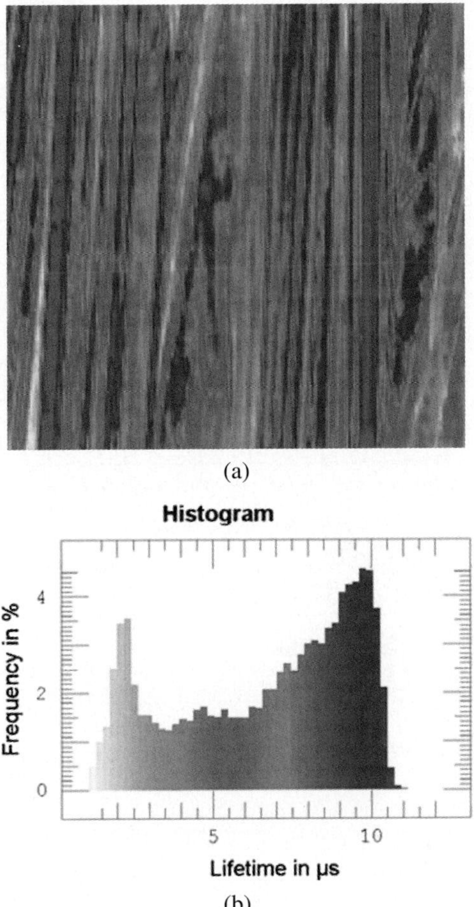

Fig. 5.10. Topography of minority carrier lifetime in EFG-ribbon-wafers. *The dark* areas show high quality material. (**a**) shows the topography (**b**) shows the statistical distribution of the data

This forms the best result within a development of several years, as indicated in Fig. 5.12.

Beside the efficiencies that can be obtained, potential cost savings in material are also very important. In EFG production the standard thickness today is 300 μm. In a pilot project, tubes with wall thicknesses around 200 μm have been manufactured and processed to solar cells. At present, a thickness of 80 μm seems to be possible. This would reduce the Si-consumption from about 7 g/Wp today to below 3 g/Wp tomorrow.

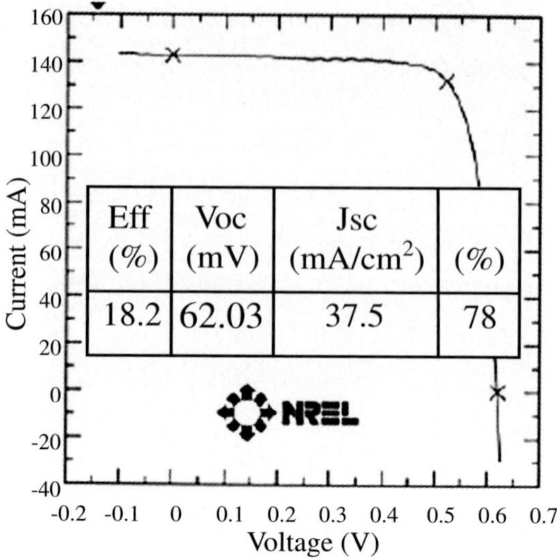

Eff (%)	Voc (mV)	Jsc (mA/cm^2)	(%)
18.2	62.03	37.5	78

Fig. 5.11. Best EFG cell showing 18.2% efficiency obtained so far

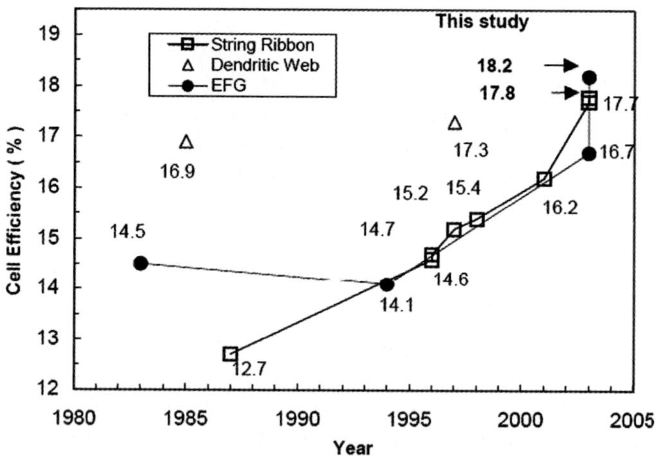

Fig. 5.12. Development of the ribbon material efficiencies

6 A Novel High-Efficiency Rear-Contact Solar Cell with Bifacial Sensitivity

R. Hezel

6.1 Introduction

At present, wafer-based silicon solar cells have a share of more than 90% of the photovoltaic market. Despite rapid growth in the manufacturing volume, accompanied by a significant drop in the module selling price, the high costs currently associated with photovoltaic power generation are one of the most important obstacles to widespread global use of solar electricity. Up to a certain level, a higher production volume is a key driver in cost reduction. However, apart from a drastic reduction of the silicon wafer thickness in conjunction with improved light-trapping schemes, innovative processing sequences combining very high solar cell efficiencies with simple and cost-effective fabrication techniques are needed to become competitive with conventional energy sources and thus to move solar energy from niche to mainstream.

The energy conversion efficiency has a great impact on the costs of a PV system. With a higher efficiency the module power density is increased, i.e. less cell and module area is required to achieve the same output power. Consequently all area-related costs are reduced, which make up more than 70% of the costs of a PV system. These include costs of the silicon feedstock, wafering, cell processing, module fabrication, installation and maintenance [1]. In particular, the silicon wafer contributes significantly to the module costs. Getting more power out of silicon is thus one of the most important challenges to realize an increase in efficiency. Reduction of the wafer thickness down to values of about $100\,\mu m$, as well as making the solar cell bifacially sensitive, are further means to reduce the cost of solar electricity.

As can be seen in Fig. 6.1, considerable progress in efficiency of crystalline silicon solar cells has been achieved in the past with laboratory cells characterized by high process complexity. A record efficiency of 24.7% has been obtained [2]. The theoretical limit of a silicon solar cell of $80\,\mu m$ thickness and with Lambertian light trapping, an efficiency of 28.8% was determined [3].

The efficiencies of the majority of industrial solar cells are presently in the range of 13%–16% including monocrystalline Czochralski-grown and cast multicrystalline silicon as well as ribbon-grown silicon. These numbers clearly indicate the enormous potential for further efficiency improvement in commercial devices.

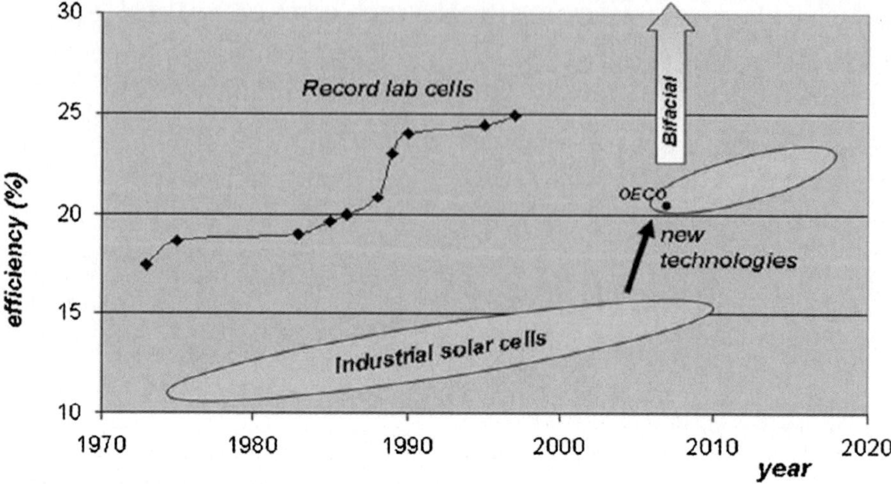

Fig. 6.1. Past, present and future of crystalline silicon solar cell efficiencies in the laboratory and in industry. Efficiencies exceeding 20% should be dominating the market in the near future. The novel bifacial OECO solar cells to be introduced in the following are potentially able to achieve effective cell efficiencies close to 35% by additionally using light impinging on the rear side

However, there are severe limitations to the standard screen printing approach [4]. Therefore it is indispensable to open up a new high-efficiency area above 20% in the near future with industrial crystalline silicon cells fabricated by novel cost-effective technologies (Fig. 6.1).

For some years promising candidates for this high-efficiency region have been commercially available. They are described in more detail in a separate section of this book. A recent comparative study of these devices including the novel obliquely evaporated-contact (OECO) solar cell should be mentioned [5].

The OECO solar cell, which will be extensively discussed in the following, is a completely different high-efficiency device characterized by a corrugated rear surface and both contact grid systems located at the rear side on the corresponding flanks of the ridges [6–8]. Bifacial sensitivity is automatically included together with the advantages of back-contact solar cells for efficiency, module fabrication and visual appearance. Efficiencies of 21.5% could already be obtained for front illumination [9]. High-efficiency and low-cost features are outlined together with the current fabrication sequence and the novel processing steps, including oblique contact-evaporation and surface passivation. The OECO cell is an all-silicon nitride-passivated device. Due to its importance to high-efficiency, the solar cells low-temperature surface passivation for front and rear side by plasma-enhanced chemical-vapor-deposited (PECVD) silicon nitride is also extensively discussed.

It should be emphasized that the bifacial sensitivity of the OECO cell with its potential for high rear-side contributions offers a simple way to effectively increase cell efficiency. Effective efficiencies close to 35% should be achievable by proper module arrangement. A variety of possible bifacial applications is presented in the course of this article. As an interesting feature, from further improvements in rear-side efficiency the front-side efficiency will greatly benefit.

6.2 Structure of the Bifacial Rear-Contact Solar Cell

Figure 6.2 shows a schematic of the novel back-collecting and bifacially sensitive obliquely evaporated-contact (OECO) solar cell using p-type silicon [7–9]. The characteristic features include:

(i)   A textured and well-passivated homogeneous front surface by PECVD silicon nitride, which simultaneously serves as antireflection layer.
(ii)   A corrugated back surface with n-contact lines (emitter contacts) on one flank and p-contact lines (base contacts) on the opposite flank of the ridges. The flanks can be vertical, as shown in Fig. 6.2, or inclined, both resulting in very low grid shading of rear illumination.
(iii) A n^+ emitter generated at the rear surface except in the vicinity of the p-contacts.
(iv)   The whole rear surface is covered by PECVD silicon nitride acting both as excellent passivation and antireflection layer for efficient utilization of light impinging on the rear side.

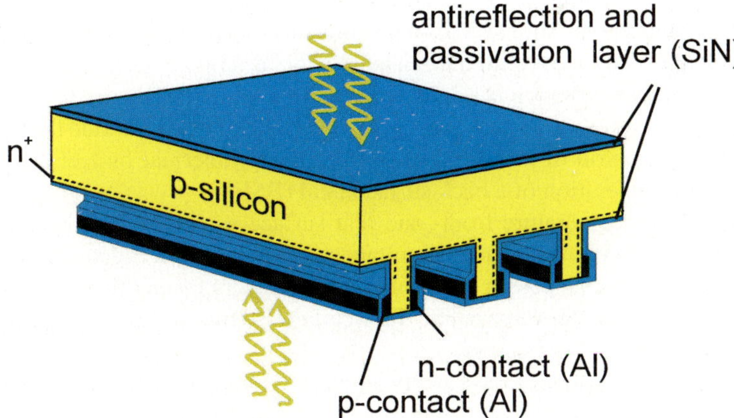

Fig. 6.2. Schematic of the high-efficiency bifacially sensitive OECO solar cell. Both contact lines are placed on the steep flanks of the ridges at the rear side. Also, light impinging on the rear side is efficiently used

6.3 High-Efficiency and Low-Cost Production Features

For advanced crystalline silicon solar cells, several efficiency-enhancing processing steps mainly focused on reducing carrier recombination are commonly applied [4, 10, 11]. Preferred implementations include: back surface field (BSF), selective emitter, floating junction and high-temperature thermal oxide passivation associated with narrow openings for point- or line-contact formation including complex alignment.

It is important to note that fabrication of the novel rear-contact OECO solar cells requires neither these costly, time- and energy-consuming high-temperature steps, nor does it require masks and alignment to achieve comparable one-sun front side efficiencies approaching 22%. A special feature of the OECO cells is their bifacial sensitivity, i.e. additional high power can be gained using the light directed onto the rear side.

Some of the unique high-efficiency and low-cost production features are:

- Absence of grid-shadowing on the front side.
- Effective cell efficiencies close to 35% are achievable due to bifacial operation, which is possible without additional processing. Rear-side efficiency can be close to that of the front side.
- The fabrication of the corrugated rear-side structure by one simple grooving step turns out to be highly cost-effective. In contrast to other approaches it allows, in a simple way, formation of both contact systems as narrow grid fingers at the corresponding flanks. By properly orienting the grooves, texturing of the flanks can be avoided in order to keep the contact area low.
- Simple and reliable separation of n- and p-contact lines, a small grid finger area as well as low metal consumption per cell are achievable by the novel self-aligned high-throughput oblique evaporation technique.
- The high-quality yet simple MIS-n^+p contact scheme gives two major advantages [12]. (i) Low-cost aluminum is applicable as contact grid metal and (ii) a selective emitter diffusion is not required to obtain high-efficiencies.
- Inherent passivation of the base contacts is provided by the rear-side design, thus replacing the boron diffusion process with its high thermal budget commonly used for the generation of a back surface field (BSF).
- Excellent low-temperature front- and rear-surface passivation is accomplished by plasma silicon nitride which simultaneously acts as antireflection coating.
- The back-contact cell design and "soft" processing are favorable for thin wafers. Substrate warpage does not occur. To a certain extent, the thinner the cells are the more efficient they become.
- The optimum base thickness is easily adjustable by the rear-side grooving process.
- Due to the special rear-side design characterized by narrow base regions without emitter coverage, lateral minority-carrier diffusion is negligible. As a consequence, in contrast to other back-contacted solar cells, neither additional lifetime requirements for the base material nor sophisticated tight rear-side patterning are of concern for the novel cells [11].

- Lower cell operating temperature and thus higher voltage results due to the "open" rear side. The long-wavelength radiation leaves the cell without being absorbed by a continuous rear metallization characteristic for most of the commercial solar cells.
- Since both contacts are on the rear side, module fabrication costs are reduced. High-throughput surface-mount automated assembly can be used.

6.4 Inherent Passivation of the Base Contacts

As a new characteristic for the back-contacted OECO solar cells, due to their geometrical arrangement at the flanks of the narrow ridges, the p-contacts collecting majority carriers are, to a large extent, screened against minority carriers without the presence of a local back-surface field. With proper cell design, the minority carriers (electrons) are, except in the V_{oc}-state, preferentially collected by the emitter running on both sides of the elevations. Thus, the carrier density in the vicinity of the base contacts is significantly reduced [7–9]. As a consequence, recombination at these contacts is sufficiently low. Therefore, in contrast to other high-efficiency solar cells, the complex formation of a local back surface field is not required. This

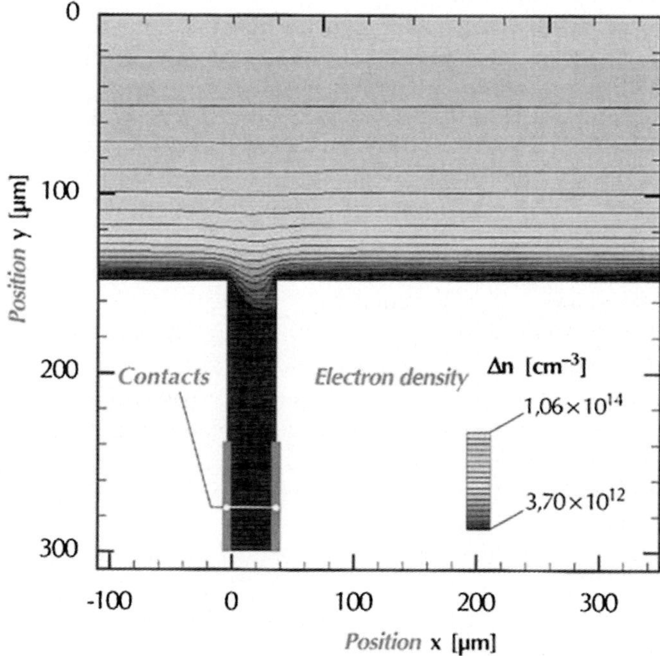

Fig. 6.3. Calculated two-dimensional electron density for a p-Si OECO solar cell under front side illumination and J_{sc} conditions. The extremely low density of electrons present in the narrow ridges results in a considerable reduction of carrier recombination at the base contacts

special feature of the back-contacted OECO cell was extensively investigated by two-dimensional calculations using DESSIS [8, 9].

As an example, Fig. 6.3 shows the calculated two-dimensional electron carrier density under front-side illumination and J_{sc} conditions for a properly designed rear-side structure with narrow ridges and wide grooves. The high injection level of $2 \times 10^{14}\,\mathrm{cm}^{-3}$ near the front surface decreases to $3 \times 10^{13}\,\mathrm{cm}^{-3}$ near the rear surface of the grooves. This behavior is characteristic for back-collecting solar cells with a planar rear side. Within the narrow ridge of the OECO cell, however, the minority carrier density is drastically reduced by more than a factor of 100 down to $2 \times 10^{11}\,\mathrm{cm}^{-3}$, leading to a considerable reduction of carrier recombination at the base contacts, which are located at the right flanks of the ridges. This shielding-effect for the minority charge carriers, acting as a kind of inherent passivation by geometric means, increases the short-circuit current density of the OECO solar cell by more than $2\,\mathrm{mA/cm}^2$ compared to a similar cell with a fully planar rear side. The fill factor is also increased by the extremely inhomogeneous minority-carrier distribution.

6.5 Processing Sequence

There are several options for the production of OECO solar cells. One example for the processing sequence is shown in Fig. 6.4, where only industrially feasible self-aligning mask-free steps are applied [8, 13]. First, the front surface of the wafer is textured with random pyramids, preferably by anisotropic etching (Fig. 6.4a). After the rear side is grooved, a diffusion barrier layer is deposited on the flanks of the ridges to prevent emitter formation in the vicinity of the base contacts (Fig. 6.4b).

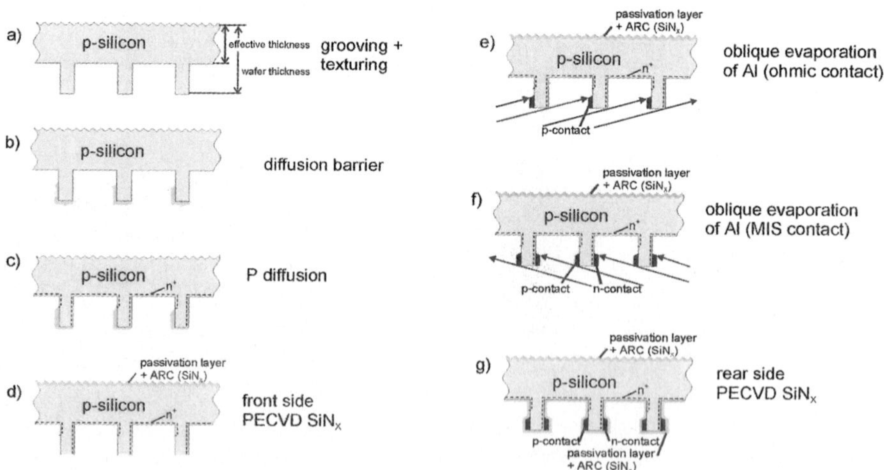

Fig. 6.4. Processing sequence for back-contacted bifacial OECO solar cells using only techniques feasible for industrial high-volume manufacturing

A conventional phosphorous diffusion follows at 890 °C to form the n^+-emitter, whereby the front side is protected against diffusion by proper positioning of the wafers (face to face) or by a diffusion barrier layer (Fig. 6.4c). A shallow emitter profile with a sheet resistivity around 90 Ω/sq is required, if comparable efficiencies for front- and rear-side illumination of the bifacial cell should be achieved. If only the efficiency for front-side illumination is to be optimized, a heavily doped emitter is preferable. Phosphorous glass and diffusion barrier are then removed. Low temperature ($<$400 °C) remote PECVD silicon nitride is used as front-surface passivation and antireflection layer (Fig. 6.4d).

Base-contact metallization is performed by oblique evaporation of aluminum (Fig. 6.4e). Ohmic contact formation and growth of an ultrathin ($\sim$1.5 nm) oxide layer is simultaneously performed by a short annealing step at 500 °C.

A high-quality metal-insulator-silicon (MIS)-n^+p contact is obtained by oblique evaporation of aluminum from the direction opposite to the p-contact (Fig. 6.4f). As a nanolayer, the thin oxide serves two main purposes [12]: (i) it prevents Al from degrading the pn-junction, so that low-cost Al instead of expensive Ag can be used for reliable emitter contacts of solar cells [14]; and (ii) the majority carriers (holes) are blocked, whereas the minority carriers (electrons) are able to pass through the insulating layer by quantum-mechanical tunneling. Thus the simple-to-fabricate "tunnel" oxide replaces the high-temperature diffusion step usually applied to form a selective emitter.

Then the whole rear surface is covered with PECVD silicon nitride as passivation and antireflection layer (Fig. 6.4g). Finally the grid fingers of each polarity have to be connected by busbars running across the contact grid. For this purpose, after selective removal of the nitride layer from the respective grid fingers, busbar formation and tabbing are simultaneously performed by attachment of metal ribbons using conductive adhesives.

In conclusion, the relatively simple fabrication process exclusively uses industrially feasible, mask- and aligning-free processing steps such as surface grooving, emitter diffusion (n^+), self-aligned metallization and low-temperature passivation by silicon nitride on the front and rear side. Toxic materials are excluded. This underlines the high potential for OECO solar cells to be fabricated economically in an environmentally benign way.

6.6 Production Technology

6.6.1 Back-Surface Grooving

As the key feature of the back-contacted OECO solar cell, a corrugated rear surface has to be provided that consists of a set of parallel grooves forming specific elevations with steep side walls for the simple mask-free and self-aligned deposition of both contact line systems by oblique vacuum evaporation.

In general, the fabrication of the distinct back surface structure can be performed by various technologies, e.g., chemical etching, laser grooving or by a grinding technology.

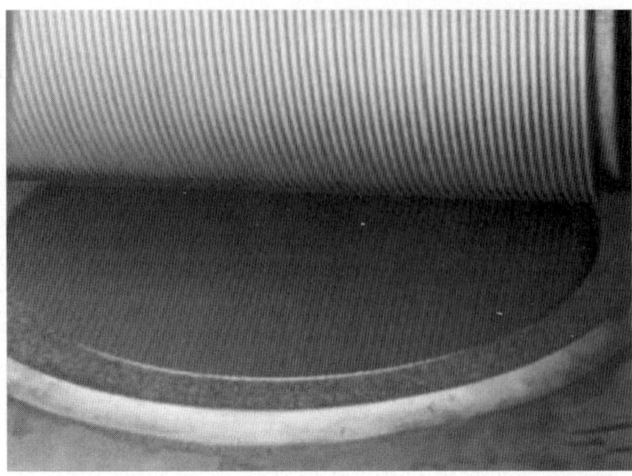

Fig. 6.5. High-throughput grinding tool for surface grooving of OECO solar cells. A $10 \times 10\,\mathrm{cm}^2$ wafer can be processed in a few seconds

The first approach, mechanical grooving with a fast rotating diamond-coated tool was developed. This method is a relatively simple and reliable process with high-throughput capabilities [15–18]. In order to demonstrate the industrial feasibility of the grinding technology, a novel high-throughput grinding system was constructed. The main feature of this equipment is a 150 mm wide grinding tool, which grooves silicon wafers up to $150 \times 150\,\mathrm{mm}^2$ with one fast stroke. A section of this grinding tool is depicted in Fig. 6.5 [19].

By optimizing tool and process parameters the effect of crystal defects induced by mechanical abrasion is minimized [20]. As demonstrated by a large number of industrial-size wafers, breakage during the grinding process is negligible.

An important advantage of grooving for high-efficiencies is worth mentioning [8]. Whereas the cell surfaces are randomly textured with pyramids, the flanks can remain flat in order to keep the contact area low. This is accomplished simply by proper orientation of the grooves so that preferential etching does not occur at the flanks. As an example, for a (100) surface, the flank orientation should be of the (110) type.

Another cost-effective way for silicon surface grooving is based on chemical etching in conjunction with the definition of an etching mask by laser ablation or screen-printing [21].

An additional approach – direct laser ablation of silicon – can be used for groove formation. This is a well-known technology that has been successfully applied to mass production of buried contact solar cells [10].

6.6.2 Metallization by Oblique Evaporation

Oblique evaporation of contacts is the crucial step both for obtaining high-efficiencies as well as for simple, low-cost and reliable processing of the OECO solar cells [7]. In general, conventional vacuum evaporation with the wafers perpendicularly oriented to the metal beam (mostly including mechanical masks or photolithography for structuring) cannot be regarded as a low-cost process for economic solar cell production. However, the situation is completely different for evaporation under a shallow angle, where the throughput of wafers can be drastically increased. The principle of the novel oblique-evaporation technique is shown in Fig. 6.6. It is based on the fact that vacuum evaporation is a directional process that allows us to make use of shadowing effects of a distinct surface structure to define the grid fingers. Using the self-shading effect, the metal fingers are deposited along the steep flanks of the ridges without any mask or alignment. The width of the fingers is simply adjusted by variation of the evaporation angle and thus the cross-section of the contact lines can be increased without significantly affecting light obscuration.

As a further, very important feature of the OECO technique, the separation of the n- and p-contact lines in order to avoid shunting is ingeniously simple and reliably accomplished without any masks or alignment [7]. As can be seen in Fig. 6.7, during evaporation first from the left side (p-contacts) and subsequently from the right side (n-contacts) even under a very shallow angle φ some metal is also deposited on the narrow tops of the ridges, thus connecting the two contact fingers. However, this metal layer is very thin (thickness $\sim a \sin(\varphi)$) compared to the grid-line thickness a and exhibits a porous columnar structure, so that it can easily be removed by a short etch without significantly reducing the thickness of the contact fingers. In the case of aluminum, the etch rate of the porous film obtained by evaporation under an angle φ of typically $4°$–$8°$ is about three times higher than that of the nearly vertically deposited grid finger material [7].

An example of a high-throughput equipment for oblique vacuum evaporation is also schematically depicted in Fig. 6.6. The wafers are arranged in a vacuum chamber closely spaced on a rotating cylinder with their surface orientation deviating only slightly from being parallel to the evaporation beam. Thus the packing density and hence throughput is up to ten times higher compared to conventional vacuum

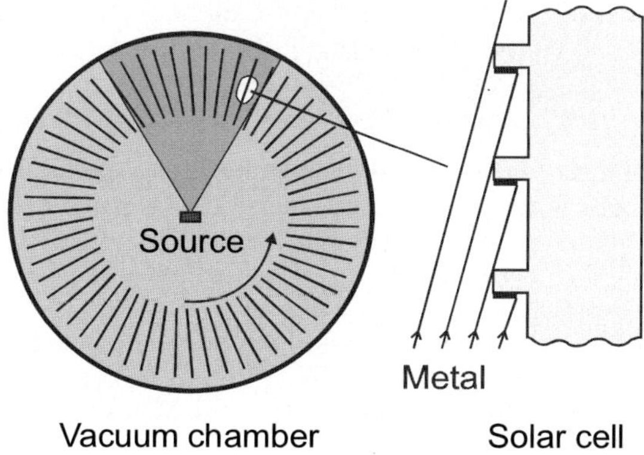

Fig. 6.6. Principle of oblique evaporation for contact metallization of OECO cells and arrangement of the wafers in the vacuum chamber. Self-alignment is provided by the shading effect of the groove tops

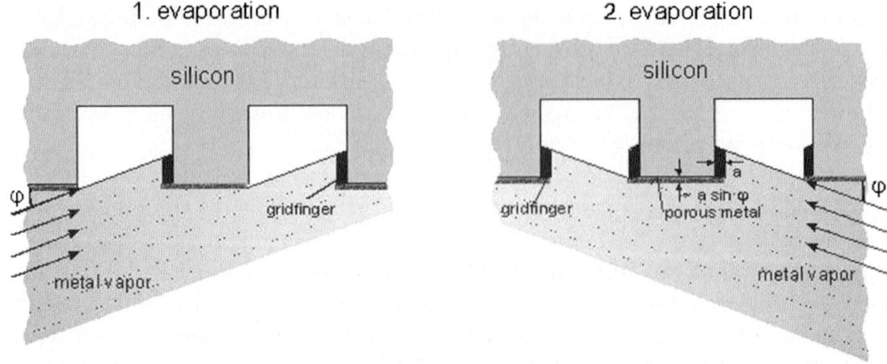

Fig. 6.7. Subsequent evaporation of both contact schemes. Separation of the n- and p-contact lines is reliably accomplished without any mask or alignment. Only a very thin porous metal film has to be removed from the ridge tops by a short etch

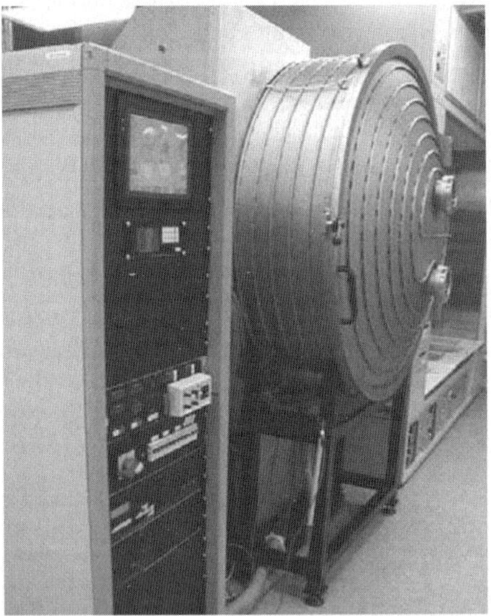

Fig. 6.8. Prototype of high-capacity oblique evaporation equipment for the metallization of OECO solar cells. Large wafer cassettes are arranged on a cylinder revolving around the evaporation source

evaporation, where the substrates are positioned perpendicular to the evaporation beam. Furthermore, metal wastage is prevented since nearly all the metal evaporated is used for the grid fingers. Electron beam or resistive heating can be applied for evaporation of the source material.

A high-capacity prototype of the evaporation equipment suitable for mass production was constructed according to the design shown in Fig. 6.8. A floor space of only $2.5\,m^2$ is required for this system, whose capacity amounts to about 1,000 wafers of $10 \times 10\,cm^2$ in size. Reliable operation was demonstrated in a pilot line [22].

6.6.3 Surface Passivation by PECVD Silicon Nitride

Passivation Mechanism and Film Properties

The achievement of high-efficiencies for crystalline silicon solar cells is highly dependent on the reduction of carrier recombination at the surface. Surfaces represent rather severe defects in the crystal structure and are the site of many allowed states within the forbidden energy gap of silicon. Excellent surface passivation achieved through the growth of dielectric films is thus of prime importance for high-efficiency solar cells. Furthermore, by passivation of the front and rear surface with dielectric layers – apart from serving as antireflection coatings – the internal optical reflection is also increased, resulting in good light-trapping properties. This is crucial to the future introduction of thinner and thus less-costly silicon substrates in solar cell manufacturing, so that lower wafer cost is not offset by efficiency losses [3].

Extrinsic silicon surface passivation by dielectric films is based upon the Shockley-Read-Hall theory [23, 24]. The recombination of charge carriers via surface states is dominated by the density of those centers that are located near the middle of the forbidden gap. The recombination rate at the silicon/insulator interface reaches its maximum value in case of depletion, when the electron and hole concentrations at the surface are equal. For strong accumulation or inversion, however, the concentration of majority or minority carriers, respectively, is prevailing. Under these conditions, the surface recombination rate is drastically reduced [3, 24]. Thus both the reduction of the surface state density and the presence of strong inversion or accumulation accomplished by fixed insulator charges can be used for surface passivation, characterized by the effective surface recombination velocity [25].

Two different techniques are hitherto applied to obtain low effective surface recombination velocities for high-efficiency solar cells [3, 24]: (i) growth of a thermal oxide film on silicon to reduce surface-state density and (ii) creation of a strong built-in electric field (high-low junction) in order to repel the minority carriers from recombination sites at the surface [26].

Thermally grown SiO_2 films provide very good surface passivation on n- and p-type Si-wafers and on phosphorous-diffused silicon wafers via an extremely low interface state density [24]. However, for solar cell application there are severe drawbacks. Due to their low refractive index of 1.46, they are not suitable for an efficient reduction of reflection losses. Furthermore, high temperature ($>1,000\,°C$) processing is required, which is an energy- and time-consuming step. Since the oxide has to be grown before metallization, complex procedures have to be applied to open the film for contacting the underlying silicon.

The most promising alternative to thermally grown SiO_2 is amorphous silicon nitride fabricated at low temperature by plasma-enhanced chemical vapor deposition (PECVD). These films, first introduced and optimized for solar cells by the author's group in 1981, reveal excellent passivation of undiffused and diffused silicon surfaces, combined with optimal antireflection properties and low temperature processing [25, 27–31]. Furthermore PECVD silicon nitride is known from IC technology for its excellent impurity barrier properties, corrosion protection of the metallization, scratch- and crack-resistance and good step coverage [32]. Chemical, mechanical, electrical as well as optical properties of SiN films depend strongly on the preparation method and the particular process parameters used. Only a few dependencies which are relevant for the OECO cell fabrication shall be discussed.

Of all deposition parameters, temperature was found to be the most important [30]. Deposition temperatures around 400 °C provide optimal surface passivation, whereas at lower and higher temperatures the passivation quality is strongly decreasing. It is well known that a high amount of hydrogen (up to 25% H) is incorporated into the plasma silicon nitride films, partially forming Si–H and N–H bonds. The films are therefore often denoted as SiN_x:H, but in this work briefly, SiN. The saturation of unsaturated dangling bonds at the silicon surface by hydrogen is responsible for strong decrease of the surface state density in the range 350 °C–420 °C [30, 33]. At higher temperatures, both N–H and Si–H contents are lost and outdiffusion of hydrogen occurs.

The good AR coating properties of SiN films are due to the fact that the index of refraction n can be varied in a wide range from 1.7 to 3.0. An increase of n, which can be accomplished e.g. by increasing the SiH_4/NH_3 gas ratio, is correlated with a shift of the film composition toward silicon-rich films [34]. Very silicon-rich SiN films with a refractive index $n > 2.3$ were found to provide optimal surface passivation [30]. The more the SiN_x:H layers tend to resemble amorphous hydrogenated silicon, the better their surface passivation properties become. However, light absorption – particularly in the short-wavelength region – increases with Si content.

As to the amount of positive charges at the Si/SiN interface, it was found that the lower the amount of Si–H bonds the higher the positive interface charge density. If the amount of charges is sufficiently high, e.g. for nitride films with a low index of refraction, inversion can be achieved, where, as mentioned above, field effect passivation plays a significant role [25]. Such inversion layers accomplished by SiN antireflection coatings were successfully applied as emitters in MIS-inversion layer solar cells with efficiencies up to 19.6% [12, 35]. The excellent stability of the inversion layer is demonstrated by these cells encapsulated in novel large-area modules and installed since 1994 in many places, e.g., in the German-Spanish 1MW PV power plant in Toledo [36, 37].

With the present OECO cells, however, inversion layer formation may cause parasitic shunting which can be avoided by applying a more silicon-rich nitride layer with its higher index of refraction. It contains fewer positive charges and surface passivation is dominated by a reduction of interface–state density via hydrogen termination of Si-dangling bonds at the silicon surface.

It should be pointed out that nitride passivation is particularly well suited for use with multicrystalline substrates due to its consistency with hydrogenation of the bulk material resulting in a significant improvement of carrier lifetime [31].

Plasma Deposition Reactors for Silicon Nitride Layers

The properties of PECVD SiN depend strongly on the design of the reactor as well as on the deposition parameters. There are two fundamentally different reactor designs, parallel-plate (often referred to as "direct") and "remote".

In the parallel-plate version, the wafer is placed onto one of the two electrodes and is thus in direct contact with the plasma. It is important to note that the surface passivation properties of the SiN films depend strongly on the plasma frequency used. In the low-frequency (LF) mode (10–500 kHz), the ions in the plasma are able to follow the excitation frequency leading to surface damage and low-quality passivation. UV stability problems are a consequence of this surface damage with direct plasma SiN films [38, 39]. In the high-frequency (HF) regime (>4 MHz, typically 13.56 MHz) bombardment of the substrate surface is minimized since the ions in the plasma cannot follow the excitation of the electromagnetic field.

The second and most successful class of plasma reactors is formed by the downstream or remote system, which was introduced into photovoltaics in 1989 by the author's group at the University of Erlangen [38]. An important feature of the remote PECVD systems is that the Si wafer is located outside the plasma region, allowing for deposition of SiN films with no surface damage to the wafers and making the frequency relatively unimportant. Ammonia (NH_3) as one of the process gases is excited outside the deposition chamber by means of microwaves and mixed with silane (SiH4) in the chamber.

Up to now, the best surface passivation quality has been achieved with remote PECVD and parallel-plate HF reactors [30]. Figure 6.9 shows a schematic of the static laboratory-type remote PECVD system with downstream geometry (Oxford Plasmalab 80). It can be seen that the wafer is located outside the plasma. A mixture of ammonia (NH_3) and nitrogen (N_2) is excited by passing through a microwave cavity and mixes with silane (SiH_4) downstream of the plasma. The reaction takes place above the substrate which is placed on a heated plate.

In-line remote PECVD systems have been available to the PV industry for several years. Up to now they have been exclusively applied for the deposition of SiN antireflection coatings and as a source of hydrogen for the bulk passivation of multicrystalline silicon solar cells. Only recently have the surface passivation properties of SiN films deposited in such a large-area industrial PECVD system (SINA, Roth and Rau) been extensively studied [40].

The machine shown in Fig. 6.10 employs a 2.45 GHz linear microwave source for plasma excitation. In this source two quartz tubes are mounted perpendicular to the wafer transport direction. Ammonia is fed into the source above the tubes, whereas silane is added below at the sides of the plasma source. The wafers are placed on a carrier for transport through the processing chamber. Load looks at either end of the processing chamber are used for loading and unloading of the

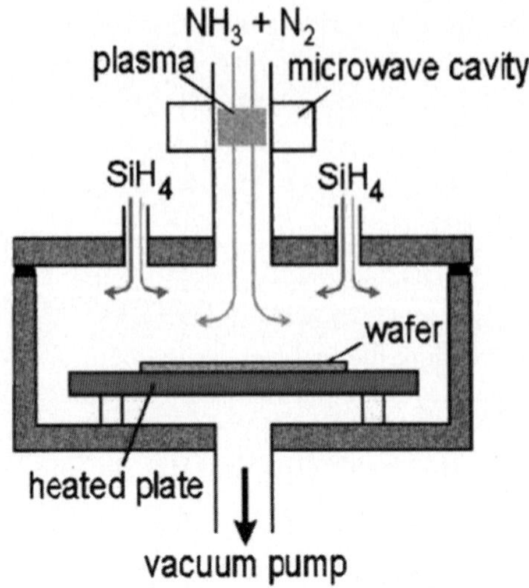

Fig. 6.9. Schematic of a static remote PECVD reactor

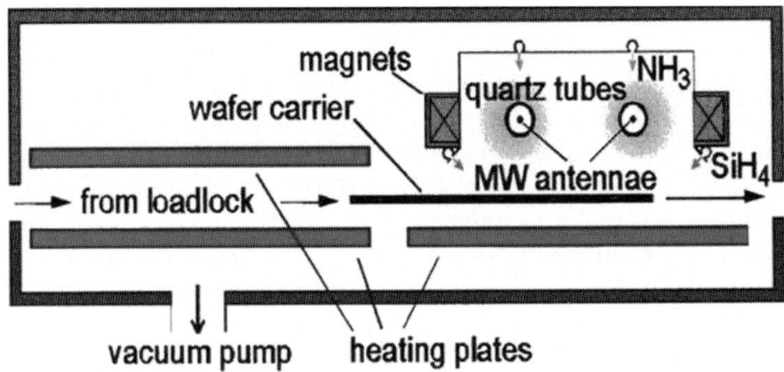

Fig. 6.10. Schematic cross-section of a microwave in-line remote PECVD system

carrier without breaking the processing vacuum. A detailed technical description of the complete inline system has been given elsewhere [40, 41].

The surface passivation properties of silicon nitride films could be optimized under dynamic deposition conditions in this reactor [40, 42]. Excellent results both on n$^+$-emitters and on low resistivity ($\sim$1 Ω cm) p-type silicon have been obtained, which are practically equivalent or even superior to those of the best laboratory reactors. It has been demonstrated that this industrial-scale, in-line deposition system is well suited for the passivation of advanced solar cells such as the OECO devices with efficiencies well above 20% [15, 22].

Front-Surface Passivation

Excellent passivation of the front surface is crucial to reach high-efficiencies, particularly for back-collecting solar cells [13]. Values of the effective front surface recombination velocity S_{eff} below 50 cm/s are required for high short-circuit current densities J_{sc} under front-side illumination. Record values below 10 cm/s could be obtained for silicon with resistivity above 1.5 Ω cm passivated by remote PECVD SiN layers [43]. However, these excellent surface recombination velocties were realized on planar silicon surfaces using silicon-rich SiN films with refractive indexes n above 2.4. The higher absorption of these films cause some losses in the short-circuit current density.

In order to achieve the highest possible cell efficiency, a layer with good optical properties and high passivation quality on a textured, low-resistivity silicon surface ($\sim$0.5 Ω cm) is required.

With the commonly used SiN antireflection film (refractive index $n = 2.05$ and thickness $d_{2.05} = 105$ nm) only $S_{\mathrm{eff}} = 240$ cm/s is achieved on a textured 0.5 Ω cm substrate. By this lower passivation quality the efficiency would be reduced by about 2% absolute. However, if a very thin silicon-rich SiN layer with $n = 2.5$ is deposited underneath, S_{eff} can be drastically reduced. This is demonstrated in Fig. 6.11 where the effective lifetime τ_{eff} and the surface recombination velocity S_{eff} are plotted as a function of the thickness $d_{2.5}$ of the silicon-rich layer, topped by a 70 nm thick nitride film with $n = 2.05$. The silicon nitride was deposited by remote PECVD at a temperature of 400 °C. The electrical properties were determined using injection dependent lifetime spectroscopy [8].

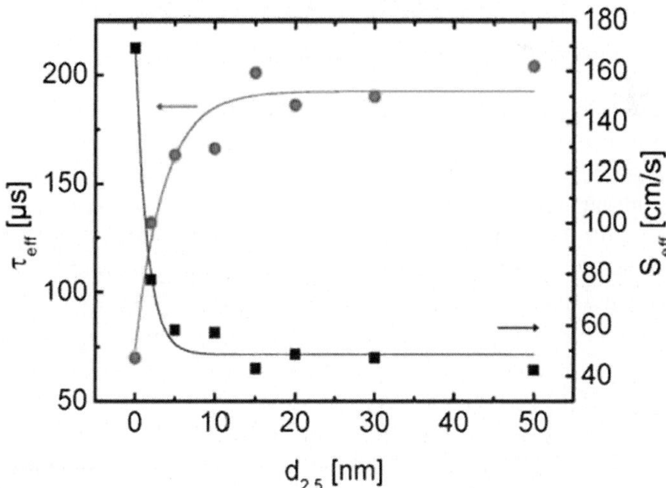

Fig. 6.11. Measured effective minority carrier lifetime τ_{eff} and surface recombination velocity S_{eff} for SiN double layers deposited at 400 °C on textured 0.5 Ω cm Si. The thickness $d_{2.5}$ of the Si-rich bottom nitride layer ($n = 2.5$) is varied, the top nitride layer ($n = 2.05$) has a constant thickness of 70 nm

As seen in Fig. 6.11, adding only a few nanometers of the silicon-rich nitride results in a steep increase in τ_{eff} up to a saturation value of about 200 µs for $d_{2.5} \geq$ 10 nm. This corresponds to an excellent surface recombination velocity of 50 cm/s. From absorption measurements it was found that for $d_{2.5} > 10$ nm more than 5% of the sunlight is absorbed in the silicon-rich nitride film, which is not tolerable for highly efficient solar cells. For $d_{2.5} \leq 5$ nm, less than 2% is absorbed [9]. This small absorption is overcompensated for by the higher passivation quality. Thus, the cell efficiency shows a maximum for $d_{2.5} = 4$ nm with a gain of 1.1% absolute.

This newly developed silicon nitride double layer electrically outperforms the formerly used single silicon nitride film while preserving the excellent optical properties. Furthermore, the costly preparation of a floating junction, including a high-temperature diffusion step, is not required.

Rear-Surface Passivation

In the earlier development stage, the whole rear surface of the OECO cells was covered by a conventional PECVD SiN layer with a refractive index $n = 2.05$. A deposition temperature of 300 °C compatible with the MIS contacts had to be used. However, as was thoroughly investigated, due to their positive interface charges, these nitride layers create a conducting inversion channel between the diffused n^+-emitter and the ohmic base contact [44]. As a consequence, lower values of the shunt resistance and fill factor resulted. It was recently demonstrated with conventional rear-SiN passivated solar cells that this parasitic shunting can be eliminated by introducing a local back surface field (LBSF) [45].

Due to the unique features of the OECO cell, the generally applied back-surface field for passivation of the base contacts is not required. Therefore, we can avoid this extra processing step for the purpose of channel stopping.

Instead, in a more elegant way via an adapted processing and a new rear passivation scheme (consisting of a SiN double layer similar to that on the front side but deposited at the lower temperature of 300 °C) the parasitic shunting could be completely suppressed [9]. Shunt resistance values above $9 \, \text{k}\Omega \, \text{cm}^2$ are achieved. Furthermore, the surface recombination velocity is reduced by nearly a factor of 10, from 2,000 cm/s for the conventional SiN layer with $n = 2.05$ to 200 cm/s for the optimized double layer with $n = 2.5/2.05$. The high shunt resistance and thus the absence of parasitic shunting achieved by the SiN double layer is attributed to the fact that in the silicon-rich first nitride layer ($n = 2.5$) much fewer fixed positive charges are present resulting in a higher inversion-channel sheet resistance.

In conclusion, applying the optimized PECVD SiN double layers to the rear side of the OECO solar cells provides a simple way to improve the passivation quality of the rear surface while also reducing the shunting effect.

6.6.4 Interconnection Technology Based on Conductive Adhesives

In contrast to the conventional metallization by screen printing, the oblique evaporation process used for the OECO cells does not provide busbars which electrically interconnect the grid fingers with each other and serve as solder areas for cell interconnection in module fabrication. Therefore, for OECO-type cells, an alternative technology is applied by which busbar formation and cell interconnection can be achieved using electrically conductive adhesives [15]. Their curing temperature is very low, typically below 200 °C, and the whole interconnection process is rather simple. After application of the adhesive – commercially available as a tape or as a one- or two-component paste – the metallic interconnectors (tabs or a prefabricated metal pattern) are attached to the cell and cured at the temperature specific for the adhesive.

This technique, already well established for chip mounting and in the automotive industry, has several advantages over traditional soldering. These advantages are particularly relevant for very thin and large as well as back-contacted silicon solar cells [46, 47]:

(i)   As a low-temperature joining technique, it avoids build-up of mechanical stress on joints and cells which ultimately may cause breakage; thus, process yield and reliability increased.
(ii) Busbar formation and cell interconnection are accomplished in one process step.
(iii) The adhesives are nonpolluting (lead free!).

Conductive adhesives suited for contacting solar cells consist of a matrix, mostly an epoxy resin, and up to 80 wt% of conductive particles varying in size from several µm to several tens of µm. Electrical conductance is through side-to-side contact of the particles suspended in the epoxy matrix. Epoxies are easy to adjust, resistant to humidity and without hazardous out-gasing.

Since long-term stability of the interconnection has been proven by accelerated aging tests for some conductive adhesives, this novel technology appears to be a promising alternative to conventional soldering [15].

6.7 Cell Results

$4\,cm^2$ solar cells were processed using 0.5 Ω cm FZ-silicon wafers with an effective base thickness of 150 µm. Only the front side was textured and, as outlined above, both sides were coated with double layer passivation stacks of PECVD silicon nitride.

The J–V curves under front- and rear-side illumination at STC (1 sun, AM1.5 G, 25 °C) are shown in Fig. 6.12 [9]. Efficiencies of 21.5% and 17.7% (independently confirmed at CalLab, Fraunhofer ISE, Germany) are achieved for front- and rear-side illumination, respectively (cell size: $2 \times 2\,cm^2$).

To our knowledge these are the highest efficiencies of back-contacted, bifacially sensitive solar cells fabricated without photolithography.

Remarkably high values of the short-circuit current density J_{sc} of $41.9\,mA/cm^2$ are achieved due to the excellent effective front-surface recombination velocity, very good optical properties and the inherent contact passivation provided by the narrow

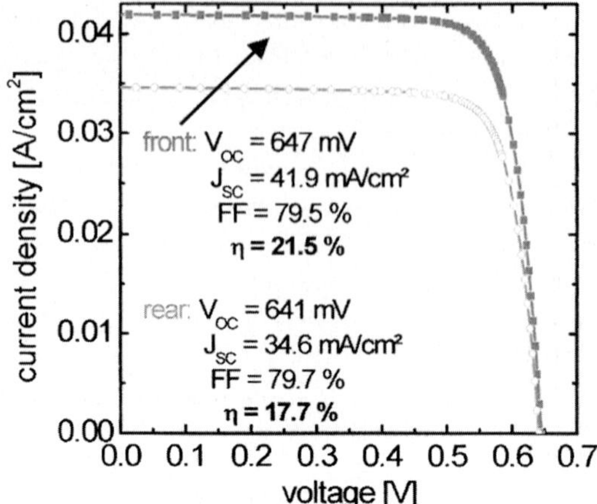

Fig. 6.12. Measured J–V-characteristics of back-contacted bifacial OECO solar cells. Efficiencies of 21.5% and 17.7% are achieved for front- and rear-side illumination, respectively

ridges. Although the rear side is not textured and both kinds of contacts are placed on this side, high J_{sc} values of 34.6 mA/cm^2 are realized under rear illumination. With a textured rear side and an optimized emitter diffusion, rear-side efficiencies up to 20% are expected.

The high fill factor of 79.5% is attributed to the absence of any parasitic shunt ($R_{sh} = 9\,\mathrm{k\Omega\,cm^2}$) and to a very low series resistance ($R_s = 0.4\,\Omega\,\mathrm{cm^2}$). The excellent quality of both surface passivations and evaporated contacts is reflected by the relatively high open-circuit voltage $V_{oc} = 647$ mV. It should be mentioned that due to the "open" rear side of the bifacial cell the operating temperature of the cell is lower compared to conventional cells with continuous rear metallization.

6.8 Efficiency Perspectives

In general, rear-contact solar cells have a key advantage. At least to a certain extent, the thinner they are, the more efficient they become. Figure 6.13 shows the efficiencies of back-collecting solar cells calculated as a function of the minority carrier diffusion length L_d for a base thickness of 50, 100, 200 and 300 μm, respectively [7]. Realistic conditions were used for the simulation, which led to efficiencies of 20.1% for $10 \times 10\,\mathrm{cm^2}$ front-collecting OECO cells and up to 21.2% for $4 \times 4\,\mathrm{cm^2}$ laboratory cells [22].

The efficiency of back-collecting solar cells depends strongly on the bulk diffusion length L_d and on the effective front-surface recombination velocity S_{front}. As can be seen from Fig. 6.13, with decreasing diffusion length the efficiency is sharply dropping, since the minority carriers generated mainly at the front side have to diffuse to the rear junction. High-efficiencies are achievable only if the bulk diffusion length strongly exceeds the base thickness. For high-quality material such as

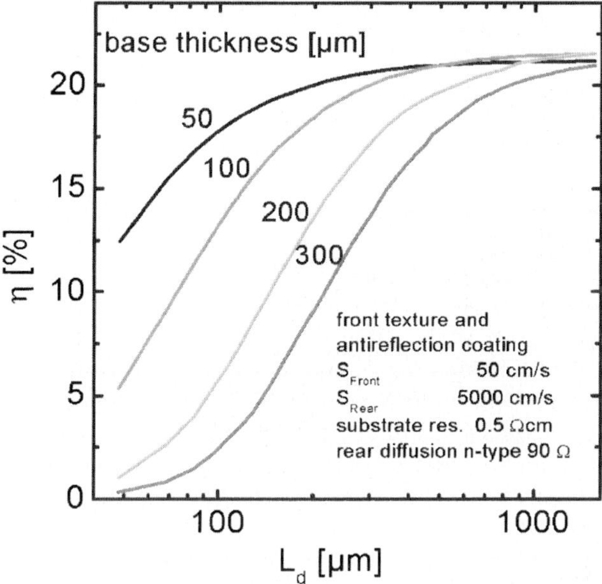

Fig. 6.13. Efficiency of back-collecting solar cells calculated as a function of the minority carrier diffusion length L_d and different base thickness. The thinner the cells, the more efficient they are

B-doped FZ–Si or Ga-doped Cz–Si with diffusion lengths above 800 μm, efficiencies approaching 23% are attainable. For material of lower quality such as B-doped Cz–Si (L_d ~250 μm) or multicrystalline silicon (L_d ~150–300 μm) the base thickness has to be reduced well below 200 μm to reach efficiencies up to 20%. Further details about these materials are presented in the following section.

Thus higher efficiencies can also be achieved for lower quality material if the base thickness is further reduced and optical confinement is provided. Efficient light trapping has recently been demonstrated for back-collecting OECO solar cells passivated on both sides by PECVD silicon nitride [48]. In the course of the rear-side grooving process of the OECO cell, the proper effective base thickness can also be adjusted. Even base thicknesses as low as 20 μm could be obtained without wafer breakage [18]. Excellent mechanical stability and flexibility is provided by the supporting ridges [49].

Thus, a starting wafer thickness down to values approaching 100 μm should be feasible in mass production with the effective base width of about 50 μm adjusted by grooving. It should again be noted that, in the case of the back-collecting OECO solar cells parallel to the reduction of the manufacturing costs by using thinner wafers, higher front-side efficiencies are realized.

For rear illumination the cells basically behave like conventional front-collecting devices. As already mentioned, efficiencies up to 20% are expected in the future despite the fact that both grid finger systems and busbars are placed on the rear side.

Shadowing by the grid fingers is almost negligible due to their vertical position on the flanks of the ridges.

6.9 Silicon Substrate Options

The high minority carrier lifetime of the silicon substrate is a prerequisite for high-efficiency solar cells. Due to the special rear-side design of the OECO cells, the requirements on the material quality are not as stringent in comparison to other back-contact solar cells, where a fraction of the minority carriers must diffuse laterally in addition to traversing the width of the cell [11].

Float-zone (FZ) silicon as the highest quality but most expensive single crystalline material has been, up to now, used mainly for laboratory devices and for niche applications to reach record cell efficiencies. However, only recently a novel photovoltaic-grade FZ–Si material was introduced for which, due to its high and stable carrier lifetime, high solar cell efficiencies can be demonstrated [50, 51]. The high production costs of FZ–Si caused by the fact that the starting material has to be in the form of an almost perfectly shaped polycrystalline rod could be drastically reduced and ingot prices comparable to those of Czochralski-grown (Cz) silicon should be within reach.

Currently, Cz-silicon is preferred for low-cost manufacturable single-crystalline silicon solar cells. Boron-doped Cz–Si has a market share up to 40% of the present world solar cell production. However, solar cells manufactured on B–Cz–Si have a serious problem: their initial efficiency degrades under illumination. For high-efficiency cells, a degradation of up to 10% relative has been reported. This is presently the main obstacle to making B–Cz–Si a perfect high-efficiency solar cell material. One approach to significantly reduce the effect of lifetime degradation on cell performance is to increase the ratio diffusion length/cell thickness by using thinner substrates; this is particularly beneficial for the back-collecting OECO solar cell [52].

The degradation effect is due to the activation of a specific metastable defect, which is correlated with the boron and oxygen concentration in the material [53]. Based on this knowledge several methods for completely eliminating the lifetime degradation in Cz–Si solar cells were proposed, whereby the two most promising approaches are (i) replacement of B with another dopant element such as Ga or P, and (ii) reduction of the oxygen concentration in the Cz material. The latter can be achieved by damping the melt flows with magnetic fields resulting in the so-called magnetic-field-assisted Cz (MCz) silicon with a very low oxygen concentration.

Surprisingly, Cz–Si doped with Ga has a stable lifetime on a much higher level than with B-doping and is thus absolutely comparable to the outstanding B-doped FZ–Si. The results of a comprehensive material study are shown in Fig. 6.14, where the efficiencies of front-collecting OECO-type solar cells on Ga-doped Cz–Si are plotted for the resistivity range of $0.08\,\Omega\,cm$ to $1.34\,\Omega\,cm$ together with some values for B-doped FZ–Si and Cz–Si [54]. Peak efficiencies of more than 21% could be obtained on $0.4\,\Omega\,cm$ Ga-doped Cz–Si as well as on $0.4\,\Omega\,cm$ B-doped FZ–Si,

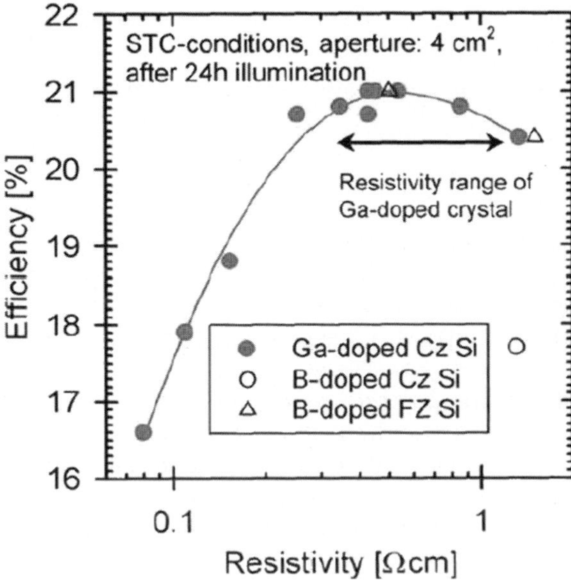

Fig. 6.14. Measured efficiencies of front-collecting OECO-type solar cells on Ga-doped Cz–Si and B-doped FZ–Si as a function of base resistivity. For both materials the same high performance is obtained. The inherent resistivity range of a Ga-doped Cz–Si crystal (see arrow) is tolerable for industrial production of high-efficiency solar cells

whereas a lower efficiency results for cells on B-doped solar grade Cz–Si mainly due to light-induced degradation.

As a consequence of the two orders of magnitude lower segregation coefficient of gallium in silicon compared to boron in silicon, the Ga-doped Cz–Si crystals exhibit a considerably higher variation in resistivity along their growth axis compared to B-doped crystals. Therefore the usability for high-efficiency solar cells of a complete 6″ Ga-doped Cz–Si crystal in the broad resistivity range between 0.25 and 1.34 Ω cm was investigated and the results are shown in Fig. 6.14. As can be seen, the efficiencies were found to reach more than 97% of the peak value, demonstrating that the inherent resistivity variations in Ga-doped Cz–Si crystals are well within the tolerable range for mass production of high-efficiency solar cells.

Other high-efficiency solar cell processes were also applied to the alternative Cz-materials at different institutes, and stable efficiencies well above 20% could be obtained on Ga-doped Cz–Si, B-doped MCz–Si and P-doped n-type Cz–Si [54–56].

In conclusion, there are several silicon material options for economic mass production of high-efficiency OECO solar cells, including B-doped Cz–Si, cast multicrystalline Si, Ga-doped Cz–Si and B-doped FZ–Si. Some alterations to the processing sequence are required for the use of n-type silicon.

As already mentioned, emphasis should be on the use of thin wafers. In addition to the high-efficiencies achievable for both sides of the bifacial OECO solar cell even with B-doped Cz–Si this is another key issue to reduce silicon consumption and thus to drastically lower the cost/kWh solar electricity.

As to the availability of silicon, unlike the case of other semiconductors, there will basically be no shortage [57, 58]. Currently, silicon feedstock production and its supply to the PV industry is not sufficient to satisfy market demand. However, there is considerable growth in the world-wide silicon supply for solar application. This is partly due to capacity expansions by existing silicon producers and to new production facilities coming online [57].

6.10 Application of Bifacial Solar Cells

6.10.1 General Applications of Bifacial Flat Panels

Since bifacial solar cell designs offer a simple way of effectively improving cell efficiency, great efforts have been made in the past regarding both development as well as application of these devices for space and terrestrial systems, including concentrators [9, 14, 25, 28, 36, 59–65].

Up to now, however, large-scale installations could not be realized since bifacial solar cells with sufficiently high rear-side efficiencies were not commercially available. To underline the potential of bifacial cells in general, and that of the OECO cell in particular, we present the following examples of the many promising applications that provide power gains per unit area of the cells in the range between 30% and 70% compared to monofacial systems. Due to the high front efficiency exceeding 21% and the expected high rear-to-front-efficiency ratio close to 0.9 with the OECO cell, an extremely high power output can be achieved [9]. It should be mentioned that the operating temperature of bifacial cells and modules is lower, resulting in a higher open-circuit voltage [64, 66]. This is attributed to the "open" rear side of the bifacial cell, through which the long-wavelength radiation not used in the silicon leaves the cell without being absorbed by the continuous rear metallization, which is typical of conventional cells. Furthermore, in case of a reduced packing density of the bifacial cells, the heat can be better dissipated within the module [64].

Low-cost installations directing light onto the rear surface of the cells are required.

Figure 6.15 (left) shows the arrangement of relatively narrow bifacial modules in a certain distance parallel to a diffusely reflecting wall, such as a white-painted building façade [64]. Both the light impinging on the front side as well as the light falling between the modules on the white wall and scattered onto the rear side is used. There is ample room for different module configurations, e.g. to represent logos etc. [64]. Figure 6.15 (right) depicts the installation of a bifacial PV module inclined to a reflecting background. Another example particularly suitable for flat roofs of private and industrial buildings and for large standalone PV power plants is to simply mount bifacial PV modules in front of a high albedo background, such as sand, gravel, concrete, snow etc. (Fig. 6.16 (left)). In this context an interesting behavior of bifacial modules in winter and particularly in high altitudes should be

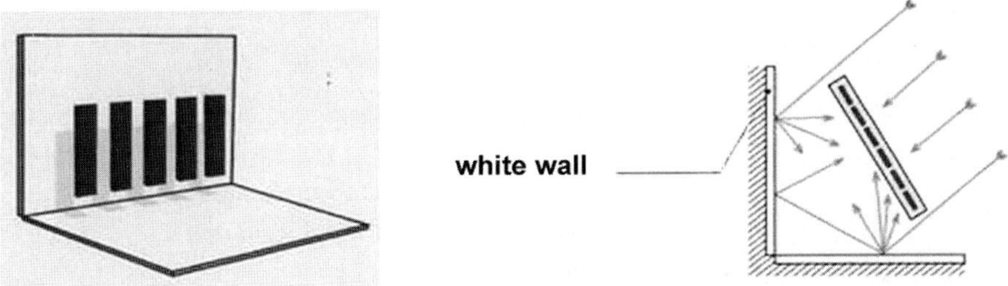

Fig. 6.15. Bifacial PV modules arranged in front of a diffusely reflecting background such as a white-painted building façade (*left*). Various arrays are possible, e.g., to represent logos etc. Installation of bifacial PV modules inclined to a white background (*right*)

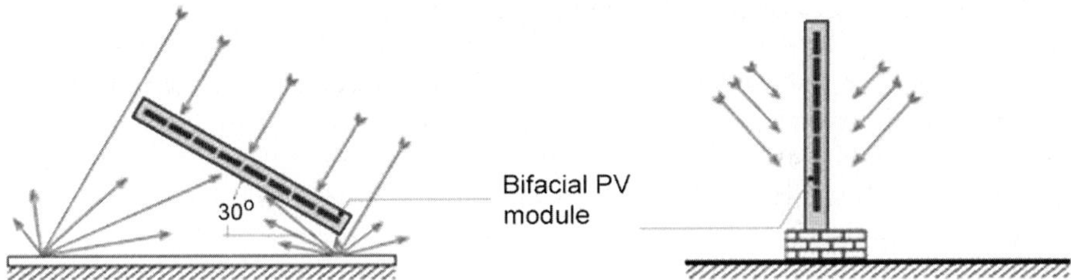

Fig. 6.16. Bifacial module on a floor consisting, e.g., of sand, gravel, concrete, snow etc. as light-scattering background (*left*). This configuration is particularly suitable for flat roofs and large standalone PV power plants. Vertical installation of bifacial modules with north–south orientation, e.g., on fences, railings or walls (*right*)

mentioned. When the front side is covered with snow and ice, electric power is still obtained by light reflected onto the rear side. As a consequence, cell and module temperature is raised thus helping to melt the front snow cover.

Further configurations with enhanced albedo for bifacial flat panels are discussed elsewhere [60, 61].

Vertical installation of bifacial modules, as shown in Fig. 6.16, is a suitable way of reducing the foundation area and of combining the panels with structural materials like fences, railings or walls. If oriented in a north–south direction, one side will be illuminated in the morning and the other side in the afternoon with a minimum at noon. As much energy output as a conventional optimally oriented PV module is delivered [63, 67]. There are several small demonstration projects including sound barriers on north–south motorways and vertical fence installations [63, 68].

6.10.2 Integration of Bifacial PV Modules in Low-Cost Concentrating Systems

The implementation of bifacial PV modules in highly reflective mirror systems is effective [60]. Figure 6.17 shows a representation of concentrators with small con-

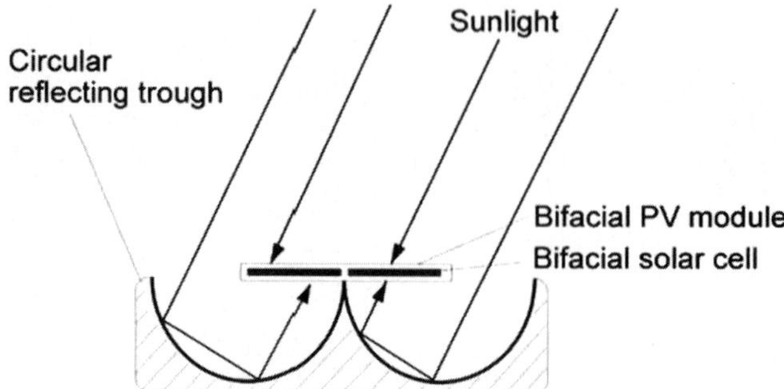

Fig. 6.17. Schematic cross-section of a static concentrator with bifacial solar cells

centration factors. The depicted Compound-Parabolic-Concentrator uses both direct and diffuse light, and all light rays either directly hit the front surface of the module or the rear side after one or more reflections [69]. Since the system tolerates a wide range of incoming light angles, tracking is not required. Several other configurations have been studied, including deviations from semicircular toward less-deep mirror structures [60, 61, 67].

6.10.3 Multifunctional Bifacial PV Elements

Bifacial PV Sun-Shading and Daylighting Element

A novel multifunctional sun-shading element was recently introduced which is based on sparsely packed, bifacially sensitive solar cells in combination with a white semi-transparent back sheet [64]. It is one part of the strategy to substitute expensive solar cells with cheap light-scattering material in order to raise the power output per cell and thus to increase the effective cell efficiency. On the other hand, apart from protecting against sun and rain, not only is sunlight collected by the front and rear surface of the cell efficiently converted into electricity, but also diffuse glare-free daylight is provided, thus preventing darkening of the room behind.

The principle is outlined in Fig. 6.18 (left). The sun-shading element consists of a set of parallel strings made up of bifacial solar cells, whereby the individual strings are arranged about one cell-width apart from each other. At about the same distance behind the module the white semitransparent reflector sheet is placed so that both the light falling directly on the front side as well as the light scattered by the sheet onto the rear side of the cell is used. There is ample room for other attractive cell arrangements within the module.

Figure 6.18 (right) shows an example of the shading element with each string consisting of 10 bifacial solar cells $10 \times 10\,\mathrm{cm}^2$ in size [14]. For comparison, two different reflector sheets made of PMMA were applied whereas the higher transmittance of the back sheet at the right-hand side can clearly be seen by the mirror image in the window behind. In this way daylighting and solar electricity generation can be varied within wide limits. From inside the room, the faint shadows cast by

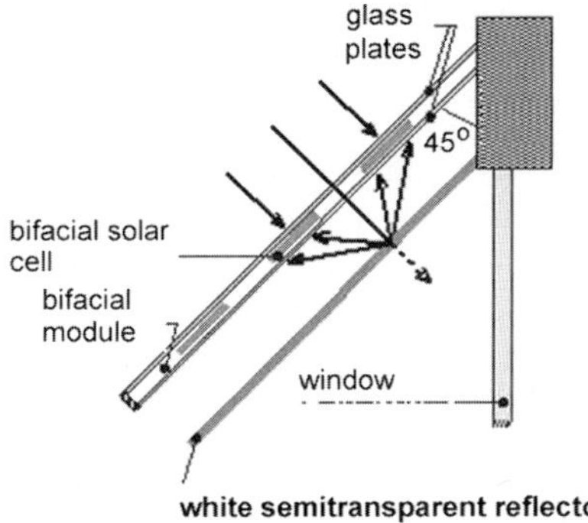

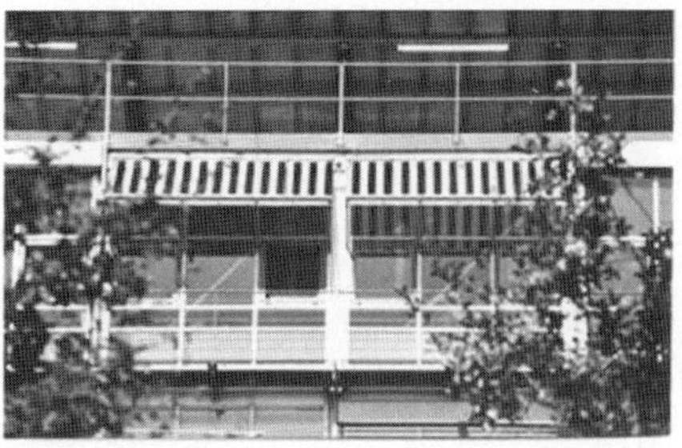

Fig. 6.18. Principle of the multifunctional PV sun-shading element with bifacial solar cells and semitransparent reflector sheet (*left*). Two prototypes of the PV element with bifacially active solar cells and different white back reflector sheets installed at a building façade (*right*). The higher transmittance of the reflector sheet of the right-hand module can clearly be seen by the mirror image in the window behind

the solar cells onto the white plate can be seen as they move according to the sun's position [64].

It's interesting to note that the power gain of the south-oriented bifacial sun shading element relative to monofacial operation was evaluated for symmetrical bifacial cells to about 50% at noon and increased up to 70% in the morning and afternoon hours, since at flat incidence relatively more light is scattered onto the rear side of the cells. Further details about the performance of these elements are presented elsewhere [64]. A broad spectrum of applications is possible, such as for shop windows, private homes, offices and industrial buildings.

Bifacial PV Facade Elements

Based on the same principle as the sun-shading module above, a bifacial PV element suitable for glass facades, entrance halls etc., is shown in Fig. 6.19.

For reflection of the light onto the rear of the cells, a white semitransparent (perforated) curtain is arranged behind the module which – besides daylighting – allows a clear view from inside through the façade. An important feature of the vertical arrangement of bifacial modules has to be mentioned. Generally for conventional PV modules placed on vertical facades, the output power is reduced by about 30% compared to the ideal inclination. This is due to the oblique incidence of sunlight. However, as shown in Fig. 6.19, this situation is favorable for the rear side of bifacial modules because, due to the shallow angle of the incoming light, a larger portion is scattered onto the back surface of the cell. Thus, for vertically oriented bifacial modules the decrease of power output by the front side is at least partly compensated by the increase in power output by the rear side.

In the case of a similar multifunctional bifacial PV façade element introduced recently, the curtain is replaced by diffusely reflecting venetian blinds arranged at

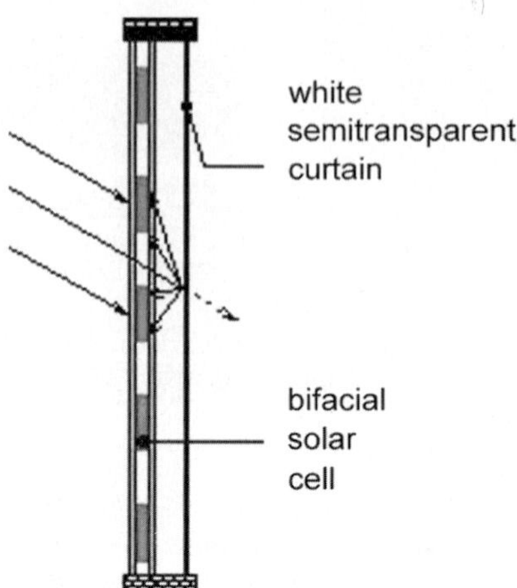

Fig. 6.19. Principle of a bifacial PV façade element. A white semitransparent curtain is arranged behind the module allowing a clear view from inside through the glass façade

a certain distance behind the module [70]. During times of high sun radiation, the blinds of a building are usually closed to avoid heating or dazzling. Here, the PV element will produce the maximum electric power on both the front and the rear side. At low radiation – like on a cloudy or rainy day – the blinds will be open and the solar cells receive light only on their front side. However, daylight will fall into the interior of the building. Varying the angle of the roller blinds, the electrical power output of the cells together with room illumination by daylight can be controlled [70].

Peak power values may particularly be realized with a similar arrangement, as shown in Fig. 6.18 but with cell size and lateral spacing reduced together with a reflector sheet attached closer to the rear side of the module. The considerably cheaper round or semicircular monocrystalline silicon wafers can be advantageously applied.

This may finally lead to a bifacial module with integrated diffuse reflector either opaque or semitransparent, which can be installed like any other conventional panel. Under optimized conditions it may provide up to 70% more power compared to a module made up of the same area of corresponding monofacial cells. With OECO cells, effective cell efficiencies approaching 35% should be within reach [9].

6.11 Conclusions

To address limits in efficiency and reduce the cost of current commercial solar cells, new cost-effective processing sequences are required. The OECO solar cells introduced in this paper are distinguished by the highest efficiencies of rear-contacted bifacially sensitive solar cells fabricated without photolithography.

Absence of shading losses on the front-side, uniform visual appearance and cost reduction in module assembly are the general advantages of rear-contact solar cells. In the future, however, further considerable cost advantages are expected for OECO cells as rear-contact devices. Particularly if lower-quality silicon can be used, reduction of the wafer thickness will result in higher front-side efficiencies. Thus, by saving expensive silicon material – which is crucial for the future of photovoltaics – cell performance is also improved. In this context, simultaneous busbar formation and cell interconnection using conductive adhesives has to be mentioned as a reliable cost-effective technique for thin OECO cells.

Together with the strength of silicon in terms of resource availability, nontoxicity and stability, the high-efficiency bifacial OECO solar cell with its economic and ecologically sound manufacturing process may significantly contribute to sustainable progress in photovoltaics. This refers to both one-sided and even more to double-sided applications, culminating in effective cell efficiencies up to 35%.

Acknowledgements. The OECO solar cell was developed at the Lower Saxonian Institute for Solar Energy Research (ISFH) at Hameln, Germany, when the author was Director of this institution and Professor of the Physics Faculty of the Hannover University. The author would like to thank J.W. Mueller, A. Merkle and all the members of the PV department at the ISFH for their valuable contributions to this work.

References

1. S.R. Wenham, M.A. Green, M.E. Watt, *Applied Photovoltaics*, Centre for Photovoltaic Devices and Systems, University of New South Wales, Sydney, Australia
2. J. Zhao, A. Wang, M.A. Green, Prog. Photovolt.: Res. Appl. **7**, 411 (1999)
3. M.A. Green, *Silicon Solar Cells: Advanced Principles and Practice* (Bridge Printery, Sydney, 1995)
4. M.A. Green, Prog. Photovolt.: Res. Appl. **8**, 127 (2000)
5. J. Bernreuter, *High, Higher, the Highest*, Photon International, May 2003 and *Hoch die Leistung*, Photon Mai 2003, Solarverlag Aachen
6. R. Hezel, Patent pending
7. R. Hezel, in *Proc. 29th IEEE Photov. Spec. Conf.*, New Orleans, 2002, p. 114
8. J.W. Müller, Dissertation, Univ. Hannover, Shaker Verlag Aachen, 2005
9. J.W. Müller, A. Merkle, R. Hezel, in *Proc. 20th Europ. Photov. Solar Energy Conf.*, Barcelona, 2005, p. 1020
10. M.A. Green, D. Jordan, Prog. Photovolt.: Res. Appl. **6**, 169 (1998)
11. K.R. McIntosh, M.J. Cudzinovic, D.D. Smith, W.P. Mulligan, R.M. Swanson, in *Proc. 3rd World Conf. on Photov. Energy Conversion*, Osaka, 2003, p. 971
12. R. Hezel, Prog. Photovolt.: Res. Appl. **5**, 109 (1997)
13. J.W. Müller, A. Merkle, R. Hezel, in *Proc. PV in Europe, Conf. and Exhibition*, Rome, p. 248, WIP, Munich, 2002
14. K. Jaeger-Hezel, W. Schmidt, W. Heit, K.D. Rasch, in *Proc. 13th Europ. Photov. Solar Energy Conf.*, Nice, 1995, p. 1515
15. A. Metz, R. Hezel, in *Proc. 17th Europ. Photov. Solar Energy Conf.*, Munich, 2001, p. 1359

16. H. Nakaya, M. Nishida, Y. Takeda, S. Moriuchi, T. Tonegawa, T. Machida, T. Nunoi, in *Proc. 17th Intern. Photov. Solar Energy Conf.*, Nagoya, 1993, p. 91
17. G. Willeke, H. Nussbaumer, H. Bender, E. Bucher, Sol. Energy Mater. Sol. Cells **26**, 345 (1992)
18. R. Hezel, R. Ziegler, in *Proc. 21th IEEE Photov. Spec. Conf.*, Louisville, 1993, p. 260
19. R. Hezel, Sol. Energy Mater. Sol. Cells **74**, 25 (2002)
20. A. Metz, R. Hezel, in *Proc. 28th IEEE Photov. Spec. Conf.*, Anchorage, 2000, p. 175
21. P. Engelhart, N.-P. Harder, T. Neubert, H. Plagwitz, B. Fischer, R. Meyer, R. Brendel, in *Proc. 21th Europ. Photov. Solar Energy Conf.*, Dresden, 2006, p. 773
22. R. Hezel, Adv. Sol. State Phys. **44**, 39 (2004); B. Kramer (Ed.), Springer, Berlin
23. W. Shockley, W.T. Read, Phys. Rev. **87**, 835 (1952)
24. A.G. Aberle, *Crystalline Silicon Solar Cells*, Centre for Photovoltaic Engineering UNSW, Sydney, NSW 2052, Australia (1999)
25. R. Hezel, K. Jaeger, J. Electrochem. Soc. **136**(2), 518 (1989)
26. J. Mandelkorn, J.H. Lamneck, J. Appl. Phys. **44**, 4785 (1973)
27. R. Hezel, R. Schoerner, J. Appl. Phys. **52**, 3076 (1981)
28. K. Jaeger, R. Hezel, in *Proc. 7th Europ. Photov. Solar Energy Conf.*, Sevilla, 1986, p. 806
29. A.G. Aberle, R. Hezel, Prog. Photovolt.: Res. Appl. **5**, 29 (1997)
30. T. Lauinger, J. Moschner, A.G. Aberle, R. Hezel, J. Vac. Sci. Technol. A **16**, 530 (1998)
31. A. Cuevas, M.J. Kerr, J. Schmidt, in *Proc. 3rd World Conf. on Photov. Energy Conversion*, Osaka, 2003, p. 913
32. A.K. Sinha, H.J. Levinstein, T.E. Smith, G. Quintana, S.E. Haszko, J. Electrochem. Soc. **125**, 601 (1978)
33. R. Hezel, K. Blumenstock, R. Schörner, J. Electrochem. Soc. **131**(7), 1679 (1984)
34. J. Robertson, Philos. May. B **63**, 47 (1991)
35. C. Peters, R. Meyer, R. Hezel, in *Proc. PV in Europe, Conf. and Exhibition*, Rome (WIP, Munich, 2002), p. 127
36. R. Hezel, W. Hoffmann, K. Jaeger, in *Proc. 10th Europ. Photov. Solar Energy Conf.*, Lisbon, 1991, p. 511
37. M. Alonso, R. Pottbrock, R. Voermans, J.J. Villard, B. Yordi, in *Proc. 12th Europ. Photov. Solar Energy Conf.*, Amsterdam, 1994, p. 1163
38. M. Rammensee, Doctoral thesis, University of Erlangen-Nürnberg, 1995
39. R. Hezel, R. Auer, M. Rammensee, *Progress in Plasma Processing of Materials* (Begell House Inc., New York, 1999), p. 891
40. J.D. Moschner, J. Henze, J. Schmidt, R. Hezel, Prog. Photovolt.: Res. Appl. **12**, 21 (2004)
41. K. Roth, F. Chen, M. Fritzsche, M. Kirschmann, J. Müller, H. Schlemm, in *Proc. 21st Europ. Photov. Solar Energy Conf.*, Dresden, 2006, p. 1137
42. J. Schmidt, J.D. Moschner, J. Henze, S. Dauwe, R. Hezel, in *Proc. 19th Europ. Photov. Solar Energy Conf.*, Paris, 2004, p. 391
43. T. Lauinger, J. Schmidt, A.G. Aberle, R. Hezel, Appl. Phys. Lett. **68**, 1232 (1996)
44. J.W. Müller, A. Merkle, R. Hezel, in *Proc. 19th Europ. Photov. Solar Energy Conf.*, Paris, 2004, p. 990
45. S. Dauwe, L. Mittelstädt, A. Metz, R. Hezel, Prog. Photovolt.: Res. Appl. **10**(4), 35 (2002)
46. J. Liu, Conductive adhesives for electronic packaging, Electrochemical Publications Ltd, Isle of Man (1999), ISBN 0-901150-37
47. J.H. Bultmann, M.W. Brieks, A.R. Burges, J. Hoornstra, A.C. Tip, A.W. Weber, Sol. Energy Mater. Sol. Cells **65**, 339 (2001)
48. J.W. Müller, A. Merkle, R. Hezel, in *Proc. 3rd World Conf. on Photov. Energy Conversion*, Osaka, 2003, p. 1399

49. L.W. Mittelstädt, A. Metz, R. Hezel, in *Proc. 16th Europ. Photov. Solar Energy Conf.*, Glasgow, 2000, p. 1340
50. J. Vedde, T. Clausen, L. Jensen, in *Proc. 3rd World Conf. on Photov. Energy Conversion*, Osaka, 2003
51. C. del Canizo et al., in *Proc. 19th Europ. Photov. Solar Energy Conf.*, Paris, 2004, p. 536
52. K.A. Münzer et al., in *Proc. 2nd World Conf. on Photov. Energy Conversion*, Vienna, 1998, p. 1214
53. K. Bothe, R. Hezel, J. Schmidt, Appl. Phys. Lett. **83**(6), 1125 (2003)
54. A. Metz, T. Abe, R. Hezel, in *Proc. 16th Europ. Photov. Solar Energy Conf.*, Glasgow, 2000, p. 1189
55. S.W. Glunz, S. Rein, J.Y. Lee, W. Warta, J. Appl. Phys. **90**, 2397 (2001)
56. J. Schmidt, Solid State Phenom. **95**, 187 (2004)
57. H.A. Aulich, F.W. Schulze, in *Proc. 21th Europ. Photov. Solar Energy Conf.*, Dresden, 2006, p. 549
58. J.H. Werner, Adv. Solid State Phys. **44**, 51 (2004); B. Kramer (Ed.), Springer, Berlin
59. A. Cuevas, A. Luque, J. Eguren, J. Del Alamo, Sol. Energy **19**, 419 (1982)
60. A. Luque, *Solar Cells and Optics for Photovoltaic Concentration* (Adam Hilger, Bristol, 1989)
61. A. Cuevas, in *Proc. 33rd Annual Conf. of the Australian and New Zealand Solar Energy Society*, Harbart, 1995, p. 983
62. A. Hübner, A.G. Aberle, R. Hezel, Appl. Phys. Lett. **70**(8), 1008 (1997)
63. T. Nordmann, A. Fröhlich, M. Dürr, A. Goetzberger, in *Proc. 16th Europ. Photov. Solar Energy Conf.*, Glasgow, 2000, p. 1777
64. R. Hezel, Prog. Photovolt.: Res. Appl. **11**, 549 (2003)
65. J. Coello, C. del Canizo, A. Luque, in *Proc. 21st Europ. Photov. Solar Energy Conf.*, Dresden, 2006, p. 1358
66. C.Z. Zhou, P.Y. Verlinden, R.A. Crane, R.M. Swanson, R.A. Sinton, in *Proc. 26th IEEE Photov. Spec. Conf.*, Anaheim, Ca, 1997, p. 287
67. A. Goetzberger, G. Walze, in *Techn. Digest of the International PVSEC-14*, Bangkok, 2004, p. 719
68. T. Joge et al., in *Proc. 29th IEEE Photov. Spec. Conf.*, New Orleans, 2002, p. 1549
69. B. Mayregger, R. Auer, N. Niemann, A.G. Aberle, R. Hezel, in *Proc. 13th Europ. Photov. Solar Energy Conf.*, Nice, 1995, p. 2377
70. R. Hezel, R. Auer, in *Proc. EUROSUN 96*, ed. by A. Goetzberger and J. Luther. International Solar Energy Society: Freiburg, 1996, p. 713

7 Commercial High-Efficiency Silicon Solar Cells

R. Hezel

7.1 Introduction

The present rapidly expanding photovoltaic market is dominated by mono- and multicrystalline silicon solar cells based upon the standard, decades-old screen-printing approach [1, 2]. Despite significant progress in both performance and cost reduction, there are limitations in efficiency that arise from using the screen-printing process to apply the front contact [1, 3].

Currently, there are three improved processing sequences for high-efficiency devices that are commercially available [1, 4]. These include the Point-Contact solar cell of Sun Power, the HIT cell of Sanyo Electric and the laser-grooved buried contact (LGBC) cell of BP Solar. Using completely different approaches in design and process technology, and deviating significantly from conventional silicon solar cells, these nonconventional cells have the potential to reach cell efficiencies beyond 20%. Details about the fabrication process are not available from the manufacturers. Basic features and properties of the high-efficiency structures are presented in the following.

7.2 The Point-Contact Solar Cell

The high-efficiency cell of Sun Power Corporation (founded 1988) is a simplified version of the highly sophisticated point-contact solar cell designed for concentrator applications. These cells were developed by Prof. Swanson together with NASA in 1973 and have been fabricated with conventional IC processing technology. They were successfully applied for niche applications, such as solar cars and solar airplanes [5].

Originally several photolithography steps were applied to define the rear features (i.e., diffusions, contact openings and fingers), so that one-sun efficiencies approaching 23% could be achieved. In order to reduce the fabrication costs and to make processing suitable for mass production, a novel screen-printing technology for masking purposes was developed [4, 6]. It is evident that these low-cost methods cannot define the rear features as tightly as photolithography, and therefore some changes in the design had to be made [6].

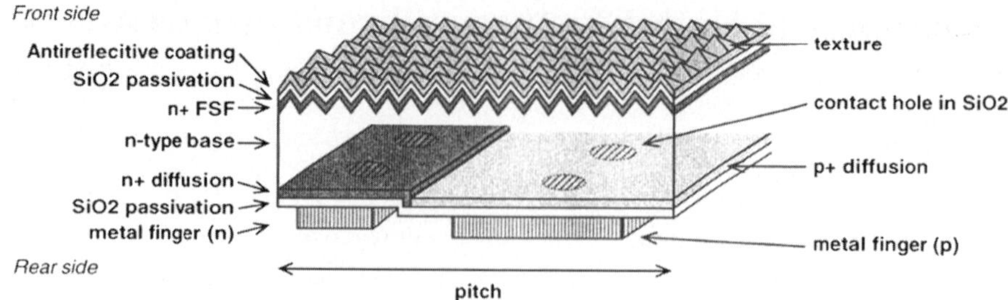

Fig. 7.1. Schematic diagram of the point-contact solar cell (Sun Power) [6]

The device is schematically depicted in Fig. 7.1. Both contact schemes are placed on the rear side. This is advantageous due to (i) improvement of efficiency since shading losses by the front grid are avoided; (ii) reduction of module fabrication costs as well as higher cell-packing density within the module; and (iii) better visual appearance of the modules due to the absence of the front metal grid.

High minority carrier lifetime and thus diffusion length is a prerequisite for any high-efficiency cell. However, back contacted solar cells are particularly sensitive to the minority carrier diffusion length, since most of the carriers are generated near the front surface and have to diffuse through the entire cell to the collecting junctions at the rear surface. Recombination of the charge carriers in the bulk should therefore be as low as possible.

Due to the relatively coarse contact geometry in the case of Sun Power's low-cost cell, some minority carriers must travel a significant lateral distance in addition to traversing the thickness of the cell to the collecting junction. As a consequence, extraordinarily high-quality silicon starting material with the lifetime >1 ms is required [6]. Low-cost photovoltaic float-zone silicon – available from Topsil – can meet these stringent lifetime requirements [7].

Furthermore, excellent front-surface passivation is provided by thermal SiO_2 together with a lightly n-doped front floating junction.

Interdigitated n^+ base and p^+ emitter diffusions and grid lines are used to collect the photogenerated carriers on the rear side. As an important high-efficiency feature, small-area contact holes are opened in the rear passivation SiO_2 film. Thus, localized point contacts are formed to reduce the metal-semiconductor contact area. This results in a low rear-surface recombination loss.

Since the back-surface has quite high reflectance due to the SiO_2 passivation layer, efficient light trapping occurs in the cell [1].

Recently the "surface polarization" effect was discovered by Sun Power in their back-contacted high-efficiency solar cells [8]. If the module is operated at a high positive voltage with respect to the ground, a negative charge is left on the antireflection coating due to the leakage current flowing from the cell through glass to the frame and ground. This negative surface charge attracts light-generated positively charged minority carriers (holes) to the surface of the n-type silicon substrate where they recombine with electrons and are thus lost.

When a module is operated at a negative voltage with respect to the ground, the surface polarization reverses and the performance of the module is not affected. Thus the surface polarization effect is completely reversible.

According to Sun Power, the polarization effect can be easily avoided by designing systems with proper grounding so that the modules only see negative voltage. Furthermore, work is under way to solve the problem by changing the cell design, so that grounding is not required.

With a cell efficiency of 22.4% Sun Power holds the record of all commercially produced silicon solar cells [9]. Modules are available with efficiencies ranging from 16.1% up to 19.3% [10].

7.3 The HIT Solar Cell

Based on experience with hydrogenated amorphous silicon films and solar cells, Sanyo Electric in 1990 launched basic research into a novel structure consisting of both monocrystalline and amorphous silicon. In 1997 a solar module with a conversion efficiency of 17.3% was commercialized. Since then considerable further progress has been made both in the laboratory and in mass production, culminating in a 21.8% efficient laboratory cell with a practical size of 100.4 cm^2 [11].

Of prime importance are (i) a high-quality amorphous-crystalline heterojunction due to the excellent surface passivation of crystalline silicon by intrinsic hydrogenated amorphous silicon (a-Si:H) layers and (ii) the use of n-type Cz–Si with its stable high minority carrier lifetime [12].

In Fig. 7.2 a schematic diagram of the HIT (Heterojunction with Intrinsic Thin Layer) solar cell is shown [13]. The cell is composed of a textured n-type Cz–Si wafer sandwiched between p/i a-Si:H films on the illuminated side and i/n a-Si:H

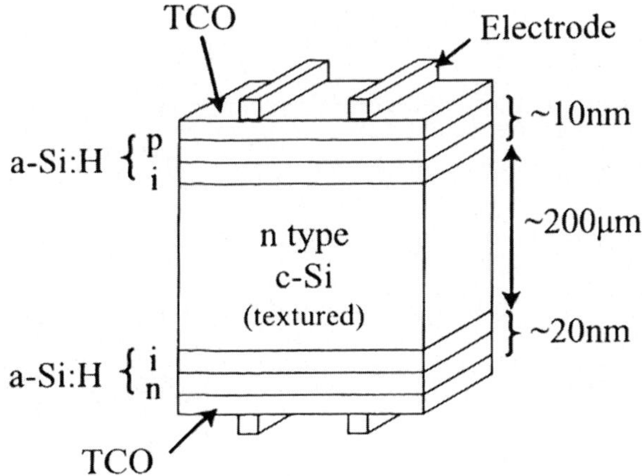

Fig. 7.2. Schematic diagram of the HIT Solar Cell (Sanyo Electric) [12]

films as a back surface field (BSF) structure on the rear side. Transparent conductive oxide (TCO) layers are deposited on both doped layers followed by a silver grid for current collection. TCO on the front side also serves as an antireflection (AR) layer. Spacing of the front grid fingers is narrower compared to conventional p/n diffused solar cells due to the relatively high sheet resistance of the TCO layer. Low-temperature processes ($<200\,^{\circ}$C) and the symmetrical structure of the HIT cells suppress both thermal and mechanical stress during production, which is advantageous for thin wafers. Furthermore, bifacial operation is possible [14].

Limitations in the short-circuit current of the cell may be given by the inherent absorption in the TCO layer and in the a-Si emitter layer. Further improvements are possible by developing high-quality widegap alloys for the reduction of the a-Si optical absorption, TCO with high carrier mobility, by optimization of the back surface field and by using finer grid-electrodes.

Very high open-circuit voltages can be obtained by plasma deposition of the intrinsic a-Si layer on a properly cleaned crystalline Si surface. Plasma and/or thermal damage to the crystalline Si surface during a-Si, TCO and Ag electrode fabrication has to be as low as possible.

For a high fill factor – in addition to a low resistance grid electrode material – a highly conductive window p-layer and a low sheet resistance of TCO is required.

A reduced temperature coefficient of $-0.33\%/\,^{\circ}$C is a further advantage of the HIT cell [15]. The output power of most conventional crystalline modules drops by 0.4% to 0.5% per $^{\circ}$C temperature increase.

At present HIT solar cell modules are commercially available with efficiencies ranging from 16.5% to 17.4%. The highest cell conversion efficiency in a mass produced HIT module is 19.5% [10].

7.4 The Buried-Contact Solar Cell

The laser-grooved buried-contact (LGBC) solar cell was introduced as a high-efficiency cell design in 1984 by M.A. Green and S. Wenham, University of New South Wales in Sydney, Australia. Manufactured by BP Solar in Spain since 1992 it was the first of the nonconventional cells to be commercialized [1, 3, 16].

The most striking feature of the buried contact cell are the fine contact lines which do not run on top of the cell surface, as is the case with conventional cells. Instead, a novel metallization scheme is applied, whereby deep and narrow grooves define the location and cross-sectional shape of the front metal conductors (Fig. 7.3). Grooves about 20 μm wide and up to 60 μm in depth are routinely obtained by using a laser scriber. Thus much higher values of the aspect ratio are obtained compared to conventional metallization. The advantages are low grid shadowing and low resistance losses in the finger metallization, boosting both short-circuit current and fill factor of the cells.

A two-step emitter is formed by heavily doping the contact region with phosphorous (n^{++} local emitter) whereas the rest of the surface is lightly diffused to obtain a shallow n^+p junction. This lowly doped n^+-emitter is effectively passivated with

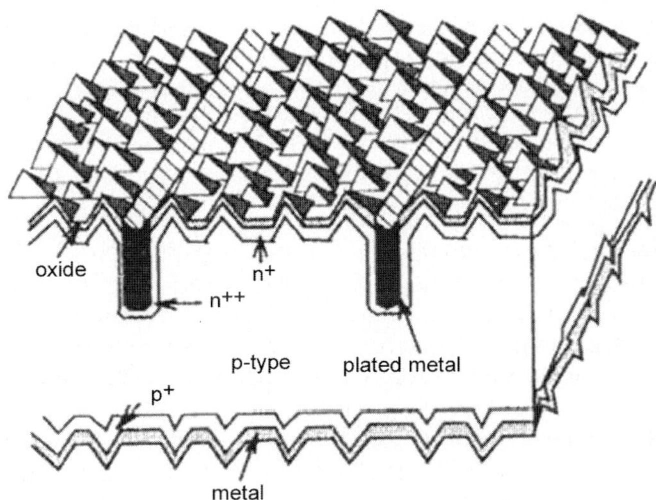

Fig. 7.3. Schematic diagram of the laser-grooved buried-contact (LGBC) solar cell (BP Solar) [17]

silicon nitride, which simultaneously serves as an excellent antireflection coating. The two-step emitter structure, together with a random pyramid textured surface, results in an optimum spectral response and minimum contact resistance of the cell. Furthermore, only a small contribution to the cell saturation current density is given, which determines the open-circuit voltage of the cell.

A p^+-region acting as back-surface field is incorporated by aluminum alloying in order to reduce recombination of the electron–hole pairs at the rear side.

The contacts on both sides of the cell are obtained by self-aligning electroless plating of nickel, followed by copper. Additional electrolessly plated layers such as silver can be applied. The insulating silicon nitride restricts the plating to the grooved areas and to the rear of the wafer.

The technology of the buried-contact cell has been described in detail elsewhere [16]. At present LGBC modules ("Saturn") produced by BP Solar are commercially available with efficiencies ranging from 13.9% to 15.5% [10].

Recently, cell efficiencies of 18.3% were obtained in a pilot line on 147.5 cm^2 boron-doped Czochralski-silicon wafers [17]. By improving the rear structure, 20.1% efficient large-area laser-grooved buried-contact solar cells were realized in the laboratory on 140 μm thick boron-doped float-zone silicon wafers [18]. The best laboratory result reported for LGBC cells (area 12 cm^2) on FZ-Si wafers was achieved in 1991 with an efficiency of 21.3% [19].

References

1. M.A. Green, *Silicon Solar Cells: Advanced Principles and Practice* (Bridge Printery, Sydney, 1995)

2. C. Podewils, Photon, Das < Solarstrom Magazin 3/2007, Solar Verlag Aachen
3. M.A. Green, Prog. Photovolt.: Res. Appl. **8**, 127 (2000)
4. J. Bernreuter, Photon International 5/2003 and Photon 5/2003, Solar Verlag Aachen
5. P.J. Verlinden et al., Prog. Photovolt.: Res. Appl. **2**, 143 (1994)
6. W.P. Mulligan, D.H. Rose, M.J. Cudzinovic, D.M. De Ceuster, K.R. McIntosh, D. Smith, R.M. Swanson, in *Proc. 19th Europ. Photov. Solar Energy Conf.*, Paris, 2004, p. 387
7. J. Vedde, T. Clausen, L. Jensen, in *Proc. 3rd World Conf. on Photov. Energy Conversion*, Osaka, 2003
8. Photon 4/2006, Solar Verlag Aachen
9. Denis De Ceuster et al., in *Proc. 22nd Europ. Photov. Solar Energy Conf.*, Milan, 2007, p. 816
10. Photon 6/2007, Solar Verlag Aachen
11. E. Maruyama et al., in *Proc. 4th World Conf. on Photov. Energy Conversion*, Hawaii, 2006, p. 1455
12. J. Schmidt, Solid State Phenom. **95–96**, 187 (2004)
13. M. Tanaka et al., in *Proc. 3rd World Conf. on Photov. Energy Conversion*, Osaka, 2003, p. 955
14. M. Taguchi et al., Prog. Photovolt.: Res. Appl. **8**, 503 (2000)
15. M. Taguchi et al., in *Proc. 31st IEEE Photov. Spec. Conf.*, 2005, p. 866
16. T.M. Bruton et al., in *Proc. 11th Europ. Photov. Solar Energy Conf.*, Amsterdam, 1994, p. 761
17. T. Bruton et al., in *Proc. 3rd World Conf. on Photov. Energy Conversion*, Osaka, 2003, p. 899
18. N. Mason et al., in *Proc. 21st Europ. Photov. Solar Energy Conf.*, Dresden, 2006, p. 521
19. J. Zhao et al., in *Proc. 22nd IEEE Photov. Spec. Conf.*, Las Vegas, 1991, p. 399

8 III–V Solar Cells and Concentrator Arrays

Z.I. Alferov, V.M. Andreev, and V.D. Rumyantsev

8.1 Introduction:
Early History of Heterostructures and III–V Solar Cells

Semiconductor heterostructures allow us to solve the problems of controlling the fundamental parameters of the semiconductor devices. These heterostructures provide the ability to change the electronic band structure, band gaps and refractive indices of the material itself during epitaxial growth, as well as to control the effective masses and mobilities of the charge carriers in it. The development of the physics and technology of semiconductor heterostructures has resulted in remarkable changes in our everyday life. Heterostructure electronics is widely used in many areas. It is hardly possible to imagine our life without double heterostructure (DHS) laser-based telecommunication systems, heterostructure solar cells (HSSCs) and light-emitting diodes (LEDs), heterostructure bipolar transistors and low-noise, high-electron mobility transistors for high-frequency applications including, for example, satellite television. Now DHS lasers exist in practically every home in CD players. Heterostructure solar cells are widely used for space and terrestrial applications.

The idea of using heterojunctions in semiconductor electronics was put forward at the beginning of the electronics era. W. Shockley, in his first patent concerned with p–n-junction transistors, proposed a wide-gap emitter to obtain unidirectional injection of charge carriers [1]. A. Gubanov was the first to analyze theoretically current–voltage characteristics of isotype and anisotype heterojunctions [2]. However, the most important theoretical investigations at this early stage of heterostructure research were done by H. Kroemer, who introduced the concept of quasi-electric and quasi-magnetic fields in a graded-band heterojunction and made an assumption that heterojunctions might exhibit extremely high injection efficiencies in comparison to homojunctions [3]. In the same period, various concepts were developed regarding application of heterostructures in semiconductor solar cells. The next important step was taken several years later when the concept of double-heterostructure lasers had been formulated independently by Alferov [4] and Kroemer [5]. In 1966, it was predicted that the density of injected charge carriers could be higher – by several orders of magnitude – than the carrier density in the wide-gap emitter ("superinjection" effect) [6]. In the same year, the main advantages of the DHS concept were summarized [7] for the use in various devices, especially lasers and high-power rectifiers.

At that time, general skepticism surrounded the possibility of creating an "ideal" heterojunction with a defect-free interface, where theoretically predicted excellent injection properties would be realized. In fact, the pioneering study of the first lattice-matched epitaxial single-crystal Ge–GaAs heterojunctions by Anderson [8] gave no proof of nonequilibrium charge carrier injection in heterostructures. Mostly owing to this general skepticism, only a few groups tried to find an "ideal couple", which seemed to be a quite difficult problem. Many conditions of compatibility between thermal, electrical, and chemical properties, as well as the crystalline and band structures of the contacting materials were to be met.

A lucky combination of properties in gallium arsenide – i.e., small charge carrier effective mass and wide energy gap, effective radiation recombination, sharp optical absorption edge due to the "direct" band structure, high electron mobility at the absolute minimum of the conduction band and its strong reduction at the nearest minimum at the (100) point – ensured this material would be under "active investigation" in different electronic devices, even at that initial stage of research. Since the maximum effect would be achieved by using it in the heterostructures with wide band-gap materials, the most promising systems considered at that time were GaP–GaAs and AlAs–GaAs. To be "compatible," materials of the "couple" must have, as the first and the most important condition, close lattice constants; therefore, heterojunctions in the AlAs–GaAs system were preferable. However, prior to starting the work on preparation and study of these heterojunctions, one had to overcome a certain psychological barrier. By that time, AlAs had long been synthesized, but many properties of this compound remained poorly studied, since AlAs was known to be chemically unstable and to decompose in moist air. The possibility of preparing the stable and applicable heterojunctions in this system seemed to lack promise.

Initially, the attempts to create double-heterostructures were related to a lattice-mismatched GaAsP system. Alferov et al. succeeded in fabricating the first DHS lasers in this system by vapor phase epitaxy. However, due to lattice mismatch, the lasing occurred only at liquid nitrogen temperature, similar to the behavior of the homojunction lasers. At the same time, it was discovered that small crystals of AlGaAs solid alloys of different compositions, which had been prepared by growing from a melt, were stable for at least two years. It immediately became clear that AlGaAs is suitable for preparing durable heterostructures and devices. Studies of the phase diagrams and growth kinetics in this system and the development of a version of the liquid-phase epitaxial growth method resulted soon in the fabrication of the first lattice-matched AlGaAs heterostructures [9, 10].

Then the progress in the semiconductor heterostructure field was very rapid. The following properties and effects had been experimentally proved: unique injection properties of a wide-gap emitter and the effect of superinjection [11]; stimulated emission at recombination [12]; the band-diagram of the AlGaAs–GaAs heterojunction and carefully studied luminescence properties [13]; and the effect of carrier diffusion in a graded-band heterostructure. At the same time, the majority of the most important devices were created, realizing many of the main advantages of the heterostructure concept: low-threshold, room-temperature lasers [14–17]; high-efficiency LEDs [10, 18]; solar cells [19]; bipolar transistors [20]; and p–n–p–n switching devices [21].

At that early stage in heterostructure physics and technology, it became clear that new lattice-matched structures were needed in order to cover a wider range of the wavelength spectrum. The first important step was in the works [22, 23], in which the various lattice-matched heterojunctions based on quaternary III–V solid solutions were proposed for independent variation of the lattice constant and the band gap. Soon, InGaAsP compositions were recognized as one of the most important materials for many different practical applications: InGaAsP/InP for lasers in the infrared intervals suitable for fiber optics communications [24]; and InGaP/InGaAsP/GaAs lasers in the visible region [25]. In the early 1970s, ideal lattice-matched heterostructures were limited to only the mentioned materials. Later this "world map" of the III–V heterostructures was drastically expanded.

Since the first solar-powered satellites, Vanguard-1 and Sputnik-3, were launched in 1958, solar cells based on Si had become the main sources of electricity on the spacecrafts. The first space arrays were based on single crystal silicon solar cells characterized by efficiency of about 10%. During the 1960s and 1970s, considerable improvements in the Si cell design and technology were introduced, which allowed increases in the efficiency up to 18%. These improvements were due to, e.g., fabrication of "violet" cells with increased short-wavelength photosensitivity, formation of so-called back-surface field, the application of photolithography to ensure optimal front grid pattern, reduction of optical losses by front surface texturing and improved antireflection coating deposition. These advanced Si cells are still used for space missions that do not strictly require III–V solar cells with their higher efficiency and better radiation stability [26, 27].

At the beginning of the 1960s, it was found that GaAs-based solar cells with the Zn-diffused p–n junction ensured better temperature stability and higher radiation resistance. One of the first scaled applications of the temperature-stable GaAs solar cells took place on the Russian spacecrafts Venera-2 and Venera-3, launched in November 1965 to the "hot" planet Venus. The area of each GaAs solar array fabricated by the Russian Enterprise KVANT for these spacecrafts was $2\,m^2$. Then the Russian moon cars were launched in 1970 (Lunokhod-1) and in 1972 (Lunokhod-2) with GaAs $4\,m^2$ solar arrays in each. The operating temperature of these arrays on the illuminated surface of the Moon was about 130°C. Therefore, silicon-based solar cells could not operate effectively in these conditions. GaAs solar arrays have shown efficiency of 11% and have provided the energy supply during the lifetime of these moon cars.

The first AlGaAs/GaAs solar cells with passivating wide bandgap window were created in 1970 [19]. In the following decades, by means of the liquid-phase-epitaxy (LPE) of AlGaAs/GaAs heterostructures [19–36], their AM0 efficiency was increased up to 18–19% [34–38] owing to the intensive investigations in the fields of physics and technology of space solar cells [39–42]. These investigations were

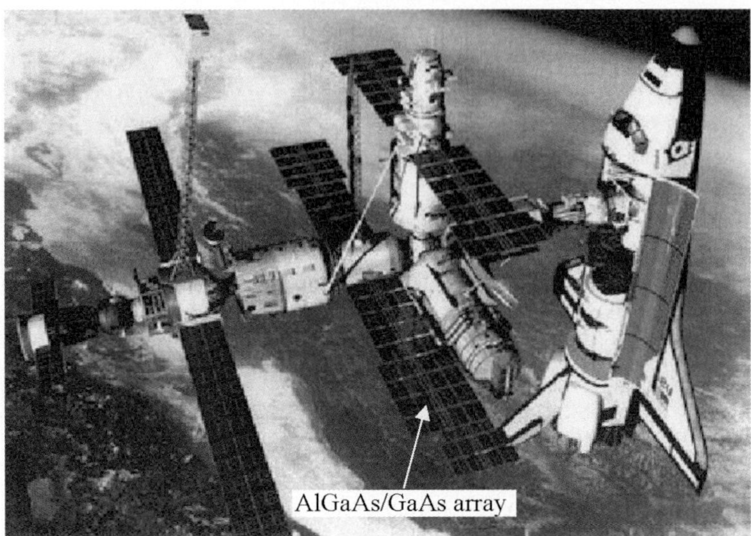

Fig. 8.1. Command module of MIR Space Station was launched into orbit on March 13, 1986, with a PV array based on AlGaAs/GaAs solar cells developed by the Ioffe Institute and fabricated in NPO Kvant. The array operated during the entire 15-year space station mission

stimulated and supported by ambitious space programs in the former USSR [33] and in the USA [26, 27].

High efficiency and improved radiation hardness of the AlGaAs/GaAs solar cells stimulated the large-scale production of AlGaAs/GaAs space arrays for the spacecrafts launched in the 1970s and 1980s. For example, an AlGaAs/GaAs solar array with a total area of $70\,\mathrm{m}^2$ was installed in the Russian space station MIR launched in 1986 (Fig. 8.1). During 15 years in orbit, the array degradation appeared to be lower than 30% under conditions that included appreciable shadowing, the effects of numerous dockings, and a challenging ambient environment. At that time, it was the best large-scale demonstration of AlGaAs/GaAs solar cell advantages for space applications. Further improvement of the LPE technology allowed obtaining [43, 44] the efficiencies of 24.6% (AM0, 100 suns) on the basis of the heterostructures with an ultra-thin AlGaAs window layer and a back surface field layer.

Since the late 1970s, AlGaAs/GaAs heterostructures were also produced by the metal organic chemical vapor deposition (MOCVD) technique [45, 46]. The advantage of MOCVD is the possibility to fabricate multilayer structures in high-yield reactors with layers of a specified composition and precise thickness that can vary from 1–10 nm to several microns. AlGaAs/GaAs heterostructures with an ultra-thin ($\sim$0.03 μm) top window layer and with a back surface wide-bandgap barrier were fabricated by MOCVD for space cells. AlGaAs/GaAs $4\,\mathrm{cm}^2$ space solar cells with efficiencies of 21% [47] and 21.7% [48] were fabricated on the base of these structures.

Enhanced light absorption was provided in the cells with an internal Bragg reflector [49–51]. This dielectric mirror increases the effective absorption length of sunlight within the long-wavelength part of the photoresponse spectrum and allows making the base layer thinner. In this case, the cell efficiency is more tolerant to reduction of the carrier diffusion length and, as a result, these cells are more radiation resistant [51].

Due to the fact that MOCVD is capable of producing single-crystal layers on silicon and germanium substrates, it has the potential for fabrication of low-cost, high-efficiency III–V solar cells on these substrates. The lattice-mismatch of 4% between Si and GaAs does not allow growing GaAs on Si with sufficient quality. However there is a progress in improving the GaAs/Si structure quality by using special structures and growth techniques: strained superlattice, thermo cyclic growth and cyclic structure annealing.

Ge is a quite good lattice-match to GaAs material. Therefore high-quality epitaxial growth of GaAs was realized by MOCVD, which is now the basic technique for growing multilayer AlGaAs/GaAs/Ge single-junction and GaInP/GaAs/Ge multijunction solar cells. This method provides epitaxial structures with good crystal quality on Ge substrates, with high productivity and good reproducibility.

Among other single-junction cells, the InP-based cells are rather promising for space applications because InP has a higher radiation resistance [27, 52, 75] than GaAs. However, there are certain obstacles for the scale application of InP-based cells in space arrays. First, there is no lattice-matched wide-bandgap window for InP to make stable passivation of the front surface. Second, it is difficult to grow this material with high quality on the Ge and Si substrates due to lattice-mismatches as high as 8% between InP and Si and 4% between InP and Ge.

Multijunction (tandem) cells ensured the further increase in III–V solar cell efficiencies. Despite a large number of theoretical studies of tandem solar cells [53–56], their efficiencies remained low for a long time, since the ohmic and optical losses in available designs were unacceptably high. Monolithic and mechanically stacked tandem cells with increased efficiencies were developed in the beginning of the 1990s. In mechanically stacked tandems with GaAs top cells and GaSb (or InGaAs) bottom cells [57–59, 62, 65–67], efficiencies exceeding 30% were achieved under concentrated sunlight. Monolithic tandem cells have been developed and fabricated by MOCVD on the structures of GaInAs/InP [64], Si/AlGaAs [68], AlGaAs/GaAs [69, 70], GaAs/Ge [71–74], GaInP/GaAs [60, 61, 63, 76, 77] GaInP/GaAs/Ge [78–84], GaInP/GaInAs [85] and GaInP/GaInAs/Ge [81, 82, 86, 87, 99–103] heterostructures.

8.2 Single-Junction AlGaAs/GaAs Concentrator Solar Cells

The creation of AlGaAs/GaAs heterostructure solar cells opened up new possibilities for increasing the efficiency of solar energy conversion. The idea of wide-band gap window was realized for solar cells, which allowed protecting the photoactive

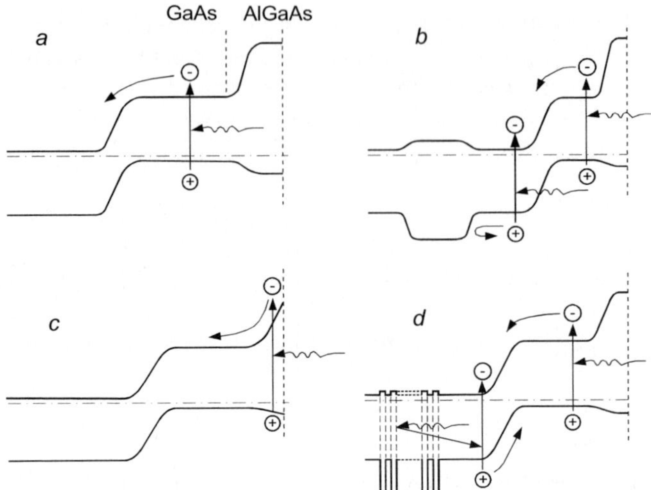

Fig. 8.2. Energy band diagrams of solar cells based on AlGaAs/GaAs heterostructures: (**a**) Structure with a p–n junction in GaAs and with a frontal wide-gap "window" of p-AlGaAs. (**b**) Structure with a back potential barrier in the n-region. (**c**) Structure with a frontal p-AlGaAs layer of variable composition. (**d**) Structure with a Bragg mirror

region of the cells against the influence of surface electronic states. Defect-free heterojunctions between AlGaAs (wide-gap window) and p–n GaAs (photoactive region) were successfully formed, which provided ideal conditions for the photogeneration of electron–hole pairs and their collection by the p–n junction. Since solar cells with a GaAs photoactive region turned out to be even more radiation-resistant, they quickly found an application in space solar arrays, despite their significantly higher cost compared to silicon cells.

First, the developments of AlGaAs/GaAs solar cells were based on relatively simple structures and technologies. Also, a relatively simple LPE technique was applied. Only one wide-gap p-AlGaAs layer had to be grown, whereas the p–n junction was formed by the diffusion of a p-type impurity from the melt into the base material of n-GaAs (Fig. 8.2(a–c)). From the middle of the 1980s, high-tech methods began to penetrate the sphere of semiconductor solar photovoltaics. The progress in the field of GaAs-based solar cells was stimulated by the application of new epitaxial techniques for heterostructure growth. The main achievement here was metal-organic chemical vapor deposition.

New technologies have led to improvements in the solar cell structure parameters. First, the wide-gap AlGaAs window was optimized, and its thickness became comparable with that of the nanosized active regions in heterolasers. The AlGaAs layer also served as the third component in the triple-layered interference antireflection coating (ARC) of a cell. A prismatic cover was applied to reduce the shadowing losses on the top grid finger contacts in concentrator solar cells (Fig. 8.3(a)). A heavily doped GaAs contact layer was grown on top of the wide-gap AlGaAs

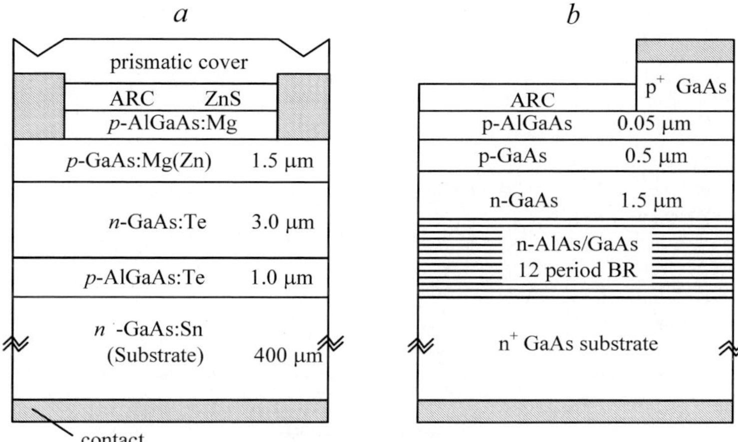

Fig. 8.3. Heterostructure of the AlGaAs/GaAs-based solar cells. (**a**) Prepared by LPE with thick (3 μm) base n-GaAs layer. (**b**) Prepared by MOCVD with internal Bragg reflector and thin (1.5 μm) base n-GaAs layer

window, and it was removed during the postgrowth treatment in the areas between the contact stripes (Fig. 8.3(b)). Second, a back (behind the p–n junction) wide-gap layer was introduced, which ensured, along with the front wide-gap layer, a double-sided confinement of photogenerated carriers within the region of light absorption (Fig. 8.2(b) and Fig. 8.3). The recombination losses of carriers before their collection by the p–n junction were reduced. At this stage of the optimization of single-junction AlGaAs/GaAs photocell heterostructures, the modified low-temperature LPE technique was still competing with the newly developed MOCVD technique.

For these structures the record efficiency of 27.8% for illumination with the concentrated (216 suns, AM1.5d) sunlight was measured in MOCVD-grown solar cells [88]. At the same time, the record efficiency of 24.6% for single-junction cells at illumination with a $100\times$ concentration of AM0 sunlight (Fig. 8.4) still belongs to LPE-grown solar cells [89, 90]. Also, the highest efficiencies for high concentration ratios in the range of 1,000–2,000 suns (AM1.5d) were measured in the LPE grown AlGaAs/GaAs single-junction cells (Fig. 8.4): 26.2% ($1,000\times$) and 25.0% ($2,000\times$) [91]. These cells can operate under ultra-high sunlight concentration with efficiency as high as 23% at 5800 suns (AM1.5d) [92].

In MOCVD-grown AlGaAs/GaAs solar cell structures, a single wide-bandgap AlGaAs layer, which forms the back potential barrier, can be replaced by a system with pairs of AlAs/GaAs layers making a Bragg mirror (Fig. 8.3(b) and Fig. 8.5) [93]. The wavelength of the reflection peak for such a mirror is chosen in the vicinity of the absorption edge of the photoactive spectrum region, so that the long-wavelength light that was not absorbed in this region can be absorbed during the second passage after reflection from the mirror (Fig. 8.2(d)). At the same time, the wide-gap mirror layers continue to serve as the back potential barrier for photogenerated carriers.

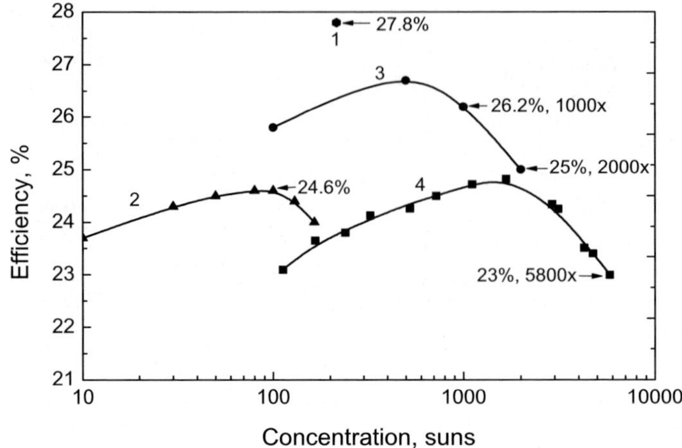

Fig. 8.4. Highest efficiencies in the MOCVD (*1*) and LPE grown AlGaAs/GaAs single-junction concentrator solar cells under AM0 (curve *2*) and AM1.5d (*1, 3, 4*) spectrum irradiation [88–92]

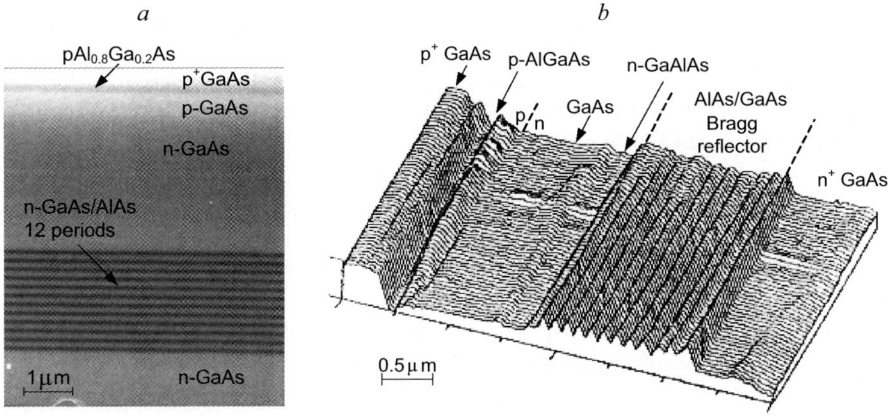

Fig. 8.5. SEM (**a**) and STM (**b**) images of the solar cell heterostructure with internal Bragg reflector

In these conditions, the thickness of the photoactive region can be reduced by half without loss of current as compared to the thickness of structures without a mirror (Fig. 8.3(b)). This factor led to a significant increase in the radiation resistance of such photocells, because the amount of lattice defects generated under irradiation by high-energy particles decreases proportionally to the thickness of the photoactive region.

More complicated structures with several Bragg reflectors [94] tuned for several IR bands of solar radiation allow us to increase the reflection of the sub-bandgap

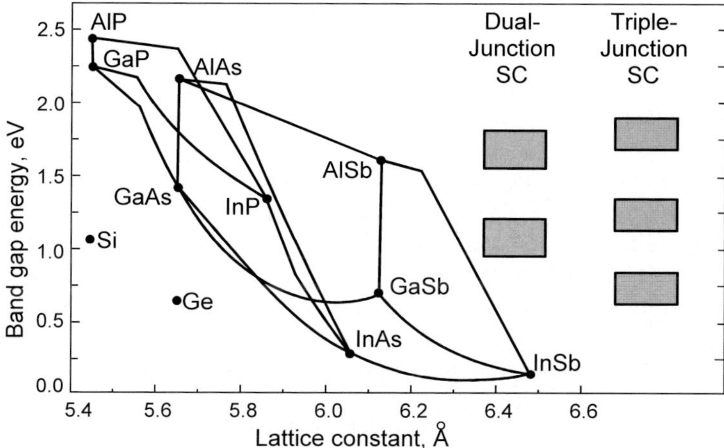

Fig. 8.6. Band gaps of III–V compounds and their solid solutions vs. the lattice constants of these materials. The optimum E_g are shown for the dual- and triple-junction solar cells

IR-radiation to reduce cell operation temperature and, as a result, to increase the cell efficiency.

8.3 Multijunction Solar Cells

The idea of tandem solar cells began to be discussed in the early 1960s and was considered to be promising. However, increasing the efficiency seemed a long way away. The situation started to change in the late 1980s, when many research groups concentrated their efforts on developing different types of multijunction solar cells. The optimal band gaps for dual and triple-junction cells are shown in Fig. 8.6.

At the first stage, the best results on efficiency were obtained through the mechanically stacked multijunction cell concept started in 1989 by Fraas and Avery; that effort resulted in a 32.6% (AM1.5D, 100×) efficient concentrator GaAs/GaSb mechanically stacked dual-junction cell [59]. However, everyone understood that the really promising cells would be those with a monolithic structure.

The first high-efficiency monolithic tandem cells were fabricated by MOCVD on GaInAs/InP [95], GaAs/AlGaAs [96]. To prepare GaInAs/InP tandem cells [95], GaInAs n- and p-layers are grown on an InP substrate to form the bottom cell. InP n- and p-layers were grown on top of this structure to form the top cell. The contacts were made according to a three-terminal scheme: one back contact covering the entire surface and two ridge-like contacts to the illuminated surface. One of them served to connect the top of the bottom cell and the back of the top cell. The cell efficiencies were 8.9% for the bottom GaInAs cell and 22.9% for the top InP cell, the total efficiency being as high as 31.8% AM 1.5 at concentration ratio of 50×.

High-efficiency AlGaAs/GaAs monolithic tandem cells have been made with GaAs bottom and $Al_{0.37}Ga_{0.63}As$ top subcells [96]. An efficiency of 27.6% measured under AM1.5G spectrum irradiation was achieved in this tandem (top cell: $E_g = 1.93$ eV). The component cells were electrically connected by a metallic contact fabricated during the post-growth processing.

Two-terminal monolithic tandem solar cells based on AlGaAs/GaAs heterostructures were fabricated by low-temperature LPE [97]. The top and bottom cells were connected by a tunnel junction formed in GaAs. The heterostructure was grown by a two-stage LPE procedure. The bottom GaAs-based cell structure was grown at the first stage. Heavily doped p^+-GaAs and n^+-GaAs layers were grown on this structure to prepare a tunnel junction. Their thickness was chosen as thin as possible (8–10 nm) to minimize the sunlight absorption losses within a GaAs-based subcell. The doping levels were as high as 10^{20} cm^{-3} when Ge or Te was added to the melt. This is quite sufficient to form a tunnel junction. The top AlGaAs layer was grown to protect the tunnel diode during the second LPE growth. Reference samples of such GaAs subcells (without p^+ and n^+ layers and with thin $pAl_{0.9}Ga_{0.1}As$ window layer) have demonstrated outdoor efficiency exceeding 27% (AM1.5, 100–300 suns). At the second stage, the top AlGaAs subcell was grown with the photoactive region made of $Al_xGa_{1-x}As$ ($x > 0.3$). These cells demonstrated rather high external quantum yield of 80–90% in the spectral range of 650–450 nm. The open-circuit voltage of 2.53 eV and the fill factor of 0.8 at 50 suns were obtained in these tandem cells. Further developments of monolithic tandem solar cells by LPE were not continued because the reproducibility of two-stage LPE progress was not ensured.

Researchers from the NREL (National Renewable Energy Laboratory, USA) were the first to obtain the sufficient efficiency increase in the monolithic dual-junction solar cells [98]. Using the MOCVD technique, they grew GaInP/GaAs structures matched by their lattice constants, in which the top photocell had a p–n junction in $In_{0.5}Ga_{0.5}P$ and the bottom one was in GaAs. The cells were electrically connected in series by means of a tunnel p–n junction specially formed between the cascades. Efficiency of 30.2% (AM1.5d, 180×) was obtained in these dual-junction cells.

At the same time, the interest in triple-junction cells was growing. As a consequence of well-directed efforts, efficiency as high as 35–40% was demonstrated in monolithic GaInP/Ga(In)As/ Ge cells [99–103].

8.3.1 GaInP/GaAs Dual-Junction Solar Cells

Figure 8.7 shows a monolithic dual-junction GaInP/GaAs cell structure. At the Ioffe Institute, such structures were grown by a low-pressure AIX 200/4 reactor equipped with EpiRas 2000TT unit (real time in-situ epitaxy monitoring tool). It should be noted that the EpiRas system provides simultaneous measurements of the different characteristic parameters by the following three methods: normalized reflection spectroscopy, reflection anisotropy spectroscopy (RAS), and emissive pyrometry. This allows us to obtain data on real temperature of the growth surface, growth rate, thickness of the layers, composition of ternary alloys, doping levels, surface reconstruction and interface quality. Permanent recording of the RAS signal during the wafer heating process makes it possible to measure the wafer deoxidation

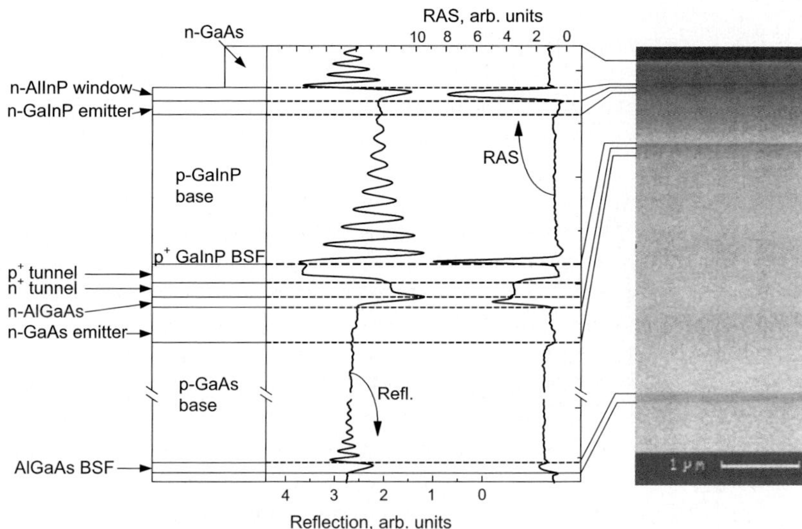

Fig. 8.7. GaInP/GaAs monolithic dual-junction cell structure: cross-sectional diagram (*left*); time-resolved curves of light reflection (at $h\nu = 2\,\text{eV}$) and RAS (at $h\nu = 3.5\,\text{eV}$) recorded during the structure growth (*in the middle*); scanning electron microscope image of the grown structure (*right*)

temperature. The surface and interface roughness can be estimated as well. Due to the difference in refraction indices of the growing materials, oscillations arise on the time-resolved light reflection curve. Attenuation of these oscillations due to an increase in absorption in the growing layer is used to determine the composition in the case of the ternary alloys, whereas the period of oscillations is used for growth rate and layer thickness calculations. Layer parameters calculated with the help of these data are in good agreement with those measured by means of the scanning electron microscopy, secondary ion mass spectroscopy (Figs. 8.7, 8.8) as well as by x-ray diffractometry, photoluminescence and other methods.

The structures of multijunction solar cells are among the most complicated of all semiconductor devices. Nevertheless, it can be "deciphered" by using the whole store of the modern diagnostic equipment. These methods allow us to obtain comprehensive information about the structure layers. However, there is a problem of precise measurements of the doping level in the thin (10–15 nm) layers of tunnel diodes.

The modes of MOVPE reactor operation were varied to adjust the conditions for growth of photoactive (AlInP, GaInP, GaAs, etc.), tunnel, buffer and spacer layers and to seek reproducible technological processes for fabrication of GaInP/GaAs dual-junction cells of p-on-n and n-on-p polarities. Since monolithic dual-junction (DJ) solar cells are two current sources connected in series, the overall current in the outer circuit will be equal to the minimum current generated in one of the junctions. The current value will be the highest one, when the photocurrent values of the top

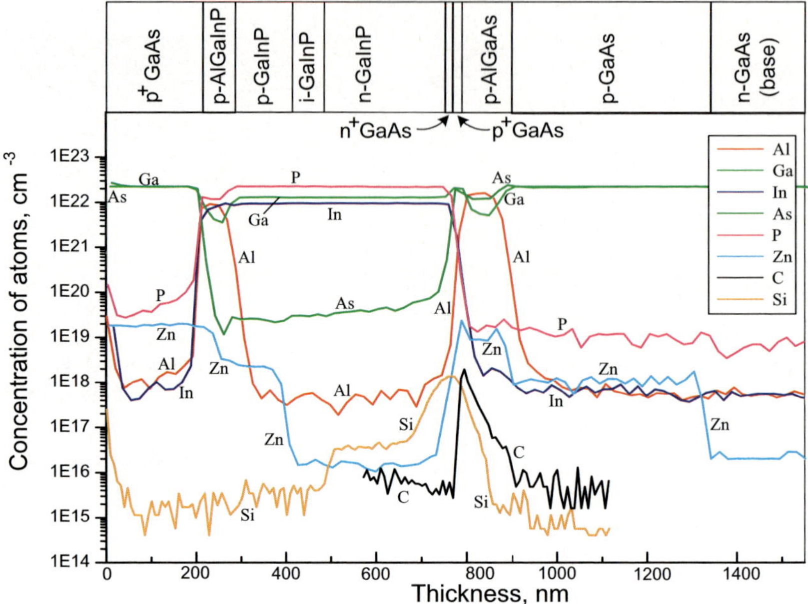

Fig. 8.8. SIMS distributions of P, As, In, Al, Ga, Zn, C, Si and structure scheme of p-on-n dual-junction GaInP/GaAs solar cell, also interpreted through use of Raman spectroscopy, SEM and EBIC methods. The structure is shown from the front surface of the top cell to the base n-GaAs layer of the bottom cell

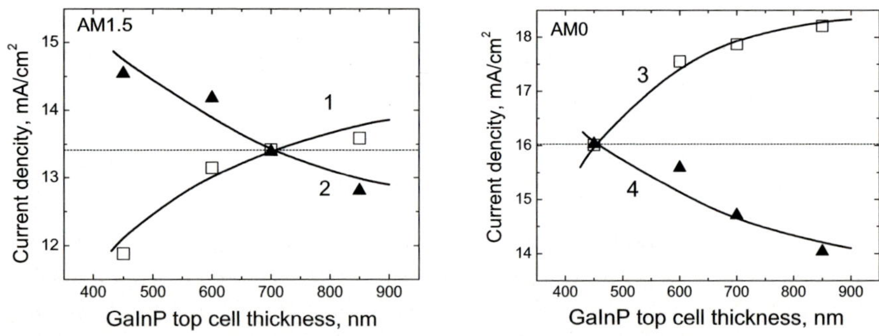

Fig. 8.9. Photocurrent densities in the GaInP top (curves *1, 3*) and GaAs bottom (*2, 4*) cells vs. thickness of GaInP cell for AM1.5 (*left*) and for AM0 (*right*) spectra [104]

and bottom cells are matched and maximal. Current matching can be achieved by varying the top cell thickness, since the amount of light absorbed by the bottom cell depends on the top cell thickness (Figs. 8.9, 8.10). In the case of the AM0 spectrum conversion, the equality in the currents of the GaInP and GaAs junctions is possible at converting the solar spectrum part with photon energies higher than 1.9 eV in the bottom GaAs junction. This is achieved by means of decreasing the top cell thick-

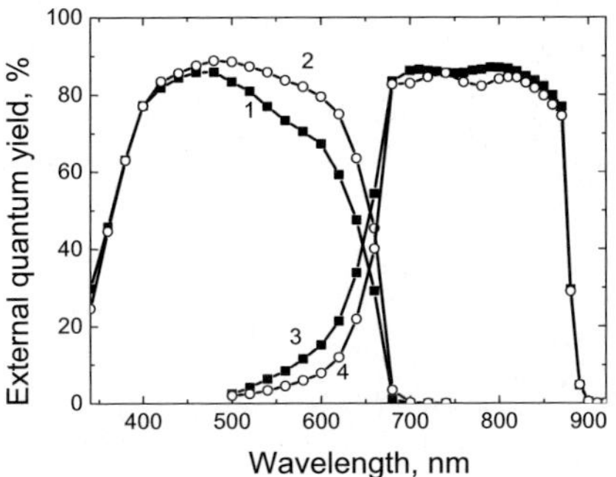

Fig. 8.10. External quantum yield in GaInP top (curves *1, 2*) and GaAs bottom (*3, 4*) cells of a dual-junction monolithic GaInP/GaAs solar cell with different thicknesses of the GaInP top cell: *1, 3* – 450 nm, *2, 4* – 700 nm [104]

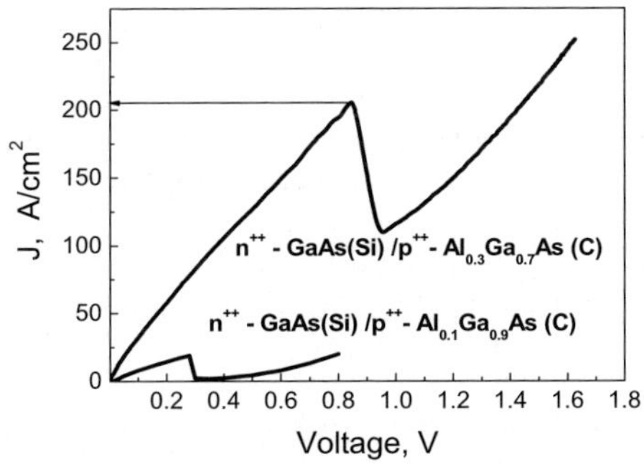

Fig. 8.11. I–V curves of tunnel diodes based on n$^+$-GaAs (Si) /p$^+$-AlGaAs (C) structures with different Al content developed for dual-junction GaAs/GaInP solar cells [104]

ness. Otherwise, at the complete absorption of photons with the energy higher than 1.9 eV by the top GaInP cell, its current will be higher than that of the bottom GaAs cell. For the terrestrial AM1.5 sunlight characterized by less ultraviolet radiation, the current correlation in a solar cell is achieved at a larger thickness of the top GaInP cell (Figs. 8.9, 8.10). At the GaInP cell thickness of 450 nm, the matching between currents of the top and bottom cells has been achieved: $J_{GaInP} = 16.01\,\mathrm{mA/cm^2}$, $J_{GaAs} = 16.03\,\mathrm{mA/cm^2}$ (AM0 spectrum). The current matching for the AM1.5d spectrum was achieved at the GaInP thickness of 700 nm: $J_{GaInP} = 13.39\,\mathrm{mA/cm^2}$, $J_{GaAs} = 13.42\,\mathrm{mA/cm^2}$ [104].

The tunnel diode for DJ concentrator solar cells should operate at high light intensity. In the growing technique for such tunnel diodes the doping p-AlGaAs layers with C was used at the smallest ratio of V/III ($<$2.5) at various Al contents. As a result of optimizing technological processes, a tunnel diode based on the n$^+$-GaAs(Si)/p$^+$-Al$_{0.3}$Ga$_{0.7}$As structure with the peak current density above 200 A/cm^2 was fabricated (Fig. 8.11); this ensured the operation of the developed DJ cells at a high concentration level.

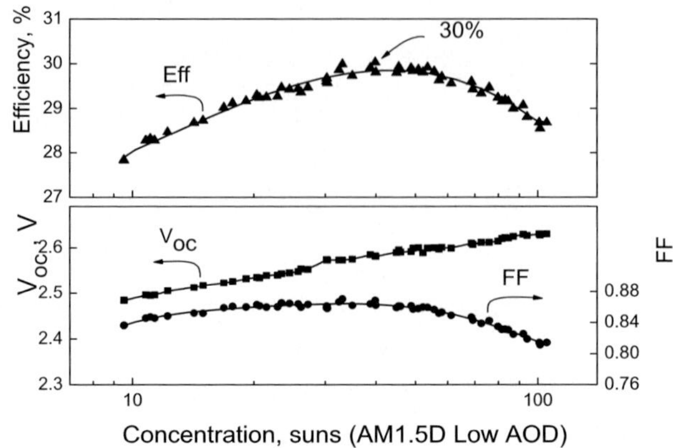

Fig. 8.12. Efficiency, V_{OC} and FF versus concentration for the n-on-p GaInP/GaAs dual-junction solar cells [104]

The I–V measurements of DJ cells under concentrated light were performed using developed at the Ioffe Institute three-channel pulsed solar simulator with a tunable blue/red ratio. Figure 8.12 shows V_{OC}, FF and efficiency values versus sunlight concentration for a terrestrial DJ cell. The maximum efficiency is above 30% at the concentration ratio of 30–50 X has been measured in this cell [104].

8.3.2 Hybrid Triple-Junction GaInP/GaAs–GaSb Monolithic/Mechanically Stacked Solar Cells

One way to increase tandem cell efficiency is the fabrication of hybrid cells with a monolithic GaInP/GaAs IR transparent top cell mechanically stacked with an IR-sensitive bottom cell. An essential aspect of this cell concept is the optical transmittance of the top cell. The interference effects in the multilayer structure and light adsorption in the GaAs substrate material result in the main optical losses of IR light passing through the top cell to the bottom one. When the top cell is operating in the mechanically stacked tandem, its transmittance could be improved in two ways: (1) thinning the GaAs substrate and (2) reducing the base doping level. For both these cases, the optimization of ARC properties on the top and bottom sides of the top cell should be done.

Because of the high light absorption by free charge carriers in the p-doped GaAs material, the DJ cell of n-on-p polarity was grown on an IR transparent n-GaAs substrate. An additional tunnel diode between the n-GaAs substrate and the n-on-p DJ cell was inserted in these structures [104]. The measured transmittance spectra for top cells as a function of substrate doping and thickness show that at simultaneous decreasing the doping level and thickness of the GaAs substrate, the interference effects become more pronounced, and the interference optical losses remain substantial in spite of transmittance improvement. Nevertheless, more than 85% of the

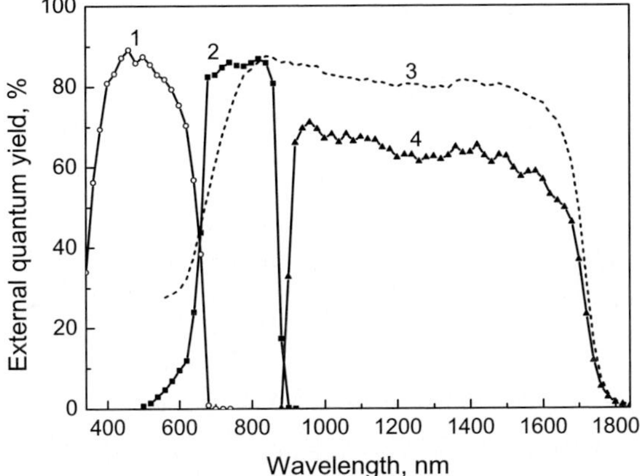

Fig. 8.13. Spectral response of a hybrid GaInP/GaAs (monolithic)/GaSb mechanically stacked triple-junction cell. Curves *1, 2*: spectra of top GaInP (*1*) and middle GaAs (*2*) sub cells. Curve *3*: GaSb cell as it is, Curve *4*: GaSb cell behind GaInP/GaAs top cell based on 380 μm thick IR-transparent GaAs substrate

infrared light passes through the InGaP/GaAs top cell and reaches the GaSb bottom cell.

Solar cells based on GaSb intended for mechanically stacked tandems were fabricated by the Zn diffusion into the n-GaSb front epitaxial layer grown by LPE on the heavily doped n^+-GaSb substrate. The GaSb cells based on epitaxial layers are characterized by the higher photosensitivity in comparison with the cells based on the "bulk" material [105, 106]. Application of the epitaxial technology for the fabrication of GaSb cells together with the optimization of the antireflection coating of both the top and bottom cells allows for gains in the external quantum yield in the spectral range of the top cell transparency; that improvement gives an increase in the generated photocurrent (Fig. 8.13). The cells with an epitaxial layer grown on a heavily doped substrate are characterized by the fill factor of 0.68–0.70, which does not decrease with the increase of light concentration up to 300 suns (Fig. 8.14). As a result these cells demonstrate higher values of the efficiency compared to those of the cells earlier fabricated by zinc diffusion into the GaSb wafer.

The maximum achieved efficiencies for the top and bottom cells arranged in a triple stack is 30.2% (40 suns) for the DJ cell and 5.9% (420 suns) for the GaSb cell. The best efficiency of 35% was obtained for GaInP/GaAs–GaSb mechanical stacks based on well-matched current top DJ cells [104]. The recent improvements of the GaSb cell show really optimistic results for it, placed behind the IR-transparent DJ cell: 17.7 mA/cm^2, FF = 0.72 and 6.2% (AM1.5D, Low AOD, 290 X) efficiency. Thus, the efficiency above 38% (AM1.5) seems to be achievable in the improved concentrator hybrid cell based on GaInP/GaAs top and GaSb bottom subcells.

Efficiency as high as 34% (15 suns, AM0) has been achieved in the hybrid triple-junction monolithic/mechanically stacked voltage-matched circuits based on

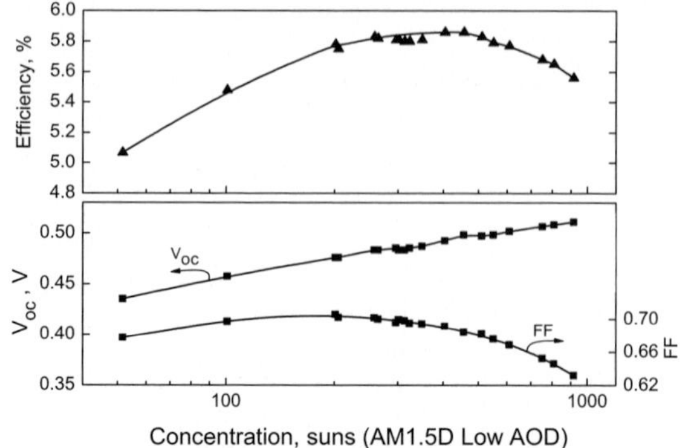

Fig. 8.14. Efficiency, V_{oc} and FF versus concentration for the GaSb bottom cell illuminated through GaInP/GaAs DJ cell with 380 μm n-GaAs ($n = 2 \times 10^{16}$ cm^3) substrate [104]

a GaInP/GaAs monolithic top cell and a GaSb bottom cell [107]. Efficiencies of 27.5% in the top GaInP/GaAs cell and of 6.5% in the bottom cell were achieved. To arrange two-terminal circuits, seven GaSb cells were connected in series ensuring output voltage (V_{mp}) slightly exceeding the V_{mp} of GaInP/GaAs cells connected in parallel.

The quadruple GaInP/GaAs–AlGaAsSb/GaInAsSb cells can ensure further efficiency increase up to 40% and more at concentrated AM1.5d sunlight. This can be achieved owing to a possible efficiency increase in the monolithic dual-junction bottom cell based on lattice-matched AlGaAsSb/GaInAsSb structures with band gaps of ∼1 eV in the top subcell and ∼0.6 eV in the bottom subcell [108].

Unfortunately, complicated assembly of the mechanically stacked cells and difficulties of heat removal from the top cell at sunlight concentration ratio exceeding 100 suns are obstacles to industrializing this approach.

8.3.3 Monolithic GaInP/Ga(In)As/Ge Triple-Junction Solar Cells

Efficiencies of 35–40% was obtained recently [99–103] in the monolithic GaInP/ Ga(In)As/Ge concentrator triple-junction cells (see Fig. 8.15). Top and middle subcells include the following layers: back-surface field (BSF) layer, base, spacer, emitter and window. The Ge-subcell consists of a base (substrate), a diffused emitter and a window. Subcells are connected in series by tunnel diodes, which in turn include highly doped thin (10–20 nm) layers. Combination of the lattice matched GaInP top cell, GaAs middle cell and Ge bottom cell divides the solar spectrum into three parts at excess photocurrent density in the Ge-cells (Fig. 8.16). Current matching can be improved if the middle cell has lower band gap (for instance, 1.2–1.3 eV) in the lattice-mismatched (metamorphic) GaInP/GaInAs/GaAs structure [87, 99, 100]. The problem of the crystal quality arises during the growth procedure development for such metamorphic solar cells. It should be noted that GaInAs with a near to ideal band gap of 1.1 eV has the lattice mismatch of 1.6% with the Ge substrate. In spite

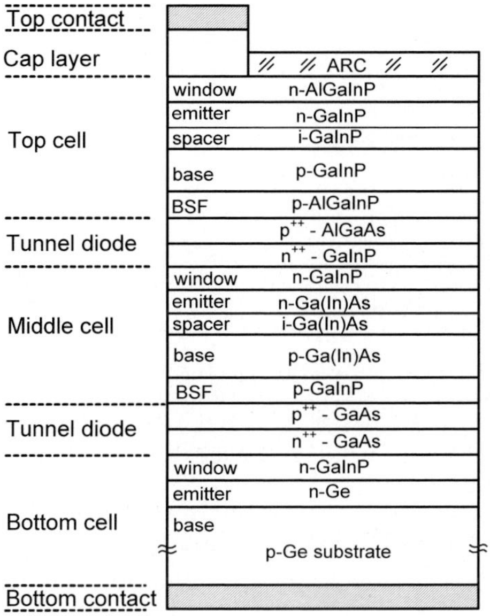

Top contact		
Cap layer		⁄⁄ ⁄⁄ ARC ⁄⁄ ⁄⁄
Top cell	window	n-AlGaInP
	emitter	n-GaInP
	spacer	i-GaInP
	base	p-GaInP
	BSF	p-AlGaInP
Tunnel diode		p^{++} - AlGaAs
		n^{++} - GaInP
Middle cell	window	n-GaInP
	emitter	n-Ga(In)As
	spacer	i-Ga(In)As
	base	p-Ga(In)As
	BSF	p-GaInP
Tunnel diode		p^{++} - GaAs
		n^{++} - GaAs
Bottom cell	window	n-GaInP
	emitter	n-Ge
	base	
		p-Ge substrate
Bottom contact		

Fig. 8.15. Typical GaInP/Ga(In)As/Ge structure of a monolithic triple-junction solar cell on p-Ge substrate

of the higher theoretical efficiency of such metamorphic cells, the achieved cell efficiencies are approximately equal to those for lattice matched cells. Nevertheless, the highest efficiency (>40%) was reached by Spectrolab, Inc. in the metamorphic $Ga_{0.44}In_{0.56}P/Ga_{0.92}In_{0.08}As/Ge$ three-junction concentrator solar cells [103].

Multijunction solar cells are characterized by a complicated structure. In a triple-junction cell, three photoactive p–n junctions are connected in series by two intermediate n^+–p^+ tunnel junctions, biased by voltage in the forward direction. Very high doping concentrations of the tunnel junction regions require small thicknesses of the corresponding layers in the structure to reduce the nonphotoactive light absorption. In addition, two enclosing barrier layers designed to minimize dopant diffusion from the n^+ and p^+ layers in both tunnel junctions should be introduced in a multijunction solar cell structure. Very often technological difficulties associated with formation of the tunnel junctions are the reason for lower conversion efficiency of a cell. This is especially true in the case of the cells intended for operation under high sun concentration conditions.

If the generated photocurrent density in a cell exceeds the density of the peak tunnel current (J_p) of one or both tunnel junctions, in this case there exists a part of the I–V curve near the open circuit voltage point, where a trace from the action of the internal tunnel diode(s) can be revealed. The J_p value is an important parameter of a cell, establishing the limit in the photocurrent density for efficient operation. Figure 8.16 shows a family of the illuminated I–V curves for a TJ cell. It was measured at different light intensities from a high-power flash solar simulator [109].

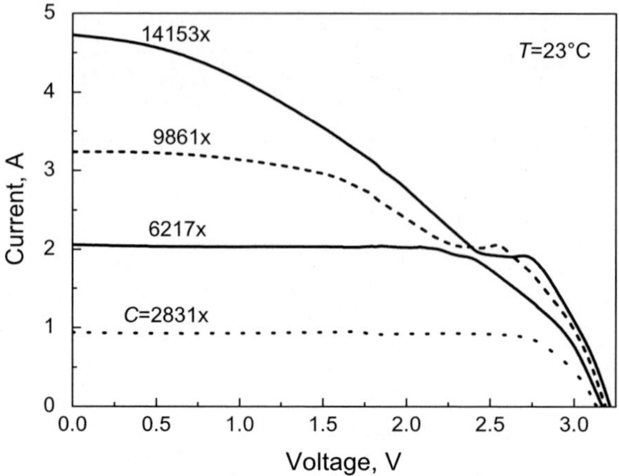

Fig. 8.16. A family of illuminated I–V curves at different light intensities from the high-power flash solar simulator for TJ cell (designated illumination area is 2 mm in diameter) [109]

A tunnel peak is revealed at sun concentration beginning from $\sim$9800$\times$. Resolution of the tunnel peaks is difficult, when I–V curves are strongly deformed due to obvious action by the cell's internal resistance. The value of J_p as high as 65 A cm^{-2} has been calculated from I–V curve for $C = 9861\times$, when considering only the designated illumination area.

The main result of Fig. 8.16 is that TJ cells can operate at illumination intensities as high as several thousand suns. Tunnel peaks have a tendency to move toward the open circuit voltage point, when illumination increases. At the same time, peak current decreases. This is probably caused by overlapping of the tunnel curves, with part of the curve related to the photoactive junctions being more vertical near the open circuit point at higher photocurrents. Other reasons may be regarded as well. Among them is a parasitic photoactivity of the tunnel junctions, when generated photocurrent reduces peak current. Another reason can be associated with the carrier transport through the cell structure, where the thickness of all the layers is smaller than the diffusion length of the photogenerated carriers, or potential barriers are not high enough. Further investigations could resolve the causes of this phenomenon.

A reduction in ohmic losses is obtained by lowering both series and sheet resistances; this ensures a high fill factor value exceeding 0.87 at concentration ratios up to 1,000 suns and FF $= 0.8$ at 4,000 suns (Fig. 8.17). Efficiencies of about 37% at 1,000$\times$, 36% at 2,500$\times$ and 34.5% at 4,000$\times$ have been measured in one of the Spectrolab's cells available in the market.

The following statements may be formulated on the basis of the presented data: heterostructures of high-efficiency, multijunction solar cells are the most complicated structures among all semiconductor devices. The confirmation of this declaration is as follows.

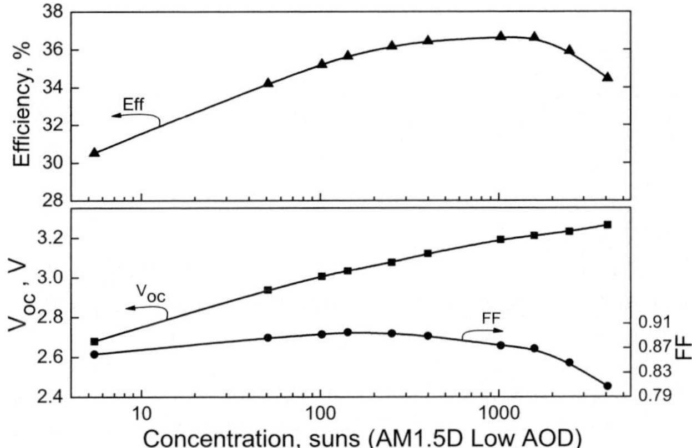

Fig. 8.17. Efficiency (Eff), fill factor (FF) and open circuit voltage (V_{oc}) vs. sunlight concentration ratio for a triple-junction GaInP/GaInAs/Ge Spectrolab's solar cell (area is $4\,mm^2$ and designated illumination area is 1.7 mm in diameter)

– Full range of the III–V materials in view of the binaries and solid alloys is involved in formation of the multijunction solar cell structure (including nitrides for advanced cells). A very wide range of the layer band gaps covering photon spectrum from UV to IR should be ensured. All the layers are lattice matched, or moderately metamorphic.

– A triple-junction cell consists of about 20 layers and the quantity of layers will be larger in advanced 4–6-junction cells, or in the cells with Bragg reflectors, as well as in the cells incorporating superlattices and quantum dots. Layer thickness is varied in a very wide range from 10 nm in the tunnel diodes up to a few micrometers in the photoactive regions.

– Doping level is varied from 10^{15}–$10^{16}\,cm^{-3}$ in the spacer layers up to 10^{19}–$10^{20}\,cm^{-3}$ in commutating tunnel diodes. A drastic change in the doping level should be ensured in the tunnel diodes and this sharpness should be conserved in the structure during further crystallization at high growth temperatures. Also, the operating capacity of the tunnel junctions should be ensured during the lifetime of outdoor cell operation at various temperatures and high photocurrent densities.

– III–V cell structures are grown on Ge substrate, being the foreign material in relation to the cell material. A number of additional technological problems are expected if the Ge substrate is substituted for the Si substrate, which is more promising from economical point of view.

– Individual cell dimensions are varied from $1\,mm^2$ in the terrestrial concentrator modules with mini-lenses up to about $30\,cm^2$ in arrays without concentration for space application. It means that extremely high quality of growth and post-growth technologies must be ensured.

- Solar cells are among such semiconductor devices which operate under difficult climatic conditions. A thin glass sheet or dielectric layer is the only barrier between the environment and the cell structure.
- In concentrator cells, optically transparent protectors and front layers are subjected to the action of highly intensive light (up to 1,000 suns and higher in the center of the focal spot), so that a radiation resistance of corresponding materials should be ensured.
- Conflicting demands on the cell structure are accompanied by a requirement to provide the lowest cell cost as an essential issue in reducing the system cost of solar electricity.

In spite of the complexity of MJ cell structures and technology, a number of new companies have been formed to organize the production of concentrator PV installations based on multijunction cells. This expansion is driven by the new perspectives for significant efficiency increase and reduction in the costs of solar electricity.

It is clear that solar cells are the key elements in the concentrator PV installations. Table 8.1 summarizes the efficiencies of terrestrial single- and multijunction III–V concentrator solar cells achieved in the period of 1989–2006. Cell producers, sunlight concentration ratios (suns), conditions at measurements (air mass) and the cell structure (type of solar cells) are shown in the table. The cells in the upper part of the table are characterized by rather high efficiency. However, in the 1990s there was no production of such cells. Getting the high-power companies (Spectrolab, AZUR Space, EMCORE Photovoltaics, Sharp, etc.) involved in "terrestrial" concentrator activity allowed for large-scale production of MJ concentrator solar cells for concentrator modules. This means that an opportunity arises for expanding the concentrator PV industry in the near future [110–114].

8.4 Concentrator PV Modules and Installations with III–V Solar Cells

The concentrator approach is the only way for large-scale use of high-efficiency III–V cells for terrestrial applications. Indeed, optical elements made of relatively cheap materials can focus the sunlight on small-area cells, which allows for drastically reduced consumption of semiconductor materials in production of the solar arrays. The costs for optical elements and mechanical sun-tracking systems are covered by the expense of the larger amount of "solar" electricity produced in higher-in-efficiency cells and owing to normal positioning of the PV modules with respect to sunrays during the daytime. For more than 30 years many research groups were engaged in developing concentrator PV systems. Under development were the solar cell structure and fabrication technology, effective concentrator optical systems, module design, and sun trackers [28, 40, 115, 116]. Interest in concentrator PV grew substantially after the higher-in-efficiency multijunction solar cells promised to achieve photovoltaic conversion efficiencies near 35–40% at high levels of sunlight concentration.

Table 8.1. Selected efficiencies of the concentrator solar cells based on III–V compounds

Year	Producer	Eff (%)	Suns	Air mass	Type of solar cell	Ref.
1989	Boeing	32.6	100	AM1.5	GaAs/GaSb, mech. stacked	[88]
1991	Spire	27.6	255	AM1.5	AlGaAs/GaAs, single-junction	[88]
1991	NREL	31.8	50	AM1.5	InP/InGaAs DJ, monolithic	[88]
1994	IOFFE	24.6	100	AM0	AlGaAs/GaAs, single-junction	[43]
1994	NREL	30.2	180	AM1.5d	GaInP/GaAs, DJ, monolithic	[88]
1999	IOFFE/IES-UPM	24.8	1,680	AM1.5d	AlGaAs/GaAs, single-junction	[92]
		23	5,800			
2001	Fraunhofer ISE	30.2	300	AM1.5d	GaInP/GaInAs DJ, monolithic	[88]
2001	IOFFE/IES-UPM	26.2	1,000	AM1.5d	AlGaAs/GaAs, single-junction	[91]
		25	2,000			
2001	JX Crystals	34	15	AM0	GaInP/GaAs-GaSb, TJ hybrid circuit	[107]
2005	Fraunhofer ISE RWE-SSP	35.2	600	AM1.5d	GaInP/GaInAs/Ge, monolithic	[111]
2006	IOFFE	35	50	AM1.5 low-AOD	GaInP/GaAs/GaSb, TJ hybrid monolithic/mech.stacked	[104]
2006	Toyota TI Sharp Corp.	38.9	489	AM1.5g	GaInP/GaInAs/Ge, TJ monolithic	[102]
2006	Spectrolab	39.3	179	AM1.5 low-AOD	GaInP/GaInAs/Ge, TJ monolithic	[88]
2006	Spectrolab	40.7	240	AM1.5 low-AOD	GaInP/GaInAs/Ge, TJ monolithic	[103]

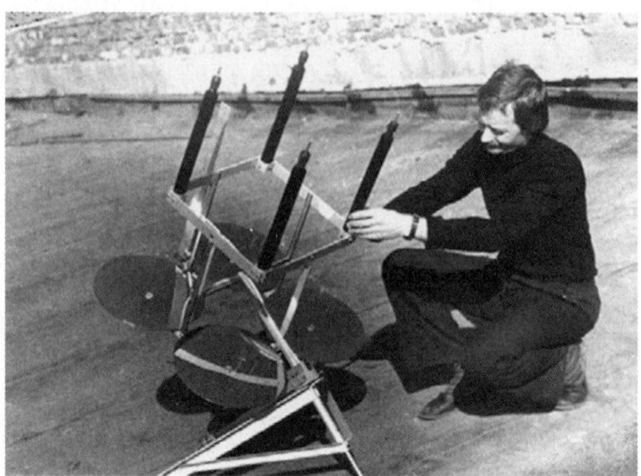

Fig. 8.18. Concentrator PV installation with four parabolic mirrors and AlGaAs/GaAs cells mounted on the heat pipes, 1981 [117]. In photo: Rumyantsev

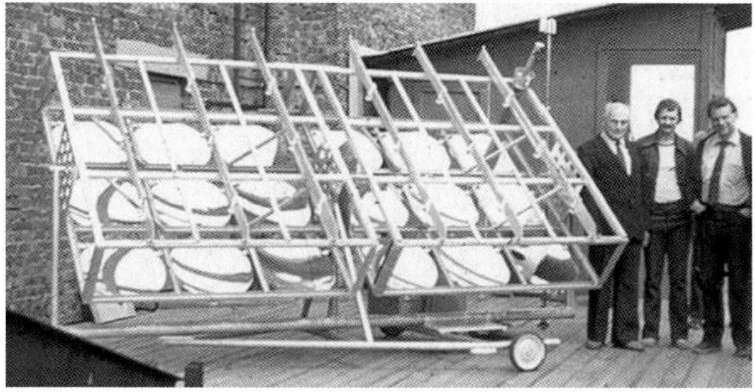

Fig. 8.19. Solar PV installation with AlGaAs/GaAs solar cells and parabolic mirrors, 1981 [118]. In photo: Alferov (*on the right*), Rumyantsev (*in the center*) and Tuchkevich, former director of Ioffe Institute

In the first concentrator modules and installations, large-area mirrors (0.5–1 m in diameter) focused the sunlight on cells of several square centimeters in area. Cooling by water or by means of thermal pipes was necessary [115–118] (see Figs. 8.18, 8.19). The appearance of Fresnel lens fabrication technology has required revision of the photovoltaic module design. Now, solar cells could be placed behind the concentrators. The module housing could serve as a protector from the environment (Fig. 8.20). Since the Fresnel lenses had smaller dimensions ($25 \times 25\,\mathrm{cm}^2$), the photocell dimensions were also decreased down to less than $1\,\mathrm{cm}^2$. The characteristics of such photocells were improved due to lower internal ohmic losses and simplified assembly. For cooling the cells, it was sufficient to use the heat conductivity of the module's metallic housing [119].

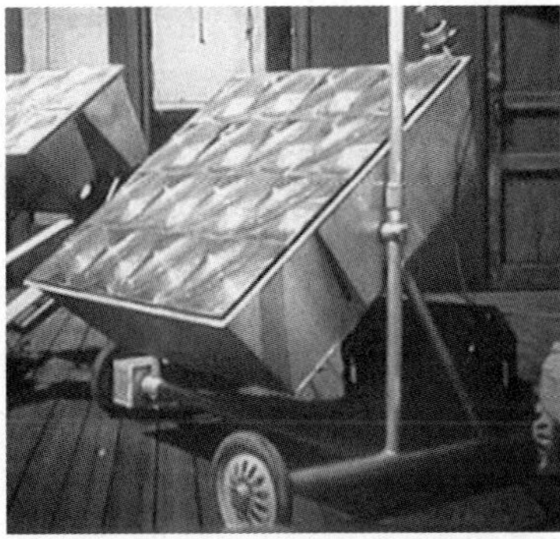

Fig. 8.20. Solar PV installation with 16 Fresnel lenses ($25 \times 25\,\mathrm{cm}^2$ each) and AlGaAs/GaAs cells, 1986 [119]

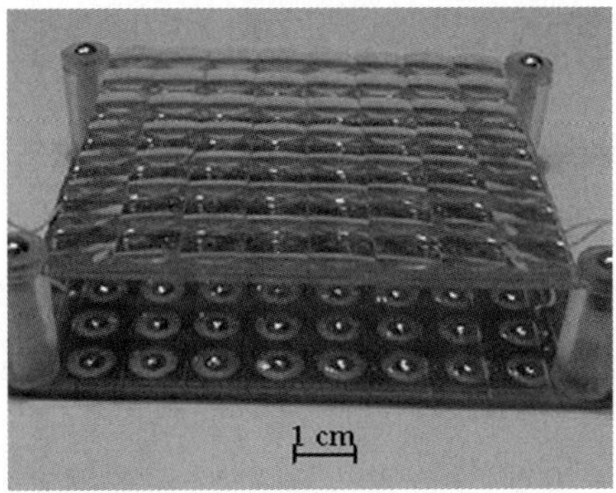

Fig. 8.21. Concentrator PV module employing small- aperture area smooth-surface lenses and AlGaAs/GaAs cells, 1989 [120, 121]

In the late 1980s, a concept was proposed that meant a radical decrease in the concentrator dimensions and retention of a high sunlight concentration ratio [120, 121]. The first experimental modules of this type consisted of a panel of lenses, each of 1×1 or $2 \times 2\,\mathrm{cm}^2$, focusing radiation on the AlGaAs/GaAs cells of submillimeter size (see photograph in Fig. 8.21). There are several advantages of a module with small-aperture area concentrators: the requirements imposed on the capability of heat-sinking material are essentially relieved such as requirements for the thermal expansion coefficient and thickness. The focal distance of lenses appears to be comparable with the structural thickness of the conventional modules without concentrators.

The advantages of the small-size concentrator cells are the following: low ohmic losses at collection of low current at nonuniform light intensity distribution and high local photocurrent density; high cell chip throughput from a wafer; and the possibility of applying the highly productive mounting methods. Somewhat later this approach resulted in creation of the "all-glass" photovoltaic modules with III–V cells and panels of small-aperture area Fresnel lenses (each lens is $4 \times 4\,\mathrm{cm}^2$). The

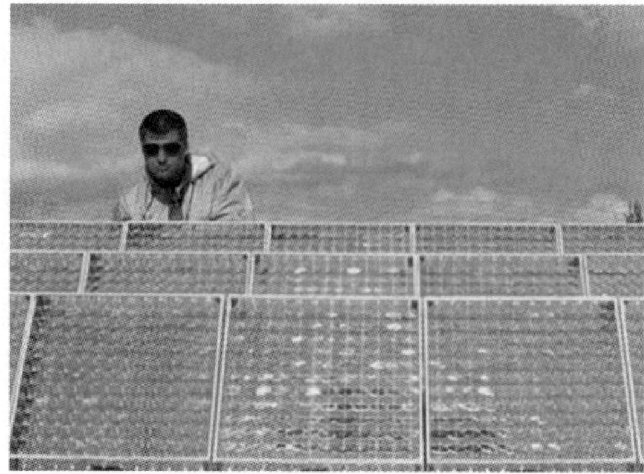

Fig. 8.22. Array of the full-size concentrator modules with small aperture area Fresnel lenses [130]

lens panels had a "glass-silicone" composite structure. This work was carried out through close cooperation between the research teams from the Ioffe Institute (St. Petersburg, Russia) and Fraunhofer Institute for Solar Energy Systems (Freiburg, Germany) [122–125].

In recent years, the team at the Ioffe Institute developed the concentrator modules [126–129], in which Fresnel lenses are arranged on a common superstrate in the form of a panel of 12×12 lenses. The cells are as small as $2 \times 2\,\mathrm{mm}^2$ and 1.7 mm in designated area diameter operating at mean concentration ratio of about $700\times$ [130] (see photograph in Fig. 8.22).

For the use of the monolithic multijunction cells, the following fundamental advantage should be noted. They operate at lower photocurrent, so that ohmic losses, say, in a five-junction cell, would be lower than the losses in a one-junction cell operating within the same spectral range by a factor of 5. Nonuniformity in the illumination distribution along the cell surface is a negative feature of concentration. For multijunction cells, an important factor is chromatic aberrations in concentrators of the refractive type. Negative influence of this type of illumination nonuniformity cannot be compensated for by using a more dense contact grid, because lateral currents arise between subcells inside the cell structure. Small-size cells have certain advantages in this respect. On the other hand, parameters of a concentrator as an element of a PV system should be optimized in the required way.

8.4.1 Concentrator Modules with Mini-lens Panels: Design and Fabrication

Comprehensive analysis has been done regarding concentration properties of the Fresnel mini-lenses operating with III–V triple-junction cells [131]. The lens profile optimization was carried out taking into account the refraction index of the lens material and its dependence on wavelength, focal distance, receiver diameter, sun illumination spectrum, and sensitivity spectra of the subcells in a multijunction cell.

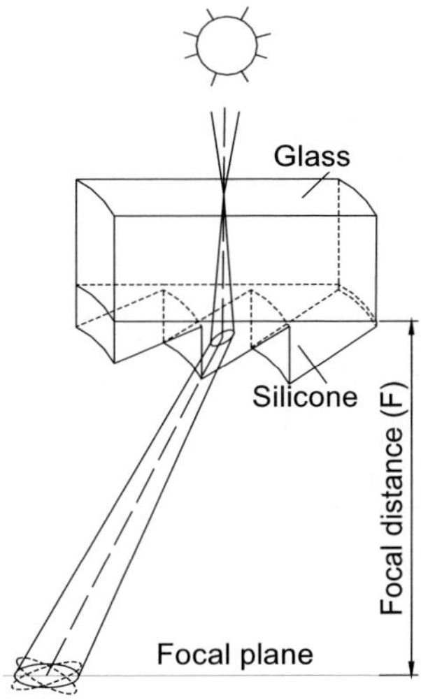

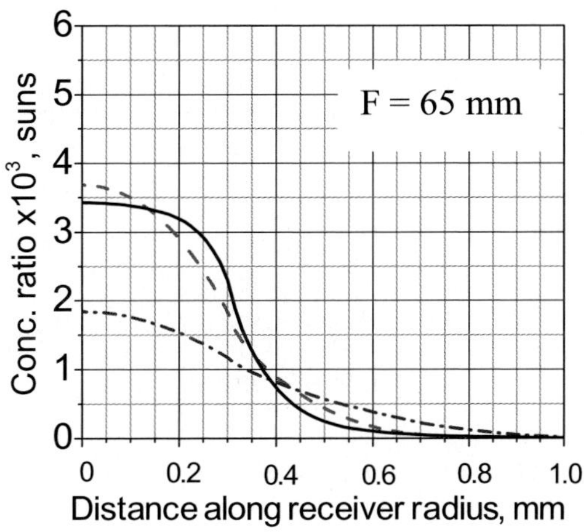

Fig. 8.23. Optical layout of a Fresnel lens fragment with a composite structure (*on the left*), and calculated light intensity distributions along the receiver diameter for spectral bands corresponding to three cascades in a triple-junction cell (*on the right*: *solid line* for top sub-cell; *dashed* and *dash-dotted lines* for middle and bottom sub-cells, respectively). Lens aperture area is $40 \times 40\,\text{mm}^2$ at focal distance F = 65 mm and groove pitch of 0.25 mm [131]

Lens structure consists of a sheet of silicate glass and refracting microprisms formed of transparent silicone on the inner side of the glass. The microprisms themselves are formed by polymerization of the silicone compound directly on the glass sheet with the use of a negatively profiled mold. The advantages of this concentrator technology are based on a high UV stability of silicone, its excellent resistance to thermal shocks and high/low temperatures, good adhesive properties in a stack with silicate glass, simplicity and very high accuracy of the formation method. Small mean thickness of the prisms ensures negligibly low absorption of the sunlight in comparison with Fresnel lenses made of bulk acrylic with a "regular" total thickness of about 3 mm.

Figure 8.23 shows the optical diagram of the Fresnel lens operation. Sunrays with divergence, corresponding to the sun disk size, are incident upon the lens surface. The overlap of the elliptical light spots from different parts of the lens forms distribution of light intensity along the focal plane. A receiver of diameter d can accept a certain part of light. This amount of light, divided by total amount of light, incident within lens aperture area and spectral range of receiver sensitivity, is defined as lens optical efficiency with respect to given receiver diameter.

Figure 8.23 (right) shows an example of light intensity distributions along the receiver radius for spectral bands corresponding to three cascades in a triple-junction cell. It is seen that a concentration ratio as high as 3,500 suns can occur in the receiver center. Averaged lens optical efficiencies versus receiver diameter for focal distances of F = 45, 65 and 85 mm are shown in Fig. 8.24 (on the left). It was

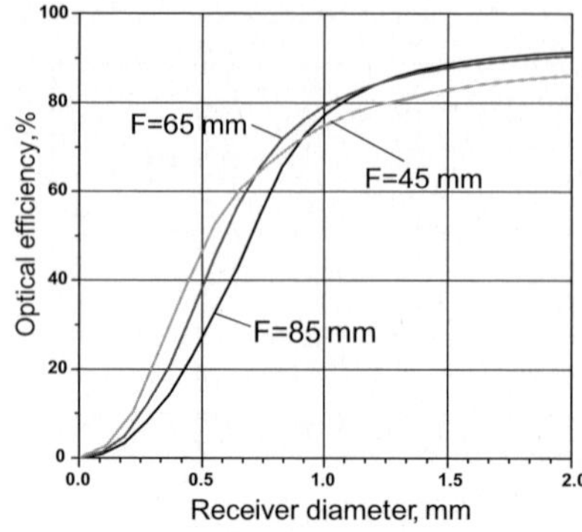

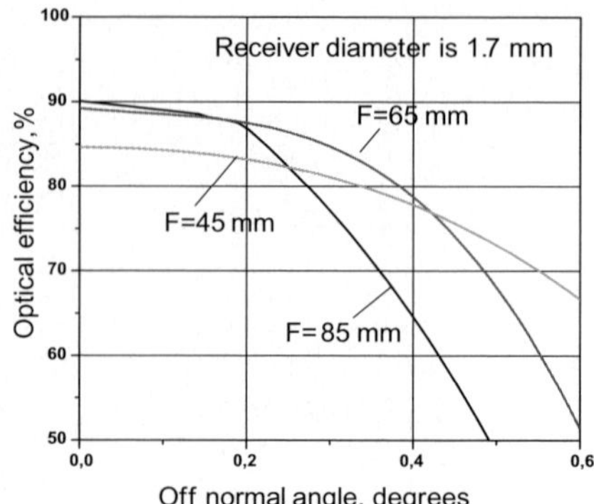

Fig. 8.24. Dependences of lens optical efficiency on receiver diameter at a normal angle of incidence (*on the left*) and those at off-normal angles for the case of 1.7 mm receiver diameter (*on the right*)

assumed in calculations that there exists a balance between photocurrents in the top and middle subcells, but an excess of photocurrent in the bottom subcell, as one can estimate from the cell photoresponse curves. Therefore, lens optical efficiency may be calculated only for top and middle subcells.

At real operation of the concentrator modules, the incidence angle of the sunrays upon the lens surface is under variation. Off-normal behavior of the concentrator systems with different focal distances, but alike receiver diameters of $d = 1.7\,\text{mm}$, is shown in Fig. 8.24 (on the right). One can see that the off-normal curve is wider for shorter focal distances, but an advantage in acceptance angle at $F = 45\,\text{mm}$ is revealed, when absolute optical efficiency is low enough – near 75%. In this case, the local concentration ratio in the center of the light spot is near 4,500 suns. In contrast, for the case of $F = 85\,\text{mm}$ concentration in the center is only 2,500 suns at the highest (among others) lens optical efficiency in the normal position. A narrower acceptance angle for lenses with long focal distance can be compensated by more accurate tracking to the sun.

A full-scale $50 \times 50\,\text{cm}^2$ module (see photograph in Fig. 8.22) includes a 144-lens panel and a corresponding quantity of properly mounted cells. The accuracy in positioning the cells is of great importance because each cell should be situated in the center of the focal spot of a corresponding lens. This accuracy has to be about $100\,\mu\text{m}$, which can be realized by using automatic processes and standard electronic industry machines. Two versions of the cell mounting are shown in Fig. 8.25.

On the left side of Fig. 8.25, flat copper plates 0.5 mm thick provide initial distribution of heat from a solar cell. In the case of the small-aperture area submodules, a very stable and cheap silicate glass may be used in a stack with a relatively thin heat sinking material (copper or steel). In spite of the low thermal conductivity of glass, waste heat can be dissipated to ambient air, as it occurs in regular flat-plate modules without concentration. Superior insulating properties of glass allow connecting the cells in an electric circuit of any configuration ensuring electrical safety of a mod-

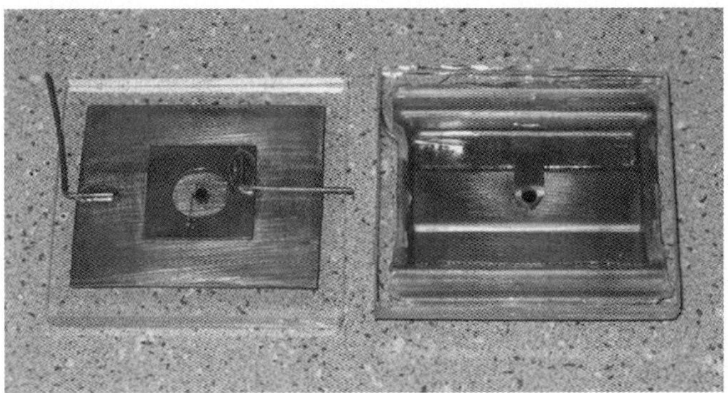

Fig. 8.25. Small-size ($2 \times 2\,\mathrm{mm}^2$) cells mounted by soldering to: flat copper plate (*left*) and trough-shaped copper plate (*right*). In the latter case, a heat-sinking trough with a string of cells can be placed behind a glass sheet

ule as a whole. Even walls of a module housing may be made of glass, justifying this approach as "all-glass" module design. On the left side of Fig. 8.25, the glass base plate also serves for hermetical sealing of the cells mounted on trough-like heat sinks. These troughs with strings of cells are glued on the outer side of the module cabinet behind the glass plate. Positioning of the troughs with mounted cells is not an elaborate procedure even when using manual fabrication techniques if a special template is applied. Hermetic sealing is provided for the thin air body inside the troughs, whereas the entire volume between the front and rear glass sheets of the module housing is connected with atmosphere. Special tubes are used to prevent dust from penetrating the module. The tubes are situated in diametrically opposite corners of module housing, thus providing an exit for condensed water. After affixing the troughs, connecting electrically the cell strings and assembling the module, the rear module side is coated with a hermetic sealing compound.

8.4.2 Outdoor Measurements of the Test Modules with Mini-lens Panels

Operational abilities of the modules of the "all-glass" design have been checked in respect to overall conversion efficiency by fabrication and outdoor measurements of test modules of reduced sizes [131]. The modules were equipped with GaInP/GaAs/Ge triple-junction cells produced by Spectrolab, Inc. In the module, described below, the cells were characterized by conversion efficiencies of 32–34% (AM 1.5d) at flash measurements with uniform distribution of incident light and the concentration ratio of about $1,000\times$.

In a module with an eight-lens panel (2×4 lenses) the cells of 2 mm in diameter were used, being connected in parallel. The sealed module was installed on a sun-tracking system. After the outdoor I–V measurement, the module was characterized indoors using a large-area flash solar tester [128] to compare corresponding results for outdoor and indoor measurements (Fig. 8.26).

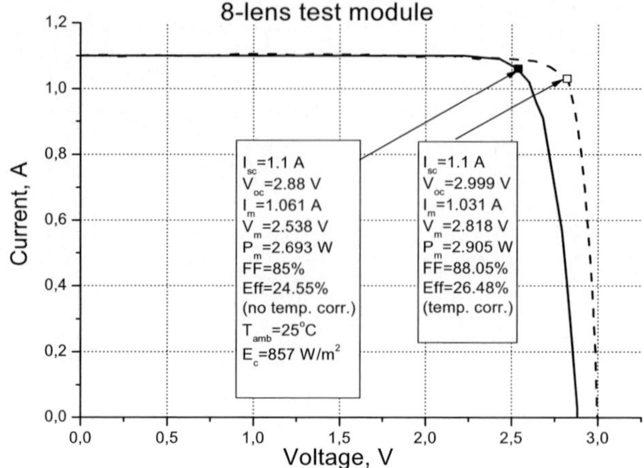

Fig. 8.26. I–V curves measured on the eight-lens test module outdoors (St. Petersburg, June 16, 2006, 16 h. 43 m., ambient $T = 25\,°C$, *solid line*) and indoors by a flash solar tester (*dashed line*). Cell temperature is about $50\,°C$ outdoors and $25\,°C$ indoors

Overall module conversion efficiency as high as 26.5% was measured at typical cell temperature of $25\,°C$ in the indoor test. It should be noted that actual outdoor efficiency for modules could exceed 28% at lower ambient temperature, or with the use of the cells with indoor efficiencies in the range of 39–40%. Applying antireflection coatings on optical elements of such a module can help to increase the overall module efficiency up to 30–32%.

Solar PV modules with small-aperture area concentrators are compact, simple in structure and are characterized by lower material consumption in comparison with previous module designs. They ensure an "ideal" situation for the conversion of sun power, when a high optical concentration of sunlight is performed, but the distributed character of heat dissipation persists, inherent in the flat-plate photovoltaic modules without concentrators.

8.5 Perspectives of the Efficiency Increase in III–V Solar Cells

Figure 8.27 demonstrates the dynamics of the efficiency increase for III–V solar cells, single-crystal Si as well as thin-film Si solar cells during the last 50 years. Further, expected efficiency increase is shown by dashed curves. It is seen that efficiencies of the cells, based on thin-film and crystalline silicon ("one-sun" and concentrator cells) have almost reached their limit. The thin-film approach is the promising way to reduce the cost of solar electricity. Concentrator III–V arrays open the same opportunity due to the possibility of realizing a cost lower than that of crystalline Si arrays at module efficiencies higher than 30%.

The experience to date in the development of the triple-junction solar cells gives us reason to hope for achieving higher efficiency in four-, five- and, maybe, even

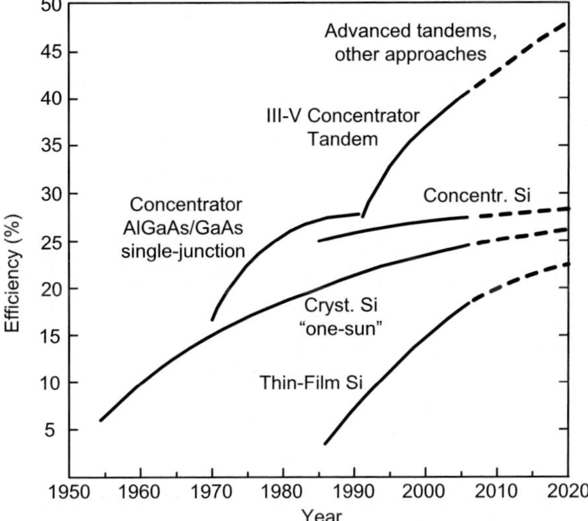

Fig. 8.27. Evolutions of achieved efficiencies till 2006 and predicted efficiencies of different types of solar cells (illumination under AM1.5 solar spectrum conditions)

more-junction structures. There are no scientific or theoretical doubts that these hopes will be justified when appropriate quality materials for intermediate cascades are found and grown. The search for these structures is under way, and several areas may be singled out. To increase the quantity of p–n junctions in MJ cells, the cost of such structures does not increase, because the total structure thickness remains the same owing to the possibility of reducing layer thickness in each cascade absorbing and converting a "narrower" part of the solar spectrum.

Complexity of the solar cell structures, namely, the multijunction structures, reduces the requirements for the bulk properties of the materials used. Indeed, the larger the number of junctions, the thinner the photoactive region in each junction and the weaker the effect of such a parameter as the minority carrier diffusion length on the efficiency of the device. The method for compensating insufficiently good bulk properties of a material by technological perfection of the multijunction cells has also begun to be used in the development of new types of thin-film solar arrays.

Solar thermophotovoltaics (TPV) [132, 133] is based on the principle of intermediate conversion of highly concentrated sunlight into radiation of a selective emitter heated up to 1200–1800 °C. At the second stage, photovoltaic conversion of this radiation occurs in a low-bandgap ($E_g = 0.5$–0.8 eV) photocell. Significant reserves for the increase in solar TPV efficiency lie in possibilities for the back effect of a photoconverter on radiation source (emitter of photons): the nonused photons can be reflected back to the radiator keeping it hot. Such a possibility is completely absent in current solar power systems. Therefore, the TPV generator is a complex system which should be more effective, if the principle of radiation recirculation is involved. A promising way for TPV converter efficiency to increase is the devel-

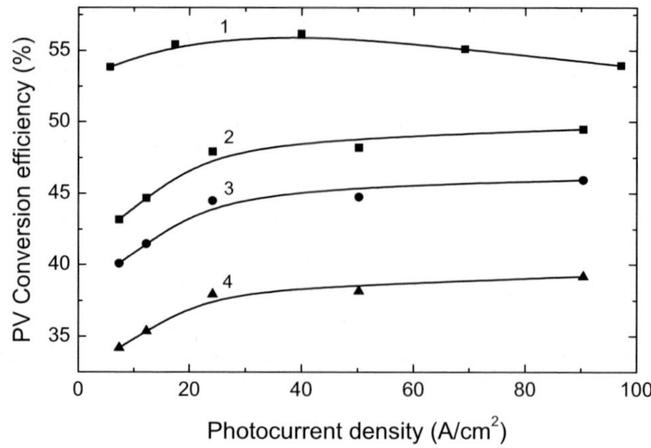

Fig. 8.28. Conversion efficiencies of GaAs (curve *1*) and GaSb (curves *2–4*) PV cells (designated illumination area is about $2\,\text{mm}^2$) as a function of the photocurrent density at monochromatic irradiation with wavelengths: *1* – 850 nm, *2* – 1680 nm, *3* – 1550 nm, *4* – 1315 nm

opment of selective emitters matched to PV cells. Such a selective emitter should radiate intensively at $h\nu > E_{\text{g}}$ and weakly at longer wavelengths. A similar role is played by an optical filter. This component is usefully included in a TPV system to return subbandgap-energy photons back to the emitter. It can be made as a dielectric stack (deposited on the cell or emitter surface, or arranged as a separate component), or as a metallic reflector on the rear surface of the cells. In other words, combining the filters, metal reflectors on the cell back and selective emitters, one has considerable room to shape the energy spectrum accepted by a cell. Theoretical conversion efficiency of the TPV approach is 84.5% and expected in practice is about 40%.

The possibility of high-efficiency PV conversion of selective radiation has been confirmed by experiments with PV conversion of the monochromatic radiation with the photon energy just a little higher than the cell band gap [134]. An efficiency of 56% was measured in GaAs-based cells under monochromatic illumination with wavelength of 850 nm, and efficiency of 49% was detected in a GaSb cell at $\lambda = 1680$ nm (Fig. 8.28).

Photocells with a graded bandgap in the photoactive region give additional possibilities for efficiency increase at a high excitation level, where the quantity of generated electron–hole pairs is higher than quantity of majority carriers. If a cell heterostructure has a gradient of the bandgap (ΔE_{g}) with a decrease in E_{g} from the front surface, the additional voltage arises owing to separation of electrons and holes, generated by photons of different energies in the different parts of the graded bandgap layer. In the case of a very high excitation level, the value of this additional voltage can be close to $\Delta E_{\text{g}}/q$ [135]. The theoretical efficiency limit in this approach is the same as for the infinite tandem cell stack. However, to use this effect, new semiconductor materials with special properties should be developed. Low-dimensional quantum well/dot structures open the door to preparation of such materials and cells. Short-period superlattices were grown by MBE for fabrication of the graded band gap layers in the laser structures [136]. Excellent heterointerface smoothness has been obtained, resulting in high internal quantum efficiency of radiation recombination. The low threshold current in these lasers was the world record for a long time and served as a good demonstration of the superlattice application for fabrication of graded bandgap layers of high quality.

Hot carrier cells should use the energy of photogenerated carries before their thermalization and collection by a p–n junction. The efficiency limit in this approach is the same as that for tandem cells. However, to realize this approach, carrier cooling rates should be reduced sufficiently, or radiative recombination rates should be sufficiently accelerated. Thus, special materials with particular band structures should be developed for these cells.

Multiple electron–hole pair cells with quantum efficiency higher than unity also allow for increase in efficiency. The theoretical efficiency for an idealized cell of such a type is the same as for the infinite tandem cell stack. Several electron–hole pairs should be generated by each incident photon in this case. The higher-than-one quantum efficiency behavior was actually found, although very close to one, for high-energy visible photons and for UV photons. However, competitive processes of the carrier energy relaxation are too efficient, which have not allowed for noticeable improvement in solar cell performance until now.

Analyzing current trends in physics of semiconductors, for instance, progress in the development of third-generation injection lasers, one finds primarily wider use of the quantum dot (QD) heterostructures [137]. A new approach involving the use of materials with QDs has been proposed for solar cell development as well: the creation of an photoactive medium with an "intermediate band" [138]. A semiconductor material for such cells should have an intermediate half-filled (or metallic) band close to the center of the forbidden gap. In addition to the conventional abandoning electrons from the valence to the conduction band by absorption of high-energy photons, abandoning to/from intermediate band to the conduction band can be realized by absorption of low energy photons. This three-photon effect ensures a better utilization of the sunlight energy. Voltage degradation is expected to be prevented by the existence of three separated quasi-Fermi levels, each one related to every existing band. The maximum efficiency of 63% was calculated for a cell with the bandgap of 1.95 eV and intermediate band Fermi level located at 0.71 eV from one of the bands. The generalization of this concept to more than two intermediate bandgaps (multiband solar cells) gives maximum theoretical efficiency as high as 86.8%, which is identical to the efficiency of a large stack of tandem cells. Low-dimensional structures can constitute a way for engineering the intermediate band concept. In addition, quantum mechanical calculations have shown that, in principle, it is possible to arrange atoms of a bulk material in such a way that it can exhibit the required intermediate band.

8.6 Conclusion

At present, III–V heterostructure solar cells are already widely used for space applications. Progress in terrestrial applications of III–V solar cells is associated with the development of cells with efficiencies exceeding 45% at the concentrated sunlight. These devices can form a technical basis for large-scale solar power engineering in the future. In this case, a considerable amount of electrical energy supplying our homes will be generated by heterostructure solar cells illuminated by the sun through the concentrators.

There are legends to the effect that, in the antique times, priests used concentrated sunlight during ritual ceremonies for setting the Holy Fire in temples. From that arose the traditional way to set the Olympic Fire. Historically, the first utilitarian use of concentrated sunlight took place for military purposes: Grecians, on Archimedes' initiative, set fire to the ships of Romans who besieged Syracuse in 212 B.C. The Grecian soldiers directed the sunbeams toward the targets using a great number of polished metallic shields. Only in recent history have people again turned to the idea of the practical application of concentrated sunlight, creating solar furnaces for highly refractory materials, as well as solar power plants with steam cycles. It might be well to point out that the direct conversion of concentrated sunlight into electric power by means of highly efficient cascade solar cells is, as we have seen from the above, one of the main ways for satisfying the power demands of the mankind. It is significant that at present there is no particular application of this technology for creating weapons – now, and also in the foreseeable future. Hence, development, harnessing and fostering widespread use of the technology are not burdened by additional risks for humanity. Quite the contrary, this will aid in reducing the presently discussed greenhouse effects.

There are other alternative, yet also promising technologies for future power generation. For example, one could use atomic energy. At the very beginning, this technology was intended to create a new type of weapon. This was soon realized with the creation of bombs with unprecedented destructive power. The military aspect of this technology remains quite actual and, for many, attractive. And this precarious situation persists today, although atomic power plants were also built during a very short period of time. Thus, hopes have arisen of creating an inexhaustible power source using thermonuclear reactions. If the risks associated with plausible catastrophes on atomic plants, and the problems of the radioactive waste burial, are added to the risk of nuclear weapon proliferation, the public anxieties connected with atomic technology development become understandable.

On the other hand, a generalized situation with energy could be outlined in the following way. Why build many dangerous nuclear reactors on our planet Earth if there already exists a huge, safe and inexhaustible reactor – the sun – which sends an abundance of power to the Earth in the form of sunlight? Our task rests "only" on the reasonable and effective use of this power.

References

1. W. Shockley, Circuit Element Utilizing Semiconductor Material. U.S. Patent 2269347, September 25, 1951
2. A.I. Gubanov, Theory of the contact between two semiconductors with different types of conduction. Zh. Tekh. Fiz. **20**, 1287 (1950)
3. H. Kroemer, Theory of a wide-gap emitter for transistors. Proc. IRE **45**, 1535 (1957)
4. Z.I. Alferov, The double heterostructure: concept and its applications in physics, electronics and technology. Les prix Nobel, Norstedts Tryckeri, Stockholm, 2001, pp. 65–93
5. H. Kroemer, A proposed class of heterojunction injection lasers. Proc. IEEE **51**, 1782 (1963)
6. Z.I. Alferov, V.B. Khalfin, R.F. Kazarinov, A characteristic feature of injection into heterojunctions. Fiz. Tverd. Tela **8**, 3102–3105 (1966) [Sov. Phys. Solid State **8**, 2480 (1967)]
7. Z.I. Alferov, Possible development of a rectifier for very high current densities on the bases of a p–i–n (p–n–n$^+$, n–p–p$^+$) structure with heterojunctions. Fiz. Tekh. Poluprovodn. **1**, 436–438 (1966) [Sov. Phys. Semicond. **1**, 358–361 (1967)]
8. R.L. Anderson, Germanium-gallium arsenide heterojunctions. IBM J. Res. Develop. **4**, 283 (1960)
9. Z.I. Alferov, V.M. Andreev, V.I. Korol'kov, D.N. Tret'yakov, V.M. Tuchkevich, High-voltage p–n junctions in Ga$_x$Al$_{1-x}$As crystals. Fiz. Tekh. Poluprovodn. **1**, 1579–1581 (1967) [Sov. Phys. Semicond. **1**, 1313–1314 (1968)]
10. H.S. Rupprecht, J.M. Woodall, G.D. Pettit, Efficient visible electroluminescence at 300 K from Ga$_{1-x}$Al$_x$As p–n junctions grown by liquid-phase epitaxy. Appl. Phys. Lett. **11**, 81 (1967)
11. Z.I. Alferov, V.M. Andreev, V.I. Korol'kov, E.L. Portnoi, D.N. Tret'yakov, Injection properties of n–Al$_x$Ga$_{1-x}$As-p-GaAs heterojunctions. Fiz. Tekh. Poluprovodn. **2**, 1016–1017 (1968) [Sov. Phys. Semicond. **2**, 843–844 (1969)]
12. Z.I. Alferov, V.M. Andreev, V.I. Korol'kov, E.L. Portnoy, D.N. Tret'yakov, Coherent radiation of epitaxial heterojunction structures in the AlAs–GaAs system. Fiz. Tekh. Poluprovodn. **2**, 1545–1547 (1968) [Sov. Phys. Semicond. **2**, 1289–1291 (1969)]
13. Z.I. Alferov, V.M. Andreev, V.I. Korol'kov, E.L. Portnoi, D.N. Tret'yakov, Recombination radiation in epitaxial structures in the AlAs–GaAs system, in *Proc. IX Int. Conf. on the Physics of Semiconductors*, Moscow, 1968, 1 (Nauka, Leningrad, 1968), pp. 504–510
14. Z.I. Alferov, V.M. Andreev, E.L. Portnoy, M.K. Trukan, AlAs–GaAs heterojunctions injection lasers with a low room-temperature threshold. Fiz. Tekh. Poluprovodn. **3**, 1328–1332 (1969) [Sov. Phys. Semicond. **3**, 1107–1110 (1970)]
15. I. Hayashi, Heterostructure lasers. IEEE Trans. Electron Devices **ED-31**, 1630–1645 (1984)
16. Z.I. Alferov, V.M. Andreev, D.Z. Garbuzov, Y.V. Zhilyaev, E.P. Morozov, E.L. Portnoi, V.G. Trofim, Investigation of the influence of the AlAs–GaAs heterostructure parameters on the laser threshold current and the realization of continuous emission at the room temperature. Fiz. Tekh. Poluprovodn. **4**, 1826–1829 (1970) [Sov. Phys. Semicond. **4**, 1573–1575 (1971)]
17. I. Hayashi, M.B. Panish, P.W. Foy, S. Sumski, Junction lasers which operate continuously at room temperature. Appl. Phys. Lett. **17**, 109–111 (1970)

18. Z.I. Alferov, V.M. Andreev, V.I. Korol'kov, E.L. Portnoi, A.A. Yakovenko, Spontaneous radiation sources based on structures with AlAs–GaAs heterojunctions. Fiz. Tekh. Poluprovodn. **3**, 930–933 (1969) [Sov. Phys. Semicond. **3**, 785–787 (1970)]

19. Z.I. Alferov, V.M. Andreev, M.B. Kagan, I.I. Protasov, V.G. Trofim, Solar-energy converters based on p–n $Al_x Ga_{1-x}$As–GaAs heterojunctions. Fiz. Tekh. Poluprovodn. **4**, 2378–2379 (1970) [Sov. Phys. Semicond. **4**, 2047–2048 (1971)]

20. Z.I. Alferov, F.A. Ahmedov, V.I. Korol'kov, V.G. Nikitin, Phototransistor utilizing a GaAs–AlAs heterojunction. Fiz. Tekn. Poluprovodn. **7**, 1159–1163 (1973) [Sov. Phys. Semicond. **7**, 780–782 (1973)]

21. Z.I. Alferov, V.M. Andreev, V.I. Korol'kov, V.G. Nikitin, A.A. Yakovenko, p–n–p–n structures based on GaAs and on $Al_x Ga_{1-x}$As solid solutions. Fiz. Tekn. Poluprovodn. **4**, 578–581 (1970) [Sov. Phys. Semicond. **4**, 481–483 (1971)]

22. Z.I. Alferov, V.M. Andreev, S.G. Konnikov, V.G. Nikitin, D.N. Tret'yakov, Heterojunctions on the base of III–V semiconducting and of their solid solutions, in *Proc. Int. Conf. Phys. Chem. Semicond. Heterojunctions and Layer Structures*, Budapest, 1970, 1, ed. by G. Szigeti (Academiai Kiado, Budapest, 1971), pp. 93–106

23. G.A. Antipas, R.L. Moon, L.W. James, J. Edgecumbe, R.L. Bell, In Gallium Arsenide and Related Compounds. Conf. Ser. IOP **17**, 48 (1973)

24. A.P. Bogatov, L.M. Dolginov, L.V. Druzhinina, P.G. Eliseev, L.N. Sverdlova, E.G. Shevchenko, Heterolasers on the base of solid solutions $Ga_x In_{1-x}As_y P_{1-y}$ and $Al_x Ga_{1-x}Sb_y As_{1-y}$. Kvantovaya Electron. **1**, 2294 (1974) [Sov. J. Quantum Electron **1**, 1281 (1974)]

25. Z.I. Alferov, I.N. Arsent'ev, D.Z. Garbuzov, S.G. Konnikov, V.D. Rumyantsev, Generation of coherent radiation in $pGa_{0.5}In_{0.5}P$–$pGa_{x\sim 0.55}In_{1-x}As_{y\sim 0.10}P_{1-y}$–$nGa_{0.5}In_{0.5}P$. Pisma Zh. Tech. Fiz. **1**, 305–310 (1975) [Sov. Phys. Tech. Phys. Lett. **1**, 147–148 (1975)]

26. D. Flood, H. Brandhorst, Space solar cells, in *Current Topics in Photovoltaics,* vol. 2, ed. by T.J. Coutts, J.D. Meakin (Academic, New York, 1987), pp. 143–202

27. S.G. Bailey, D.J. Flood, Space Photovoltaics. Prog. Photovolt.: Res. Appl. **6**(1), 1–14 (1998)

28. V.M. Andreev, V.A. Grilikhes, V.D. Rumyantsev, *Photovoltaic Conversion of Concentrated Sunlight* (Wiley, New York, 1997)

29. H.J. Hovel, J.M. Woodall, High-efficiency AlGaAs–GaAs solar cells. Appl. Phys. Lett. **21**, 379–381 (1972)

30. V.M. Andreev, T.M. Golovner, M.B. Kagan, N.S. Koroleva, T.A. Lubochevskaya, T.A. Nuller, D.N. Tret'yakov, Investigation of high efficiency AlGaAs–GaAs solar cells. Sov. Phys. Semicond. **7**(12) (1973)

31. Z.I. Alferov, V.M. Andreev, G.S. Daletskii, M.B. Kagan, N.S. Lidorenko, V.M. Tuchkevich, Investigation of high efficiency AlAs–GaAs heteroconverters, in *Proc. World Electrotechn. Congress*, Moscow, 1977, Section 5A, report 04

32. H.J. Hovel, *Semiconductors and Semimetals*, ed. by Willardson, R.K., Beer, A.C. Solar Cells, vol. 11 (Academic, New York, 1975)

33. V.M. Andreev, III–V heterostructure photovoltaics in Russia, in *Proceedings of 17th European Photovoltaic Solar Energy Conference*, 2000, pp. xxxi–xxxii

34. J.M. Woodall, H.J. Hovel, An isothermal etchback-regrowth method for high efficiency $Ga_{1-x}Al_x$As–GaAs solar cells. Appl. Phys. Lett. **30**, 492–493 (1977)

35. V.M. Andreev, V.R. Larionov, V.D. Rumyantsev, O.M. Fedorova, S.S. Shamukhamedov, P AlGaAs–pGaAs–nGaAs solar cells with efficiencies of 19% at AM0 and 24% at AM1.5. Sov. Tech. Phys. Lett. **9**(10), 537–538 (1983)

36. H.J. Hovel, Novel materials and devices for sunlight concentrating systems. IBM J. Res. Dev. **22**, 112–121 (1978)
37. E. Fanetti, C. Flores, G. Guarini, F. Paletta, D. Passoni, High efficiency 1.43 and 1.69 eV band gap $Ga_{1-x}\,Al_x\,As$–GaAs solar cells for multicolor applications. Solar cells **3**, 187–194 (1981)
38. R.C. Knechtly, R.Y. Loo, G.S. Kamath, High-efficiency GaAs solar cells. IEEE Trans. Electron Dev. **ED-31**(5), 577–588 (1984)
39. H.S. Rauschenbach, *Solar Cell array Design Handbook. The Principles and Technology of Photovoltaic Energy Conversion* (Litton Educational Publishing, New York, 1980)
40. A. Luque, *Solar Cells and Optics for Photovoltaic Concentration* (Adam Hilger, Bristol, 1989)
41. L.D. Partain (ed.), *Solar Cells and Their Application* (Wiley, New York, 1995)
42. P.A. Iles, Future of photovoltaic for space applications. Prog. Photovolt.: Res. Appl. **8**, 39–51 (2000)
43. V.M. Andreev, A.B. Kazantsev, V.P. Khvostikov, E.V. Paleeva, V.D. Rumyantsev, M.Z. Shvarts, High-efficiency (24.6%, AM0) LPE grown AlGaAs/GaAs concentrator solar cells and modules, in *Conf. Record First World Conference on Photovoltaic Energy Conversion*, 1994, pp. 2096–2099
44. V.M. Andreev, V.D. Rumyantsev, A^3B^5 based solar cells and concentrating optical elements for space PV modules. Solar Energy Mater. Solar Cells **44**, 319–332 (1996)
45. R.D. Dupuis, P.D. Dapkus, R.D. Vingling, L.A. Moundy, High-efficiency GaAlAs/GaAs heterostructure solar cells grown by metalorganic chemical vapor deposition. Appl. Phys. Lett. **31**, 201–203 (1977)
46. N.J. Nelson, K.K. Jonson, R.L. Moon, H.A. Vander Plas, L.W. James, Organometallic-sourced VPE AlGaAs/GaAs concentrator solar cells having conversion efficiencies of 19%. Appl. Phys. Lett. **33**, 26–27 (1978)
47. J.G. Werthen, G.F. Virshup, C.W. Ford, C.R. Lewis, H.C. Hamaker, 21% (one sun, air mass zero) 4 cm^2 GaAs space solar cells. Appl. Phys. Lett. **48**, 74–75 (1986)
48. S.P. Tobin, S.M. Vernon, S.J. Woitczuk, C. Baigar, M.M. Sanfacon, T.M. Dixon, Advanced in high-efficiency GaAs solar cells, in *Conf. Record 21st IEEE Photovoltaic Specialists Conference*, 1990, pp. 158–162
49. S.P. Tobin, S.M. Vernon, M.M. Sanfacon, A. Mastrovito, Enhanced light absorption in GaAs solar cells with internal Bragg reflector, in *Conf. Record 22nd IEEE Photovoltaic Spesialists Conference*, 1991, pp. 147–152
50. V.M. Andreev, V.V. Komin, I.V. Kochnev, V.M. Lantratov, M.Z. Shvarts, High-efficiency AlGaAs–GaAs solar cells with internal Bragg reflector, in *Conf. Record First World Conference on Photovoltaic Energy Conversion*, 1994, pp. 1894–1897
51. M.Z. Shvarts, O.I. Chosta, I.V. Kochnev, V.M. Lantratov, V.M. Andreev, Radiation resistant AlGaAs/GaAs concentrator solar cells with internal Bragg reflector. Solar Energy Mater. Solar Cells **68**, 105–122 (2001)
52. M. Yamaguchi, Space solar cell R&D activities in Japan, in *Proceeding 15th Space Photovoltaic Research and Technology*, 1997, pp. 1–10
53. C.C. Fan, B.-Y. Tsaur, B.J. Palm, Optimal design of high-efficiency tandem cells, in *Conf. Record 16th IEEE Photovoltaic Specialists Conf.*, 1982, pp. 692–698
54. M.A. Green, *Solar Cells* (Prentice-Hall, New Jersey, 1982)
55. M.F. Lamorte, D.H. Abbott, Computer modeling of a two-junction, monolithic cascade solar cell. IEEE Trans. Electron. Dev. **ED-27**, 231–249 (1980)
56. M.B. Spitzer, C.C. Fan, Multijunction cells for space applications. Solar Cells **29**, 183–203 (1990)

57. L.M. Fraas, High-efficiency III–V multijunction solar cells, in *Solar Cells and Their Applications*, ed. by L.D. Partain (Wiley, New York, 1995), pp. 143–162
58. R.K. Jain, D.J. Flood, Monolithic and mechanical multijunction space solar cells. J. Solar Energy Eng. **115**, 106–111 (1993)
59. L.M. Fraas, J.E. Avery, J. Martin, V.S. Sundaram, G. Giard, V.T. Dinh, T.M. Davenport, J.W. Yerkes, M.J. O'Neil, Over 35-percent efficient GaAs/GaSb tandem solar cells. IEEE Trans. Electron. Dev. **37**, 443–449 (1990)
60. S.R. Kurtz, D. Myers, J.M. Olson, Projected performance of three- and four-junction devices using GaAs and GaInP, in *Proc. 26th IEEE Photovoltaic Specialists Conf.*, 1997, pp. 875–878
61. M. Yamaguchi, Multi-junction solar cells: present and future, in *Technical Digest 12th International Photovoltaic Solar Energy Conference*, 2001, pp. 291–294
62. A.W. Bett, F. Dimroth, G. Stollwerk, O.V. Sulima, III–V compounds for solar cell applications. Appl. Phys. **A69**, 119–129 (1999)
63. M. Yamaguchi, A. Luque, High efficiency and high concentration in photovoltaics. IEEE Trans. Electron Devices **46**(10), 41–46 (1999)
64. M.W. Wanlass, J.S. Ward, K.A. Emery, T.A. Gessert, C.R. Osterwald, T.J. Coutts, High performance concentrator tandem solar cells based on IR-sensitive bottom cells. Solar Cells **30**, 363–371 (1991)
65. V.M. Andreev, L.B. Karlina, A.B. Kazantsev, V.P. Khvostikov, V.D. Rumyantsev, S.V. Sorokina, M.Z. Shvarts, Concentrator tandem solar cells based on AlGaAs/GaAs–InP/InGaAs (or GaSb) structures, in *Conf. Record First World Conference on Photovoltaic Energy Conversion*, 1994, pp. 1721–1724
66. V.M. Andreev, V.P. Khvostikov, E.V. Paleeva, V.D. Rumyantsev, S.V. Sorokina, M.Z. Shvarts, V.I. Vasil'ev, Tandem solar cells based on AlGaAs/GaAs and GaSb structures, in *Proc. 23d International Symposium on Compound Semiconductors*, 1996, pp. 425–428
67. V.M. Andreev, R&D of III–V compound solar cells in Russia, in *Technical Digest of 11th International Photovoltaic Solar Energy Conference*, 1999, pp. 589–592
68. M. Umeno, T. Kato, M. Yang, Y. Azuma, T. Soga, T. Jimbo, High efficiency AlGaAs/Si tandem solar cell over 20%, in *Conf. Record First World Conference on Photovoltaic Energy Conversion*, 1994, pp. 1679–1684
69. B.-C. Chung, G.F. Virshup, M. Ladle Ristow, M.W. Wanlass, 25.2%-efficiency (1-sun, air mass 0) AlGaAs/GaAs/InGaAsP three-junction, two-terminal solar cells, in *Conf. Record 22nd IEEE Photovoltaic Specialists Conference*, 1991, pp. 54–57
70. V.M. Andreev, V.P. Khvostikov, V.D. Rumyantsev, E.V. Paleeva, M.Z. Shvarts, Monolithic two-junction AlGaAs/GaAs solar cells, in *Proc. 26th IEEE Photovoltaic Specialists Conference*, 1997, pp. 927–930
71. M.L. Timmons, J.A. Hutchley, D.K. Wagner, J.M. Tracy, Monolithic AlGaAs/Ge cascade cell, in *Proc. of 21st IEEE Photovoltaic Specialists Conference*, 1988, pp. 602–606
72. S.P. Tobin, S.M. Vernon, C. Bajgar, V.E. Haven, L.M. Geoffroy, M.M. Sanfacon, D.R. Lillington, R.E. Hart, K.A. Emery, R.L. Matson, High efficiency GaAs/Ge monolithic tandem solar cells, in *Proc. 20th IEEE Photovoltaic Specialists Conference*, 1988, pp. 405–410
73. P.A. Iles, Y.-C.M. Yeh, F.N. Ho, C.L. Chu, C. Cheng, High-efficiency (>20% AM0) GaAs solar cells grown on inactive Ge substrates. IEEE Electron Device Lett. **11**(4), 140–142 (1990)

74. S. Wojtczuk, S. Tobin, M. Sanfacon, V. Haven, L. Geoffroy, S. Vernon, Monolithic two-terminal GaAs/Ge tandem space concentrator cells, in *22nd IEEE Photovoltaic Specialists Conference*, 1991, pp. 73–79
75. P.A. Iles, Y.-C.M. Yeh, Silicon, gallium arsenide and indium phosphide cells: single junction, one sun space, in *Solar Cells and Their Applications*, ed. by L.D. Partain (Wiley, New York, 1995), pp. 99–121
76. J.M. Olson, S.R. Kurtz, A.E. Kibbler, P. Faine, Recent advances in high efficiency GaInP$_2$/GaAs tandem solar cells, in *Proc. 21st IEEE Photovoltaic Specialists Conference*, 1990, pp. 24–29
77. K.A. Bertness, S.R. Kurtz, D.J. Friedman, A.E. Kibbler, C. Kramer, J.M. Olson, High-efficiency GaInP/GaAs tandem solar cells for space and terrestrial applications, in *Conf. Record First World Conference on Photovoltaic Energy Conversion*, 1994, pp. 1671–1678
78. P.K. Chiang, D.D. Krut, B.T. Cavicchi, K.A. Bertness, S.R. Kurtz, J.M. Olson, Large area GaInP/GaAs/Ge multijunction solar cells for space application, in *Conf. Record First World Conference on Photovoltaic Energy Conversion*, 1994, pp. 2120–2123
79. P.K. Chiang, J.H. Ermer, W.T. Niskikawa, D.D. Krut, D.E. Joslin, J.W. Eldredge, B.T. Cavicchi, Experimental results of GaInP$_2$/GaAs/Ge triple junction cell development for space power systems, in *Conf. Record 25th IEEE Photovoltaic Specialists Conference*, 1996, pp. 183–186
80. R.R. King, N.H. Karam, J.H. Ermer, M. Haddad, P. Colter, T. Isshiki, H. Yoon, H.L. Cotal, D.E. Joslin, D.D. Krut, R. Sudharsanan, K. Edmondson, B.T. Cavicchi, D.R. Lillington, Next-generation, high-efficiency III–V multijunction solar cells, in *Proceedings of 28th IEEE Photovoltaic Specialists Conference*, 2000, pp. 998–1005
81. R.R. King, C.M. Fetzer, P.C. Colter, K.M. Edmondson, J.H. Ermer, H.L. Cotal, H. Yoon, A.P. Stavrides, G. Kinsey, D.D. Krut, N.H. Karam, High-efficiency space and terrestrial multijunction solar cells trough bandgap control in cell structures, in *Proc. 29th IEEE Photovoltaic Specialists Conference*, 2002, pp. 776–779
82. R.R. King, R.A. Sherif, D.C. Law, J.T. Yen, M. Haddad, C.M. Fetzer, K.M. Edmondson, G. Kinsey, H. Yoon, M. Joshi, S. Mesropian, New horizons in III–V multijunction terrestrial concentrator cells research, in *Proceedings of 21st European Photovoltaic Solar Energy Conference*, Dresden, 2006, pp. 124–128
83. P.K. Chiang, C.L. Chu, Y.C.M. Yeh, P. Iles, G. Chen, J. Wei, P. Tsung, J. Olbinski, J. Krogen, S. Halbe, S. Khemthong, Achieving 26% triple junction cascade solar cell production, in *Proc. 28th IEEE Photovoltaic Specialists Conference*, 2000, pp. 1002–1005
84. H.Q. Hou, P.R. Sharps, N.S. Fatemi, N. Li, M.A. Stan, P.A. Martin, B.E. Hammons, F. Spadafora, Very high efficiency InGaP/GaAs dual-junction solar cell manufacturing at Emcore Photovoltaics, in *Proc. 28th IEEE Photovoltaic Specialists Conference*, 2000, pp. 1173–1176
85. A.W. Bett, F. Dimroth, G. Lange, M. Meusel, R. Beckert, M. Hein, S.V. Riesen, U. Schubert, 30% monolithic tandem concentrator solar cells for concentrations exceeding 1000 suns, in *Proc. 28th IEEE Photovoltaic Specialists Conference*, 2000, pp. 961–964
86. F. Dimroth, U. Schubert, A.W. Bett, J. Hilgarth, M. Nell, G. Strobl, K. Bogus, C. Signorini, Next generation GaInP/GaInAs/Ge multijunction space solar cells, in *Proc. 17th European Photovoltaic Specialists Conference*, 2001, pp. 2150–2154
87. R.R. King, M. Haddad, T. Isshiki, P. Colter, J. Ermer, H. Yoon, D.E. Joslin, N.H. Karam, Metamorphic GaInP/GaInAs/Ge solar cells, in *Proc. 28th IEEE Photovoltaic Specialists Conference*, 2000, pp. 982–985

138   Z.I. Alferov et al.

88. M.A. Green, K. Emery, D.L. King, Y. Nishikawa, W. Warta, Solar cell efficiency tables (version 29). Prog. Photovolt.: Res. Appl. **15**, 35–40 (2007)
89. V.M. Andreev, A.B. Kazantsev, V.P. Khvostikov, E.V. Paleeva, V.D. Rumyantsev, M.Z. Shvarts, High-efficiency (24.6%, AM0) LPE grown AlGaAs/GaAs concentrator solar cells and modules, in *Proceedings of 1st World Conference on Photovoltaic Energy Conversion*, Hawaii, 1994, pp. 2096–2099
90. S.G. Bailey, D.J. Flood, Space photovoltaics. Prog. Photovolt.: Res. Appl. **6**, 1–14 (1998)
91. C. Algora, E. Ortiz, I. Rey-Stolle, V. Diaz, P. Pena, V.M. Andreev, V.P. Khvostikov, V.D. Rumyantsev, A GaAs solar cell with efficiency of 26.2% at 1000 suns and 25.0% at 2000 suns. IEEE Trans. Electron Devices **48**(5), 840–844 (2001)
92. V.M. Andreev, V.P. Khvostikov, V.R. Larionov, V.D. Rumyantsev, E.V. Paleeva, M.Z. Shvarts, C. Algora, 5800 Suns AlGaAs/GaAs concentrator solar cells, in *Technical Digest of the International Photovoltaic Science and Engineering Conference*, Sapporo, Japan, 1999, pp. 147–148
93. M.Z. Shvarts, O.I. Chosta, I.V. Kochnev, V.M. Lantratov, V.M. Andreev, Radiation resistant AlGaAs/GaAs concentrator solar cells with internal Bragg reflector. Solar Energy Mater. Solar Cells **68**, 105–122 (2001)
94. V.M. Andreev, I.V. Kochnev, V.M. Lantratov, S.A. Mintairov, V.D. Rumyantsev, M.Z. Shvarts, Ultra-violet sensitive infra-red reflective AlGaAs/GaAs solar cells with two Bragg reflectors, in *Proc. of the 16th European Photovoltaic Solar Energy Conference*, Glasgow, 2000, pp. 1019–1021
95. M.W. Wanlass, J.S. Ward, K.A. Emery, T.A. Gessert, C.R. Osterwald, T.J. Coutts, High performance concentrator tandem solar cells based on IR-sensitive bottom cells. Solar Cells **30**, 363–371 (1991)
96. B.-C. Chung, G.F. Virshup, S. Hikido, N.R. Kaminar, 27.6% efficiency (1 sun, air mass 1.5) monolithic $Al_{0.37}Ga_{0.63}As/GaAs$ two junction cascade solar cell with prismatic cover glass. Appl. Phys. Lett. **55**, 1741–1743 (1989)
97. V.M. Andreev, V.P. Khvostikov, E.V. Paleeva, V.D. Rumyantsev, S.V. Sorokina, M.Z. Shvarts, V.I. Vasil'ev, Tandem solar cells based on AlGaAs/GaAs and GaSb structures, in *Proc. 23rd International Symposium on Compound Semiconductors*, St. Petersburg, Russia, Sept. 23–27, 1996
98. D.J. Friedman, S.R. Kurtz, K.A. Bertness, A.E. Kibbler, C. Kramer, J.M. Olson, D.L. King, B.R. Hansen, J.K. Snyder, GaInP/GaAs monolithic tandem concentrator cells, in *Proceedings of the 1st World Conference on Photovoltaic Energy Conversion*, Waikoloa, Hawaii, USA, 1994, pp. 1829–1832
99. R.R. King, D.C. Law, C.M. Fetzer, R.A. Sherif, K.M. Edmondson, S. Kurtz, G.S. Kinsey, H.L. Cotal, D.D. Krut, J.H. Ermer, N.H. Karam, Pathways to 40%-efficient concentration photovoltaics, in *Proc. 20th European PVSEC*, Barcelona, Spain, 2005, pp. 6–10
100. F. Dimroth, R. Beckert, M. Meusel, U. Schubert, A.W. Bett, Metamorphic $Ga_yIn_{1-y}P/Ga_{1-x}In_xAs$ tandem solar cells for space and for terrestrial concentrator applications at C > 1000 suns. Prog. Photovolt.: Res. Appl. **9**(3), 165–178 (2001)
101. D.J. Aiken, M.A. Stan, S.P. Endicter, G. Girard, P.R. Sharps, A loss analysis for a 28% efficient 520x concentrator module, in *Proceedings of the IEEE 4th World Conference on Photovoltaic Energy Conversion*, Hawaii, 7–12 May 2006, pp. 686–689
102. M. Yamaguchi, Y. Okada, A. Yamamoto, T. Takamoto, K. Araki, Y. Ohshita, Novel materials and structures for high efficiency multi-junction solar cells, in *Proceedings at the 21st European Photovoltaic Solar Energy Conference*, Dresden, 2006, pp. 53–56

103. R.R. King, D.C. Law, K.M. Edmondson, C.M. Fetzer, G.S. Kinsey, D.D. Krut, J.H. Ermer, R.A. Sherif, N.H. Karam, Metamorphic concentrator solar cells with over 40% conversion efficiency, in *Proceedings for 4th International Conference on Solar Concentrators (ICSC-4)*, El Escorial, Spain, 2007, pp. 5–8
104. M.Z. Shvarts, P.Y. Gazaryan, V.P. Khvostikov, V.M. Lantratov, N.K. Timoshina, InGaP/GaAs–GaSb and InGaP/GaAs/Ge–InGaAsSb hybrid monolithic/stacked tandem concentrator solar cells, in *Proceedings at the 21st European Photovoltaic Solar Energy Conference*, Dresden, 2006, pp. 133–136
105. V.M. Andreev, V.P. Khvostikov, V.D. Rumyantsev, O.A. Khvostikova, P.Y. Gazaryan, A.S. Vlasov, N.A. Sadchikov, S.V. Sorokina, Y.M. Zadiranov, M.Z. Shvarts, Termophotovoltaic converters with solar powered high temperature emitters, in *Proceedings of the 20th European Photovoltaic Solar Energy Conference*, Barcelona, June 2005, pp. 8–13
106. V.M. Andreev, A.S. Vlasov, V.P. Khvostikov, O.A. Khvostikova, P.Y. Gazaryan, N.A. Sadchikov, Sun powered TPV converters based on GaSb cells, in *Proceedings at the 21st European Photovoltaic Solar Energy Conference*, Dresden, 2006, pp. 35–38
107. L.W. Fraas, W.E. Daniels, H.X. Huang, L.E. Minkin, J.E. Avery, M.J. O'Neill, A.J. McDanal, M.F. Piszczor, 34% efficient InGaP/GaAs/GaSb cell-interconnected-circuits for line-focus concentrator arrays, in *Proceedings of the 17th European Photovoltaic Solar Energy Conference*, Munich, 2000, pp. 2300–2303
108. V.M. Andreev, V.P. Khvostikov, V.D. Rumyantsev, S.V. Sorokina, M.Z. Shvarts, Single-junction GaSb and tandem GaSb/InGaAsSb & AlGaAsSb/GaSb thermophotovoltaic cells, in *Proc. of the 28th IEEE PVSC*, Alaska, September, 2000, pp. 1265–1268
109. V.M. Andreev, E.A. Ionova, V.R. Larionov, V.D. Rumyantsev, M.Z. Shvarts, G. Glenn, Tunnel diode revealing peculiarities at I–V measurements in multijunction III–V solar cells, in *Proceedings of the IEEE 4th World Conference on Photovoltaic Energy Conversion*, Hawaii, 2006, pp. 799–802
110. Z.I. Alferov, V.M. Andreev, V.D. Rumyantsev, III–V heterostructures in photovoltaics, in *Concentrator Photovoltaics*, ed. by A. Luque and V. Andreev. Springer Series in Optical Sciences, vol. 130 (2007)
111. A.W. Bett, F. Dimroth, G. Siefer, Multi-Junction concentrator solar cells, in *Concentrator Photovoltaics*, ed. by A. Luque and V. Andreev. Springer Series in Optical Sciences, vol. 130 (2007)
112. M. Yamaguchi, K. Araki, T.T. Takamoto, Concentrator solar cell modules and systems developed in Japan, in *Concentrator Photovoltaics*, ed. by A. Luque and V. Andreev. Springer Series in Optical Sciences, vol. 130 (2007)
113. N.H. Karam, R.A. Sherif, R.R. King, Multijunction concentrator solar cells, an enabler for low-cost concentrating photovoltaic systems, in *Concentrator Photovoltaics*, ed. by A. Luque and V. Andreev. Springer Series in Optical Sciences, vol. 130 (2007)
114. M. Yamaguchi, K. Araki, T.T. Takamoto, Concentrator solar cell modules and systems developed in Japan, in *Concentrator Photovoltaics*, ed. by A. Luque and V. Andreev. Springer Series in Optical Sciences, vol. 130 (2007)
115. G. Sala, A. Luque, Past experiences and new challenges of PV concentrators, in *Concentrator Photovoltaics*, ed. by A. Luque and V. Andreev. Springer Series in Optical Sciences, vol. 130 (2007)
116. V.D. Rumyantsev, Terrestrial concentrator PV systems, in *Concentrator Photovoltaics*, ed. by A. Luque and V. Andreev. Springer Series in Optical Sciences, vol. 130 (2007)
117. Z.I. Alferov, V.M. Andreev, Kh.K. Aripov, V.R. Larionov, V.D. Rumyantsev, Pattern of autonomous solar installation with heterostructure solar cells and concentrators. Geliotechnica **2**, 3–6 (1981). Appl. Solar Energy, **2** (1981)

118. Z.I. Alferov, V.M. Andreev, Kh.K. Aripov, V.R. Larionov, V.D. Rumyantsev, Solar Photovoltaic installation with 200 Watt output based on AlGaAs-heterophotocells and reflective concentrators. Geliotechnika **6**, 3–6 (1981). Appl. Solar Energy, **6** (1981)

119. A.A. Vodnev, A.V. Maslov, V.D. Rumyantsev, Sh.Sh. Shamukhamedov, Experience on creation of the solar installations based on AlGaAs/GaAs-photocells with concentrators, in *Sunlight Concentrators for Photovoltaic Power Installations*, ed. by V.A. Grilikhes, Leningrad, Energoatomizdat, 1986, pp. 25–29 (in Russian)

120. V.M. Andreev, A.A. Alaev, A.B. Guchmazov, V.S. Kalinovsky, V.R. Larionov, K.Y. Rasulov, V.D. Rumyantsev, High-efficiency AlGaAs-heterophotocells operating with lens panels as the solar energy concentrators, in *Proc. of the all-Union Conference "Photovoltaic phenomena in semiconductors"*, Tashkent, 1989, pp. 305–306 (in Russian)

121. V.M. Andreev, V.R. Larionov, V.D. Rumyantsev, M.Z. Shvarts, High-efficiency solar concentrating GaAs–AlGaAs modules with small-size lens units, in *11th European Photovoltaic Solar Energy Conference and Exhibition – Book of Abstracts*; abstract No. 1A. 15, Montreux, Switzerland, 12–16 October, 1992

122. Project: INTAS96-1887, 1997–2000 years, Photovoltaic installation with sunlight concentrators. Final Report, 2000

123. V.D. Rumyantsev, M. Hein, V.M. Andreev, A.W. Bett, F. Dimroth, G. Lange, G. Letay, M.Z. Shvarts, O.V. Sulima, Concentrator array based on GaAs cells and Fresnel lens concentrators, in *Proceedings of the 16th European Photovoltaic Solar Energy Conference and Exhibition*, Glasgow, United Kingdom, 1–5 May 2000

124. V.D. Rumyantsev, V.M. Andreev, A.W. Bett, F. Dimroth, M. Hein, G. Lange, M.Z. Shvarts, O.V. Sulima, Progress in development of all-glass terrestrial concentrator modules based on composite Fresnel lenses and III–V solar cells, in *Proceedings of the 28th PVSC*, Anhorage, Alaska, 2000, pp. 1169–1172

125. A.W. Bett, C. Baur, F. Dimroth, G. Lange, M. Meusel, S. van Riesen, G. Siefer, V.M. Andreev, V.D. Rumyantsev, N.A. Sadchikov, FLATCON^{TM} – modules: technology and characterization, in *Proceedings of 3rd World Conference on Photovoltaic Energy Conversion 3O-D9-05*, 2003

126. V.M. Andreev, E.A. Ionova, V.D. Rumyantsev, N.A. Sadchikov, M.Z. Shvarts, Concentrator PV modules of "all-glass" design with modified structure, in *Proceedings of 3rd World Conference on Photovoltaic Energy Conversion 3P-C3-72*, 2003

127. Z.I. Alferov, V.D. Rumyantsev, Trends in the development of solar photovoltaics, in *Next Generation Photovoltaics*, IoP, 2004, pp. 19–49

128. V.D. Rumyantsev, N.A. Sadchikov, A.E. Chalov, E.A. Ionova, D.J. Friedman, G. Glenn, Terrestrial concentrator PV modules based on GaInP/GaAs/Ge TJ cells and minilens panels, in *Proceedings of the IEEE 4th World Conference on Photovoltaic Energy Conversion*, Hawaii, 2006, pp. 632–635

129. V.D. Rumyantsev, A.E. Chalov, E.A. Ionova, V.R. Larionov, N.A. Sadchikov, V.M. Andreev, Practical design of PV modules t for very high solar concentration, in *Proc. on CD of the Third Int. Conf. on Solar Concentrators for the Generation of Electricity or Hydrogen*, Scottsdale, Arizona, May 2005

130. V.D. Rumyantsev, N.A. Sadchikov, A.E. Chalov, E.A. Ionova, V.R. Larionov, V.M. Andreev, G.R. Smekens, E.W. Merkle, Pilot installation with "all-glass" concentrator PV modules, in *Proceedings at the 21st European Photovoltaic Solar Energy Conference*, Dresden, 2006, pp. 2097–2100

131. V.D. Rumyantsev, A.E. Chalov, N.Y. Davidyuk, E.A. Ionova, N.A. Sadchikov, V.M. Andreev, Solar concentrator modules with fresnel lens panels, in *Proc. of the Fourth Int. Conf. on Solar Concentrators for the Generation of Electricity or Hydrogen*, El Escorial, Spain, 2007, pp. 33–36

132. P.A. Davies, A. Luque, Solar thermophotovoltaics: brief review and a new look. Solar Energy Mater. Solar Cells **33**, 11–22 (1994)
133. V. Andreev, V. Khvostikov, A. Vlasov, Solar thermophotovoltaics, in *Concentrator Photovoltaics*, ed. by A. Luque and V. Andreev. Springer Series in Optical Sciences, vol. 130, 2007
134. V.M. Andreev, V.A. Grilikhes, V.P. Khvostikov, O.A. Khvostikova, V.D. Rumyantsev, N.A. Sadchikov, M.Z. Shvarts, Concentrator PV modules and solar cells for TPV systems. J. Solar Energy Mater. Solar Cells **84**, 3–17 (2004)
135. Z.I. Alferov, V.M. Andreev, Yu.M. Zadiranov, V.I. Korol'kov, N. Rahimov, T.S. Tabarov, Photo-EMF in $Al_xGa_{1-x}As$ graded band-gap heterostructures. Pisma Z. Tech. Fiz. **4**, 369–372 (1978) [Sov. Tech. Phys. Lett. **4**(4), 149–150 (1978)]
136. Z.I. Alferov, A.M. Vasiliev, S.V. Ivanov, P.S. Kop'ev, N.N. Ledentsov, M.E. Lutsenko, B.Y. Melser, V.M. Ustinov, Reducing the threshold in GaAs–AlGaAs DHS SCH quantum well lasers ($j_{th} = 52$ A/cm^2, $T = 300$ K) with quantum well restriction by short period superlattice of variable period. Pisma Z. Techn. Fiz. **14**, 1803–1806 (1988) [Sov. Tech. Phys. Lett. **14**, 782 (1988)]
137. Z.I. Alferov, N.A. Bert, A.Y. Egorov, A.E. Zhukov, P.S. Kop'ev, A.O. Kosogov, I.L. Krestnikov, N.N. Ledentsov, A.V. Lunev, M.V. Maksimov, A.V. Sakharov, V.M. Ustinov, A.F. Tsatsul'nikov, Y.M. Shernyakov, D. Bimberg, An injection heterojunction laser based on arrays of vertically coupled InAs quantum dots in a GaAs matrix. Fiz. Tekh. Poluprovodn. **30**, 351–356 (1996) [Semiconductors, **30**, 194–196 (1996)]
138. A. Marti, L. Guadra, A. Luque, Intermediate-band solar cells, in *Next Generation Photovoltaics. High Efficiency trough Full Spectrum Utilization*, ed. by A. Marti, A. Luque (Institute of Physics, Bristol, 2004), pp. 140–164

9 The Economic Perspective: Is Concentrator PV Capable of Breaking the Economic Barrier

E.W. Merkle, R. Tölle, and M. Sturm

PV will contribute to the new energy mix only if we manage the transition from a subsidy-driven to a cost-effective method of producing solar electricity

9.1 Climate Change and Depletion of Fossil fuels

The provision of clean, sustainable energy is the paramount issue of this century! Due to the discussion of climate change and the depletion of natural energy sources, there is worldwide support for renewable energy.

The International Energy Agency (IEA) predicts a significant increase in worldwide energy demand. Due to the depletion of fossil resources and the problems of climate change, this demand will have to be satisfied by renewable energy sources in the future.

Only the energy of the sun – 15,000 times the amount which is needed – has the potential to meet the demand. It is obvious that within a few decades solar energy has to replace all fossil fuels.

According to industry analysts, The growing concern about climate change due to CO_2 emissions combined with the steep rise in prices for fossil fuels will lead to much higher growth in PV installations in the following decades.

9.1.1 Photovoltaic as Part of Global Energy Trends

The perspectives of the global PV markets are subordinate to the long-term energy perspectives. It is a fact that all fossil energy sources, to varying extents, are unsustainable.

The UN Climate Report makes clear that the growing use of climate-destroying energy sources on an industrial level and also by private households demands a redirection of climate politics. Furthermore it can be stated that the specific sourcing cost of fossil energy sources rise disproportionate.

In many cases, access to the still-existing fossil resources is possible only in politically unstable regions with unsatisfactory production infrastructure.

Considering this background photovoltaic is one of the sustainable options for generating energy besides wind, hydro- and geothermal energy, biomass or the conventionally based generation of energy.

The goal of 20% renewable energies, which was decided on the EU Climate summit, will be a great catalyst for the PV industry, raising it far above average development potential. The expected rise in prices of conventionally generated electricity makes photovoltaic an increasingly competitive form of sustainable energy generation.

9.1.2 Growth Perspective of Photovoltaic

The growth forecasts for PV have been surpassed by the actual growth for the last decade.

With a current market of around 2 Gigawatt (GW), forecasts for the year 2030 currently range from a market volume of 170 up to 1,000 GW of installations per year with a sales volume of $500 to $2,000 billion per annum in 2030.

The latter figures were published by Rogol of Photon Consulting, a leading PV analyst [2]. The more conservative figures were published by research analysts from the capital market environment (e.g., Bank Sarasin [3]).

Even the conservative figures estimate a 100-fold growth of the industry within the next 22 years.

By then the market share of PV-produced electricity, which is now only 0.2%, will be in the range of 20 to 40%.

The drivers of this extraordinary growth perspective are the following:

1. The steep rise in costs of conventional energy and reduction of costs of solar power
2. Direct or feed-in subsidies
3. PPA (power purchase agreement) and reverse metering
4. New markets
5. Trading of CO_2 credits

Here, we analyse all five drivers for the future growth of the PV industry.

Steep Rise in Energy Costs and Reduction of Costs of Solar Power

During the last few years, a steep rise in the cost of energy has taken place. Due to growing demand and depletion of fossil fuels this increase will most likely accelerate.

In contrast to this rise, there is a similar steep drop in the price of PV-produced electricity – an 85% reduction between 1982 and 2007. Even the rather conservative Deutsche Bank predicts that solar power will be cheaper than other sources of energy within a decade [1].

Both developments lead to a convergence, as shown in Fig. 9.1.

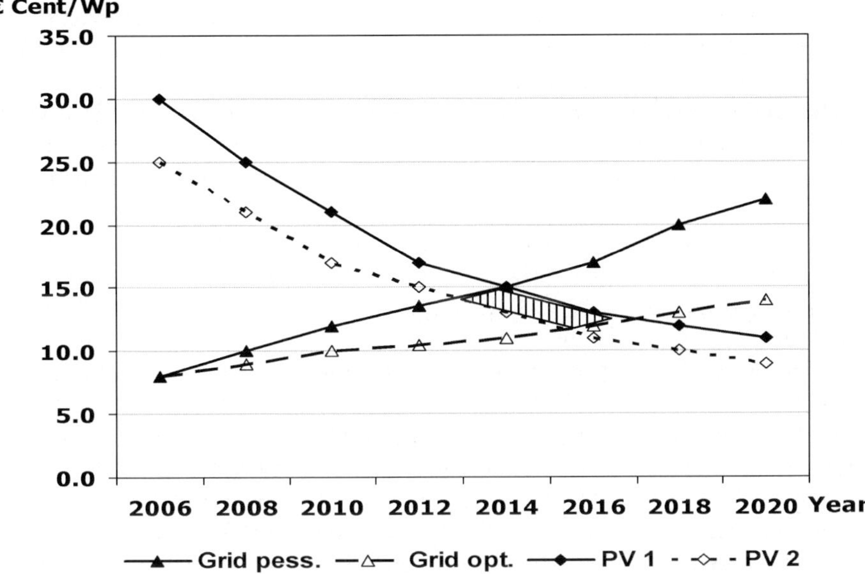

Fig. 9.1. Depending on optimistic (PV 2) and pessimistic (PV 1) scenarios, "grid parity" will be reached in most countries with high sun exposure, i.e. $>1500\,\mathrm{kWh}$ per m^2 and year, between 2,013 and 2,017. Source: IEA, own calculations

Direct or Feed-in Subsidies

The growth of PV installations started with incentive programs for rooftop installations in Japan and Germany. While those direct subsidies were related only to the initial investment, the real success story started with the inauguration of the Renewable Energy Law (EEG) in 1999 and revised in 2003. Through this law, a feed-in tariff of more than 0.5 EUR was given to the investors for each kWh produced by PV in Germany. This law was so successful that more than 50% of all worldwide PV installations in 2006 were in Germany. This law has meanwhile been copied, with local adaptations, by close to 60 nations. The feed-in tariff remains stable and is guaranteed for 20 years once the installation is connected to the grid. But the tariff was lowered annually by 5–6.5% in the past few years and the digression of the feed-in tariff will accelerate in the coming years. This system is giving security to investors at a level similar to real estate investments, but also poses a strong incentive to lower the prices of PV systems. Whereas in the first stage mostly small rooftop installations were built, the focus has changed to large field installations in Germany and recently in other European markets like Spain and Italy.

Power Purchase Agreement (PPA) and Reverse Metering

A big advantage of PV is the production of energy at the place where it is needed. Here a tremendous market is foreseen. In the western states of the U.S., two systems are in operation. PPAs have been brought into public focus through retail outlets like Wal-Mart. They signed a 10–20 year agreement to buy the electricity produced by the solar panels at a fixed price. The owners are capital investors. This model will become more and more profitable as PV module prices decrease. With thin-film modules a return on investment (ROI) of 7% can be realized without subsidies. More than 100 cities in the U.S. and Hawaii already operate these PPAs.

A second and similar system was put into operation mainly for homeowners: reverse metering. With this system a private homeowner can feed the electricity produced by his PV modules back into the grid. The meter then runs backwards, for example, during daytime hours when nobody is at home and not much electricity is used. On sunny days in Arizona, California and other sun-belt states, homeowners produce all the electricity they need for the evening hours. Because demand in electricity frequently peaks during hot summer days around noon time, utilities need not invest into additional power plant capacity once this system reaches a critical volume of several 10,000 homes.

In a growing number of states like Arizona and California, where state rebates and federal tax credits can be added, PV systems at the presently high price of around $6,500 U.S. already generate an ROI of up to 7%. If prices continue to go down, PV will become a mainstream investment for millions of households. Already premiums are being paid for houses with solar installations.

New Markets/New Regulations

New markets will arise when alternatives for fossil fuels must be found. PV installations can replace millions of diesel generators all around the world. Electricity and thus the chance for a civilized life can be brought to 2–3 billion people who do not currently have access to the grid. New thin-film modules with sizes of $260 \times 220 \, cm^2$ enable use in buildings. Those building-integrated PV systems (BIPV) will have a tremendous market. Most buildings can generate most of their electricity though integration into walls or semitransparent modules instead of shaded solar glass. The costs may even be less than standard glass windows once a critical volume for those modules is achieved. The German government is currently discussing a new regulation, which would require new buildings to produce 15% of their energy requirement by renewable energy sources. This new regulation will jump start the BIPV market.

A huge demand will come once plug-in hybrid cars become popular. With the solar energy generated through a solar roof on the carport or shaded parking area, most of the energy can be generated needed to power a car for 95% of its use (daily mileage 50 miles).

There will be many new markets coming up once a change in thinking has taken place and energy prices keep sky rocketing and climate problems reach new heights.

Trading of CO$_2$ Credits

The trading of CO$_2$ credits is becoming more popular in the world. The simple fact that PV systems produce CO$_2$-free electricity may have an additional market value, thus promoting the investments into PV power installations.

In the following sections the authors present their own opinion about the future potential of three different PV technologies, i.e. the first-generation crystalline silicon flat plate, the second-generation thin-film and the third-generation concentrator PV (CPV) technologies. Within this article CPV refers only to high-concentration technologies above 500× based on III–V compound solar cells. The potential of low-to-medium silicon concentration technologies (below 100×) would require an article in itself, since the technological variations are huge and complex.

9.2 Cost Reduction as the Major Target

9.2.1 Cost Potentials of the Current Technologies

Ever the first modern silicon wafer-based solar cell was developed 50 years ago, the perception has been that using it to produce electricity would be expensive.

However, these rather high costs are due to the fact that the industry has not reached its stage of maturity yet. Small business units are still prevailing. Only recently have large industrial units been built, achieving considerable reductions in costs.

However, the different technologies have different potentials for cost reduction.

1. The first generation: Silicon flat-plate technology, which has used the abundant supply of off-quality silicon wafers for decades, now suffers from high prices of feedstock and a large number of production processes.
2. The second generation: Thin-film technology has better options to reduce costs due to low material consumption (1% of first-generation use of semiconductor material) and automatic coating processes.
3. The third generation: Concentrator technology (CPV) has the lowest material consumption and also excellent options for fully automated production lines.

The raw material consumption necessary for 100 GWp assumed for 2020 of the different PV generations is shown in Table 9.1 and is compared to the 2006 world total production of the same material.

In the case of CPV, the worldwide Germanium reserves are currently estimated at 8,200 metric tons. According to Umicore, the market leader in Germanium refining, all waste streams in the Germanium production are recycled [4]. The recycling of end-of-lifetime CPV modules is needed to extend the Germanium reach. From all the technologies described in Table 9.1, the third-generation CPV has the second lowest raw material capacity expansion requirements after the second-generation amorphous silicon thin-film technology. For all technologies shown in Table 9.1 only the bulk semiconductor material has been taken into account, since the bulk

Table 9.1. Projected semiconductor raw material consumption in 2020 for different PV technologies

	Raw material	2006 World production total	2020 Raw material needed for 100 GWp PV
1st Generation	c-Si	40,000 t/a	600,000 t/a
2nd Generation	a-Si/μc-Si	20,000 t/a	20,000 t/a
	CdTe	300 t/a	5,000 t/a
	CIGS	300 t/a	3,000 t/a
3rd Generation	Ge	100 t/a	600 t/a

material amount is the cost driver. All other materials – such as the front and back electrodes, buffer layers and the very thin junction material in the case of concentrator solar cells – have been neglected.

9.2.2 Thin-Film PV in Comparison to Crystalline Silicon PV: Advantages in Price, Performance and Large Size

Although conversion efficiencies are not as high as crystalline silicon PV, thin-film PV shows superior performance in hot and overcast climates because of the multiple p/n-junctions that can absorb different wavelengths of sunlight. Thin film layers can be deposited on large glass substrates, a technology introduced by Applied Materials on 5.7 m^2 large modules. This module size is ideal for incorporation into building-integrated photovoltaic (BIPV). The incremental costs of the system are reduced, the building owner is provided with energy and cost savings, and return on investment is increased. BIPV enables thin-film PV to serve as a platform for products that cannot easily be created with conventional crystalline silicon PV.

Thin-film PV will likely win over crystalline silicon PV for projects in locations where space is not a constraint, due to its lower cost and the ability to use large plots of land. Emerging economies that establish solar programs will be drawn to the cost savings of thin-film PV as well, unless feed-in tariffs are set high enough to suit crystalline silicon costs, as is currently the case in, e.g., Spain, Italy and Greece. In Germany, however, all major multi-MWp power plant projects in 2008 will use thin-film technology because of price pressure from the digression of the EEG. Thin-film PV also works better in Germany due to the comparatively low insulation in comparison to the Mediterranean countries.

Besides these side advantages of thin-film PV, the most important argument will be the lower price in the market due to a more favorable cost structure. Table 9.2 illustrates the expected module production cost for crystalline silicon PV, CdTe, and a-Si technologies in 2007 and 2010.

Although we expect polysilicon cost/watt to decrease by about 50% until 2010 and nonpolysilicon costs to decrease by about 20%, c-Si modules still remain more expensive than thin-film products. Crystalline silicon PV modules involve a series of production steps and costs that can each be performed in-house or by a third

Table 9.2. Module cost analysis: crystalline vs. thin-film 2007E and 2010E

($ per Watt)	2007E			2010E		
	c-Si	a-Si	CdTe	c-Si	a-Si	CdTe
Polysilicon	1.65			0.85		
Ingot / Wafering	0.35			0.25		
Solar Cells	0.25			0.20		
Modules	0.45	2.00	1.25	0.40	1.25	0.90
Total Cost	$2.70	$2.00	$1.25	$1.70	$1.25	$0.90

Source: Company reports and CIBC World Markets Corp

party. Since a-Si and CdTe production processes are continuous and all executed by the manufacturing firm, the pricing is not broken down into different steps; only the cost of producing the module is measured. With regards to CdTe module costs, we use First Solar's projected cost of $0.70/W in 2010 as recently reported in Photon International. However, we believe $0.90/W is more likely in 2010 and that First Solar will achieve its goal of $0.70/W in the following years.

9.2.3 CPV in Comparison to Crystalline Silicon Flat-Plate PV

Of the three generations, CPV exhibits the steepest increase in efficiency of all three generations. Therefore the steeper learning curve opens the potential for faster cost reduction. The overall higher efficiency potential of CPV leads to a cost reduction of all BOS (balance of system) components. Even at the currently low production volume of concentrator solar cells the cost of the concentrator solar cell per Wp under high concentration is already only around one third of the crystalline silicon cell cost. But one obviously has to take the increased complexity of the concentrator portion of system cost, i.e. the optics as well as the tracker, into account. For comparison the LED industry, which uses technologies similar to concentrator solar cells, has achieved 90% price reductions of LEDs within six years through mass production and learning curve effects. Since LED manufacturers are still profitable, it has to be assumed that the cost reduction will be very similar. This shows the enormous potential of the steep CPV learning curve. If CPV manages to create a learning curve similar to LED technology, then solely the concentrator solar cell cost under concentration can drop below 10 €ct/Wp in the near future.

9.2.4 Conclusion: Cost Potential to Reach "Grid Parity"

All three technologies show considerable potential for cost reduction. However, the second- and third-generation technologies – with low consumption of expensive semiconductor material and the option for fully automated production processes – show a much greater potential to considerably lower the costs of PV systems. CPV uses approximately 1,000 times less, and thin-film 100× less semiconductor material in comparison to crystalline silicon. But the market for CPV is geo-

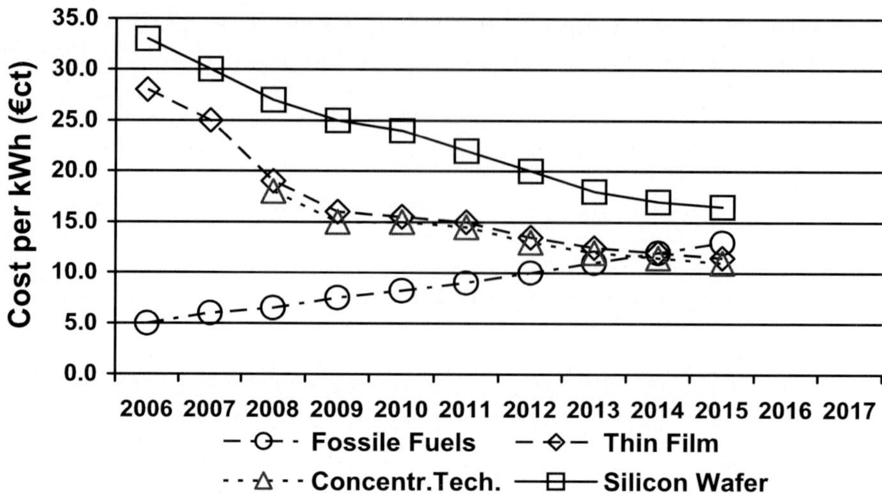

Fig. 9.2. Costs per KWh produced in sun-rich areas with the three PV generations. Source: IEA and company calculations

graphically limited to the sun-belt region on Earth and the technology is applicable only to large-scale power plants. In comparison, thin-film technologies are best suited for BIPV applications as well as power plant applications, in which there are no area constraints. Crystalline silicon, however, can be applied in all markets.

Grid parity will be achieved by these technologies within the next five to nine years. In our view the first-generation crystalline silicon technology might have difficulties following the cost reduction curves of the second and third generation, unless step changes in efficiency or cheaper feedstock sources can be realized. Sanyo's HIT as well as Sunpower's back contact cell concepts show that step changes in efficiency in the first generation are still possible, and initial results using metallurgical-grade silicon are promising. Another possible step for crystalline silicon might be application to low- and medium-concentration systems, which would reduce material consumption significantly. If those technologies are combined with increased pressure from reduced feed-in tariffs, then the first generation might also be able to reach grid parity faster than shown in Fig. 9.2.

The cost potential of the three technologies is shown in Fig. 9.2.

Table 9.1 shows that the amount of semiconductor material necessary to produce 100 GWp of power is 600,000 t/a in the case of crystalline silicon flat-plate technology, but only 600 t/a for germanium as used in CPV systems. At a concentration factor of 100, which is technically still feasible for silicon, the raw material requirement would be reduced to 6,000 t/a. At 100 GWp production volumes the cost will be driven by the material cost. Therefore crystalline silicon flat plate has an inherent disadvantage in comparison to thin-film and CPV technologies as long as silicon feedstock prices are high. CPV especially has the overall lowest semiconductor material requirement of all PV technologies, but this comes with the added cost of both optical and tracking systems.

9.3 Meeting the Tremendous Growth Perspective

9.3.1 Growth Beyond all Imagination

The latest market forecast by M. Rogol of Photon Consulting expects the world market to hit 14 GWp by 2010 [2]. At 45% CAGR (compound annual growth rate) the market would be in excess of 40 GWp by 2013!

To satisfy this enormous demand, the industry will have to change considerably. Investments in the sub-GWp manufacturing capacity are common today (e.g. 250 MWp, Conergy; 500 MWp, SolarWorld and Solon for 2010; First Solar expects 900 MWp for 2009), but in the future multi-GWp facilities are mandatory. REC, one of the largest silicon producers from Norway has already announced construction of a 1.5 GW facility in Singapore – all in first-generation technology. In comparison to today's production processes, the industry will have to change the way it is thinking about manufacturing expansions. Logistic problems will play a much more important role in the future. Production lines, which fully integrate all process steps virtually from sand for solar glass production until the delivery of modules to the sites for power plants, will have to become mainstream in the future. Enormous quantities have to be moved in those factories. To ship 1 GW of modules, approx. 10,000 containers are needed. This means about 40 containers a day or one full 40-ft container every 15 minutes during daytime.

Companies need an enormous volume just to defend their market share.

Two simple examples (based on conservative market expectations) are given below to explain this fact:

1. According to the latest Sarasin Forecast, in 2020, the world market will be at 65 GWp (Study Nov. 2007 [3]). Ten percent of the market share represents a production capacity of 6.5 GWp. At the average forecast of 50% CAGR, the company would have to add 3.25 GWp of additional production capacity in 2021 just to maintain market share!
2. Let's say a company plans to acquire 10% of the market share in 2030. Given the conservative estimate of 180 GWp for the market, the companies needs a production capacity of 18 GWp. At 33% CAGR the company would have to add 6 GWp of additional production capacity in 2031 just to maintain market share!

9.3.2 Multi-GWp Capability

A GE-Matrix can be used to assess the future potential of the different PV technologies. For this one needs to assess the technological readiness of all candidates. To assess the technological readiness, one has to distinguish between material availability and actual manufacturability in the GWp range. Manufacturability issues include in-line process capability, material logistics as well as number of devices handled per MWp.

The current three generations of PV technologies – i.e. crystalline flat-plate, thin-film technologies as well as concentrator PV – can be viewed along a two-axis coordination system, i.e. the technological multi-GWp capability and their cost reduction potential, as shown in Fig. 9.3.

Today's dominating silicon flat-plate technology has much higher technological barriers to overcome compared to the second- and third-generation technologies. The fact that thin-film technologies currently grow faster than crystalline silicon and that in markets with high price pressure like Germany, large PV power plants are realized only in thin-film technologies confirm that the market believes in the superior cost-reduction potential of thin-film technologies. A similar development can be expected when CPV technologies start to enter the market.

All thin-film (TF) technologies have a high cost reduction potential, but non-silicon technologies like CIS and CdTe use rare metals like indium and tellurium, which are a significant constraint for their muli-GWp capabilities. All silicon technologies have the advantage of using the second-most abundant element on Earth and therefore have basically unlimited supplies of raw materials. But crystalline silicon flat-plate has the disadvantage, in comparison to TF technologies, that it uses approximately 100 times more semiconductor material and needs to handle 100 times more devices per MWp.

CPV has the lowest semiconductor material consumption per Wp and the highest efficiency potential of all technologies, which shows up in the highest cost re-

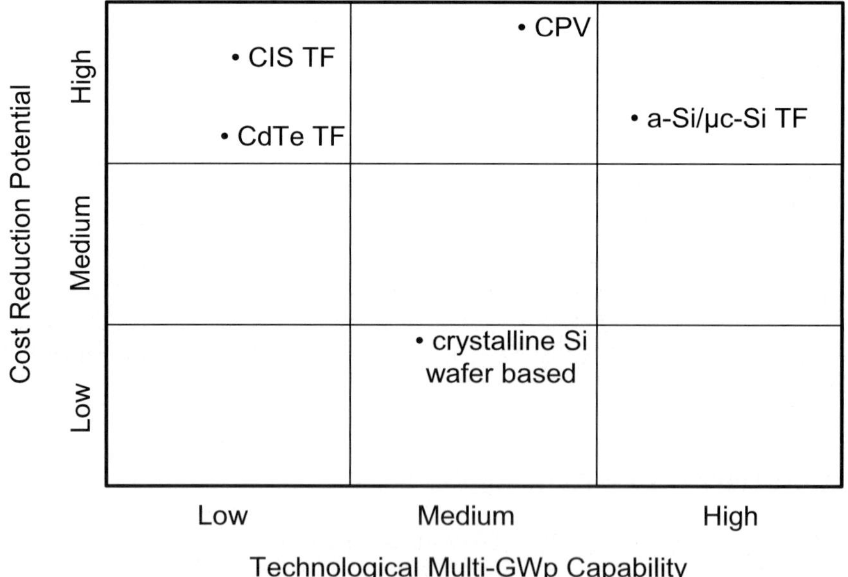

Fig. 9.3. Assessment of the technological readiness of different PV technologies

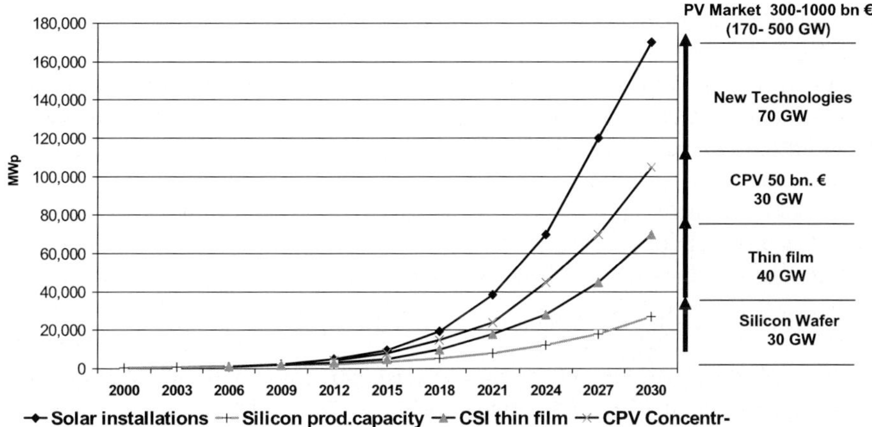

Fig. 9.4. Conservative estimate of PV world market development to 2030 distinguished between different technologies

duction potential. However, at present the technology requires the handling of even more devices per MWp than crystalline silicon, which impacts on its multi-GWp capability. Therefore, from Fig. 9.3 we can conclude that the two technologies with the best multi-GWp capability and the highest cost reduction potential are silicon-based thin-film and concentrator PV, albeit for different reasons (as explained earlier).

9.3.3 The Market in 2030:
Will There Be a Winning Technology?

The prediction of the growing worldwide energy demand requires the PV industry to prepare for enormous growth. A conservative estimate of a market demand of 170 GWp in 2030 is shown in Fig. 9.4.

In comparison to today's market, in which the silicon flat-plate technology still dominates and has around 90% market share, we expect the market to change in the future. Both thin-film and CPV technologies will gain significant market share due to their superior multi-GWp capabilities, i.e. their cost-reduction potential as well as their multi-GWp manufacturability. But in general all three generations will prevail due to the fact that they serve partly different markets and applications. It is also anticipated that a large part of the future growth up to 2030 will come from technologies which are still to be developed.

9.4 Cost Barriers for Leaving the Niche

9.4.1 Explosive Growth of PV – Low Rate of Innovation

Installations of photovoltaic power systems have achieved tremendous growth rates in Germany and Japan, with high double-digit growth rates for many years. These two countries alone account for 88% of installed systems. Other countries in Europe and around the world are only slowly catching up.

The growth of the PV industry is strongly related to public subsidies for either investments or for each unit of electricity fed into the grid. One of the "success stories" is the German EEG, which strongly supports the production of solar energy fed into the grid. Similar laws have been passed by other European governments. Feed-in laws are even on the way to becoming adopted worldwide. Although this policy has proven to be successful in bringing a small-scale industry to an industrial level, it has shortcomings, too. The most important are:

- Prices are much higher in countries with high subsidies.
- There is no real pressure on prices and costs.
- No innovation is required to reach a comfortable profit and relax on the pillow provided by subsidies.
- Lack of innovation shows serious side effects with the shortage of silicon halting some of the growth expectations.
- No serious alternative to the high-price silicon-wafer technology has been investigated after 2004.
- Thin-film technology has tried to solve this problem for the last 15 years, with thus far limited success; in 2007, however, thin-film has grown faster than crystalline silicon for the first time.

In case of a significant cut in subsidies the market for PV systems will break down because its economic viability so far is based on subsidies.

9.4.2 High Growth at High Price Levels – the Problem of a Subsidized Industry

Most of today's PV technology concepts have been started without the shortcomings mentioned above.

This is true for the traditional flat-plate solar industry, which started with a feed-stock that was available in large enough quantities for a long time. However, any serious forecast will project that permanent subsidies cannot be the solution to the energy problems the world is facing. The basic problem is that the dominating flat-plate silicon technology is consuming huge quantities of expensive semiconductor material to collect the sun's energy at low-density levels. It is very hard to believe that there will be enough low-cost, high-purity silicon to cover the 100 to 500 times higher demand in the year 2030 or 2050. The investment costs for solar silicon production facilities are above 100 million Euro per 1,000 tons annual capacity and the high consumption of energy for the complex production process limit the price reduction potential.

Different but similar problems in concept can be seen in other areas of the PV industry. Looking into concentrator PV concepts we have to conclude that most of today's CPV prototypes have been developed by research institutes, mostly subsidized through government projects.

Basic errors in concept are:

- Materials which are either not suitable or too expensive for mass production cost targets.
- High consumption of material in relation to the peak production of power.
- High maintenance costs.
- Lack of concerns for the necessities of mass production processes, long-term stability and the standard qualification procedures.

9.4.3 Solar Energy: Abundant Quantity but Low Density

The main reason for the high costs of today's solar installations is the poor use of the huge but dispersed solar resource. Traditional flat-plate silicon has shown a very poor increase in efficiency over the last 50 years, from 6% reached by Bell Laboratories in 1955 to an average of less than 14% in today's installations. The PV industry has failed to prove their capability of providing a competitive system for the production of electricity. The respectable growth of the industry was achieved only through huge subsidies.

PV will pick up the role it has to play in the energy sector only if new technologies and innovations emerge with the potential for high conversion rates of the solar spectrum and a high cost-reduction potential. CPV under certain conditions has this potential.

9.5 The Learning Curve of CPV: Quick or Slow

9.5.1 Concentration on the Strength Factors

CPV will be successful only if it concentrates its activities on some basic principles:

Replace expensive semiconductor material through inexpensive optics and use a module construction concept suitable for mass production. Use wherever possible proven commercial manufacturing technologies instead of relying on prototyping. Always calculate the cost down to the complete system. Do not stop at the module. Only the complete system cost allows us to assess the cost of electricity generation. Have the application and the market in mind, not just the technology.

However, we cannot see that the CPV concepts on the market follow this approach very well. In spite of almost 20 years of developments and huge amounts of public-sponsored research and development, no concept is really ready for industrial mass production with a serious potential of reducing costs below the one Euro per watt target for modules.

9.5.2 Learning from the LED and Photonic Industries

The LED industry has been developing at a remarkable technological rate of innovation. The first white LEDs were introduced in 1996 with an efficiency of approximately 5 lumen per watt. This efficiency is comparable to the Edison light bulb around the year 1880. During the following 90 years the efficiency of the incandescent lamp has increased at a poor rate of less than 1% per year, reaching little over 10 Lm/W in 1970.

The technological development of the white LEDs shows a completely different picture, one of fast development: 108 Lm/W were reached by Osram in 2005 after only nine years; 200 Lm/W are expected for 2012. Since LEDs use basically the same – only in reverse – principle, they show up a technological pathway which is suitable for CPV.

LEDs and concentrator solar cells are, in principle, the same device. An LED produces light from electricity, whereas a concentrator solar cell produces electricity from sunlight. When a concentrator solar cell is run in reverse, it emits light and glows red. Both devices are produced by the same production technology: MOCVD (metal organic vapor deposition). Whereas the worldwide demand for space and concentrator solar cells is covered by approximately five MOCVD reactors, the largest LED manufacturer in the world runs 115 such reactors in production alone. Even today the efficiency increase in concentrator solar cells is remarkable. But in comparison to what was achieved in LED manufacturing, it looks rather mediocre. The cost reductions in the LED industry of 90% over a six-year period were achieved by a combination of efficiency gains and economy of scales from volume production. There is no technological reason why the same result cannot be achieved in concentrator solar cell production. Even at today's low production volume for concentrator solar cells, those cells are already at one third of the cost per watt in comparison to silicon solar cells. With the cost reduction potential shown in the LED industry, the concentrator solar cell cost can be decreased to a few cents per watt. When tight cost control is applied in the selection of module materials and concept, then a concentrator module price below one Euro per watt can be achieved. Together with the balance of system cost this would be sufficient to reach grid parity in the sun-belt region on earth.

9.5.3 Solar*Tec AG's Approach to CPV

SolarTec AG is currently developing its proprietary third-generation CPV technology in close collaboration with the Ioffe Institute in St. Petersburg, Russia. Ioffe's original idea of using micro Fresnel lenses and micro solar cells has been adopted by SolarTec, but the all-glass module design has been replaced by materials that are easier to adapt to volume manufacturing.

Key features of the SolarTec approach are:

1. The micro Fresnel lens approach with micro concentrator cells allow the application of a simple, passive heat-sink technology, which leads to similar cell temperatures under operation as can be observed for standard silicon flat-plate modules.
2. A short focal distance increases the acceptance angle of the module, which is a very important parameter for the overall, yearly performance ratio of the system, and reduces the specification for the tracker accuracy. The short focal

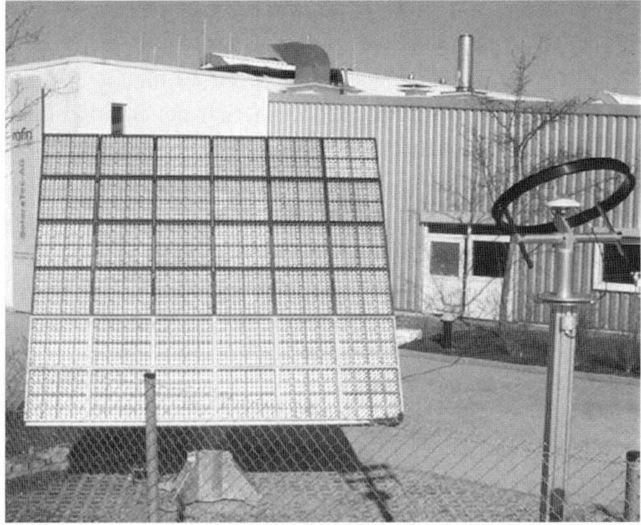

Fig. 9.5. SolarTec AG's test tracker with CPV modules and weather station in front of the R&D facility in Aschheim near Munich, Germany

distance also reduces the amount of material required for the housing frame of the module and reduces the overall weight of the module, which also decreases tracker specifications. But the reduced focal distance comes at the cost of a slightly reduced theoretical maximum optical efficiency of the Fresnel lens.

3. The Fresnel lens array is produced by injection moulding, a technology well known for volume production in other industries.
4. A high concentration ratio of $700\times$ reduces the cell area and therefore the semiconductor material consumption.
5. The module housing is also produced by injection moulding of low-cost, environmentally enduring plastic material, which reduces the module weight in comparison to most other materials and allows for optimal fit of thermal expansion coefficients between the front glass and the module frame, which is required for the module's long lifetime.
6. Each single solar cell is measured and binned according to its electrical parameters in order to reduce mismatch losses during interconnection.
7. High accuracy pick-and-place technology, frequently used in the LED industry, has been adapted for the production of the receivers.
8. Standard bonding technology has been adapted for the automated interconnection of all solar cells. Bond wires and bond parameters have been optimized together with the solar cell metallization with respect to resistance losses and adhesion properties in collaboration with SolarTec's subsidiary ENE, which provides the concentrator cells.
9. Process control tools have been developed for each process step to assure the highest quality during production.

10. SolarTec has an in-house tracker development, which realizes the required accuracy at low cost.
11. SolarTec's own PV power plant business, which has already realized more than 10 MWp of power plants with conventional first-generation silicon flat-plate modules in 2007 and plans to increase this business to more than 70 MWp in 2008, ensures that the overall system for CPV is designed for highest performance ratio.

SolarTec is currently preparing for certification according to IEC 62108, which is a necessity for the sale of CPV power plants to investors.

The result of SolarTec's and Ioffe's joint effort on the development of the technology can be seen in Fig. 9.5, which shows a fully functional test tracker at SolarTec's R&D facility in Aschheim near Munich, Germany.

References

1. Fortune, 15 Oct. 2007, p. 62
2. Rogol, Solar Annual 2007, Photon Consulting, Solar Verlag, 2007
3. Sarasin, Solar Energy 2007, Bankhaus Sarasin, 2007
4. Umicore, The role of the germanium substrate manufacturer in the CPV market, Ralf Dessein, CPV Workshop, Marburg 2007

10 Fluorescent Solar Energy Concentrators: Principle and Present State of Development

A. Goetzberger

10.1 Principle

The use of transparent sheets doped with fluorescent dyes for the concentration of sunlight was suggested first in the 1970s [1, 2]. The principle itself is much older; it was first used in scintillation counters for atomic physics [3, 4]. Although significant advances were made in early work, after some years further progress was limited by the materials available at that time – in particular the dyes – and interest was dormant for decades. Only recently new progress in materials as well as theoretical advances rekindled interest. In this article the historic work and the present state of the art will be reviewed.

Figure 10.1 shows the principle of the fluorescent concentrator, sometimes also called the luminescent solar concentrator: I represent an incident beam of light interacting with a dye molecule dissolved in a matrix of index of refraction n. The incident light will be absorbed and emitted at a different wavelength. (In the normal case of Stokes fluorescence, the emitted wavelength will be shifted to a longer wavelength.) If the probability of emission is equal in all directions, part of the light will leave the transparent medium (F_1) while another part (F_2) will be reflected back because it intersects the surface at an angle leading to total internal reflection. It is important to note that this reflection is in principle *lossless*. Thus the captured light is guided within the transparent sheet which will be also called the collector. Concentrated light can thus be obtained at the edge of the concentrator. The edges of the concentrator not contacted by solar cells have to be covered with mirrors. The fraction of light contained in the concentrator can be quite high. The fluorescent concentrator is the only concentrator known that can achieve high values of concentration without tracking. In contrast, concentrators based on geometric optics have to be tracked in order to achieve concentration of more than about 2 and they can only use direct sunlight. This is a fundamental limitation following from nonimaging optics.

In [5, 6] it has been shown that loss due to light leaving the concentrator through the two boundary planes is given by:

$$L = 1 - (n^2 - 1)^{1/2}/n \qquad (10.1)$$

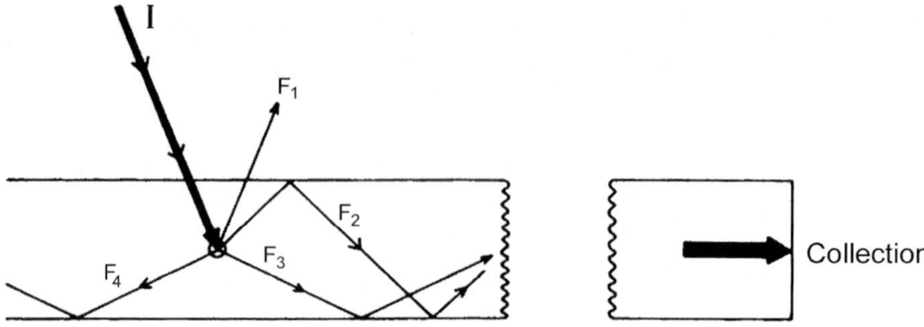

Fig. 10.1. Principle of fluorescent collection. Dye molecule D interacts with incoming light beam I. Secondary beams are partly lost (F_1) and partly guided in transparent material (F_2–F_4)

where n is the index of refraction of the concentrator. For $n = 1.5$ for instance, $L = 0.2546$, for $n = 2$, L is 0.134 (it will be shown below that by optimized design of concentrators these losses can be reduced significantly). The solid angle determined by the onset of total internal reflection is called the loss cone.

A basic requirement for efficient collection is that the incident wavelength has to have a short absorption length, the emitted wavelength a very long absorption length. This is accomplished by selecting a dye whose absorption and emission wavelengths are well separated. Also the fluorescence efficiency has to be high. The latter requirement is more easily met than the former. Quite a number of dyes are known having a fluorescence efficiency of close to 100%. New dyes with better spectral properties and stability are being developed by the chemical industry. The emission and absorption characteristics are not only dependent on the nature of the molecule but also on that of the solvent. The material of the collector has to be highly transparent and a good solvent for dyes. Plastics, glass, or organic solvents contained between plastic or glass sheets are possible candidates for this purpose. It is also possible to apply the dye dissolved in a thin film on the surface of a completely transparent sheet.

Although prices for solar cells have come down considerably in recent years, the cells are still the most expensive part of a flat plate solar generator.

Fluorescent concentrators have the following advantages:

- Concentration of Sunlight without tracking
- Concentration of direct *and* diffuse light. The concentrators are particularly well adapted to overcast conditions that occur frequently in temperate climates
- Possibility of spectrum splitting use of several sheets doped with different dyes shown below

A single semiconductor can never convert sunlight with the highest possible efficiency because quanta with higher energy than the band gap lose their energy by thermalization and those with lower energy are not absorbed. Therefore multijunction cells employing different semiconductors achieve the highest efficiency today.

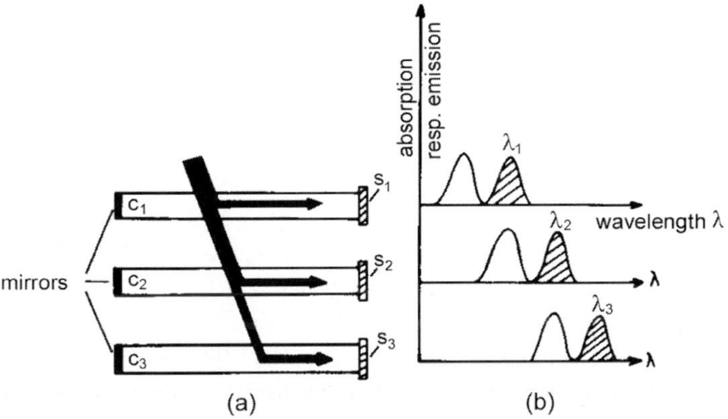

Fig. 10.2. (**a**) Fluorescent concentrator stack. Collectors c_1, c_2, c_3 are combined with solar cells S_1, S_2, S_3 of different bandgaps. (**b**) Absorption and emission (*shaded*) spectra of dyes in c_1–c_3, λ_1–λ_3 are peak emission wavelengths of c_1–c_3

They consist of complex layers of III–V compounds but are very expensive and so they can only in be used concentrating systems.

10.2 Concentrator Stacks

Fluorescent concentrators offer the possibility to separate different portions of the solar spectrum just like multijunction cells and concentrate them at the same time [2]. Figure 10.2(a) shows a stack of three collectors c_1–c_3 contacted by three different solar cells S_1–S_3. The ideal absorption and emission spectra of the fluorescent molecules in the collectors are sketched in Fig. 10.2(b). Because every collector is fully transparent to the unabsorbed part of the spectrum a rather complete separation of the solar spectrum is possible in this manner. The solar cells S_1–S_3 have band gaps adjusted to the emission bands of the collectors. A more detailed analysis carried out below demonstrates that the theoretical energy conversion efficiency is greater than 30% versus 24% for single junction silicon cells (for AM 1.5).

1. Quantum Efficiency of Fluorescent Concentrators

1.1 *Quantum Efficiency of Sequential Stack*

For the calculation of quantum efficiency we put aside the energy loss due to Stokes shift and are only interested in quantum losses. It is assumed that the quantum efficiency of fluorescence is 100%. Reflection losses can be minimized with antireflection layers but even without antireflection coatings the stack offers possibilities for minimizing reflection losses.

Much progress has occurred with antireflective coatings in the last 30 years. They have become more efficient and also more economical. Although such coatings have a lower index of refraction than the collector sheet they do not interfere with total internal reflection because only the difference between medium in which the light is emitted and air is of importance.

For collector stacks the following facts apply: The spectral range for these antireflective coatings becomes narrower and therefore easier to realize for the lower plates of the stack. It can be seen that whereas c_1 has to be transparent for the entire solar spectrum, c_3 only has to operate in the long wavelength range. An additional possibility is use of photonic structures to decrease the loss cone angle as will be described below.

Now the quantum efficiency for a stack of collectors will be calculated. Again normal incidence is assumed. The procedure applied here is the following: The incident spectrum is assumed to be divided into m parts such that each part contains an equal number of photons. This requirement is convenient for computation but not necessary for practical applications. An advantage of the stack is the fact that one half of the escape cone losses of the preceding plate are recovered by the following one. This is seen from Fig. 10.2(b). Collector c_1 emits at wavelength λ_1. If the absorption band of c_2 is arranged as shown in Fig. 10.2(b), c_2 absorbs not only the solar radiation at the wavelength band λ_1 coming from above but also the radiation emitted by the dye in c_1 in the direction of c_2. The same is true for the lower parts of the stack. A recursion formula will now be derived for the quantum efficiency of a stack versus the number of collector plates in the stack. The symbols used in this calculation are given in Fig. 10.3.

The incident radiation S suffers reflection losses R at every interface traversed. Loss of fluorescent radiation not retained in the collectors is indicated by L. As was pointed out already, the loss cone losses directed towards c_2 are recoverable. A minor detail, also indicated in Fig. 10.3 is the fact that reflection of this radiation in leaving c_1 does not have to be taken into account because exactly the same loss occurs at the top surface of the collector thus cancelling the former loss (dashed lines in Fig. 10.3).

Let S_1 be the amount of radiation entering collector c_1 at the absorption band of this collector and C_1 be radiation collected there $S_2, \ldots, S_m$ and $C_2, \ldots, C_m$ are defined accordingly. Then $S_1(\lambda_1) = (1 - R)/m$

$$C_1 = S_1(1 - L).$$

The amount of radiation entering the second collector in the appropriate band is one mth of the incident spectrum attenuated by reflection (multiple reflections are neglected) and augmented by half of the loss from the preceding collector attenuated by reflection upon entering the second collector and so on:

$$S_2(\lambda_2) = (1 - R)^3/m + (1 - R)S_1L/2; \qquad C_2 = S_2(1 - L);$$

$$S_3(\lambda_3) = (1 - R)^5/m + (1 - R)S_2L/2; \qquad C_3 = S_3(1 - L);$$

$$S_4(\lambda_4) = (1 - R)^7/m + (1 - R)S_3L/2; \qquad C_4 = S_4(1 - L);$$

$$\vdots$$

$$S_m(\lambda_m) = (1 - R)2m-1/m + (1 - R)S_{m-1}L/2; \qquad C_m = S_m(1 - L).$$

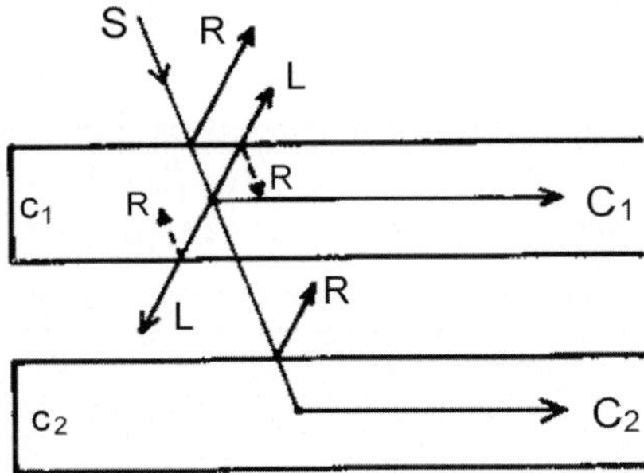

Fig. 10.3. Definition of quantities used in calculation of quantum efficiency. For details see text

Table 10.1. Quantum efficiency η_Q of collector stack

m	1	2	3	4
η_Q	0.7126	0.7299	0.7204	0.7030

The quantum efficiency is the sum:

$$\eta_Q = \sum_{k=1}^{m} C_k.$$
(10.2)

Equation (10.5) will now be evaluated for a realistic case. A common high transparency plastic like Plexiglas with an index of refraction of 1.49 without antireflection coating and $L = 0.2587$.

Obviously the stacking of collectors does not degrade quantum efficiency.

It should be pointed out that the order of dyes in the different sheets as shown in Fig. 10.2 can also be reversed – the longest wavelength on top and the highest at the bottom. This may be advantageous. In this case a band pass mirror as described in the next section can be applied.

10.3 Light Guiding by Photonic Band Pass Mirrors

The loss of fluorescent light through the surfaces of the collector can be entirely avoided by covering the front surface with a wavelength selective mirror (hot mirror) [7, 8]. This mirror should have the following properties:

- A sharp cut-off edge at the onset-wavelength of the dye's emission. All light below this wavelength should be transmitted, all above should be reflected.
- Near 100% reflection for light coming from all directions.

A band pass mirror with non-ideal properties can been realized with commercial hot mirrors [8, 9]. Better results can be expected from photonic structures. First experiments with Rugate structures have shown promising results [10]. It features a continuously varying refractive index profile in contrast to the discrete structure

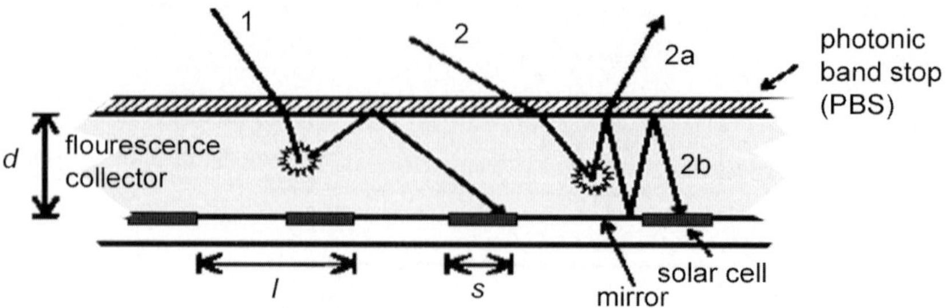

Fig. 10.4. Optimal design of fluorescent collector with band pass mirrors [9]. The coverage factor $f = s^2/l^2$

of normal Bragg reflectors. This results in the suppression of side loops, which would cause unwanted reflection and loss of usable radiation. In [9, 11] it was shown that the ultimate efficiency limits of fluorescent concentrators can only be reached with selective mirrors. On the other hand, light within the loss cone has a long path length before reaching the edges of the concentrator. In this case an arrangement as depicted in Fig. 10.4 is more advantageous.

10.4 Factors Determining Energy Efficiency of Fluorescent Concentrators

For the energy conversion efficiency all energy losses in the collection process have to be taken into account. These are in detail

R Surface reflection coefficient. This is either the Fresnel reflection coefficient or a lower value if an antireflection coating is applied

η_{abs} Absorption efficiency of the dye due to its absorption spectrum with respect to the solar spectrum

η_{qua} Quantum efficiency of dye

η_{stok} "Stokes efficiency"; $(1 - \eta_{stok})$ is the energy loss due to Stokes shift

η_{trap} Efficiency of light trapping by total internal reflection (Loss cone)

η_{dye} Efficiency of light conduction limited by self-absorption of dye

η_{mat} "Matrix efficiency"; $(1 - \eta_{mat})$ is the loss caused by light scattering or absorption in the matrix. η_{dye} and η_{mat} determine the mean free path of the emitted light in the collector

η_{tref} Efficiency of light guiding by total internal reflection. This depends on the surface quality of the matrix

The overall optical efficiency can then be written as:

$$\eta_{opt} = (1 - R)\eta_{abs}\eta_{qua}\eta_{stok}\eta_{trap}\eta_{dye}\eta_{mat}\eta_{tref}. \tag{10.3}$$

These loss factors will now be discussed.

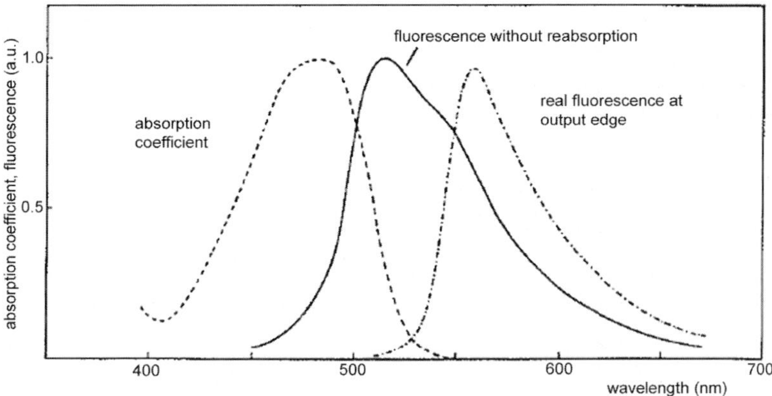

Fig. 10.5. Absorption and emission spectrum of typical dye. Output spectrum is modified by reabsorption

The *surface reflection loss R* is usually the Fresnel reflection loss. It is given by $[(n-1)/(n+1)]^2$ where n is the refractive index. For most transparent materials it amounts to about 4% per surface. It can be minimized by employing an antireflection coating. If it has a sooth surface it will not interfere with total internal reflection.

The *absorption loss* η_{abs} is determined by the fraction of the solar spectrum absorbed by the dye. Practically all dyes absorb only part of the solar spectrum. It is possible to incorporate more than one dye into a collector, leading to a cascade of absorption and reemission. A disadvantage is that at every emission part of the radiation escapes through the loss cone. If the dyes are located very close to one another radiationless energy transfer can occur via the Förster mechanism. Therefore doping of a thin surface region of the collector with a high concentration of dyes may have advantages.

The *quantum efficiencies* η_{qua} of the dyes can vary considerably. Only dyes with efficiency close to unity are usable. Fortunately dyes with such efficiency and good stability are available but this refers only to the visible range.

The *Stokes loss* η_{stok} is caused by the frequency shift between absorbed and emitted light. It is inherent in the fluorescence process. On one hand this shift should be small to minimize the energy loss, on the other it should be large enough to avoid overlap of absorption and emission loss (related to η_{dye}).

The light trapping efficiency η_{trap} is given by L (from (10.1)). It increases with increasing refractive index of the collector material. In practice there are only little differences of available materials.

η_{dye} designates the efficiency limitation caused by *self absorption of the dye*. All known dyes have a certain overlap of absorption and emission spectrum as shown in Fig. 10.5. Also shown in this Figure is how the spectrum is modified by multiple reabsorption and emission. The spectrum at the output is then red shifted. It has also been found that dyes cause a very small absorption within the emission region and beyond [12]. This absorption is difficult to determine but can have great influence on the overall efficiency. A further effect causing unwanted absorption are photodegradation products caused by degradation of dyes [13]. These products can be annealed by heating in the dark.

η_{mat} is the *efficiency due to scattering or absorption in the matrix*. It depends strongly on purity and preparation of the matrix.

Total internal reflection is theoretically lossless but in practice it depends on the surface finish of the matrix. This loss η_{tref} can in principle be completely avoided by employing a reflecting band pass filter at the surface of the collector as pointed out above. Ideally this filter should also serve as an antireflection coating for the wavelength region absorbed by the dye to reduce R.

10.5 Theoretical Limits of Concentration and Efficiency

10.5.1 Limit of Concentration

Let us first consider a conventional concentrator based on geometric optics. In this case the concentration is limited by the conservation of étendue or Liouville's theorem which relates the beam divergence at the input and output aperture. The most efficient concentrator is the Compound Parabolic Concentrator (CPC) that can approach the theoretical limits.

The concentration ratio C is given (for three dimensions) by:

$$C \le \frac{n \sin^2 \theta_2}{\sin^2 \theta_1} \tag{10.4}$$

where C is the concentration factor, θ_1 = input angle of light, and θ_2 = output angle at receiver. If diffuse light is to be concentrated, $\theta_1 = 90°$ and therefore the maximum concentration is limited to n^2 which is about a factor of two for most available transparent materials.

On the other hand, geometrical concentration can be very effective at very small input angles. For solar radiation the limiting input angle is given by the viewing angle of the sun. Therefore tracking concentrators for direct radiation permit very high concentration.

The maximum concentration of the fluorescent concentrator has been determined by Yablonovitch [14] and Smestad et al. [7]. They point out that because of the energy loss due to the Stokes effect the system operates like an optical heat pump. The radiance at a given energy is increased by changing some of the incoming energy to heat.

For fluorescent concentrators the concentration factor is determined by:

$$C \le \frac{(\nu_2)}{(\nu_1)} \exp\left(\frac{h(\nu_1 - \nu_2)}{KT}\right) \tag{10.5}$$

where ν_1 = frequency of absorbed light, ν_2 = frequency of emitted light. The concentration factor depends only on the magnitude of the Stokes shift. So concentration occurs at the sacrifice of energy efficiency.

10.5.2 Limit of Efficiency

The limits of efficiency were examined by Rau et al. [9], Glaeser and Rau [10] and Markvart et al. [15, 16]. They showed that the detailed balance principle introduced into solar cell physics by Shockley and Queisser [17] can also be used for the fluorescent concentrator-solar cell system. They investigated a single stage concentrator and found that very high efficiency is possible provided the concentrator surface is covered by a perfect band pass mirror. In [9, 10] Monte-Carlo simulations were employed to obtain relations between efficiency, band gap energy and coverage fraction. In Fig. 10.6 are presented the results of these calculations.

The simulated efficiencies for a fluorescent concentrator ($f = 1$) *with PBS* (open squares) follow the radiative Shockley–Queisser efficiency limit η_{rad} (solid line) when calculated with reference to the photonic threshold energy E_{th}. The efficiencies *without PBS* (open circles) are at about $0.88 \times \eta_{\mathrm{rad}}$ (dashed line) calculated with reference to the band gap energy $E_{\mathrm{g}} = E_{\mathrm{th}} - 0.2$ eV of the underlying solar cell. (b) Efficiencies for a band gap energy $E_{\mathrm{g}} = 1.12$ eV and threshold energy $E_{\mathrm{th}} = 1.32$ eV for ideal (rad.) and non-ideal (nonrad.) solar cells. *Without* photonic band stop (PBS) the efficiencies degrade monotonically with decreasing coverage fraction f (full and open circles, for the radiative and the non-radiative case). *With* PBS the system's efficiency drops much slower for an ideal solar cell (open squares) and even achieves an optimum at $f \approx 10^{-2}$ in the non-radiative case (full squares).

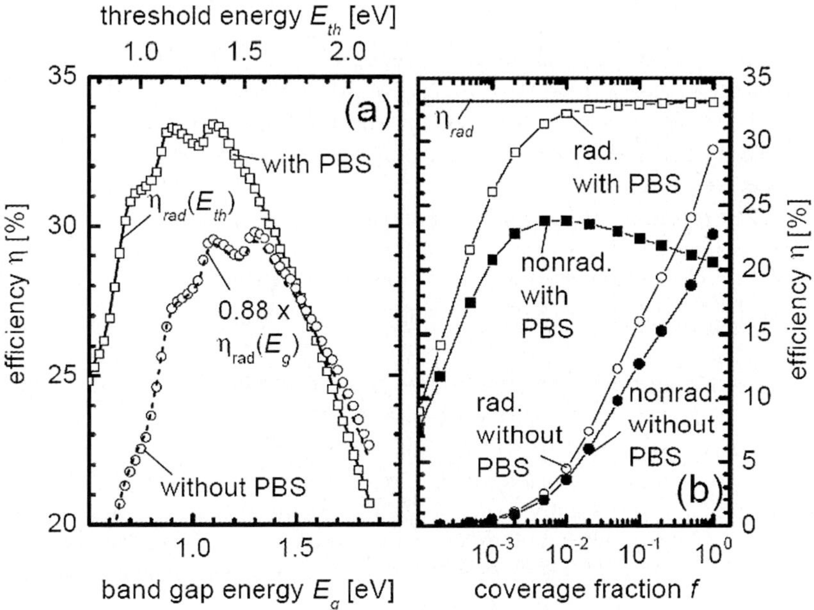

Fig. 10.6. Monte-Carlo simulations [9, 10]. For explanations see text

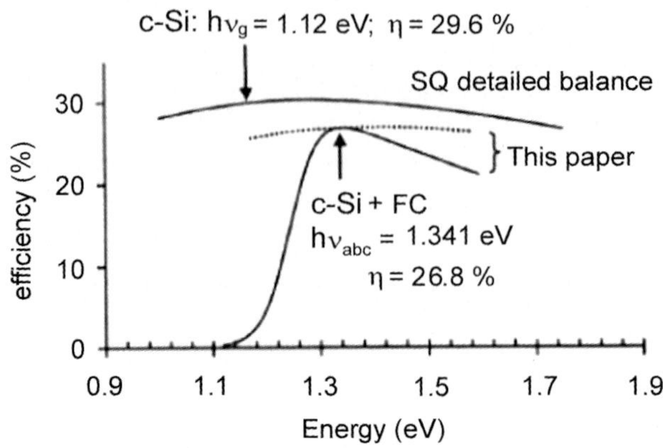

Fig. 10.7. Conversion efficiency of an ideal Si cell with and without a fluorescent concentrator

Comparable results were obtained by Markvart [15, 16] as shown in Fig. 10.7. It is seen that ideal efficiency is 26.8% vs. 29.6% without concentrator.

10.6 Improvements of Basic Design

10.6.1 Optical Concentrators at the Collector Output

This is a very old proposal [18]: At the edge of a collector plate a concentrating element (taper or more effective a CPC) is attached before the solar cell (Fig. 10.8). The additional concentration possible in this manner is given by (4). This additional concentration rests on two facts: The divergence angle of incoming rays is limited by the onset angle of total internal reflection and can then further be converted to 90°. The collector material can be made of a material of higher index of refraction than the collector material. A concentration factor between 1.5 and 2 is thus possible.

10.6.2 Combination of Fluorescent Collector with Large Area Si-Solar Cell

Because at present no dyes emitting in the IR with acceptable properties are available, a good compromise is the following concept [10] (Fig. 10.9).

A fluorescent concentrator doped with a dye emitting in the red or orange is equipped with a GaInP cell that has its maximum response in this range. The collector is transparent to all radiation not absorbed by the dye that is converted by a large area silicon cell at the bottom. Figure 10.10 shows the efficiencies of the silicon cell alone and the combined system. The silicon cell *without the concentrator had an efficiency of 16.7%. Under the fluorescent concentrator the efficiency dropped to 14.0%. The total system efficiency was 17.7%, which is significantly higher than the silicon solar cell alone.*

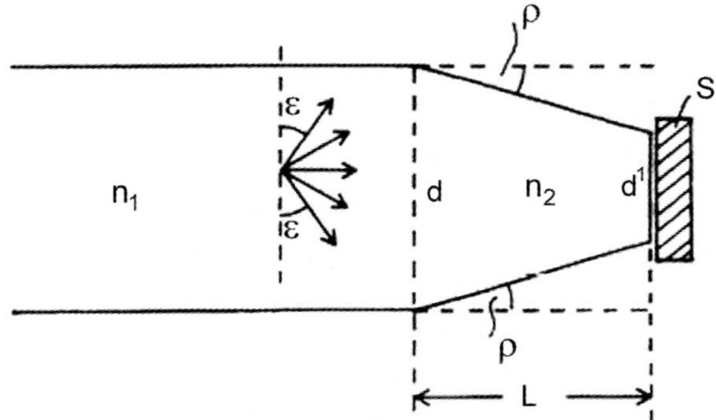

Fig. 10.8. Fluorescent collector with two stage concentration by attached taper with refractive index $n_2 > n_1$

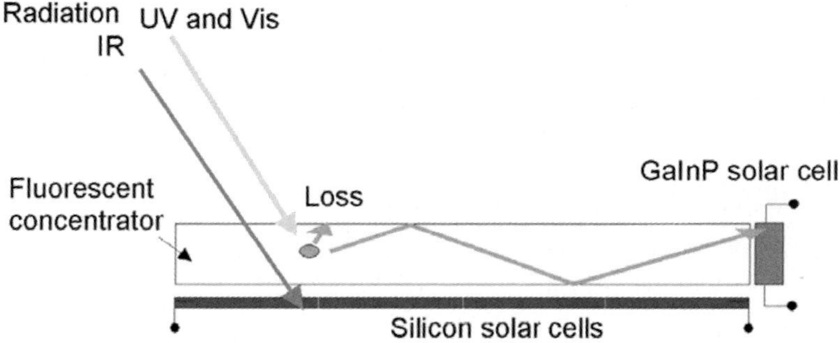

Fig. 10.9. Combination of a short wavelength fluorescent concentrator with attached GaInP cell and Si bottom cell [10]

10.6.3 Combination of Fluorescent Concentrator with Up-Conversion

Recently great progress has been achieved with up-converters – compounds that combine two or more quanta to a higher energy quantum [19].

This effect can also be useful for fluorescent concentrators as indicated in Fig. 10.11.

Below the fluorescent collector an up-converter and a mirror is arranged. The spectral properties of the fluorescent collector and the up-converter are shown below. The dye in the collector shifts the absorbed wavelength range to longer wavelength above the band energy of the solar cell. So the photons emitted downwards are converted by the up-converter to shorter wavelength to be reabsorbed by the collector. Furthermore the collector is transparent to the solar spectrum within the emission range of the dye in the collector. These photons will also be converted to higher wavelengths.

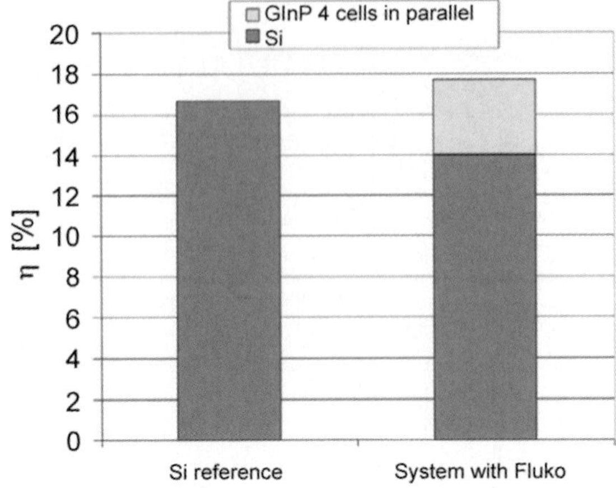

Fig. 10.10. Efficiency of silicon cell alone and of total system

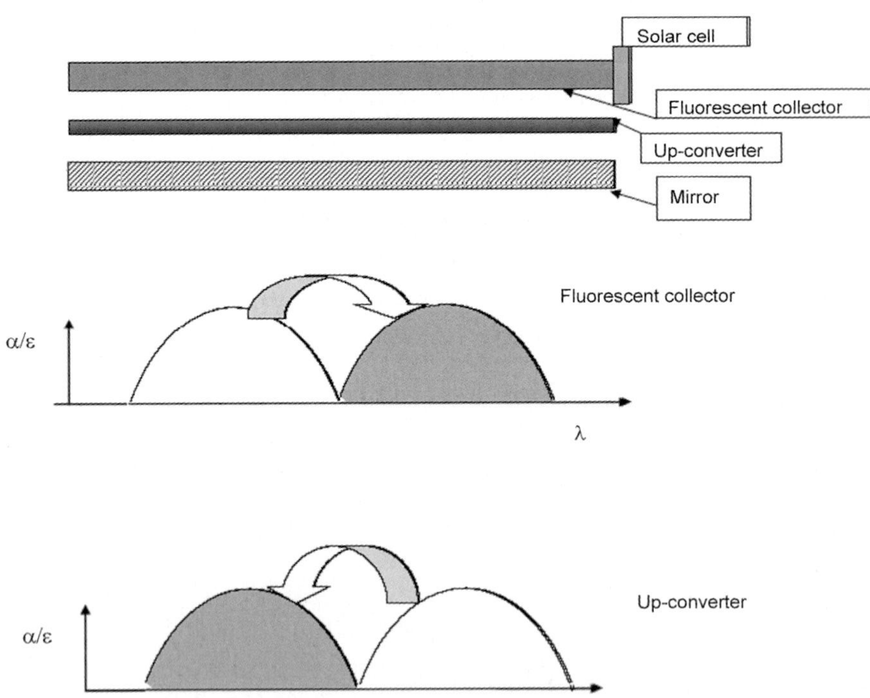

Fig. 10.11. Fluorescent collector combined with up-converter. For explanation of function see text

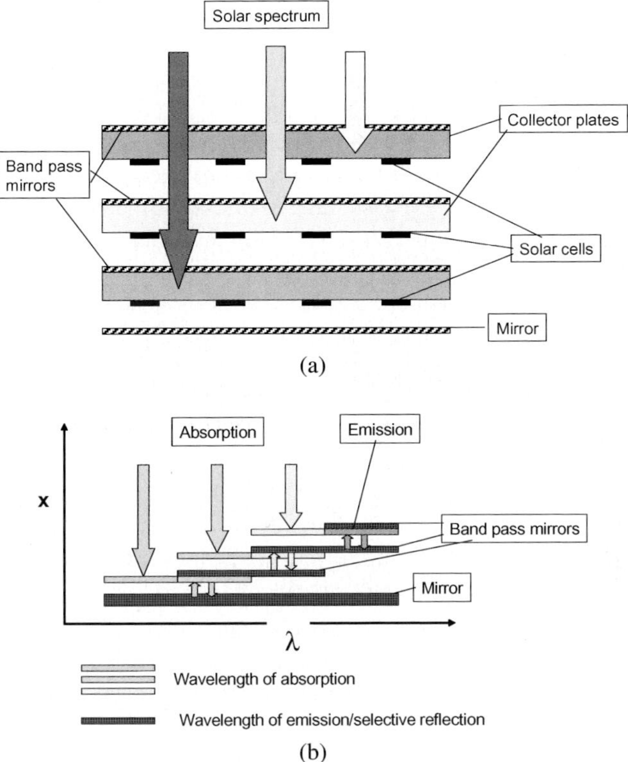

Fig. 10.12. Fluorescent collector stack with band pass reflectors. (**a**) Geometrical arrangement, (**b**) wavelength representation

Table 10.2. Electrical efficiencies for 40×40 cm^2 collectors with Si and GaAs cells. Highest efficiency of 4.0% was obtained with a double stack and GaAs cells

Dimension (cm^3)	Absorption range (nm)	Efficiency		
		Si	(%)	GaAs
$40 \times 40 \times 0.3$	360–550	2.1		2.5
$40 \times 40 \times 0.3$	490–610	1.4		2.5
Stack of both	360–610	3.0		4.0

10.6.4 Combination of Collector Stack with Band Pass Mirror

The collector stack can also be combined with a band pass mirror as described in Sect. 10.3 if conditions are chosen appropriately. For this purpose the following conditions apply:

- Longest wavelength dye on top
- Solar cells placed below each other
- Transparent electrical connections

In Fig. 10.12(a) the stacking of the collectors is sketched, in Fig. 10.12(b) we see the wavelength diagram. Consider the top plate: The dye absorbs in the yellow and emits in the red. (In reality it would be infrared.) The upper mirror reflects the emitted radiation but is transparent for all other wavelengths, downward emitted radiation is reflected by the lower mirror which extends into this wavelength region as indicated by the short arrows. The lower plates operate in the same manner.

The collector stack with band pass mirrors offers intriguing prospects: It is the only device that can concentrate diffuse radiation and could also approach highest conversion efficiency. While the original fluorescent concentrator shown in Fig. 10.2 has a theoretical efficiency of about 30%, the new design can go much higher. From Fig. 10.7 we derive that a one plate concentrator with a silicon cell has a theoretical efficiency of 90% of the thermodynamic efficiency. A collector stack is a spectrum splitting device and can now achieve an efficiency close to that of a multi-junction cell. If we assume the theoretical efficiency to be 60%, the multi-stage fluorescent concentrator has a theoretical efficiency of 54%.

Obviously, many difficulties have to be overcome to reach this goal, such as: Near ideal band pass mirrors are needed, the dyes should have well defined absorption bands without absorption in the shorter wavelengths and appropriate wide gap solar cells have to be available. In addition the cost should be competitive.

10.7 Experimental Results

10.7.1 Results of the Initial Period

Experimental work can be divided into two periods: The initial period from 1977 to about 1985 and the more recent period which started about 2000. The older results are still meaningful because they represent benchmarks to be reached and exceeded in present work. The most interesting parameters are the overall electrical efficiency and the long term stability of the collectors. These are in turn influenced by the properties of matrix and dye. In comparing efficiencies the dimensions of the samples are very important. Results of the early period are summarized in review papers by Wittwer et al. [20] and Zastrow [21].

The efficiency of 4% is still the highest value that has been realized for such a large area. The second most important issue is stability of the collector dye-system under illumination. It could be observed that by continued development the stability of the dyes improved during the course of the work. A representative measurement is shown in Fig. 10.13. The cumulative illumination corresponds to more than two years of outdoors exposure. Also clearly seen is the recovery of fluorescence during periods of darkness.

A problem that continues to limit efficiency is the lack of useful long wavelength dyes. They still have low quantum efficiency and are not very stable. Figure 10.14 gives a compilation of quantum efficiencies found until 1984. It is evident that there is a general tendency is towards lower efficiency when emission wavelength increases.

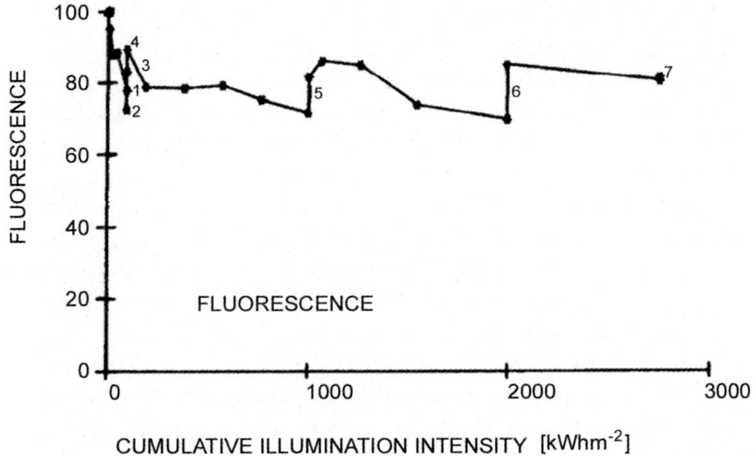

Fig. 10.13. Fluorescence during long term light exposure in kWh/m^2. Fluorescence is normalized to maximum value

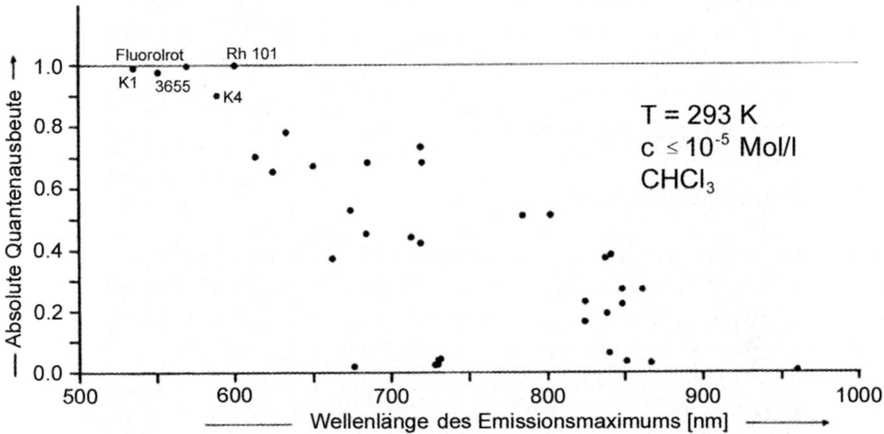

Fig. 10.14. Quantum efficiencies of different dyes vs. peak emission wavelength

10.7.2 Recent Experimental and Theoretical Work

L. Danos et al. [22] characterized fluorescent concentrators based on solid, liquid and Langmuir Blodget films. A. Chatten et al. [23] have developed a self-consistent 3D thermodynamic model for planar concentrators, modules and stacks. The results for test concentrators containing both quantum dots and organic dyes as the luminescent species show excellent agreement with experiment.

Organic dyes are still the best choice for fluorescent concentrators as shown in [24]. In this paper by Richards and McIntosh collectors doped with multiple dyes were investigated by ray tracing using experimental data from newly available dyes. In such a collector multiple dyes are absorbed and reemitted by increasingly longer

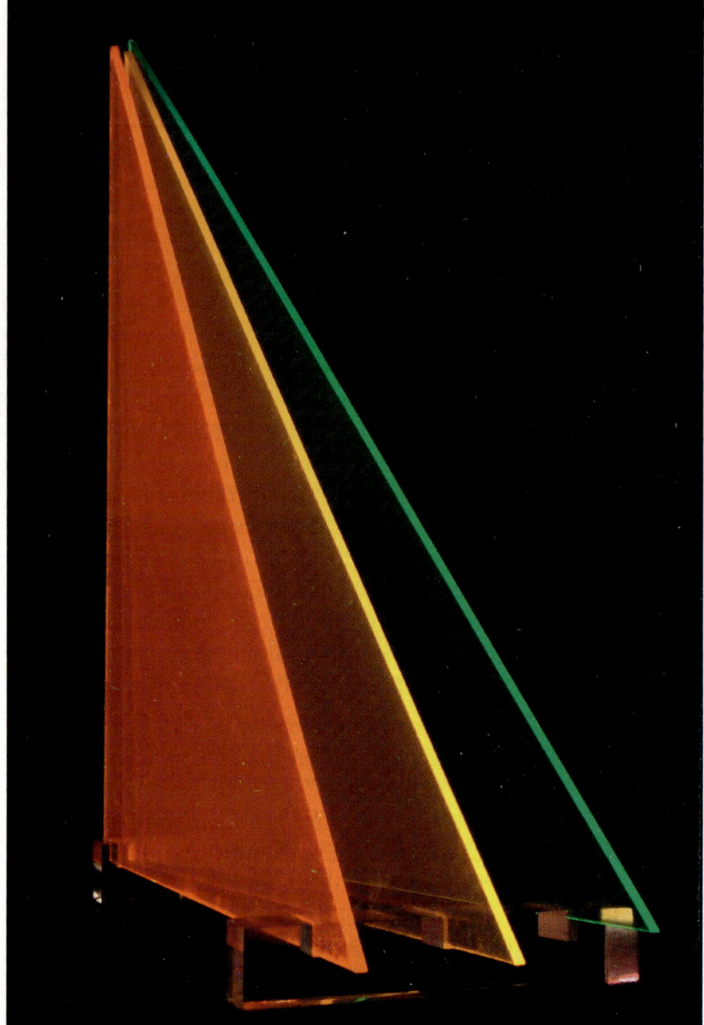

Fig. 10.15. Three PMMA plates doped with different color dyes. These plates are about 25 years old but not degraded, they were however mostly stored in the dark. Although the light output looks very spectacular only part of the light arriving at the edges is emitted because a big part is reflected back by total internal reflection

wavelength dyes. In this manner a large part of the solar spectrum is absorbed and emission occurs at a wavelength which is more suitable for silicon cells. They found that a mixture of five dyes including a near IR dye of 85% quantum efficiency gave the best result of 44% electrical efficiency. Only radiative transfer and high efficiency solar cells were studied. They also state that all dyes show photostability under sunlight for at least 10 years. Lower stability was found by Reda with more conventional dyes [25].

A new possibility to obtain better performing luminescing centers consists in quantum dots as has been pointed out by Barnham et al. [26]. These are nanometer sized semiconductor crystallites. Because they are anorganic there is hope that they exhibit greater light stability than organic dyes. Another advantage is that the absorption threshold can be tuned by choice of the dot diameter. Furthermore, Chatten et al. [27] showed by a thermodynamic model that the red shift of emission is related to the spread of quantum dot sizes.

In view of these advantages there is considerable interest in developing fluorescent concentrators doped with quantum dots. Numerous investigations were carried out in recent years. Mainly quantum dots based on CdS were used. Schüler [28] applied the dots by the sol-gel technique to glass surfaces but also core-shell quantum dots consisting of CdSe cores with CdS or ZnS shell were studied [29, 30]. So far the quantum dots show continued improvement but quantum efficiency is not yet as high as for the best organic dyes. Also some instability has been observed.

Further, it should be remarked that fluorescent concentrators have applications beyond photovoltaics. They have been in use for advertising for many years. They can also be used in green houses to convert the green light to red light which can be better absorbed by plants [20]. Application for daylighting has been studied in the early days [31] and recent work with newer dyes appears very promising [12].

Finally in Fig. 10.15 I present a photograph of three collector plates as they appear in daylight.

References

1. W.H. Weber, J. Lambe, Appl. Opt. **15**, 2299 (1976)
2. A. Goetzberger, W. Greubel, Solar energy conversion with fluorescent collectors. Appl. Phys. **12**, 123 (1977)
3. W.A. Shurcliff, R.C. Jones, J. Opt. Soc. Am. **39**, 912 (1949)
4. J.B. Birks, *The Theory and Practice of Scintillation Counting* (Pergamon, London, 1964)
5. G. Keil, J. Appl. Phys. **40**, 3544 (1969)
6. G. Keil, Nucl. Instrum. Methods **87**, 111–123 (1970)
7. G. Smestad, H. Riess, R. Winston, E. Yablonovitch, Sol. Energy Mater. **21**, 99 (1990)
8. B.S. Richards, A. Shilav, R. Corkish, 19. EU PV Sol. En. Conf. 113 (2004)
9. U. Rau, F. Einsele, G.C. Glaeser, Appl. Phys. Lett. **87**, 171101 (2005)
10. J.C. Goldschmidt, S.W. Glunz, A. Gombert, G. Willeke 21, EU PV Sol. En. Conf. 107 (2006)
11. G.C. Glaeser, U. Rau, Proc. SPIE **6197**, 143 (2006)
12. A.A. Earp, G.B. Smith, P.D. Swift, J. Franklin, Sol. Energy **76**, 655 (2004)
13. A. Zastrow, H.R. Wilson, K. Heidler, V. Wittwer, A. Goetzberger, *6th EU PV Conf. 202* (1983)
14. E. Yablonovitch, J. Opt. Soc. Am. **70**, 1362 (1980)
15. T. Markvart, J. Appl. Phys. **99**, 026101 (2006)
16. T. Markvart, L. Danos, P. Kittidachachan, R. Greef, *20. EU PV Sol. En. Conf. 171* (2005)

17. W. Shockley, H.J. Queisser, J. Appl. Phys. **32**, 510 (1961)
18. A. Goetzberger, O. Schirmer, Appl. Phys. **19**, 53 (1979)
19. S. Balushev, T. Miteva, V. Yakutin, G. Nelles, A. Yasuda, G. Wegner, Appl. Phys. Lett. **14**, 143903 (2006)
20. V. Wittwer, W. Stahl, A. Goetzberger, Sol. Energy Mater. **11**, 187 (1984)
21. A. Zastrow, SPIE **2255**, 534 (1993)
22. L. Danos, P. Kittidachachan, P.J.J. Meyer, R. Greef, T. Markvart, *21. EU PV Sol. En. Conf. 443* (2006)
23. A.J. Chatten, D.J. Farrell, B.F. Buxton, A. Büchtemann, K.W.J. Barnham, *21. EU PV Sol. En. Conf. 315* (2006)
24. B.S. Richards, K.R. McIntosh, *21. EU PV Sol. En. Conf. 185* (2006)
25. S.M. Reda, Sol. Energy **81**, 755 (2007)
26. K. Barnham, J.L. Marques, J. Hassard, P. O'Brien, Appl. Phys. Lett. **76**, 1197 (2000)
27. A.J. Chatten et al., Sol. Energy Mater. Sol. Cells **75**, 363 (2003)
28. A. Schüler, M. Python, M. Valle del Olmo, E. de Chambrier, Sol. Energy **81**, 1159 (2007)
29. S.J. Gallagher, B. Norton, P.C. Eames, Sol. Energy **81**, 813 (2007)
30. S.J. Gallagher, B.C. Rowan, J. Doran, B. Norton, Sol. Energy **81**, 540 (2007)
31. A. Zastrow, V. Wittwer, Proc. SPIE **653**, 93 (1986)

11 Hybrid Photovoltaic/Thermal Collector Based on a Luminescent Concentrator

V. Petrova-Koch and A. Goetzberger

11.1 Introduction

The efficiency of a single-junction PV cell – for example, a c-Si solar cell – has a theoretical limit of around 27%–30% [1]. This means that, in the best-case scenario, the device harvests around one-fourth of the solar energy. This relatively low efficiency is due to the impossibility of converting the broad solar spectrum with one semiconductor material. The single-junction cell represents a relatively narrow band, two-terminal device. The spectrally distributed solar radiation requires, in principle, a many-terminal or multijunction device in order to reach a high conversion efficiency. When the single junction is replaced by a multijunction cell in practice, efficiency rises substantially (to about 40% in the last few years, for the triple-junction III–V-based PV cells [2]). But even then it remains relatively low.

The introduction of an intermediate band into the semiconductor band gap [3], or solar thermophotovoltaics [4] are other innovative ways to increase the efficiency of a PV cell, but again the efficiency improvement is about the same.

Concentration of solar radiation is a prerequisite to achieve these high efficiencies. [5], and concentrator photovoltaics (CPV) have good prospects for terrestrial applications. There are two principally different ways to concentrate solar radiation. One is CPV based on geometrical optics using, for example, an array of Fresnel lenses with a tracking system [5], and is suitable for concentration of direct solar radiation only. The other type of CPV is based on the luminescent concentrator (LuCo), which is the only device known with a chance to concentrate not only direct but also diffuse solar radiation without need of a tracking system [6].

Hybrid solar collectors are an attractive approach to harvesting electricity and heat simultaneously. This will reduce the cost of the modules, and will increase significantly the total efficiency of the system. Numerous attempts have been made in the past to develop such collectors, but there was little commercial success.

In principle, all the absorbed solar radiation which does not undergo conversion to electricity in a solar cell gets converted to heat. It is well known that the conversion efficiency of a solar cell drops as temperature increases. The temperature dependence depends on band gap: Solar cells with a large band gap are less sensitive than those with lower gap. Therefore crystalline Si has a higher temperature coefficient than amorphous silicon.

The common practice is to integrate the solar module into the thermal absorber. This concept causes the well-known discrepancy that higher absorber temperature is not compatible with good performance of the solar cells. Furthermore, the solar cells do not provide a selective surface that is best for the absorber. As a result, hybrid collectors provide only relatively low temperatures. Nevertheless, many applications can be envisioned for such collectors. There is an IEA task 35 (PV/T) that is devoted to the promotion of hybrid collectors. The most recent information on this subject can be found at its website [7].

11.2 PV/T Hybrid Collector Based on a Luminescent Concentrator

If a luminescent concentrator is used in a PV/T hybrid collector, it offers a unique possibility to separate electrical and thermal conversion spectrally and in space. The incident solar radiation is split by the luminescing plate spectrally and spatially into two parts, as shown in Fig. 11.1.

The collector is constructed like a common thermal collector with the addition of a luminescing concentrator plate inserted between the cover glass and the absorber. Silicon PV Cells (mono- or bifacial, as presented in Chaps. 6 and 7) are positioned on one or several side edges of the plate. The other edges of the plate are mirrored. The luminescent plate is assumed to be doped with one or several dyes that transform the solar radiation into the red or near infrared fluorescence or phosphorescence that is best used by the silicon solar cell. It is possible to use a single dye or quantum dots with a broad absorption spectrum or a multistage sequence of dyes. The solar cells are positioned outside of the collector and thus are not exposed to high temperature.

The thermal energy reaching the absorber comes from several sources:

- The luminescent plate acts as a heat source because heat is generated by Stokes losses in the plate. Dependent on the temperature difference between LuCo plate

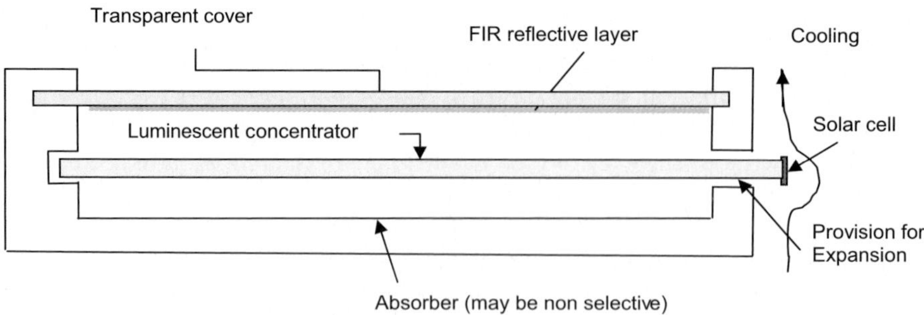

Fig. 11.1. The concept of a PV/T hybrid collector based on the luminescent solar concentrator

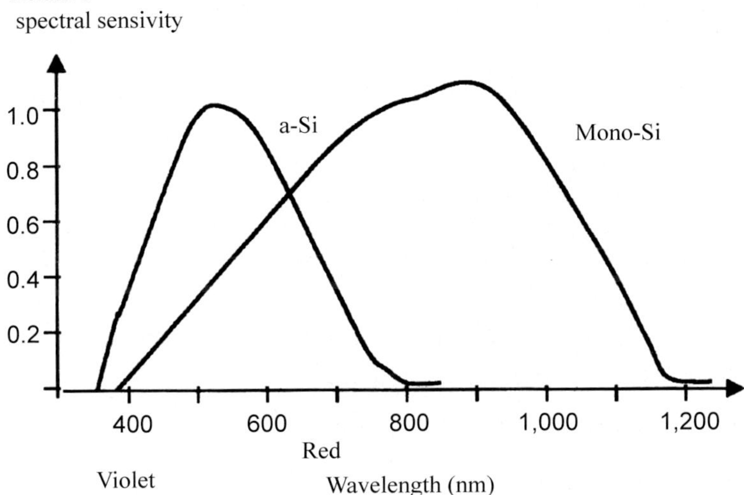

Fig. 11.2. Spectral response curves of amorphous and crystalline silicon

and absorber thermal radiation and heat flowing by conduction and convection reaches the absorber. Nonselectivity of the absorber may be advantageous.

- The luminescent plate is transparent to the infrared part of the solar spectrum. This radiation reaches the absorber directly. Onset of transmission of the LuCo plate is at the long wavelength edge of the dye absorption.
- As pointed out in the preceding article, about 25% of luminescent radiation is emitted to the outside of the plate. One half of this radiation emitted downwards will also reach the absorber. If radiation is reabsorbed by the same or other dyes in the matrix, the loss is repeated.

In order to reduce heat losses through the front plate its inside can carry an FIR reflecting coating.

The PL spectrum of the luminescent concentrator should be designed to match the spectral sensitivity curve of the solar cells (Fig. 11.2). By making use of only this part of the solar spectrum, heating of the cell will be suppressed substantially. Both crystalline and amorphous silicon are feasible. In the amorphous case, a larger part of the long wavelength spectrum would be transmitted to the absorber. From an efficiency standpoint, however, crystalline silicon is preferred.

A very rough estimate of the efficiency of the LuCo hybrid collector is now possible.

The PV efficiency can be expected to be between 5% and 10%, referred to as total collector area. This depends on the availability of suitable dyes.

The thermal efficiency of the collector (excluding system efficiency) can be expected to be between 50% and 60% in the temperature range used for water heating.

The advantages of the LuCo hybrid collector are as follows:

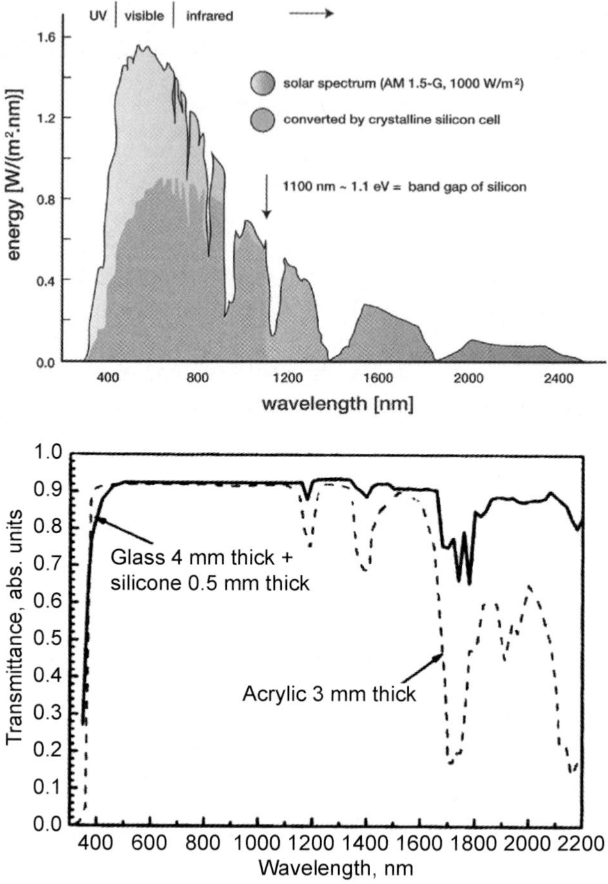

Fig. 11.3. A typical transmittance spectrum of a solar glass plate compared with that of an acrylic plate with similar thickness together with the terrestrial solar AM1.5 spectrum [5]

- High combined thermal plus electrical conversion efficiency.
- High geometrical PV concentration, thus the cost of solar cells is reduced.
- Solar cells can operate at close to ambient temperature.

Several difficulties associated with this concept should not be overlooked. They refer mostly to materials such as:

Thermal stability of the LuCo plates. So far only plastic materials have been used because very high transparency is required. Polycarbonate rather than PMMA is advised. Even better would be glass if it can be made with comparable transparency. It should be noted that the dye does not have to be distributed throughout the matrix but can also be incorporated in a thin surface film at much higher concentration, as reported recently in Scince [8].

For the present application, transparency of the matrix in the near infrared is important because it has to be transmitted within the matrix to the solar cell. Figure 11.3 shows the solar spectrum and transparency of glass and acrylic. Glass is more transparent than plastic beyond 1,200 nm.

11.3 Conclusions

This chapter describes a novel concept for a PV/T hybrid based on the luminescent solar energy collector, particularly suitable for application with highly efficient c-Si solar cells, mono- or bifacial. This collector separates electrical and thermal conversion and thus allows the solar cells to operate at lower temperature while the thermal absorber is at high temperature.

References

1. A. Goetzberger, V.U. Hoffmann, in *Photovoltaic Solar Energy Generation*. Springer Series Optical Science, vol. 12 (2005), p. 58
2. A.W. Bett, F. Dimroth, G. Siefer, Multi-junction concentrator solar cells, in *Concentrator Photovoltaics*. Springer Series in Optical Sciences, vol. 130 (2007), p. 67
3. A. Luque, A. Marti, A metallic intermediate band high efficiency solar cell, in *Prog. Photovoltaics*, vol. 9 (2001), pp. 73–86
4. V. Andreev, V. Khvostikov, A. Vlasov, Solar thermophotovoltaics, in *Concentrator Photovoltaics*. Springer Series in Optical Sciences, vol. 130 (2007), p. 175
5. V.D. Rumyantsev, Terrestrial concentrator PV systems, in *Concentrator Photovoltaics*. Springer Series in Optical Sciences, vol. 130 (2007), p. 150
6. A. Goetzberger, Fluorescent Solar Energy Concentrator: Present State of Development. Chapter in this book
7. www.iea-shc.org
8. M.J. Curie, J.K. Mapel, T.D. Heiden, Sh. Goffri, M.A. Baldo, *High Efficiency Organic Solar Concentrator for Photovoltaics in Scince*, vol. 321 (2008), p. 226

12 Installation Concept and Future Applications

O. Mayer

12.1 PV from the Customer Perspective

With annual growth rates exceeding 30%, photovoltaic (PV) energy is now firmly established as a decentralized source for generating power. Due in particular to German legislation promoting renewable energies (Renewable Energy Sources Act/EEG), PV has in recent years made triumphant advances.

If one considers the technology currently in deployment (in 2008), the following is ascertainable:

Roof-mounted installation is used for the vast majority of PV systems (that is to say, the system is mounted on top of an existing roof). The preponderance of this method is due to the current preference for "retrofitting" PV systems onto existing roofs. In such cases, dual functionalities are not exploited.

The criterion for a PV system is the maximum possible degree of generator efficiency. This is necessitated by the target of obtaining the maximum possible packing density on a limited roof area in order to reap maximum energy yields.

For the time being, building-integrated PV (BIPV) continues to play a subordinate role.

Consideration of the product range available at present (in 2008) shows that the majority of products consist of flat PV modules in which the blue silicon cells are clearly visible; when installed on a roof, the aesthetic effect is not particularly pleasing (Fig. 12.1).

This understandable lack of attention to aesthetic considerations was also expedient in view of the time frame in which the technology was developed. The target was to introduce and advance PV as a power-generation technology. In order to ensure competitive ability with existing systems, efficiency was the primary concern.

However, now that even the general public is familiar with PV technology, the target course of PV must be altered. Until now, the direction taken by PV was "dictated" by engineers in line with the following objectives:

High efficiency
High reliability
Simple installation
Low costs/Wp

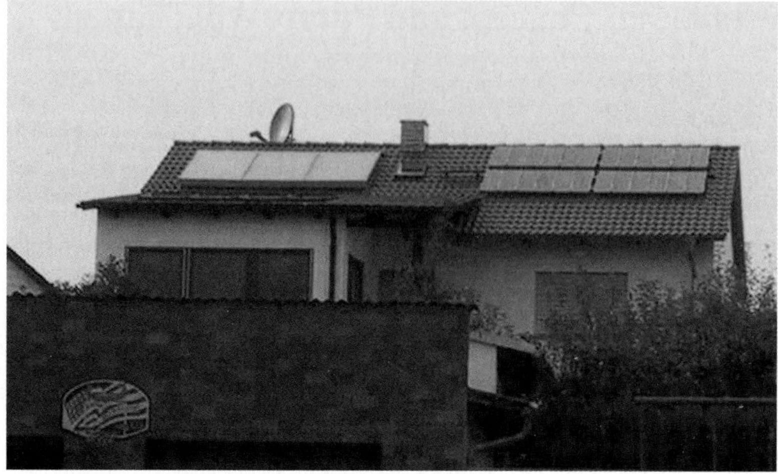

Fig. 12.1. Typical roof-mounted installation of a solar-thermal and PV system. (Source: Mayer, private photograph)

"Maximum output on the smallest space" – the perspective of the power engineer – was decisive in the development process. In view of the fact that contemporary PV systems are no longer in their technological infancy, the technology must be viewed from a new perspective. The crucial question to be asked is:

What do customers want, and for what are they willing to pay?

This question may be viewed analogously with developments in the automobile industry. While technical attributes (performance, reliability, costs, and so forth), were formerly crucial selling points for vehicles, contemporary advertising promotes wholly different characteristics (motoring experience, emotion, safety, and so forth). It is universally assumed that the performance attributes of a car are delivered automatically, and need not be queried. For the manufacturer, this leads to the question of how his or her product can be distinguished from those of the competition – the question of the differentiators or Unique Selling Points (USPs).

The KANO model (Fig. 12.2) reflects this view of customer satisfaction. Many functionalities are taken as given, and not even addressed by the customer. If only these functionalities are delivered, then customer satisfaction is scarcely achievable (red arrow). Performance characteristics desired by and imaginable to the customer lead to customer satisfaction (yellow arrow). The truly interesting attributes, however, are those which surpass the customer's conceptions and are unexpected (green arrow). They are the ones which produce enthusiasm for the product and amount to a differentiator, or unique selling point (USP). However, it must be noted that in the course of time such attributes likewise turn into ones which are automatically expected and assumed to be given.

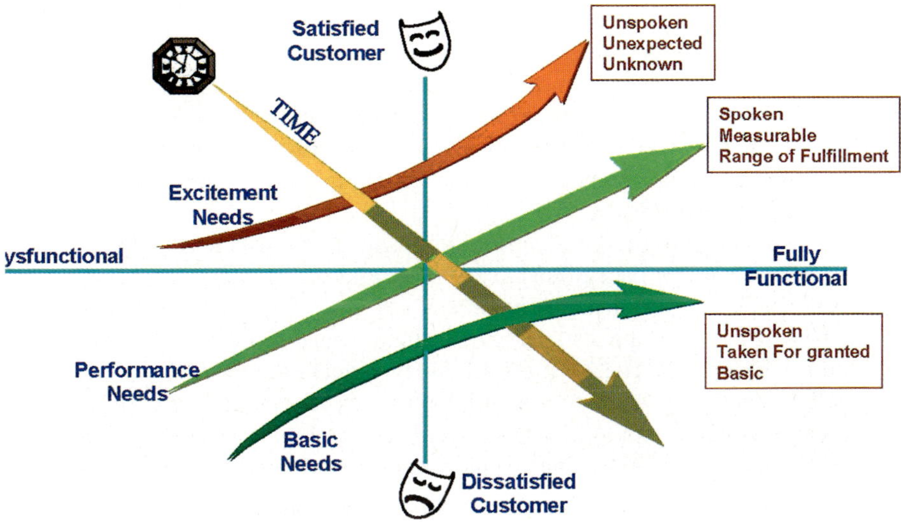

Fig. 12.2. KANO model for customer requirements. (Source: SixSigma, modified)

If one considers those applications at present feasible for PV as systems technology, there exist a number of customer requirements that do not simply translate into €/Wp. Figure 3.2 shows an overview of possible applications of PV.

When a PV system is used to feed energy to the grid in accordance with the EEG, the foremost concern is to obtain the maximum possible power yield per capital investment (distributed over the life of the system). In comparison with the efficiency of the modules, this aspect attributes a new status to parameters such as useful life of the components, costs of the balance of system (BOS), and maintenance costs. Efficiency is not directly relevant, but becomes significant due to the limited space for the installation (e.g. roof area). All these variables –and not just the cell/module efficiency – must be cooptimized.

In the case of standalone systems, a high peak output (depending on application) may be necessary alongside a high energy yield – for example, if information is required to be transmitted at a specific, periodic time or, like in the case of a pumping system, high midday water requirements simultaneously entail the need for disinfecting.

Other applications such as motor vehicles offer only very limited space on which to generate power. Therefore, the high efficiency of PV cells/modules becomes the dominant parameter. This is especially true when the power requirement is predefined by the existing ventilation system, for example in the case of vehicle air-conditioning systems.

When PV is used to provide power in extraterrestrial applications, the important aspects in addition to high efficiency are useful life, maintenance-freedom (reliability), and low weight. These parameters may well be more important than high efficiency, since the advantage gained by the latter is questionable if reliability is low. Due to technical considerations and the costs, the possibility of repairs in outer space is more or less ruled out.

When PV is used in the form of facade elements, then this technology competes with other facade constructions, whereby the comparative costs per square meter are decisive. The fact that a PV facade also allows electricity to be generated is, in this case, a secondary sales argument – a unique selling point (USP) or "differentiator" over competitive products.

When PV is deployed as an architectural element, the efficiency aspect moves almost entirely into the background. The dominant aspects are aesthetic in nature: the "look" and the impression are crucial.

In the case of other applications (garden lights, pond fountains, etc.), the flexibility of PV is decisive. The PV must be able to adapt to the product requirements, above all in regard to form and color. High efficiency is secondary in importance.

In the case of concentrator systems, a high degree of thermal endurance must be guaranteed, and tracking mechanism and inverter performance have to comply with precision requirements.

Especially relevant in the case of PV water supply are the costs per cubic meter of water. While cell/module efficiency likewise plays a role, it is merely one aspect among several (drilling costs, space requirement, reliability, 24-hour maximum permissible failure duration, BOS, etc.).

12.2 PV Deployment Today

Contemporary terrestrial PV systems may be divided into the following groups:

- Nondomestic stand-alone systems
- Domestic standalone systems
- Grid-connected centralized PV systems
- Grid-connected decentralized PV systems

Figure 12.3 shows the development of PV in countries which are members of the International Energy Agency. Grid-connected systems represent the largest share.

12.2.1 Nondomestic Standalone Systems

Nondomestic standalone systems are mainly systems supplying electricity to villages in regions formerly lacking grid electricity. Solar generators and/or wind-turbine systems are deployed as power generators, and an energy-management system provides the grid supply to a village, for example (Fig. 12.4).

In such applications a subordinate role is played by space requirements or aesthetics. At the present time, there is little demand for multifunctional characteristics; with such systems, the crucial criterion is price per Wp.

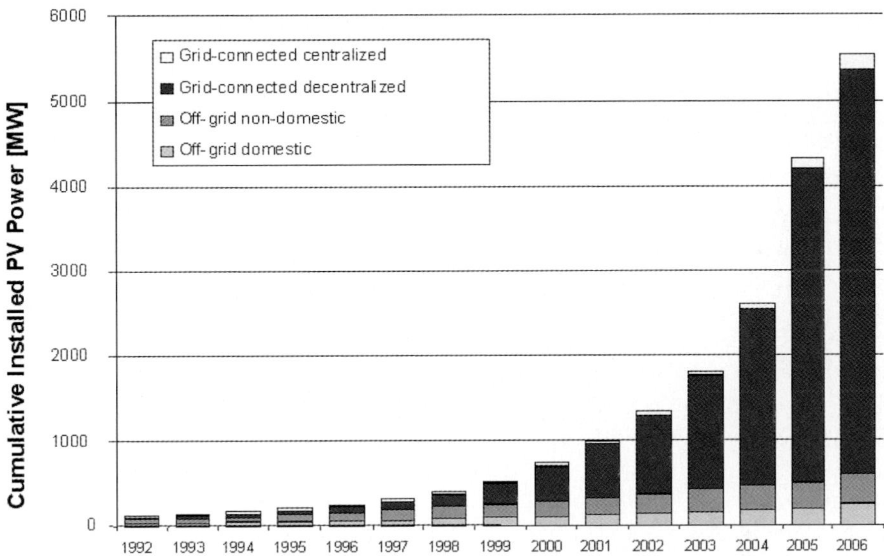

Fig. 12.3. Different applications of PV and installed Power (based on IEA data). (Source: IEA)

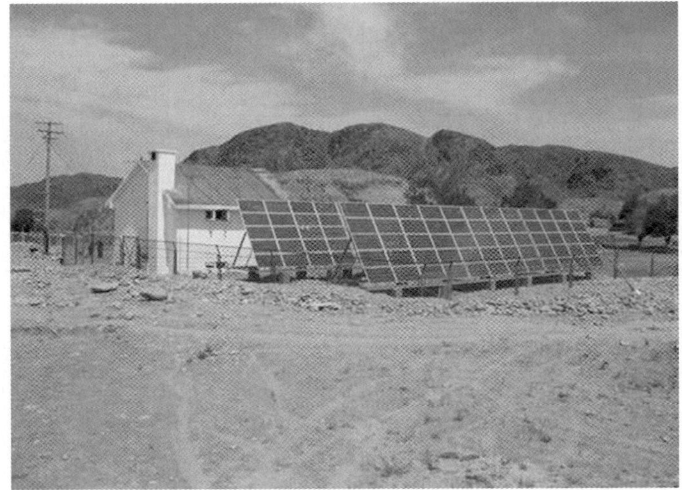

Fig. 12.4. PV generator for a village electricity supply. (Source: SMA)

12.2.2 Domestic Standalone Systems

Domestic standalone systems are also knows as solar home systems (SHS). These small PV systems are mainly used to supply homes with light, radio, and possibly also television (Fig. 12.5). With a generator output of generally 10 W to 200 W,

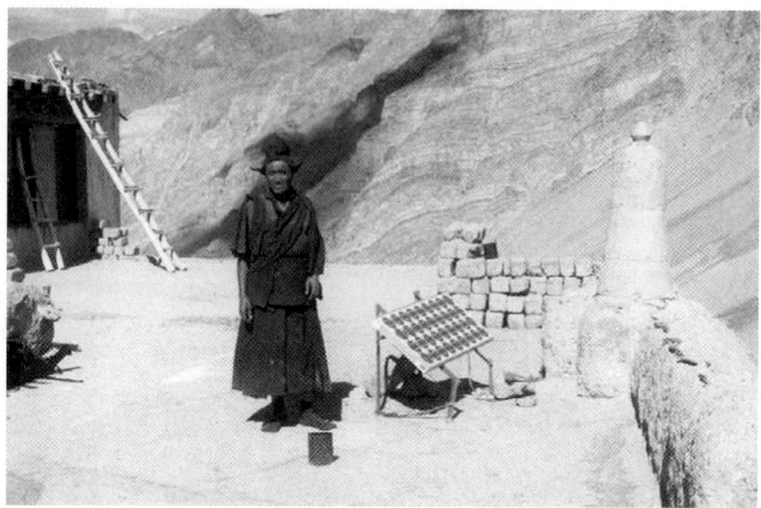

Fig. 12.5. SHS in Tibet. (Source: LBST)

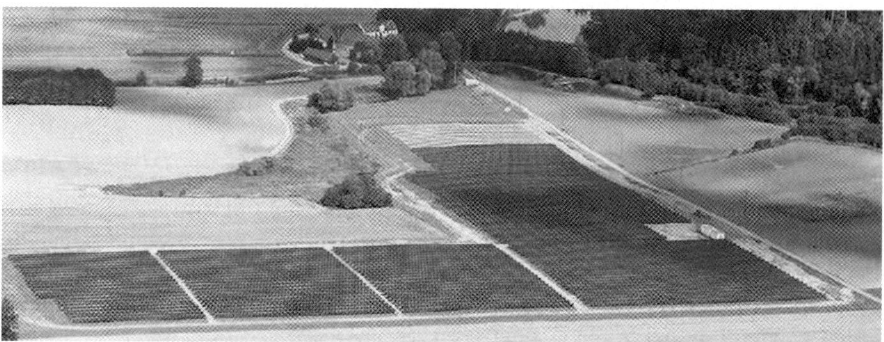

Fig. 12.6. Central PV field in Germany. (Source: Shell Solar)

they take the place of petroleum lamps or battery-driven equipment. The price paid for the supply of nonphotovoltaic electric current is on the order of 8 to 10 dollars per month. Once again, price is the decisive criterion in determining the expedience of substituting a SHS. Aesthetics or multifunctionality remain secondary considerations.

12.2.3 Grid-Connected Central PV Systems

Figure 12.6 shows a central PV field of the kind typically installed in Europe (Germany or Spain) at the present time. These systems are generally operated like power stations. The functionality required is above all high power density (high efficiency, low space requirements). As yet, aesthetic requirements are not relevant, although the optical impression will become increasingly important as these systems increase in number.

12.2.4 Grid-Connected Decentral Systems

The vast majority of photovoltaic applications are installed in the form of grid-connected decentral systems. These systems are for the most part roof-mounted installations (Fig. 12.7(a)). This mode of installation offers several advantages:

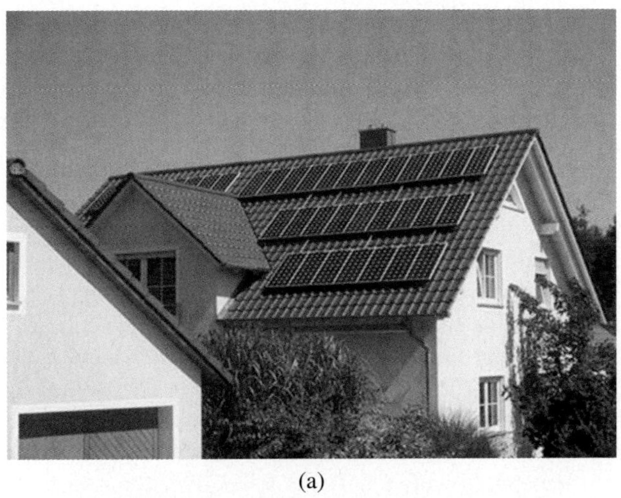

(a)

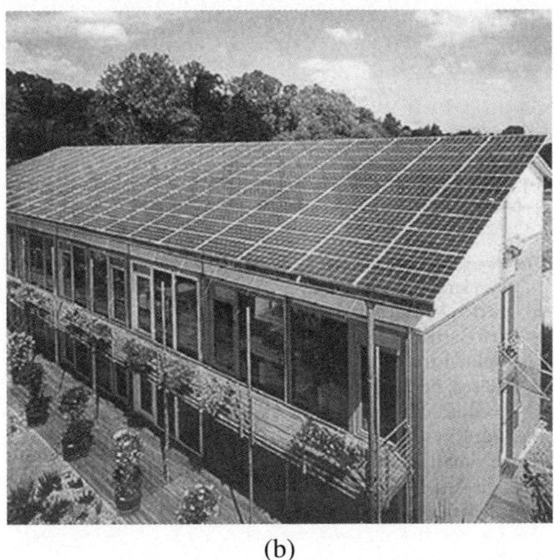

(b)

Fig. 12.7. (**a**) Roof-mounted PV System. (Source: Mayer, private photograph.) (**b**) Roof-integrated. (Source: Photon)

- The waterproofness of the roof is not dependent on the PV.
- Easier compliance with fire-protection or building regulations for roofs.
- Subsequent installation is simple.
- The generator size can be chosen without reference to the roof area.

In order to reduce costs, however, multifunctional usage of the PV modules is expedient, for example simultaneously as substitute roofing material and as power generator. This method simultaneously reduces roofing costs and the expenditure for electricity which would otherwise be purchased at commercial rates (including the cost saved on the normal roof tiling, Fig. 12.7(b)). However, contemporary systems continue to be based on the predominant consideration of *primarily* generating electric energy. All other functionalities are viewed as less important.

The possibility of introducing a dual-layered perspective is particularly manifest in the case of the decentral grid-connected systems, that dual perspective can be summed up as

"Power engineer" ↔ "Aesthete / Architect".

The "power engineer" discerns in photovoltaics above all the potential for generating electricity. The main criteria are high power density, optimum positioning, high system yield, low maintenance costs, long useful life, and so on. The objective is to produce the lowest possible energy costs in order to be able to compete with current electricity prices. Little consideration is given to optical characteristics, aesthetics, and so forth.

The "aesthete/architect" focuses on these otherwise secondary attributes, with electricity production being of subordinate importance. Solar panels are viewed as a desirable design element allowing a building to be given a particular optical effect. Figure 12.8 shows the example of a house into which the conventional PV modules have been integrated in optically compatible form.

If generation of electricity no longer occupies the foreground of considerations, then other criteria must be applied when evaluating a system. If PV is used as a facade element, the €/kWh relationship becomes less important than the cost per

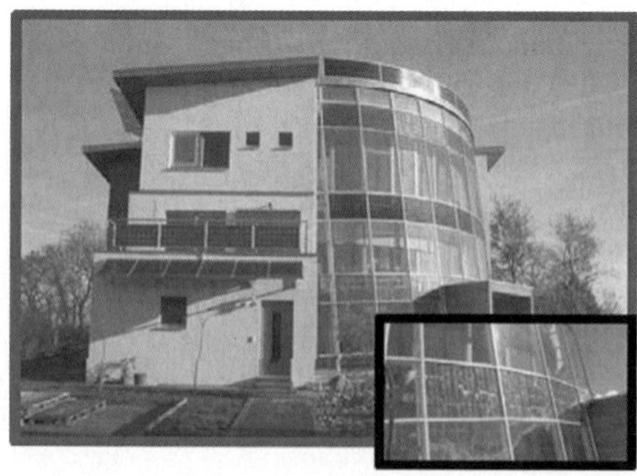

Fig. 12.8. Facade-integration of conventional PV modules. (Source: Photon)

square meter in comparison with other facade elements. Power generation is viewed as a cost-reducing factor not given in the case of conventional facade elements, with which no savings are made over the course of time. Thus, the efficiency of the system is not critically important, but the overall costs must add up:

$$\text{Invest}_{\text{PV facade}} - \text{Power yield}_{\text{useful life}} \cdot \text{€/kWh}$$
$$< \text{Invest}_{\text{conventional facade}} \cdot F_{\text{aesthetic impression}}.$$

$F_{\text{aesthetic impression}}$ is here a quality factor dealing with the optical impression:

$$F_{\text{aesthetic impression}} = \frac{\text{Evaluation of PV facade}}{\text{Evaluation of conventional facade}}.$$

In this way, the multifunctionality of PV modules widens the spectrum of market approaches when energy generation is no longer in the foreground. Figure 12.9 illustrates the functions of a PV facade element as a substitute for conventional elements.

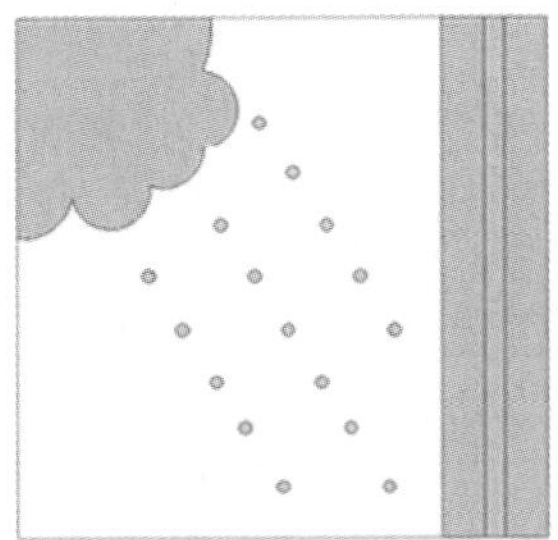

Basic functions of the external covering of the building: weatherproofness (rain, wind, . . .)

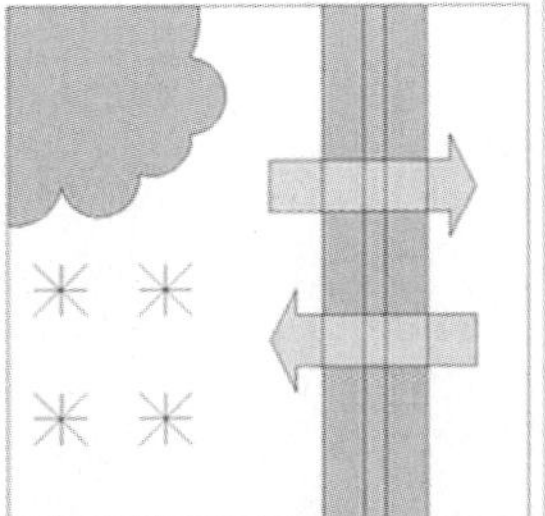

Physical functions: Thermal insulation, soundproofing, damp proofing, fire protection

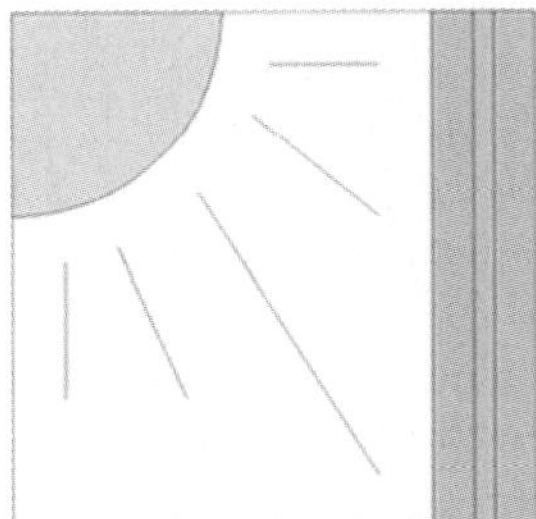

Energy conversion

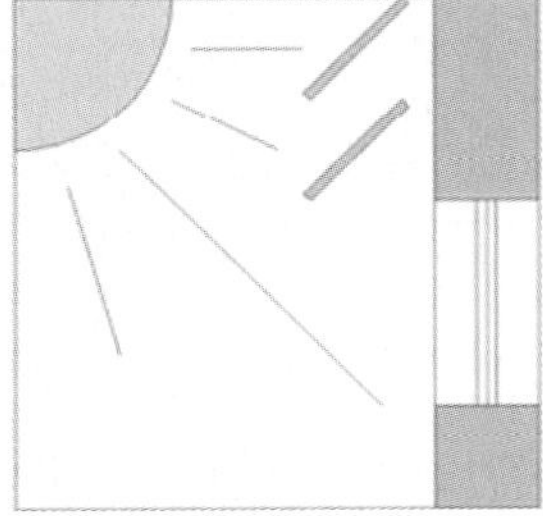

Sun and visibility protection, light deflection, electromagnetically design

Fig. 12.9. Multifunctionality of PV facades. (Source: Ingrid Lützkendorf, IFF Weimar)

The PV module must assume basic functions of the external covering of the building; these functions include weatherproofing, protection against mechanical impacts (e.g. hailstones), optical impression, and so forth. Alongside these basic functions, a number of physical functions must be given. Thermal protection and damp proofing are essential to the energy use, fireproofing is a safety consideration, and soundproofing heightens the quality of life. In locations close to airports, and particularly in the case of tall buildings, it may be important to consider electromagnetic damping properties in order to reduce radar radiation.

Contemporary PV modules are not designed for the above-mentioned functionalities. For more than 20 years now, form and structure have been dictated by the need to obtain maximum yields from minimal space. All the same, such modules are being deployed as facade elements after undergoing slight alterations. Thanks to resourceful architecture combined with considerable efforts, such attempts are rewarded with success. However, present-day modules are less suitable for widespread deployment as facade elements that also work as decentral grid-connected systems, since they lack the functionalities necessary for this purpose.

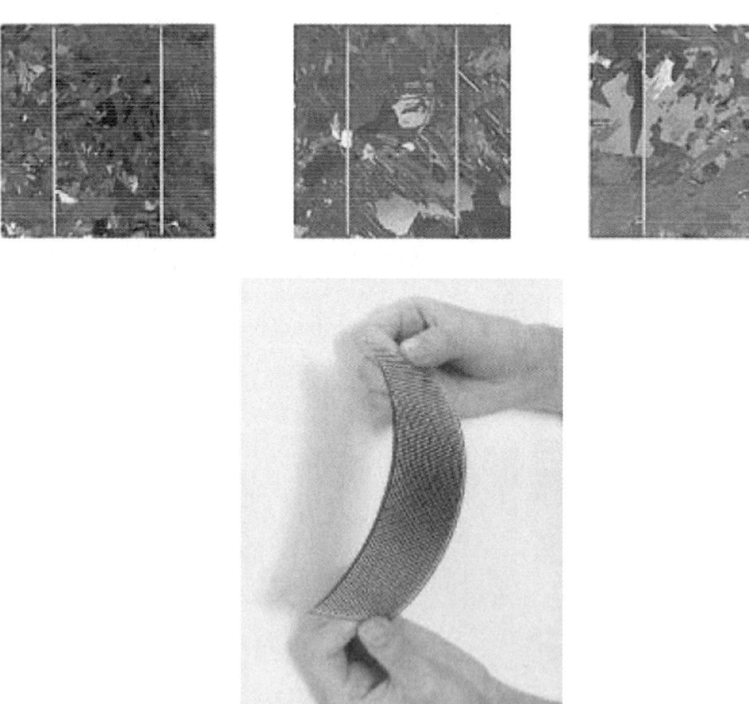

Fig. 12.10. Colored PV cells/Spherical cells. (Source: Sunways, Nikkei BP)

12.3 PV Developments in the Future

Since contemporary PV modules are not purpose-designed for deployment as facade elements, new criteria are necessary for this application. The main requirements may be seen to be coloration and shaping.

The market already offers solutions in regard to coloration (Fig. 12.10). Special coatings allow colored cells to be produced, whereby efficiency is reduced at the same time.

These cells continue to be flat. In the future, reduced cell thickness could produce flexible cells adaptable to curve forms. Another alternative is represented by spherical cells, which are embedded in a matrix. In this case, the matrix can likewise comply with a predefined form.

13 Design Rules for Efficient Organic Solar Cells

Z. Zhu, D. Mühlbacher, M. Morana, M. Koppe, M.C. Scharber, D. Waller,
G. Dennler, and C.J. Brabec

13.1 Introduction

There has been an intensive search for cost-effective photovoltaics since the development of the first solar cells in the 1950s [1–3]. Among all the alternative technologies to silicon-based pn-junction solar cells, organic solar cells are the approach that could lead to the most significant cost reduction [4]. The field of organic photovoltaics (OPV) is composed of organic/inorganic nanostructures, like the dye-sensitized solar cell, multilayers of small organic molecules and mixtures of organic materials (bulk-heterojunction solar cell). A review of several so-called organic photovoltaic (OPV) technologies was recently presented [5].

Unlike conventional inorganic solar cells, light absorption in organic solar cells leads to the generation of excited bound electron–hole pairs (often called excitons). To achieve substantial energy-conversion efficiencies, these excited electron–hole pairs need to be dissociated into free charge carriers with a high yield. Excitons can be dissociated at interfaces of materials with different electron affinities, by electric fields or the dissociation can be trap- or impurity-assisted. Blending conjugated polymers with high electron affinity molecules like C_{60} (bulk-heterojunction solar cell) has proven to be an efficient way for rapid exciton dissociation. Conjugated polymer/C_{60} interpenetrating networks exhibit an ultra-fast charge transfer ($\sim$40 fs) [6, 7]. As there is no competing decay process of the optically excited electron–hole pair located on the polymer, in this time regime an optimized mixture with C_{60} converts absorbed photon to electron with an efficiency close to 100% [8]. Besides the efficient charge carrier generation process, the bulk-heterojunction solar cell has attracted a lot of attention because of its potential to be a true low-cost photovoltaic technology. It is believed that a simple coating or printing process will allow a roll-to-roll manufacturing of flexible, lightweight PV modules which should allow for cost-efficient production and the development of products for new markets, e.g. in the field of portable electronics. One major obstacle to an immediate commercialization of the bulk-heterojunction solar cell are the relatively small device efficiencies demonstrated up to now [5]. The best energy conversion efficiencies published for small-area devices are in the range of 5–6% [9–12]. A detailed analysis of state-of-the-art bulk-heterojunction solar cells [8] reveals that efficiency loss stems primarily from the low open-circuit voltage (V_{oc}) delivered by these devices under illumination. Typically, organic semiconductors with a bandgap of about 2 eV are applied as photoactive materials but the observed open circuit voltages are only in the range between 0.5 V and 1 V.

Here, we discuss the design rules for polymer donors, allowing high power efficiencies when processed in composites with a prototype acceptor PCBM ([6, 6]-phenyl-C_{61}-bytric acid methyl ester). Specifically, one class of low bandgap donors will be discussed in more detail, as we outline the important interplay between material design, synthesis, optical, morphological and transport related properties to the power conversion of solar cells. The chapter is closely related to a series of papers on these topics, which were published recently [13–16].

13.2 Material Design Rules for Donors in Single-Junction Solar Cells

In Fig. 13.1 the open circuit voltage of different bulk-heterojunction solar cells is plotted versus the oxidation potential of the conjugated polymers used in these devices. More than 26 different polymeric donors from various material classes (thiophenes, fluorenes, phenylene-vinylenes…) were investigated in bulk-heterojunction (BHJ) composites with PCBM. A linear relation between V_{oc} and the conjugated

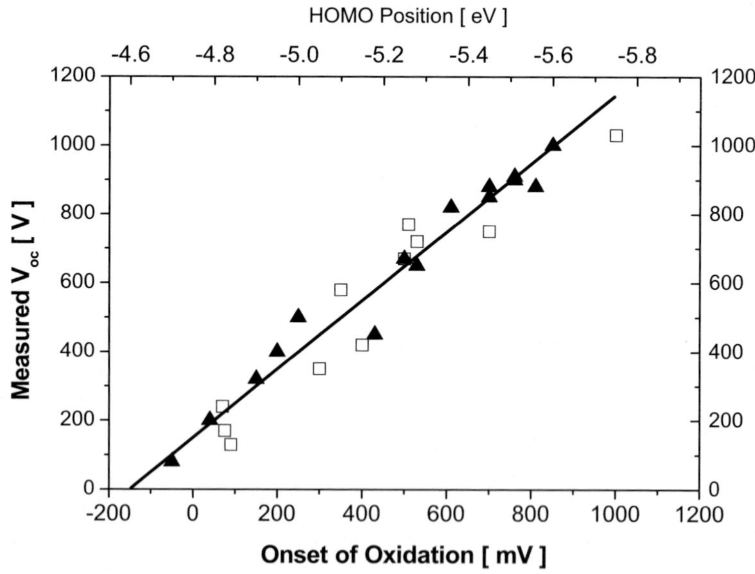

Fig. 13.1. Open-circuit voltage of different bulk heterojunction solar cells plotted versus the oxidation potential/HOMO position of the donor polymer used in each individual device. The straight line represents a linear fit with slope 1

polymer oxidation potential is found, with an x-axis offset of $-140\,\mathrm{mV}$, corresponding to a HOMO level of 4.6 eV. The offset suggests that the donor materials with lower lying HOMOs will not function in solar cells with PCBM. The LUMO of PCBM is assumed with 4.3 eV, and the difference between the PCBM LUMO and the smallest polymer HOMO value represents the energy which is obviously lost during the photo-induced charge-generation process. In our case, this number is 0.3 eV. According to Fig. 13.1 the open circuit voltage of a conjugated polymer/PCBM solar cell can be estimated by

$$V_{\mathrm{oc}} = \left| E_{\mathrm{HOMO}}^{\mathrm{Donor}} \right| - \left| E_{\mathrm{LUMO}}^{\mathrm{PCBM}} \right| - 0.3\,\mathrm{V}. \tag{13.1}$$

Based on this finding one can calculate the efficiency of a bulk-heterojunction solar cell solely as a function of the bandgap and the lowest unoccupied molecular orbital (LUMO) level of the donor. For simplicity we assume a constant external quantum efficiency of the solar cell for photon energies equal to or larger than the bandgap energy of the donor and neglect possible contribution to the short-circuit current from photons absorbed by the fullerene. Under these assumptions the short circuit current is calculated by

$$i_{\mathrm{sc}} = e \cdot \int_{E_{\mathrm{g}}}^{\infty} \mathrm{EQE}(E) \cdot n_{\mathrm{AM1.5}}(E)\,\mathrm{d}E, \tag{13.2}$$

where e is the electric charge of an electron, $n_{\mathrm{AM1.5}}$ is the number of photons arriving on the surface of the earth under AM1.5 illumination, E is the photon energy and E_{g} corresponds to the bandgap energy of the donor polymer. For simplicity, the calculations assumed an $\mathrm{EQE}(E) = 0.65$ for energies larger than E_{g} and a FF of 0.65, values which are typical for optimized devices [17]. In combination with (13.1) and (13.2) the efficiency of a bulk-heterojunction device given by

$$\begin{aligned}
\eta &= \frac{i_{\mathrm{sc}} \cdot V_{\mathrm{oc}} \cdot \mathrm{FF}}{P_{\mathrm{light_in}}} \\
&= \frac{e \cdot \int_{E_{\mathrm{g}}}^{\infty} 0.65 \cdot n_{\mathrm{AM1.5}}(E)\,\mathrm{d}E \cdot (|E_{\mathrm{HOMO}}^{\mathrm{DONOR}}| - |E_{\mathrm{LUMO}}^{\mathrm{ACCEPTOR}}| - 0.3) \cdot 0.65}{P_{\mathrm{light_in}}}, \tag{13.3}
\end{aligned}$$

where $P_{\mathrm{light\_in}}$ is the incident light power per unit area. The result is shown in Fig. 13.2 as a contour plot where the x and y axis are the bandgap and the LUMO level of the donor and the contour lines indicate constant power conversion efficiencies.

Figure 13.2 shows that the donor LUMO-level determines the maximum energy conversion efficiency of a bulk-heterojunction device. Surprisingly the variation in the efficiency is rather small upon changing the bandgap of the donor when the LUMO level is kept constant. The relative position of the polymer's LUMO is much more relevant to achieving highest efficiencies. For energy conversion efficiencies exceeding 10%, the donor polymer must have a bandgap $<1.74\,\mathrm{eV}$ and a LUMO level $<-3.92\,\mathrm{eV}$ always assuming a fill factor (FF) and the average EQE equal to 0.65. Again the calculated value is almost constant upon decreasing the donor bandgap down to 1.3 eV.

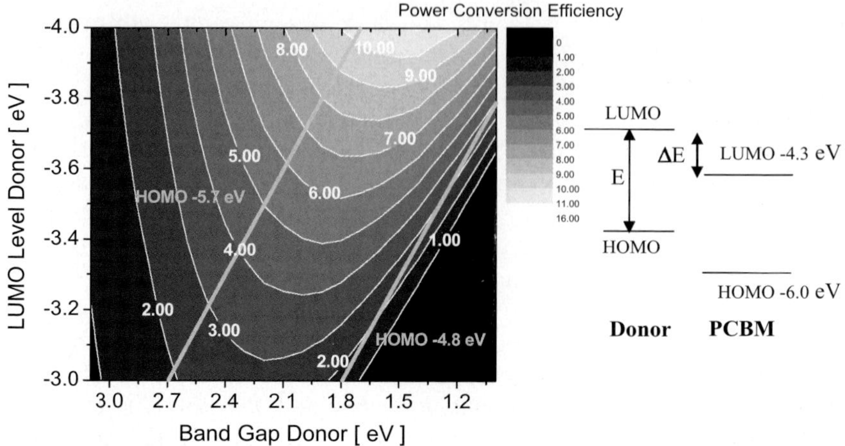

Fig. 13.2. (*Left*) Contour plot showing the calculated energy conversion efficiency (contour lines and colors) versus the band gap and the LUMO level of the donor polymer according to the model described earlier. Straight lines starting at 2.7 eV and 1.8 eV indicate LUMO levels of −5.7 eV and −4.8 eV, respectively. (*Right*) Schematic energy diagram of a donor PCBM system

Besides a reduction of the bandgap, new donor materials must be designed to optimize the LUMO as this parameter dominantly drives the solar cell efficiency.

It is important to note that an optimized open-circuit voltage is a prerequisite to achieve certain device efficiencies; however, it is not sufficient. In addition, the charge carrier mobility of electrons and holes in the donor acceptor blend must be high enough to allow an efficient charge extraction and an electrical fill factor (FF) of 0.65. The relation between charge carrier mobility and FF can be deduced from a recently presented model [17]. The main feature of this extended pn-junction model is that the photocurrent is dominantly field driven. For devices with an active layer thickness of several hundred nanometers, mobilities of $\sim 10^{-3}$ cm^2/Vs are required to prevent significant electrical and recombination losses. The model can also be used to analyze V_{oc} losses of bulk heterojunction solar cells. The overall theoretical limit of the open-circuit voltage is given by the difference between the acceptor LUMO level and the donor HOMO level, which also defines the built-in field V_{BI}. As discussed earlier and shown in Fig. 13.1, we find deviations of the theoretical maximum V_{oc} in the order of 0.3 V.

In Fig. 13.3 the current voltage curve of a poly-3-hexyl-thiophene/PCBM bulk-heterojunction solar cell acquired in the dark (full line) and the idealized field-driven photocurrent are plotted. The superposition of both curves gives the current–voltage curve under illumination. The open-circuit voltage of the solar cell is defined as the voltage which compensates the current flow through the external circuit (indicated by the vertical line in Fig. 13.3). Figure 13.3 shows that a main loss mechanism for V_{oc} is dominated by the dark current–voltage curve of the diode which is determined by the ideal factor n and the reverse dark current i_0 of the diode. This loss is typi-

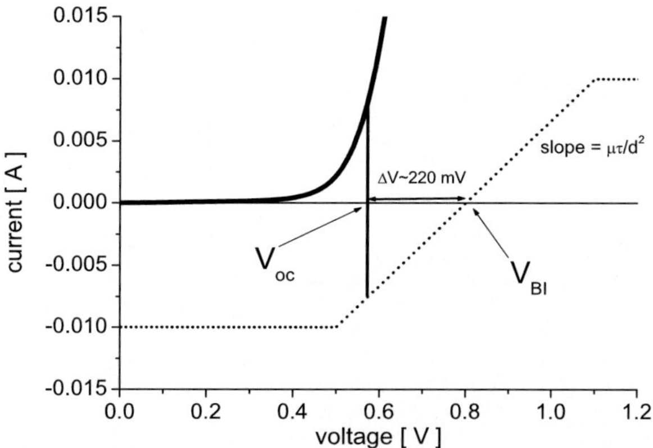

Fig. 13.3. Current-voltage curve of poly-3-hexyl-thiophene (P3HT)/PCBM solar cell measured in the dark (*full line*) and field-driven photocurrent (*dotted line*). VBI is given by ELUMO (PCBM) minus EHOMO (P3HT) $(-4.3\,\mathrm{V}-(-5.1\,\mathrm{V})) = 0.8\,\mathrm{V}$

cally of the order of 200 mV. A smaller part of the V_{oc} loss can originate from the fact that the photocurrent in bulk-heterojunction devices is dominantly field-driven. The open-circuit voltage depends on the slope $(=\mu\tau/d^2)$ of the field-driven current around V_{BI}. A steeper slope moves the V_{oc} closer to V_{BI}.

In summary, OPV can easily reach 10% efficiency with the outlined BHJ concept. There is a distinct relation between energy conversion efficiency of a bulk-heterojunction solar cell, bandgap and the LUMO level of the donor, which can be summarized in a 2D contour diagram.

Most interestingly, these investigations give a fundamental insight into the losses of BHJ solar cells and clearly outline how to go beyond 10% efficiency. First, the EQE and the FF have to be improved. There have been reports on so-called hero solar cells with a maximum EQE of more than 80%, and a FF of more than 70% has been published as well. Obviously, there is still significant potential to improve the performance of single-junction cells by further fine tuning on the EQE and FF values. Second, BHJ solar cells exhibit two quite fundamental losses – on the one hand the energetic loss due to the photo-induced charge transfer, on the other hand the V_{oc} losses due to dark current contributions. One might be interested in understanding the efficiency potential of single-junction cells in dependence on these two losses, and that is plotted in Fig. 13.4. Here, the CT loss as well as the V_{oc} loss were modeled with 0.25 V each. The calculations were run for a FF of 0.7 and an EQE of 90%. Both are challenging but realistic values for fully optimized organic solar cells. The loss-free scenario yields a maximum possible efficiency of about 30%. Each loss reduces the efficiency potential by about 5% points, so that in the case of CT and V_{oc} losses, a maximum efficiency of about 20% can be expected. A reduction in the optimum bandgap accompanies these losses. Although the loss-free case shows little sensitivity to the bandgap of the donor, a clear maximum in the 1.5 eV (900 nm regime) is observed for the scenario with V_{oc} and CT losses.

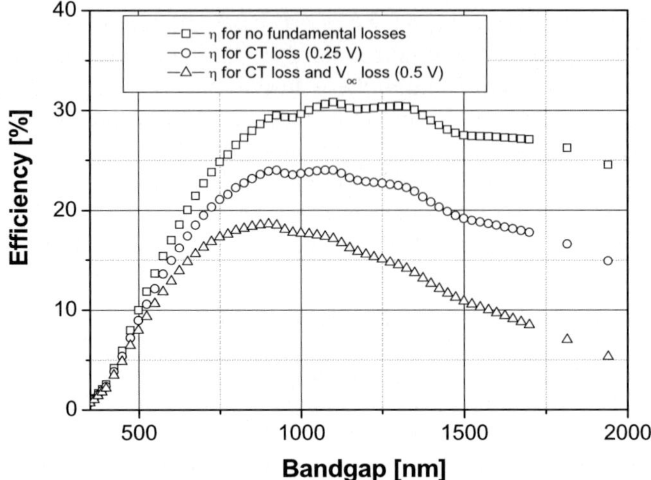

Fig. 13.4. Efficiency of organic BHJ independent of the donor's bandgap. The three different curves assume (**a**) the loss-free case (*top curve*), (**b**) energetic losses (0.25 eV) due to the photo-induced charge transfer (CT) (*middle curve*) and (**c**) losses due to CT and the V_{OC} (0.5 V) (*lower curve*)

In summary, today's single-junction organic solar cells have the performance potential to overcome 10% by fine tuning the material properties of the donor. Increasing the FF to over 70% and the EQE to 90% will pave the way to 20% power efficiency; for 30% power efficiency, though, the two fundamental losses – the V_{OC} as well as the CT loss – have to be overcome. Compared to today's efficiency of 5% [18–22], there is still some development to be done.

13.3 Toward Novel Polymeric Donors: Poly-Cyclic-Bridged-DiThieno Copolymers (PCPDT)

After more than 10 years of trying to find acceptors better than PCBM, all the alternative approaches – including other fullerenes, TiO2, ZnO, n-type polymers, and small molecular acceptors – did not outperform PCBM, despite their large potential for future performance improvements. Following the design rules discussed in the previous section, there is a huge demand for polymers with a bandgap between 1.3 and 1.6 eV. Besides bandgap, several other characteristics of conjugated polymers, including HOMO/LUMO levels and carrier mobility, need to be optimized simultaneously in order to achieve high photovoltaic performance [13]. In general, the gap between the HOMO of the electron donating polymer and the LUMO of the electron acceptor should be maximized in order to increase the open-circuit voltage, and at the same time the bandgap of the polymer should be minimized to increase photon absorption and thus short-circuit current. In addition the LUMO of the polymer (donor) should be positioned above the LUMO of the fullerene derivative (acceptor) by at least 0.2–0.3 eV to ensure efficient electron transfer. All of that was discussed in the previous section. In addition to these design rules, a high charge-carrier mobility of holes and electrons is essential for efficient charge extraction and a good fill factor. To prevent significant photocurrent loss in cells with an active layer thickness of several hundred nanometers, a carrier mobility of 10^{-3} cm^2 V^{-1} s^{-1} is desired.

In the next two sections we will review a novel class of low bandgap polymers which has a high potential to fulfill all our requirements for higher efficiencies.

13.3.1 Structural and Optical Properties of PCPDT

The employment of materials absorbing the red and near-IR part of the solar spectrum has been one of the fundamental strategies in improving the performance of organic solar cells [23, 24]. It has been well known that coupling together electron-donors and acceptors leads to effective expansion of absorption wavelength. For example, the electron withdrawing 2, 1, 3-benzothiadiazole when coupled with electron-donating thiophenes or pyrroles resulted in a number of low-bandgap polymers [25–36]. Many structures have been designed and investigated, but most of them delivered only very low device performance [37–46]. The photovoltaic performances of these polymers is typically lower than 1%, significantly inferior to what is realized with a prototype wide bandgap polymer, poly-(3-hexylthiophene) (P3HT), and only a few polyfluorene-based copolymers showed efficiencies over 1%. One of the main reasons for this, we believe, is that these polymers usually lack solubility and their building blocks do not provide suitable anchoring sites for solubilizing side chains without causing further twisting between adjacent repeating units; this causes loss of conjugation. The carbon-bridged 4H-cyclopenta[2, 1-b:3, 4-b′]dithiophene was found to be a superior building block for conjugated polymers due to the forced co-planarity of the two thienyl subunits [47, 48]. The 4-carbon of the 4H-cyclopenta [2, 1-b:3, 4-b′]dithiophene can be readily functionalized by alkyl groups to increase solubility without causing additional twisting of the repeating units in the resulting polymers. In order to further increase the absorption wavelength and lower the bandgap of the polymer, a polymer containing the combination of cyclopentadithiophene as electron-donating and 2, 1, 3-benzothiadiazole as electron-accepting units (7, Fig. 13.5) was designed and synthesized.

The absorption spectra of the polymer 8 ($M_{\mathrm{n}} = 28$ kDa) was recorded in both solution and solid state (Fig. 13.6). The optical band gap at solid state was estimated to be 1.4 eV from its absorption edge. It has a HOMO level of -5.3 eV and a LUMO level of -3.55 eV and bandgap of 1.75 eV as determined by cyclic voltammetry.

These physical parameters make this polymer a very promising material for high-performance organic solar cells though it is noted that there is a transmission window in the solid-state absorption spectrum of 8 around 500 nm which will reduce light harvesting, and, consequently cell performance. To increase light harvesting across the solar spectrum in the visible region, further random polymers copolymers 9(a–d) were prepared. The copolymer of bithiophene and cyclopenta[2, 1-b;3, 4-b′]dithiophene (10) was also synthesized for comparison purposes.

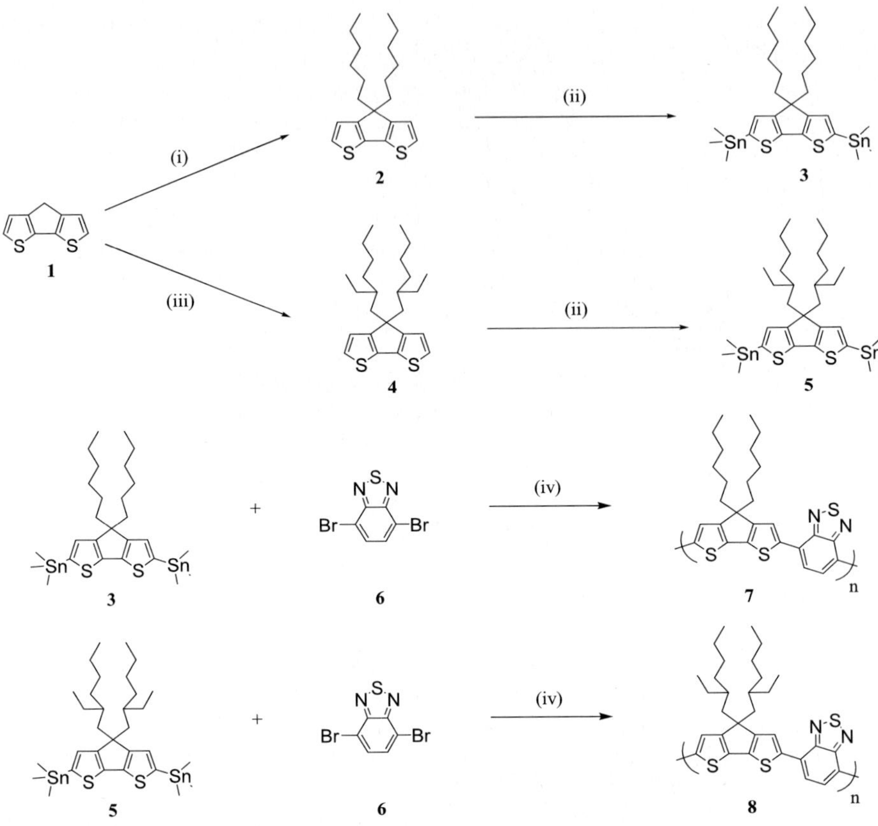

Fig. 13.5. Synthesis of poly[2, 6-(4, 4-dialkyl-4H-cyclopenta[2, 1-b; 3, 4-b$'$]dithiophene)-*alt*-4, 7-(2, 1, 3-benzothiadiazole)]

These polymers are shown in Fig. 13.7 and their corresponding optical properties compiled in Fig. 13.6. As expected, the incorporation of unbridged [2, 2$'$]bithiophene shifts the absorption maxima to the shorter wavelength region. With a ratio of the two electron-donating units, (4, 4-bis-(2-ethylhexyl)-4H-cyclopenta[2, 1-b;3, 4-b$'$]dithiophene) and 5, 5$'$-[2, 2$'$]bithiophene, between 2:1 and 1:2, the copolymer absorption covers broad range of the visible spectrum, and the dominant task – to find absorbers covering the whole visible spectrum – can be fulfilled by blends of these polymers.

An additional attractive feature of these polymers is that they have significantly higher absorptivity than the well-known regio-regular P3HT polymer. The optical densities of these polymers in chlorobenzene are normalized to the same polymer concentration (1 g/L) and their comparison is shown in Fig. 13.8. As can be seen from the spectra, the polymers 8–10 not only absorb at longer wavelength, but also exhibit higher absorptivity than P3HT. Electrochemical analysis (cyclic voltammetry) was conducted on these polymers to determine their LUMO and HOMO positions. All the polymers (8–10) have a HOMO of between −3.25 eV and −3.38 eV.

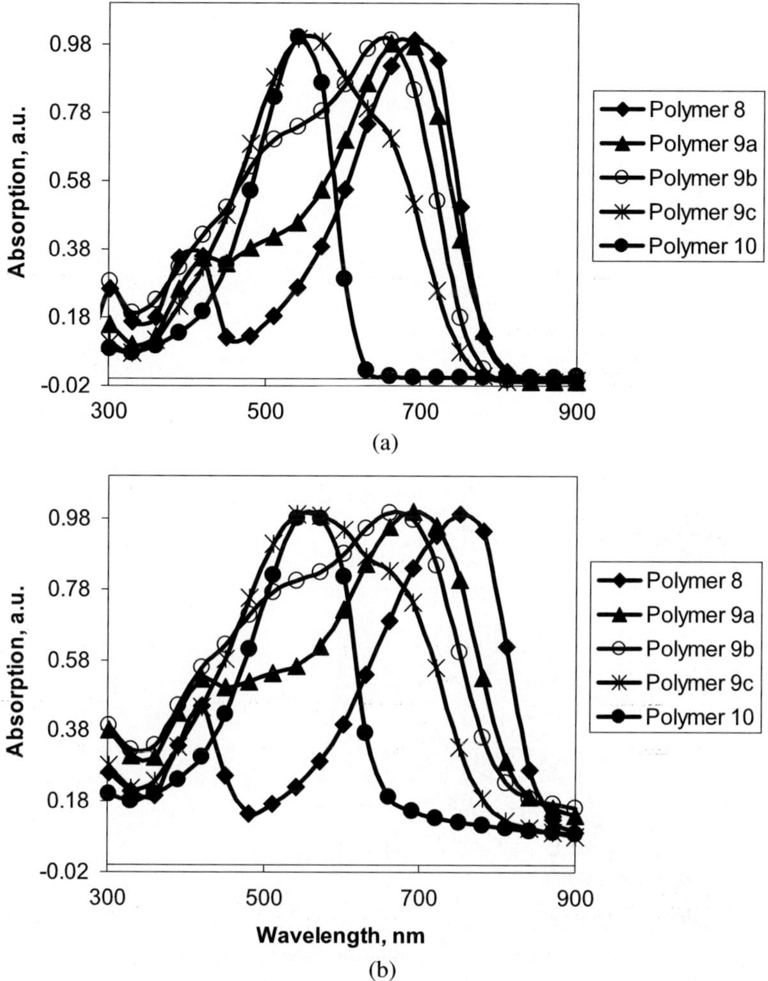

Fig. 13.6. The normalized absorption spectra of the polymers in chloroform (**a**) and in solid state (**b**)

The LUMOs of all the benzothiodiazole containing polymers (8, 9a–c) are around −3.55 eV. The LUMO of polymer 10 is around −3.0 eV. All these characteristics of PCPDT copolymers are within the desirable range for an ideal polymer for organic photovoltaic applications.

13.3.2 Transport and Electrical Properties of PCPDT-BT

The optical and electrochemical properties of the PCPDT copolymers, especially of the copolymer with benzothiadiazole (PCPDT-BT), clearly point to the potential of this material and presented the current limitations with respect to the power conversion efficiency. For high solar cell performance, the electrical transport properties of

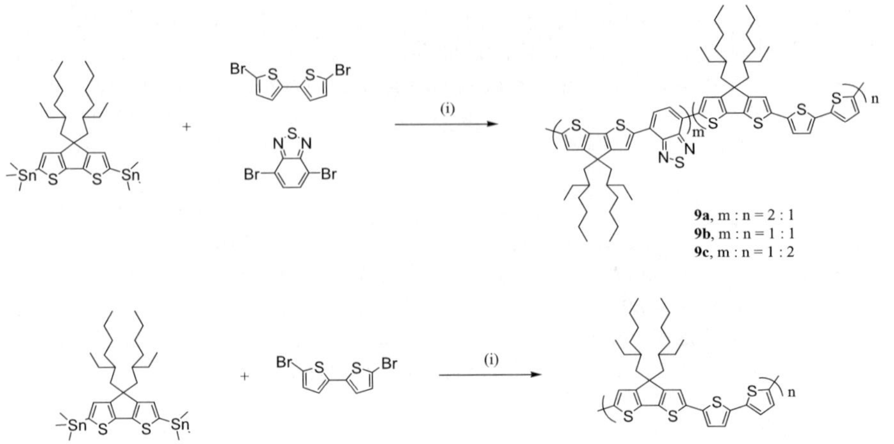

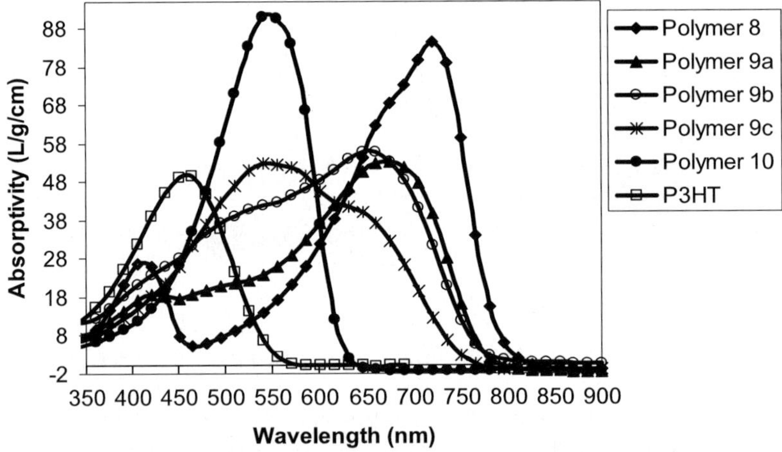

Fig. 13.7. The synthesis of both [2, 2′]bithiophene and cyclopenta[2, 1-b; 3, 4-b′]dithiophene containing copolymers

Fig. 13.8. A comparison of the absorptivity of the polymers with that of region-regular P3HT. All spectra were recorded in chlorobenzene

the donor/acceptor blend have to be sufficient to guarantee recombination-free transport. On the one hand, the ambipolar mobility and the related carrier drift length need to be larger than the device thickness. On the other hand, defects, traps and isolated or strongly phase-separated domains may significantly reduce the carrier lifetime as well. Recent steady-state and transient photoconductivity studies [49] on PCPDT-BT and PCPDT-BT:PCBM films in direct comparison with a P3HT reference system have confirmed efficient photogeneration of charges in the PCPDT-BT:PCBM blend and showed evidence of a quite comparable, though slightly lower carrier lifetime compared to the one in P3HT:PCBM blends. Besides, lifetime, mobility and transport is equally important. Both of these parameters are related to the morphology of the donor–acceptor network. Transport losses, morphological as well as trap-induced, can be investigated by bipolar field effect transistor measurements (OFET). Phase separation and subsequent crystallization can be investigated by X-ray spectroscopy.

The grazing incidence X-rays spectroscopic profiles in thin films of PCPDT-BT (Fig. 13.9) show three distinct peaks at $2\theta \sim 24\,\mathrm{deg}$, $2\theta \sim 9.6\,\mathrm{deg}$ and $2\theta \sim 3\,\mathrm{deg}$, respectively, whose intensity is rather low. The higher angle peak corresponds to a distance of approximately $3.7\,\mathrm{\AA}$ that can be assigned to the π-orbital stacking between chains. Interestingly this lattice distance is the same as found for P3HT films [50]. The higher intensity $9.6\,\mathrm{deg}$ peak corresponds to a distance of $9.15\,\mathrm{\AA}$. In RR-P3HT this peak corresponds to the interchain spacing between chains interdigitated through the side chains. The XRD pattern of PCPDT-BT could therefore correspond to a lamellar structure similar to the one found in P3HT with the lamellae being perpendicular to the substrate. The intensity of the π-stacking peak is, however, much lower with respect to ordered RR-P3HT samples (not shown). This could be due to a rather low crystalline fraction present in the PCPDT-BT film measured. However, since a π-stacking perpendicular to the substrate cannot be detected by a θ–2θ scan, the possibility of having a significant volume of lamellar structure parallel to the substrate cannot be excluded. The third peak whose intensity is rather high corresponds to a spacing of $\sim 37\,\mathrm{A}$, indicating the presence of a significant long-range order.

The dynamics of film drying in relation to the crystalline order was investigated for drop-cast films dried in nitrogen atmosphere at room temperature versus $80\,^{\circ}\mathrm{C}$. Interestingly the slowly drying films showed a smaller signal at $2\theta \sim 24^{\circ}$, which suggests a lower degree of π-orbital delocalization. In addition, films prepared from a bend of PCPDT-BT:PCBM $= 1{:}1$ were also studied to observe the changes induced in the polymer crystalline structure upon the addition of PCBM in Fig. 13.9(b). Interestingly, in this case a faster dying ($80\,^{\circ}\mathrm{C}$) reduces the intensity of the π-stacking peak in the blend. In both cases the long-range order peak at low incidence angles is strongly reduced in films dried at $80\,^{\circ}\mathrm{C}$. The data presented here seem to indicate a rather low crystalline order in PCPDT-BT, in comparison with that observed in high-mobility conjugated homopolymers like RR-P3HT [51], which is only slightly dependent on the film processing conditions. However, the high in-plane hole mobility observed in this material poses new questions concerning the relation between morphology and charge transport associated with the structure of alternating donor–acceptor copolymers.

The transport of pristine PCPDT-BT was investigated by the field-effect transistor method (FET), and the hole mobility was deduced from the slope of the transfer-characteristic [52] using a DC dielectric constant of $\varepsilon_r = 2.7$ that was determined from MOS capacitance measurements, and is in the range 5×10^{-3}–$2 \times 10^{-2}\,\mathrm{cm^2/Vs}$ ($C_{\mathrm{ox}} \sim 1.4 \times 10^{-4}\,\mathrm{F/m}$).

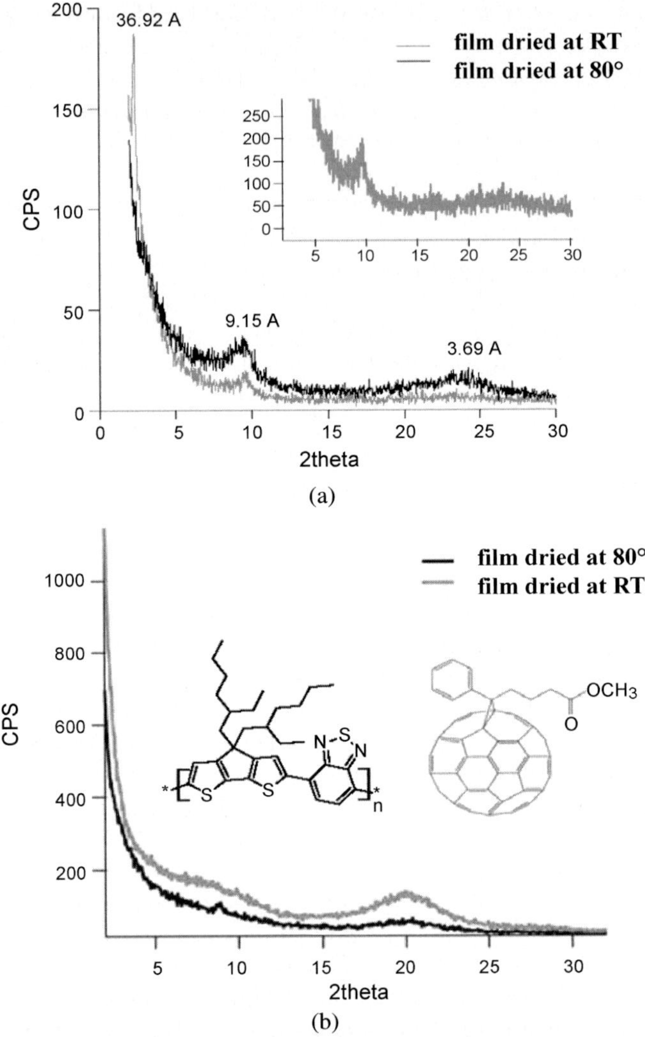

(a)

(b)

Fig. 13.9. (a) XRD pattern of a pristine PCPDT-BT film drop-cast from chlorobenzene slowly dried at room temperature (*grey line*) in N2 atmosphere compared to a film dried at 80 °C (*black line*). (b) XRD pattern of a PCPDT-BT:PCBM = 1:1 film drop-cast from chlorobenzene slowly dried at room temperature (295 K, *grey line*) in N2 atmosphere compared to a film dried at 80 °C (*black line*). The inset shows the chemical structure of PCPDT-BT (*left side*) and PCBM (*right side*)

As already known from other polymers, the processing conditions can influence the transport properties. Drying time, choice of the solvent, drying temperatures, etc. – all these parameters are known to impact the mobility of organic semiconductors. From the XRD data discussed in the previous paragraph, a dependence of

Table 13.1. Field-effect mobility data for films obtained using different coating process and temperature

Coating process	Hole mobility (cm^2/Vs)
Drop cast – r.t. drying	1.7×10^{-3}
Drop cast – 80 °C drying	1.8×10^{-3}
Spin coated – r.t. drying	5.1×10^{-3}
Spin coated – 80 °C annealing	4.2×10^{-3}

Table 13.2. Field-effect mobility data for PCPDTBT films cast using different solvents

Solvent	μ_h (cm^2/Vs)	μ_e (cm^2/Vs)
CHCl$_3$ – pristine	6×10^{-3}	2×10^{-5}
CHCl$_3$ – blend	4.8×10^{-3}	4×10^{-5}
oDCB – pristine	5×10^{-3}	9×10^{-5}
oDCB – blend	5.5×10^{-3}	4.5×10^{-4}
toluene – pristine	1.5×10^{-2}	2×10^{-4}
toluene – blend	5×10^{-3}	2×10^{-5}

the intermolecular order on the coating and drying process is expected. FETs were produced according to the conditions of the X-ray samples, and the data are summarized in Table 13.1, while Table 13.2 summarizes the impact of the solvent on the mobility. It is found that drop cast films show an almost three times lower mobility than the spin cast ones, while overall the mobility is only slight dependent on the processing and drying conditions. Also, fast and slow drying solvents do give quite comparable mobility. Highest mobility was observed for toluene-based solutions. Electron mobility of the pristine polymer is typically two orders of magnitude lower than the hole mobility.

By using the same solvents used for the pristine materials, we investigated OTFTs from blend solutions of PCBM:PCPDT-BT with a weight ratio of 1:1. The bipolar mobility was calculated as described in [53] from the measured transfer characteristics in the saturation region. The results are reported in Table 13.2 and depicted in Fig. 13.10. One can observe that the hole mobility in the blend is almost independent of the processing solvent while its value is very close to the pristine material. Considering the electron transport, we found that the blend processed from oDCB represents the only case that shows electron mobility above 10^{-4} cm^2/Vs, while μ_e in the toluene blend is even lower compared to the pristine material. In blended films cast from CHCl$_3$ or toluene the electron field-effect mobility is up to two orders of magnitude lower than that for the holes.

The presence of a homogeneously mixed PCBM phase can cause a reduction of the hole mobility. This happens due to a reduced volume occupied by the polymer in combination with changes in the molecular arrangement of the polymer chains due to the presence of PCBM. The lack of changes on μ_h in our case suggests two main possibilities: (a) polymer segregation at the bottom interface inducing a low density of PCBM at the bottom interface or (b) a rather homogeneous molecular mixing of PCBM with the polymer matrix. An investigation of the field effect

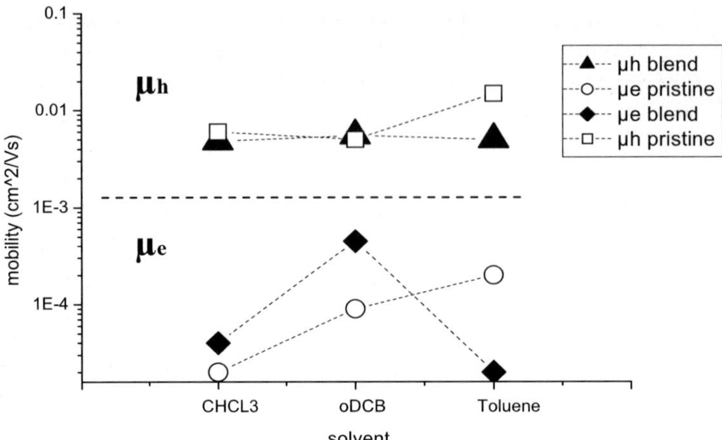

Fig. 13.10. Comparison of electron and hole mobility in pristine PCPDTBT and in blend with PCBM (1:1 ratio) for different solvents

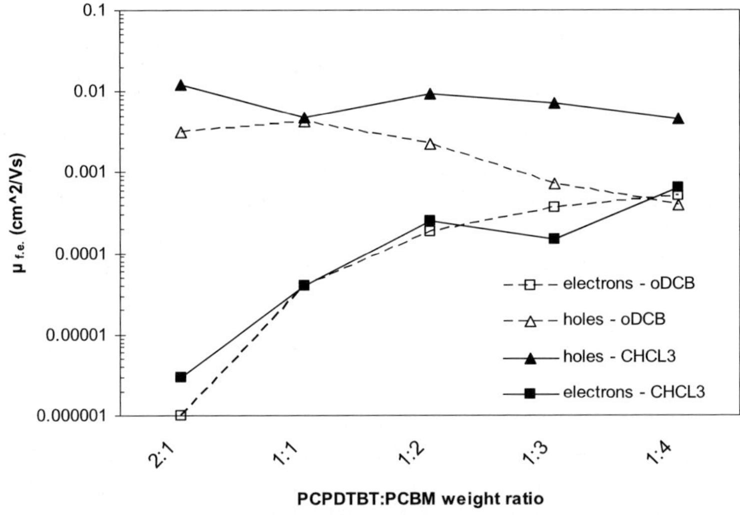

Fig. 13.11. Comparison of electron and hole field effect mobility in PCPDTBT:PCBM blend with different polymer:fullerene weight ratios for different solvents: oDCB and chloroform

mobility of holes and electrons versus the polymer:fullerene ratio for films spin-cast and doctor-bladed from various solvents helps to distinguish between these two phenomena. The results (Fig. 13.11) relative to spin-coated films clearly show that the high fullerene content in the blend is required to achieve a sufficient electron mobility to reduce transport losses. We found that the electron mobility matches the hole mobility at a fullerene weight content that is at least four times higher than the polymer content which indicates a rather homogeneous mixing of PCBM in the polymer matrix. In this case the field-effect mobility of both charge carriers is balanced and is in the range 4×10^{-4}–7×10^{-4} cm^2/Vs when oDCB is used as solvent. Generally, in the range of investigated ratios the hole mobility only varies slightly with the PCBM content. The optimal composition for charge transport is found at 1:4 ratios, which is an important design rule to optimize the performance of solar cell devices from these composite.

In summary, PCPDT-BT is one of the highly promising low-bandgap polymers with good optical and electrical properties. Following the design rules for efficiency prediction, this polymer has the potential to show a performance around 7%, with more at reasonable FF and EQE values. Morphology investigations, however, open up the concern of a poor electron percolation of the PCBM network with respect to the holes of the polymer, resulting in a design rule that demands high fullerene contents, around 80wt.%, to overcome the electron transport limitation and to achieve optimal performances.

13.4 Photovoltaic Performance of PCPDT-Based Solar Cells

In this section we present and discuss the device performance of PCPDT-BT:PCBM composites. Before embedding them into devices, the thin-coated films were investigated by absorption and luminescence spectroscopy (Fig. 13.12). The solid-state absorption peaks at 775 nm (1.6 eV) and has an onset at approximately 890 nm (1.40 eV) with a strong tailing in the solid state, which makes determination of the onset difficult. Interestingly, PCPDT-BT exhibits a quite strong bathochromic shift in the absorption of approximately 70 nm between solution and solid-state films. Such shifts [54] have been frequently observed for rigid conjugated polymers with

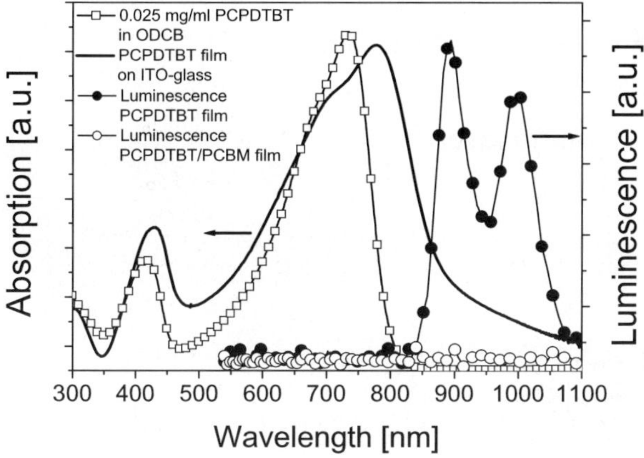

Fig. 13.12. Comparison of solid state absorption (*black line*) and solution absorption (*open squares*) to the solid state luminescence of PCPDTBT and the luminescence quenching for the blend with PCBM, EgOpt ~ 1.38 eV

a strong interchain interaction and are a sign of two-dimensional stacking and extension of the conjugation over two dimensions. As expected from the small optical bandgap, the photoluminescence of PCPDTBT lies in the infrared (IR), between 1.2 eV and 1.4 eV and can be almost completely quenched by addition of PCBM. Very efficient photoluminescence (PL) quenching is the signature of the ultrafast photo-induced charge transfer from PCPDTBT to PCBM, a prerequisite for efficient solar cells, in good accordance with the position of the electrochemical levels as depicted in Fig. 13.13(a).

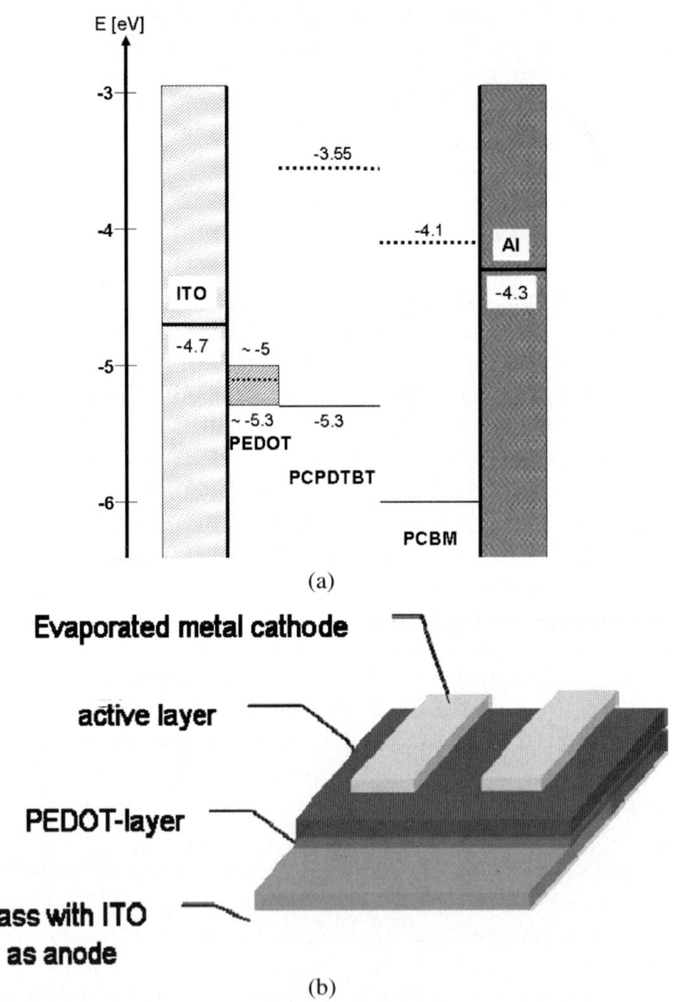

Fig. 13.13. (a) Energy scheme for a PCPDTBT/PCBM device; (b) build-up of device layers and (c) comparison of device characteristics PCPDTBT/PC61BM and PCPDTBT/PC71BM

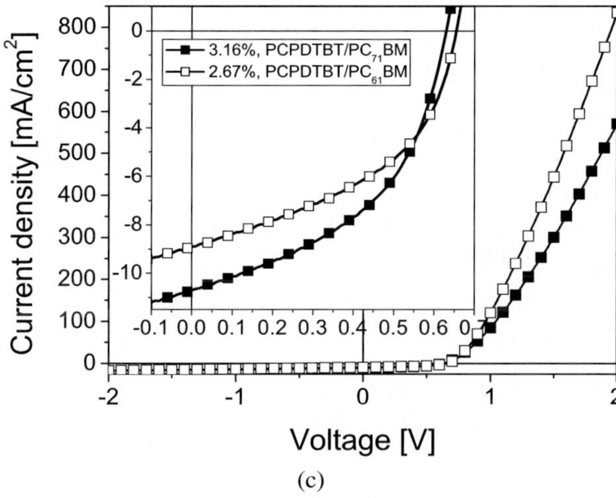

Fig. 13.13. Continued

Photovoltaic devices were produced according to the scheme shown in Fig. 13.13(b). The active layer, processed from solutions with and without additives like mono or dithiols, was embedded between PEDOT and LiF/Al [14] or TiOx/Al [11, 12] interfaces. ITO on glass was used as a transparent bottom electrode. Figure 13.13(c) shows the current voltage (jV) characteristics of PCPDTBT/PC$_{61}$BM and PCPDTBT/PC$_{71}$BM devices. Under AM1.5 illumination of 100 mW/cm^2, outstanding high photocurrents up to 10 mA/cm^2 [14] are reached for the blend with PC$_{61}$BM and more than 15 mA/cm^2 [11, 12] are observed for blends with PC$_{71}$BM. PC$_{71}$BM was used to further broaden the effectively used spectral range for the photocurrent, as can be seen from the EQE spectra shown in Fig. 13.14(a).

A clear additional contribution arising from PC$_{71}$BM around 500 nm results in an additional peak of the photocurrent spectrum reaching 35% EQE in the case of semiconductors layers processed without additives. Clearly, the usage of PC$_{71}$BM accounts for the higher I_{SC} of the PCPDTBT/PC$_{71}$BM device. The open-circuit voltage V_{OC} is typically at 650 mV; the highest observed values were close to 700 mV. These values fulfill the expectations derived from the position of the electrochemical potentials.

While the observed photocurrent and also the photovoltage are already satisfyingly high, the low fill factor (FF) of the device limits the overall performance. From the high-injection currents at low voltages and the good diode behavior (see Fig. 13.13) the presence of a large serial resistivity can be ruled out as responsible for the limitation of the FF. In addition, the high mobilities of PCPDTBT and PCBM allow exclusion of transport limitation of the individual components. In accordance to the earlier discussions, two possible underlying mechanisms with relevance to this observation are suggested: first, and most likely, an unfavorable morphology of the polymer/fullerene blend leads to recombination. The slope of

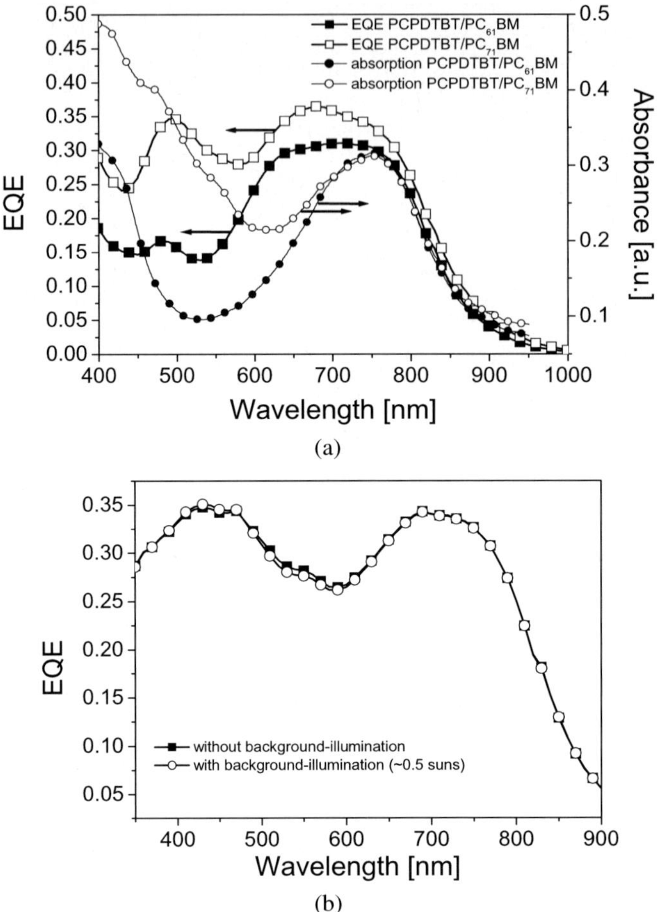

Fig. 13.14. (a) EQE and absorption spectra of a blend of PCPDTBT/PC$_{61}$BM and PCPDTBT/PC$_{71}$BM, the EQE shows similar differences as the absorption profile for the two blends. (b) EQE of a typical blend of PCPDTBT/PC$_{71}$BM with and without background light. (c) EQE of typical blends of PCPDTBT/PC$_{71}$BM under reverse bias. (d) Temperature dependence of the photocurrent of a typical PCPDTBT/PCBM solar cell

the photocurrent curve under reverse bias then indicates that higher electrical fields are necessary to collect the charge carriers and in that way diminish the recombination losses. This recombination can be of first or of second order. Second, the close energetic proximity of the donor and acceptor LUMO levels ($\sim$3.55 eV for PCPDTBT and $\sim$4.1 eV for PCBM, respectively; see Fig. 13.13(a)) may diminish the selectivity of the metal electrode contacts, lowering the diode quality by loss mechanisms such as enhanced interface recombination or tunnel injection under reverse bias. In addition, the slightly unfavorable field dependence of the PCPDT-BT composites suggests transport-induced losses in the low field regions, i.e., close

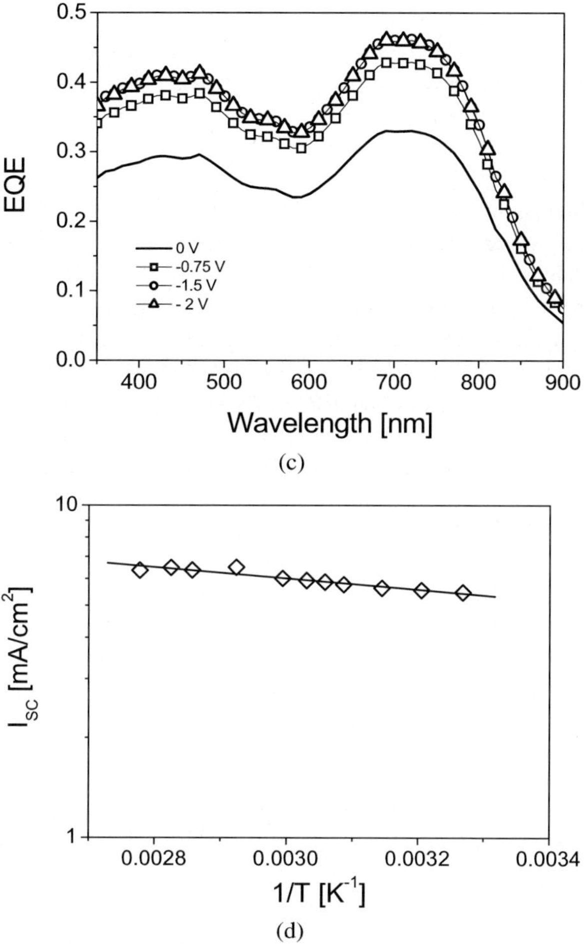

Fig. 13.14. Continued

to and around V_{oc}. In order to learn more about the recombination mechanisms in PCPDTBT/PCBM composites, white-light bias and field-dependent EQE measurements were executed and analyzed on typical PCPDTBT/PC$_{71}$BM devices. The EQE of a PCPDTBT/PC$_{71}$BM device (Fig. 13.14(a)) has two dominant features – a near-IR peak between 700 nm and 800 nm as well as a UV/Vis peak around 500 nm. The onset of photocurrent starts beyond 900 nm is in excellent agreement with the optical data. The EQE is absolutely symbatic and peaks at ∼38% in the 700–800 nm region. Using dithiol as an additive to the semiconductor blends, EQE values as high as 50% could be demonstrated, which is by far the highest value for any organic low bandgap material [11, 12].

While the near-IR peak is unambiguously identified with the PCPDTBT absorption, the UV/Vis peak is dominated by the absorption of the fullerene PC$_{71}$BM or

$PC_{61}BM$. The reduced absorption of $PC_{61}BM$ in the 500 nm region leads to reduction of the photocurrent by approximately 40 to 50%. Figure 13.14(b) shows the spectral shape of the EQE with background illumination. In case of classical second-order recombination dominating the device performance of PCPDTBT/PCBM, one would expect a major difference between these two measurement conditions. Due to charge density under white light bias that is orders of magnitude larger, the presence of bimolecular recombination would lead to a reduction of the EQE. This effect is not observed and we can safely conclude that second-order recombination mechanisms are not relevant at Jsc. Figure 13.14(c) shows the field dependence of the EQE. A white light background bias is applied to compensate for the influence of photoconductivity. Under reverse bias, the EQE continuously rises and saturates at a bias of approximately -2 V. At that bias level, the EQE has increased by a factor of approximately 1.5, from 35% to almost 50%. In parallel, the quasi-steady state photocurrent at -2 V is a factor of 10 higher than under I_{SC} conditions. This phenomenon, which is a peculiar property of most BHJ solar cell systems, is called photo shunting and was introduced in detail recently [55]. Such a strong photo shunt effect as observed for $PCPDTBT/PC_{71}BM$ devices indicates a nonselective electrode interface.

In addition, the temperature dependence of $PCPDTBT/PC_{71}BM$ devices was studied. From previous studies it is well known that the photocurrent of polymer/fullerene solar cells is determined by the choice of the polymer. For instance, devices from MDMO-PPV/PCBM [56] show distinct positive temperature dependence while devices from P3HT/PCBM [57] can be almost temperature independent. Figure 13.14(d) shows the temperature dependence of the photocurrent of PCPDTBT/$PC_{71}BM$ devices. We chose an Arrhenius-like plot to quantitatively evaluate the temperature dependence. Figure 13.14(d) clearly indicates that $PCPDTBT/PC_{71}BM$ devices have a quite strong temperature dependence of the photocurrent, comparable to earlier observations for MDMO-PPV/PCBM devices. It is a clear indication that transport on one or both of the materials in the composite suffer from the presence of shallow traps, likely connected to enhanced energetical disorder in the blend.

Taking into account all data acquired so far, the efficiency of PCPDT-BT/PCBM cells can be predicted quite well once the morphology is optimized. The EQE under reverse bias as well as the recently published model [11, 12] suggest short-circuit currents on the order of 17 mA/cm^2. In combination with more selective electrodes, a polymer with such a high mobility will show FF higher than 0.6. Together with a V_{oc} of 700 mV, these parameters qualify PCPDTBT as a candidate for exceeding 7% efficiency [11, 12, 14]. For a polymer closely related to PCPDT, with a similar structure, indeed better performance was observed. The NREL certificate shown in Fig. 13.15 rates this polymer at over 5%. Here, the current densities of 15 mA/cm^2 and the FF of 61% are already quite close to the expected maximum. Only the slightly lower V_{oc} of 580 mV reduces the efficiency to the 5–6% regime instead of the 6–7% regime.

Konarka Technologies
Organic Cell

Device ID: LS1

Jul 12, 2007 13:58

Spectrum: AM1.5-G (IEC 60904)

Device Temperature: 25.0 ± 1.0 °C

Device Area: 0.685 cm^2

Irradiance: 1000.0 W/m^2

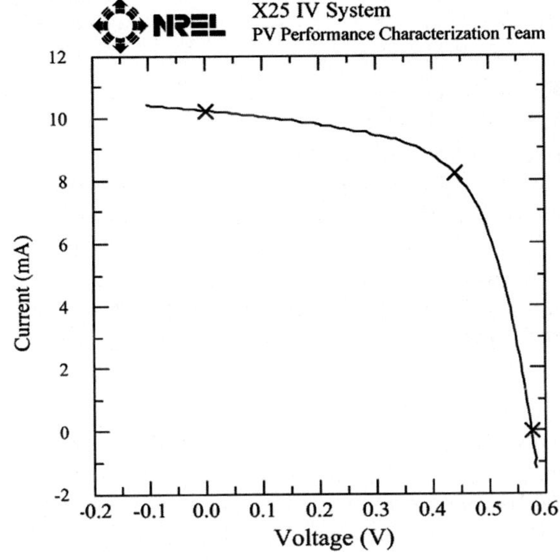

V_{oc} = 0.5756 V

I_{sc} = 10.218 mA

J_{sc} = 14.917 mA/cm^2

Fill Factor = 61.05 %

I_{max} = 8.2047 mA

V_{max} = 0.4376 V

P_{max} = 3.5908 mW

Efficiency = 5.24 %

Fig. 13.15. NREL certificate for a polymer/fullerene solar cell using a low-bandgap polymer as donor

13.5 From Single-Junction to Multijunction Solar Cells

With the existence of a well-performing low-bandgap polymer, the realization of multijunction solar cells becomes possible. The PCPDT-BT series, with a bandgap of about 1.4 eV, is certainly suitable for the incorporation into multijunction solar cells. Another reason why PCPDT-BT perfectly suits the tandem approach is the reduced transport properties induced by a nonideal morphology, which limits the active layers thickness to below 200 nm and external quantum efficiencies (EQE) less than 35% [14] and 50%, respectively [11, 12]. Thus, combining P3HT and PCPDTBT in a series connected tandem solar cells appears likely to push forward the performance of devices based on the individual materials. There has been

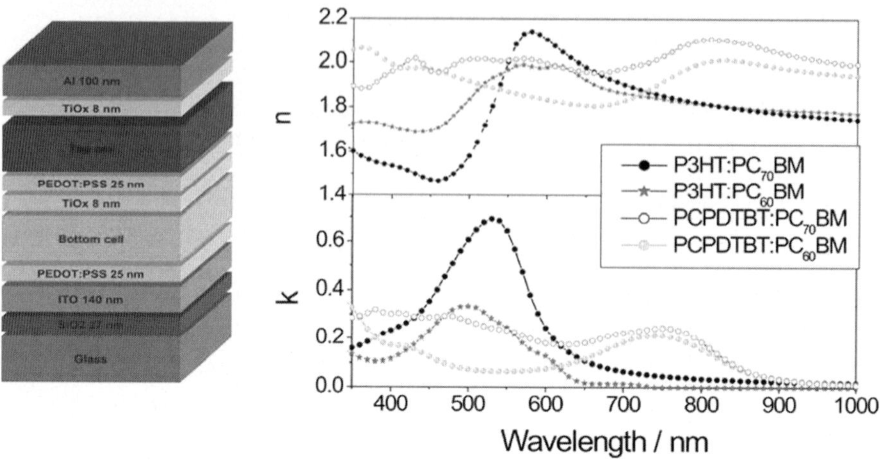

Fig. 13.16. Scheme of the structure of the tandem cells simulated, and real and imaginary parts of the complex refractive indexes of the various active materials used for the simulations

tremendous progress in the design and in the realization of tandem cells. While the first tandem concepts and interfacial layers suffered from either high absorption, nonideal transport properties, or recombination losses [58–60] leading to either unmatched current densities or to low FF, Kim et al. [61] recently presented a tandem architecture with which he reported an FF of more than 65% and efficiencies as high as 6.5%. The structure of a tandem cell from Kim, based on two half cells with P3HT and PCPDT-BT, respectively, is shown in Fig. 13.16. It is composed of a thick (thicker than the coherence length of the light) glass substrate, followed by 27 nm of SiO_2, 140 nm of indium tin oxide (ITO), 25 nm of poly(3, 4-ethylenedioxythiophene) doped with poly(styrene sulfonate) (PEDOT:PSS), a variable thickness bottom active layer, 8 nm of sol-gel TiOx, 25 nm of PEDOT:PSS, a variable thickness top active layer, 8 nm of sol-gel TiOx, and finally 100 nm of Al. The optical parameters of the four active blends that have been treated are displayed in Fig. 13.16. The TiOx/PEDOT layer is called the recombination layer, and serves the function to interconnect the two half cells in series.

It appears that the usage of PC70BM instead of PC60BM permits enlarging the imaginary part of the complex refractive index and therefore the extinction coefficient of the blends, especially in the range 350–700 nm. It is interesting to note that the PCPDTBT:PC60BM blend shows a minimum in absorption at 550 nm, exactly where the P3HT:PC70BM shows a maximum.

Looking to the structure of the tandem cell, one immediately realizes that the low bandgap polymer is the front absorber, while the wide bandgap polymer is the back absorber. This is opposite to inorganic solar cells, where the wide bandgap absorber is always placed in front. However, due to the specific optical absorption profiles of the two polymers, it turns out that the configuration with the wide bandgap polymer as the front absorber allows higher performance compared to the other layer

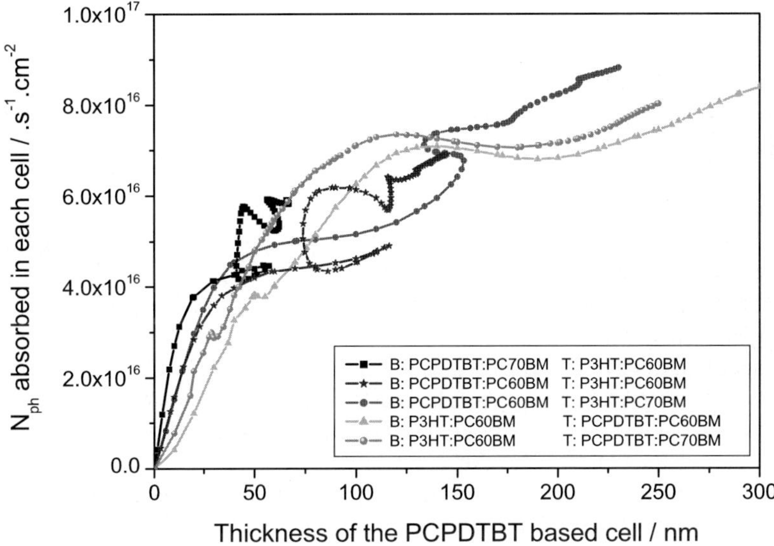

Fig. 13.17. Number of photons absorbed in both active layers (isoline 1) versus the thickness of the PCPDTBT based active layer for various material combinations under AM1.5G

architecture. The optical methodology used to analyze and predict the tandem architecture is close to the approach employed by Persson et al. [62] and is described in detail elsewhere [63]. For each active layer couple, the thickness of both the bottom (between 0 and 300 nm) and the top (between 0 and 600 nm) active layers and calculated the number of photons absorbed (N_{ph}) in those layers under AM1.5G. The design rule for tandem cells requires that the current density in the two half cells needs to be identical. Under the assumption of identical quantum efficiencies, the number of absorbed photons N_{ph} in each layer has to match. The pairs of film thicknesses, where the N_{ph} in both layers is identical, is called the isoline 1. Valuable information can be deducted from the N_{ph}, plotted versus the thickness of the single layers as shown in Fig. 13.17. This one displays the N_{ph} along the isolines 1 versus the thickness of the PCPDTBT-based cell. This way of plotting was chosen because PCPDT-BT cannot be processed in thick layers without losing its performance. As such, it is more critical to optimize the thickness of this cell. This plot yields quite unusually shaped curves, since N_{ph} of a single film thickness of the PCPDT-BT layer can be matched by multiple layer thicknesses of the P3HT layer due to optical interference effects. The precise information on the absorbed photon density now allows us to distinguish and rate the first and the last cases. Specifically one case, where PCPDT-BT/PC60BM is used as the bottom layer and P3HT/PC70BM is used as the top layer appears to be the most promising for reasonable thicknesses of the PCPDT-BT layer – between 130 and 230 nm. Under these conditions, the number of absorbed photons becomes maximized, which should be reflected in higher current densities compared to the other scenarios.

Having established and verified the optical model for organic tandem cells, one is able to answer the question of the ultimate efficiency potential of these two materials. According to the above calculations, the blends chosen by Kim et al. to realize their highly efficient organic tandem cell is the very one identified here as being the most promising by optical simulation. The combination of film thicknesses chosen for the realization of the tandem cell were about 135 nm for the PCPDT-BT layer and 155 nm for the P3HT layer, resulting in an absorbed photon density of 7.3×10^{16} photons s^{-1} cm^{-2}. Assuming an IQE of 100%, this N_{ph}, folded with the solar spectrum, would yield a short-circuit current density of 11.7 mA cm^{-2}, while the current reported for this device is about 7.8 mA cm^{-2}. This indicates that the limiting subcell driving the Jsc in the tandem has an IQE of 67%, a value in good accordance with the IQE values we have determined for PCPDTBT:PC60BM single devices. Hence this suggests that the performance of the device is limited by the PCPDTBT subcell and one can not expect efficiencies beyond 7% for this combination. Assuming an EQE of over 50% and an IQE of about 85% as was reported for PCPDT-BT when processed with additives [11, 12], one calculates a short-circuit current density of almost 10 mA cm^{-2} for the tandem cell. With a FF of 0.65 and a V_{oc} of 1.2 V, an efficiency of nearly 8% is expected for such a tandem cell.

Finally, it is interesting to discuss the efficiency potential of tandem cells versus single-junction solar cells. Again, we discuss this by way of a simplified picture, where we assumed fixed FF and fixed EQE values. The same model as suggested in the first part of this paper was expanded to tandem cells. In order to fulfill the tandem design rule – i.e. matching of the current densities – it is necessary to describe the integrated AM1.5 photon density by a linear fit. Using a simple linear fit, and again assuming that the EQE has a rectangular profile, the current density can be given as a function of the bandgap. In order to calculate the maximum possible efficiency of a tandem cell in dependence of the lower bandgap absorber, the tandem design rule was applied. Each of the half cells was assigned to absorb half of the photon density compared to the single-junction solar cell. The bandgap of the wide-bandgap material was calculated according to matching the photon density of the low bandgap solar cell to the current density. The V_{oc} was calculated directly from the bandgap, assuming the CT and V_{oc} losses of 0.5 V as assumed above. One has to keep in mind that the linear fit of the integrated photon density does deviate from the real situation, especially at very low and very high wavelengths. Nevertheless, the model is very useful to understand how a tandem cell can reach higher efficiencies compared to single junction cells. Figure 13.18 summarizes the scenario by plotting the maximum possible efficiency of single-junction solar cells versus the bandgap and of tandem junction solar cells versus the bandgap. In the case of the tandem junction solar cell, the bandgap is, of course, the bandgap of the low bandgap absorber, while the bandgap of the wide bandgap absorber is calculated to fulfill the current matching condition. As such, the calculated tandem efficiency can be regarded as the highest possible tandem efficiency which can be gained with that low bandgap polymer. Figure 13.18 clearly points out that tandem cells benefit from even lower bandgap polymers as single-junction solar cells. While the efficiency of

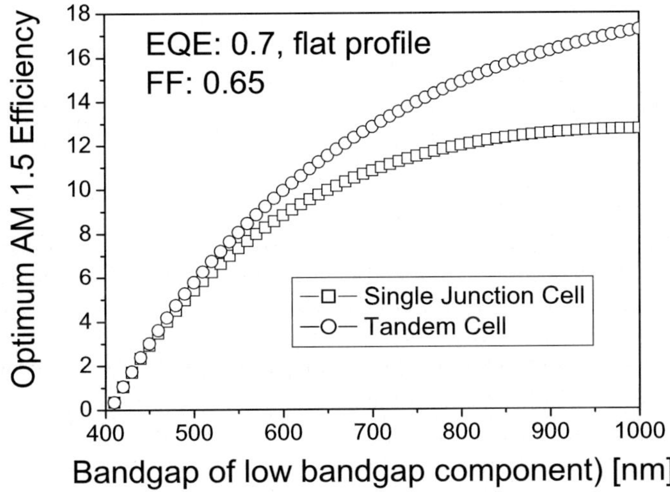

Fig. 13.18. Plot of the max efficiencies for single-junction cells versus tandem cells versus the bandgap of the low-bandgap absorber

single-junction solar cells flattens out at a bandgap of about 900–950 nm, the tandem efficiency still would further increase with lower bandgaps. Also interesting to note is that the tandem cell has nearly no benefit compared to single-junction solar cells for polymers with a bandgap below 600–650 nm.

13.6 Summary

Organic bulk heterojunction solar cells have overcome the 5% efficiency barrier, with current efficiencies rated between 5–6%. For single-junction BHJ solar cells, there are no obstacles to prevent reaching the 10% milestone. To increase the efficiency beyond 10% cell efficiency, various scenarios are currently being discussed and developed. Tandem cells certainly have the potential to reach efficiencies of up to 15%. An alternative path is to reduce the current intrinsic losses of the single-junction solar cells. One the one hand, the energy losses of about 0.25 eV are due to the photo-induced charge transfer. On the other hand the V_{oc} losses of about 0.25 V are due to the dark current injection. Overcoming each of these losses would significantly increase the efficiency potential of the organic solar cells. Assuming no energetic losses at all, an FF of 0.7 and a rectangular EQE as high as 90%, the maximum efficiency of almost 30% is predicted for a bandgap between 1–1.25 eV. All of these approaches rely on high-performing, low-bandgap polymers and underline the importance and necessity of developing such polymers. Copolymers from bridged bithiophenes and acceptors, the so-called PCPDT-X series, may be the polymers that enable these new efficiency concepts.

References

1. D.M. Chapin, C.S. Fuller, G.L. Pearson, J. Appl. Phys. **25**, 676–677 (1954)
2. M.D. Archer, R.R Hill (eds.), *Clean Electricity from Photovoltaics*. Series on Photoconversion of Solar Energy, vol. 1 (Imperial College Press, London, 2001)
3. A. Goetzberger, C. Hebling, Sol. Energy Mater. Sol. Cells **62**, 1–19 (2000)
4. C.J. Brabec, J. Hauch, P. Schilinsky, C. Waldauf, MRS Bull. **30**(1), 50–52 (2005)
5. Organic-based photovoltaics. MRS Bull. **30**(1), 10–52 (2005)
6. N.S. Sariciftci, L. Smilowitz, A.J. Heeger, F. Wudl, Science **258**, 1474 (1992)
7. C.J. Brabec, G. Zerza, N.S. Sariciftci, G. Cerullo, S. DeSilvestri, S. Luzatti, J.C. Hummelen, Chem. Phys. Lett. **340**, 232–236 (2000)
8. P. Schlinsky, C. Waldauf, C.J. Brabec, Appl. Phys. Lett. **81**, 3885–3887 (2002)
9. J. Xue, S. Uchida, B.P. Rand, S.R. Forrest, Appl. Phys. Lett. **85**, 5757–5759 (2004)
10. L. Schmidt-Mende et al., Adv. Mat. **17**, 813–815 (2005)
11. J. Peet, J.Y. Kim, N.E. Coates, W.L. Ma, D. Moses, A.J. Heeger, G.C. Bazan, Nat. Mater. **6**, 497 (2007)
12. J.Y. Kim, K. Lee, N.E. Coates, D. Moses, T.-Q. Nguyen, M. Dante, A.J. Heeger, Science **317**, 222 (2007)
13. M. Scharber, D. Mühlbacher, M. Koppe, P. Denk, C. Waldauf, A.J. Heeger, C.J. Brabec, Adv. Mater. **8**, 789 (2006)
14. D. Muehlbacher, M. Scharber, M. Morana, Z. Zhu, D. Waller, R. Gaudiana, C.J. Brabec, Adv. Mater. **18**, 2884–2889 (2006)
15. Z. Zhu, D. Waller, R. Gaudiana, M. Morana, D. Mühlbacher, M. Scharber, C.J. Brabec, Macromolecules **40**(6), 1981–1986 (2007)
16. M. Morana, Z. Zhu, D. Waller, R. Gaudiana, M. Scharber, C.J. Brabec, Adv. Funct. Mat. **18**, 1757–1766 (2008)
17. P. Schilinsky, C. Waldauf, J. Hauch, C.J. Brabec, J. Appl. Phys. **95**, 2816–2819 (2004)
18. Konarka NREL certificate from July 2005, October 2006 and August 2007
19. Plextronics NREL certificate from August 2007
20. W. Ma, C. Yang, X. Gong, K. Lee, A.J. Heeger, Adv. Funct. Mater. **15**, 1617 (2005)
21. M. Reyes-Reyes, K. Kim, D.L. Carrol, Appl. Phys. Lett. **87**, 083506–08350611 (2005)
22. G. Li, V. Shrotriya, J. Huang, Y. Yao, T. Moriarty, K. Emery, Y. Yang, Nat. Mater. **4**, 864 (2005)
23. C. Winder, N.S. Sariciftci, Mater. Chem. **14**, 1077–1086 (2004)
24. B.P. Rand, J. Xue, F. Yang, S.R. Forrest, Appl. Phys. Lett. **87**, 233508/1–233508/3 (2005)
25. E. Bundgaard, F.C. Krebs, Macromolecules **39**, 2823–2831 (2006)
26. F. Huang, L. Hou, H. Shen, J. Jiang, F. Wang, H. Zhen, Y.J. Cao, Mater. Chem. **15**, 2499–2507 (2005)
27. M. Velusamy, K.R.J. Thomas, J.T. Lin, Y.C. Hsu, K.C. Ho, Org. Lett. **7**, 1899–1902 (2005)
28. R. Yang, R. Tian, J. Yan, Y. Zhang, J. Yang, Q. Hou, W. Yang, C. Zhang, Y. Cao, Macromolecules **38**, 244–253 (2005)
29. Q. Hou, Q. Zhou, Y. Zhang, W. Yang, R. Yang, Y. Cao, Macromolecules **37**, 6299–6305 (2004)
30. F. Huang, L. Hou, H. Wu, X. Wang, H. Shen, W. Cao, W. Yang, Y. Cao, J. Am. Chem. Soc. **126**, 9845–9853 (2004)
31. M. Chen, E. Perzon, M.R. Andersson, S. Marcinkevicius, S.K.M. Jonsson, M. Fahlman, M. Berggren, Appl. Phys. Lett. **84**, 3570–3572 (2004)
32. D. Muhlbacher, H. Neugebauer, A. Cravino, N.S. Sariciftci, Synth. Met. **137**, 1361–1362 (2003)

33. C.J. Brabec, C. Winder, N.S. Sariciftci, J.C. Hummelen, A. Dhanabalan, P. Van Hal, R.A.J. Janssen, Adv. Funct. Mater. **12**, 709–712 (2002)
34. Q. Hou, Y. Xu, W. Yang, M. Yuan, J. Peng, Y. Cao, J. Mater. Chem. **12**, 2887–2892 (2002)
35. H.A.M. Van Mullekom, J.A.J.M. Vekemans, E.W. Meijer, Chem. Eur. J. **4**, 1235–1243 (1998)
36. M. Karikomi, C. Kitamura, S. Tanaka, Y. Yamashita, J. Am. Chem. Soc. **117**, 6791–6792 (1995)
37. J. Roncali, Chem. Rev. **97**, 173–205 (1997)
38. S.E. Shaheen, D. Vangeneugden, R. Kiebooms, D. Vanderzande, T. Fromherz, F. Padinger, C.J. Brabec, N.S. Sariciftci, Synth. Met. **121**, 1583–1584 (2001)
39. C. Winder, G. Matt, J.C. Hummelen, R.A.J. Janssen, N.S. Sariciftci, C.J. Brabec, Thin Solid Films **403–404**, 373–379 (2002)
40. A. Dhanabalan, J.K.J. Van Duren, P.A. Van Hal, J.L.J. Van Dongen, R.A.J. Janssen, Adv. Funct. Mater. **11**, 255–262 (2001)
41. A.P. Smith, R.R. Smith, B.E. Taylor, M.F. Durstock, Chem. Mater. **16**, 4687–4692 (2004)
42. X. Wang, E. Perzon, F. Oswald, F. Langa, S. Admassie, M.R. Andersson, O. Inganaes, Adv. Funct. Mater. **15**, 1665–1670 (2005)
43. X. Wang, E. Perzon, J.L. Delgado, P. De la Cruz, F. Zhang, F. Langa, M.R. Andersson, O. Inganas, Appl. Phys. Lett. **85**, 5081–5083 (2004)
44. F. Zhang, E. Perzon, X. Wang, W. Mammo, M.R. Andersson, O. Inganaes, Adv. Funct. Mater. **15**, 745–750 (2005)
45. L.M. Campos, A. Tontcheva, S. Guenes, G. Sonmez, H. Neugebauer, N.S. Sariciftci, F. Wudl, Chem. Mater. **17**, 4031–4033 (2005)
46. E. Perzon, X. Wang, S. Admassie, O. Inganäs, M.R. Andersson, Polymer **47**, 4261–4268 (2006)
47. M. Kalaji, P.J. Murphy, G.O. Williams, Synth. Met. **101**, 123 (1999)
48. C.A. Mills, D.M. Taylor, P.J. Murphy, C. Dalton, G.W. Jones, L.M. Hall, A.V. Hughes, Synth. Met. **102**, 1000–1001 (1999)
49. C. Soci, I.-W. Hwang, D. Moses, Z. Zhu, D. Waller, R. Gaudiana, C.J. Brabec, A.J. Heeger, Adv. Funct. Mater. **17**, 632–636 (2007)
50. T. Erb, U. Zhkavhets, G. Godch, S. Raleva, B. Stuhn, P. Schilinsky, C. Waldauf, C.J. Brabec, Adv. Funct. Mat. **15**, 1193–1196 (2005)
51. R.A. Street, J.E. Northrup, A. Salleo, Phys. Rev. B **71**, 165202 (2005)
52. G. Horowitz, J. Mater. Res. **19**, 7 (2004)
53. M. Morana, P. Koers, C. Waldauf, M. Koppe, D. Muehlbacher, P. Denk, M.C. Scharber, D. Waller, C.J. Brabec, Adv. Funct. Mat. **17**(16), 3274–3283 (2007)
54. P.J. Brown, D.S. Thomas, A. Köhler, J.S. Wilson, J.-S. Kim, C.M. Ramsdale, H. Sirringhaus, R.H. Friend, Phys. Rev. B **67**, 0642031 (2003)
55. P. Schilinsky, C. Waldauf, J. Hauch, C.J. Brabec, J. Appl. Phys. **95**, 2816 (2004)
56. E. Katz, D. Faiman, S.M. Tuladhar, J.M. Kroon, M.M. Wienk, T. Fromherz, F. Padinger, C.J. Brabec, N.S. Sariciftci, J. Appl. Phys. **90**, 5343 (2001)
57. I. Riedel, V. Dyakonov, Phys. Stat. Sol. A **201**, 1332 (2004)
58. A. Hadipour, B. de Boer, J. Wildeman, F.B. Kooistra, J.C. Hummelen, M.G.R. Turbiez, M.M. Wienk, R.A.J. Janssen, P.W.M. Blom, Adv. Funct. Mater. **16**, 1897 (2006)
59. J. Gilot, M.M. Wienk, R.A.J. Janssen, Appl. Phys. Lett. **90**, 143512 (2007)
60. G. Dennler, H.-J. Prall, R. Koeppe, M. Egginger, R. Autengruber, N.S. Sariciftci, Appl. Phys. Lett. **89**, 073502 (2007)

61. J.Y. Kim, K. Lee, N.E. Coates, D. Moses, T.-Q. Nguyen, M. Dante, A.J. Heeger, Science **317**, 222 (2007)
62. N.-K. Persson, O. Inganas, Sol. Energy Mater. Sol. Cells **90**, 3491 (2006)
63. G. Dennler, T. Ameri, C. Waldauf, P. Denk, K. Hingerl, K. Forberich, A.J. Heeger, C.J. Brabec, J. Appl. Phys. **102**, 123109 (2007)

Index

Printing: Krips bv, Meppel, The Netherlands
Binding: Stürtz, Würzburg, Germany